ROUTLEDGE INTERNATIONAL HANDBOOK
OF CLINICAL SUICIDE RESEARCH

Suicide remains one of the most pressing public health concerns across the world. Expensive in terms of the human cost and associated suffering, the economic costs, the social costs and the spiritual costs, it affects millions of people every year.

This important reference work collects together a wide range of research on suicide and suicide prevention, in order to guide future research and provide guidance for professionals about the best way to respond meaningfully to suicidal patients. Responding to the need for multi-disciplinary and international research to deepen our understanding of suicide, it demonstrates where our knowledge is firmly evidence-based and where new areas for research are emerging, as well as highlighting where we know little.

Divided into six parts, each with its own editorial introduction and commentary, the *Routledge International Handbook of Clinical Suicide* explores research with and about survivors of suicide and Indigenous populations. The other sections look at suicide-focused research in psychiatric nursing, psychiatry, psychology, and social work and allied health. This book will be of interest to all advanced students, practitioners and scholars interested in suicide and its impact and prevention.

John R. Cutcliffe holds Adjunct Professor of Nursing positions at the University of Ottawa, Canada; the University of Coimbra, Portugal and the University of Malta. He is also the CEO of Cutcliffe Consulting, which provides consulting services to higher education and mental healthcare facilities.

José Carlos Santos is Adjunct-Professor at the Nursing School of Coimbra, Portugal.

Paul S. Links is Professor and Chair in the Department of Psychiatry at the Schulich School of Medicine & Dentistry, the University of Western Ontario, and Chief of Psychiatry at the London Health Sciences Centre and St. Joseph's Health Care, London, Ontario, Canada.

Juveria Zaheer is a Psychiatrist and Research Fellow at the Centre for Addiction and Mental Health in Toronto, Ontario, Canada.

Henry G. Harder is Professor and Chair of the School of Health Sciences at the University of Northern British Columbia, Canada.

Frank Campbell is the Senior Consultant for Campbell and Associates Consulting, LLC. Dr Campbell is former president of the American Association of Suicidology (AAS).

Rod McCormick is Associate Professor of Counselling Psychology at the University of British Columbia, Canada.

Kari Harder is an Analyst at Northern Health, Canada.

Yvonne Bergmans is Suicide Intervention Consultant at the Suicide Studies Research Unit, St. Michael's Hospital, Toronto, Canada.

Rahel Eynan is an Associate Researcher with the Lawson Health Research Institute at the University of Western Ontario, Canada.

ROUTLEDGE INTERNATIONAL HANDBOOK OF CLINICAL SUICIDE RESEARCH

Edited by John R. Cutcliffe, José Carlos Santos,
Paul S. Links, Juveria Zaheer, Henry G. Harder,
Frank Campbell, Rod McCormick, Kari Harder,
Yvonne Bergmans and Rahel Eynan

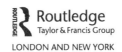

Routledge
Taylor & Francis Group

LONDON AND NEW YORK

First published 2014
by Routledge
2 Park Square, Milton Park, Abingdon, Oxfordshire OX14 4RN

Simultaneously published in the USA and Canada
by Routledge
711 Third Avenue, New York, NY 10017

First issued in paperback 2016

Routledge is an imprint of the Taylor & Francis Group, an informa business

British Library Cataloguing in Publication Data
A catalogue record for this book is available from the British Library

Library of Congress Cataloging in Publication Data
Routledge international handbook of clinical suicide research /
edited by John R. Cutcliffe ... [et al.].
p. ; cm.
International handbook of clinical suicide research
Includes bibliographical references.
I. Cutcliffe, John R., 1966– II. Title: International handbook of clinical suicide research.
[DNLM: 1. Suicide—psychology. 2. Internationality. 3. Suicide—prevention & control. WM 165]
RC480.6
362.28—dc23
2013011294

ISBN 13: 978-1-138-69043-1 (pbk)
ISBN 13: 978-0-415-53012-5 (hbk)

Typeset in Bembo
by Keystroke, Station Road, Codsall, Wolverhampton

For Dr Chris Stevenson

Every now and then an individual comes along who makes the world a better place

I have dedicated this book to Dr Chris Stevenson. Every now and then an individual comes along who makes the world a better place. She is one such person. Whether it is in her ability and willingness to convey warmth, acceptance, understanding or compassion; or her rapier-like wit and ability to embrace the quirky aspects of life; or her academic and clinical insight, imagination and sound ethical thinking, time spent in Chris's company is time well-spent indeed.

Chris has been an influence for almost all of my academic life. From the formative meetings at mental health conferences in the United Kingdom, to her examination of my doctoral thesis, to co-authorship of numerous papers and as joint investigators in pioneering, federally funded research in the United Kingdom and Ireland, I have both witnessed and benefited from her unfaltering commitment to fairness and academic rigor.

The lessons learned are innumerable, the belly-deep laughter is with me today, her patience – a balm for my own intermittent psychache. And even now, as Chris approaches the end of her physical journey, she is still teaching me things, still grounding me, still helping me laugh and see the funny side.

Chris has helped me understand that bereavement and loss, as with so many life experiences, have an existential duality. They are (sometimes simultaneously) immensely painful and yet emancipating, opportunities for growth. They are not to be avoided (as if we could!) or denied, they are to be experienced; they are meaning-making experiences.

So even though at times it seems like the world will be a more monochromatic place after Chris has gone (physically), the world will reverberate with the ripples of her presence, her contributions and her love for years to come.

And with apologies to Ridley Scott . . . "I will see you again . . . but not yet."

CONTENTS

FIGURES

TABLES

CONTRIBUTORS

Editors

Yvonne Bergmans is a Lecturer at the University of Toronto, Canada. She received her BSW from Ryerson University, Canada, in 1995 and her MSW in 1997 from the University of Toronto. Yvonne works as the Suicide Intervention Consultant at the Suicide Studies Research Unit of the Arthur Sommer Rotenberg Chair in Suicide Studies at St Michael's Hospital in Toronto. Since 1998, she has developed, coordinated and facilitated a 20-week Psychosocial/ Psychoeducational Group Intervention for Persons with Recurrent Suicide Attempts (PISA)/Skills for Safer Living (SFSL). Yvonne regularly provides workshops and staff education in working with the chronically suicidal individual for community organisations, including school personnel and front line staff at community agencies. She provides ongoing training, consultation and supervision for professionals in the PISA/SFSL intervention in Ontario, British Columbia and Ireland. She continues to be involved in a number of research projects at the Suicide Studies Research Unit, investigating interventions and the needs for individuals who experience suicide-related thinking and behaviours.

Frank Campbell, PhD, LCSW, CT is a licensed Clinical Social Worker and a Certified Thanatologist, having served as Executive Director of the Baton Rouge Crisis intervention Center and the Crisis Center Foundation in Louisiana, USA. He is currently Senior Consultant for Campbell and Associates Consulting where he consults with communities and on Forensic Suicidology cases. It was due to his more than twenty years of working with those bereaved by suicide that he introduced his Active Postvention Model (APM) most commonly known as the LOSS Team (Local Outreach to Survivors of Suicide). His work with survivors and victims of trauma has been featured in three Discovery Channel documentaries. The APM concept involves a team of first responders who go to the scene of a suicide and provide support and referral for those bereaved by the suicide. The goal has been to shorten the elapsed time between the death and survivors finding the help they feel will help them cope with this devastating loss. The Active Postvention Model has shown to have a positive impact on both the team members (most often bereaved individuals who have gotten help and now provide the installation of hope to the newly bereaved) as well as the newly bereaved. The model has now been replicated in countries as diverse as Australia, Singapore, Northern Ireland, Canada and America.

Dr Campbell is a past president of the American Association of Suicidology (AAS) and has received the Roger J. Tierney award for service and the Louis I Dublin Award in 2010 for his contributions to the field of Suicidology. Campbell was also selected by the International Association of Suicide Prevention (IASP) to receive the Dr Norman Farberow award for his international contributions on behalf of those bereaved by suicide. He was Social Worker of the Year in Louisiana and the first John W. Barton Fellow selected in his hometown of Baton Rouge. To find out more about his work in the field of Suicidology you can visit his website: www.lossteam.com.

John R. Cutcliffe holds Adjunct Professor positions at the University of Ottawa, Canada; the University of Coimbra, Portugal; and the University of Malta. He has previously held two endowed professorial research chairs: the David G. Braithwaite Research Chair at the University of Texas and the Acadia Professorship in Psychiatric and Mental Health Nursing at the University of Maine, both in the United States of America. John's clinical background is in nursing, having completed his psychiatric nurse education and then his general nurse education in the United Kingdom. His research interests focus on hope, suicide and clinical supervision and mental health more broadly, and he was recognised by the federal government of Canada and cited as one of the top 20 Research Leaders of Tomorrow for his research focusing on hope and suicidology. He has published extensively – over 275 papers, chapters, editorials/abstracts and 11 books – and his work has been translated into German, Japanese, Dutch, Spanish, Mandarin Chinese, Portuguese and Turkish. He has over $4,500,000 dollars of extra-mural research funding as Primary/Co-Investigator and his research findings, particularly those pertaining to suicide and hope, are now found in best practice guidelines in many parts of the world. He is currently working with colleagues from Dublin City University (Ireland), the University of Coimbra (Portugal) and Vestfold University College (Norway) on an international program of research focusing on suicide. He has served as the national Canadian Representative for the International Association of Suicide Prevention and the Director of the International Society of Psychiatric Nurses: Education and Research division: he is the Associate Editor for the highest-ranked *Psychiatric/Mental Health Nursing Journal*, as well as serving on the boards of eight other health or education-focused journals. In 2012, was invited by the Director of Medicine at Yale University to join the first international advisory board on Clinical Supervision.

José Carlos Santos is Adjunct-Professor at the Nursing School of Coimbra, Portugal. He has a background in nursing and experience in general and psychiatric hospitals. He completed his nursing degree, his mental health specialisation and his Master's degree in Coimbra, and his Doctoral degree in Oporto University, Portugal. He is a researcher of the Health Sciences Research Unit – Nursing (UICISA-E), hosted by the Nursing School of Coimbra. He is the coordinator of the project, "Prevention of suicidal behaviours" with three main areas: adolescents – prevention of suicidal behaviours in schools; families – prevention of suicides with the families; and professionals – guidelines and tools to prevent suicides. He is also co-investigator in a project on literacy and mental health.

He was the past President of the Portuguese Society of Suicidology (2011–2013); Member of the Horatio Expert Panel (European Association for Psychiatric Nurses); Member of the Portuguese National Council of Mental Health; Member of the National Expert Team for the National Plan of Suicide Prevention. He is also the Chairman of the Supervisory Board of the Honor Society of the Nursing School of Coimbra, chapter of Sigma Theta Tau International. He has published books, papers, chapters, abstracts/conference proceedings in Portuguese and

English. He is a board member of the following nursing journals: *International Journal of Mental Health*, *Referência*, *Revista de Investigação em Enfermagem* and *Revista Sinais Vitais*. His interests are more related to suicidal behaviors and their impact on the family, society and professionals, liaison psychiatry and, more broadly, psychiatric/mental health nursing.

Rahel Eynan is an Associate Researcher with the Lawson Health Research Institute at the University of Western Ontario. She has worked at the Suicide Studies Research Unit with the Arthur Sommer Rotenberg Chair in Suicide Studies at St Michael's Hospital for 14 years. Dr Eynan received her BA from York University, an MA from Concordia University, and a PhD in Medical Science from the University of Toronto. Over the years Dr Eynan has been involved with advocacy and programs in mental health services. She served as a Board Member and Vice-President of Madison Avenue Housing and Support Services, Inc., an organisation dedicated to providing supportive housing for individuals with severe and persistent mental illness, and for many years served as a Director on the Board of Distress Centres Ontario. Dr Eynan is the former President of the Ontario Association for Suicide Prevention and for ten years had a Lieutenant Governor of Ontario appointment to the Board of Directors of the Ontario Mental Health Foundation.

Henry G. Harder is Professor and Chair of the School of Health Sciences at the University of Northern British Columbia. He is a registered psychologist. Dr Harder has been working in the field of rehabilitation and disability management for over 20 years. His research interests are in disability issues, workplace mental health, suicide prevention and Aboriginal health. He is a Canadian Institutes of Health Research-funded scholar. Dr Harder is a published author and has made presentations and conducted workshops throughout Canada, the United States, Europe and Australia. He is a member of the College of Psychologists of British Columbia, Network Environments for Aboriginal Research in BC, the Canadian Psychological Association, the American Association of Marriage and Family Therapy, the International Society of Physical and Rehabilitation Medicine, and other professional organisations.

Kari Harder graduated from the University of Northern British Columbia, Canada, with an MSc in Community Health. From there she went on to conduct Aboriginal research with Carrier Sekani Family Services (CSFS), where she looked at the diet of the Carrier Sekani people, and conducted several evaluations of CSFS programs. She is now currently working at Northern Health as an Analyst.

Paul S. Links is Professor and Chair, Department of Psychiatry, Schulich School of Medicine & Dentistry, the University of Western Ontario and Chief of Psychiatry, London Health Sciences Centre and St Joseph's Health Care, London, Ontario. Prior to coming to Western University, Dr Links was holder of the Arthur Sommer Rotenberg Chair in Suicide Studies, University of Toronto, for three terms. This Chair was the first in North America dedicated to suicide research. Dr Links was the former President of the Canadian Association for Suicide Prevention (CASP) and former President of the Association for Research on Personality Disorders. Also he was the Acting Psychiatrist-in-Chief of the St Michael's Hospital's Mental Health Service from January to June 2011. Dr Links served as the Editor of the *Journal of Personality Disorders* from 2009–2011. He is currently on the Editorial Board of the *Canadian Journal of Psychiatry*. He has published over 125 articles in scientific journals and three books. As an investigator, he has received research grants from many agencies, including Health and Welfare Canada, the Ontario Ministry of Health, the Ontario Mental Health Foundation, the Canadian Institutes of Health Research, and the Workplace Safety and Insurance Board of Ontario. In October 2009, Dr Links was awarded the CASP Research Award for outstanding contributions to the field of suicide research in Canada. Dr Links' clinical experience and expertise developed from working with both acutely suicidal and persistently suicidal individuals (those who face a life-and-death struggle on a daily basis and are at high risk of taking their own lives).

Rod McCormick is Associate Professor of Counselling Psychology in the Department of Educational and Counselling Psychology and Special Education at the University of British Columbia, Canada. He is a member of the Mohawk Nation (Kanienkehake). He is also a consultant specialising in assisting Aboriginal and non-Aboriginal organisations with Aboriginal mental health program development/evaluation and training. Dr McCormick has conducted many research projects examining successful healing approaches used by Aboriginal peoples and has presented and/or published numerous papers pertaining to Aboriginal mental health and healing.

Juveria Zaheer is a psychiatrist and research fellow at the Centre for Addiction and Mental Health, University of Toronto, Ontario. She graduated from her psychiatry residency at the University of Toronto in June 2012 and has worked in the CAMH Emergency Department as a staff psychiatrist and the interim ED Clinic Head from December 2012 to April 2013. She is completing her Master's degree focusing on qualitative research methodology and her research interests include cross-cultural suicide prevention, critical discourse analysis and program evaluation.

Contributors

Douglas Abbott is currently the Professor of Child, Youth & Family Studies at the University of Nebraska-Lincoln, USA. He received a bachelor's degree in human biology from Oregon State University in 1974, a Master's degree in child development from Brigham Young University in 1979, and a doctorate in Child & Family Studies from the University of Georgia in 1983.

Regina T. P. Aguirre is an Assistant Professor of Social Work at the University of Texas at Arlington, USA, where she teaches research and human behavior. She is a licensed master social worker-advanced practitioner (LMSW-AP) in the state of Texas. Regina's areas of focus are suicide bereavement and the relationship between trauma and suicidality.

Munazzah Ambreen is actively involved in qualitative and quantitative research in mental health and is affiliated to the Hospital for Sick Children, Toronto, Canada, and the Centre for Addiction and Mental Health in Toronto. She completed her medical training in Pakistan and has a Master's in Human Genetics from McGill University, Canada.

Tanetta Andersson, PhD, is a Visiting Assistant Professor of Sociology at Trinity College, Hartford, Connecticut, USA. Her future research plans in this area include examining the under-theorisation of grief among emotions in collective health mobilisation (i.e., suicide prevention movement) and exploring the visual elements of constructing suicide loss survivor identity through sub-cultural identity theory.

Jesmin Antony is currently a research coordinator with the Knowledge Translation program at St Michael's Hospital, Toronto, Canada. She holds a BHSc from McMaster University and an MSc from the University of Toronto, and completed her graduate work with the Arthur Sommer Rotenberg Chair in Suicide Studies.

Marla Buchanan (Arvay) is an Associate Professor in the Department of Educational and Counselling Psychology and Special Education in the Faculty of Education at the University of British Columbia, Canada. She is currently the Director of Graduate Programs for her department. She is a faculty member in the Counselling Psychology Program and an Associate Member of the Department of Family Practice and Community Medicine at UBC. Her research interests are in the field of traumatic stress studies. She has conducted a national survey on secondary traumatisation among health care providers in Canada. She has worked internationally, providing trauma treatment and psycho-educational services regarding traumatic stress reactions. She currently teaches and is a clinical supervisor of Master's and doctoral students in the Counselling Psychology Program at UBC.

Ken Balderson is a staff psychiatrist, Medical Director of the Inpatient Mental Health Unit at St Michael's Hospital, Toronto, and an Assistant Professor, Department of Psychiatry, University of Toronto, Canada. His clinical work is in general and HIV psychiatry, and he provides mental health consultation in Nunavut. He is also physician lead responsible for developing and implementing Medication Reconciliation at St Michael's.

Catherine Cheng, B. Phil, M. Phil, is currently enrolled in the PhD program in Sociology in the University of Toronto, Canada.

Amy H. Cheung, M.D., MSc. is Associate Professor, Department of Psychiatry, University of Toronto, and works at Sunnybrook Health Sciences Centre, Toronto, Canada.

Vincenzo De Luca is Assistant Professor at CAMH, Department of Psychiatry, University of Toronto, Canada.

Samanthika Ekanayake, works at Health Systems and Health Equity Research, Centre for Addiction and Mental Health, Toronto, Canada.

Alan Fung is a psychiatrist at North York General Hospital, Toronto and Assistant Professor in the Department of Psychiatry at the University of Toronto, Canada.

Fredricka L. Gilje holds PhD, Master's and Bachelor of Science degrees in nursing with a specialty in psychiatric mental health nursing. During 1993–94, she engaged in a Fulbright Fellowship for post-doctoral study at the University of Tromsø, Norway. Nursing faculty positions she has held were located in institutions of higher education in North Dakota, Washington, and Alaska, as well as Montana. In 2012, she retired as a faculty member in the College of Nursing, Montana State University, USA. She has also served as a visiting professor in Norway, Sweden, Finland and China. She has authored or co-authored more than 38 publications in various nursing journals. Dr Gilje serves as a member of the board of directors of the Montana Chapter of the American Foundation for Suicide Prevention, the Suicide Prevention Coalition of Yellowstone Valley and St John's Lutheran Ministries of Billings, Montana. She is on the advisory board of DARTHART, a global youth network for post traumatic stress recovery for youth trauma survivors. She is a certified by the QPR Institute of Spokane, Washington, as a Gatekeeper Instructor in suicide prevention education.

Evelyn Gordon, PhD, MSc is a Lecturer in Psychotherapy and Mental Health Nursing at Dublin City University, Ireland. She is a registered psychiatric nurse (RPN), psychotherapist (FTAI / ICP) and psychotherapy supervisor (FTAI).

Travis Holyk is the Director of Research and Policy Development for Carrier Sekani Family Services, an organisation responsible for health, social, research and legal services for the First Nations people of the Carrier and Sekani territory (North Central British Columbia). As the Director of Research, he currently oversees a number of research grants held by the agency as well as university–agency research partnerships. Current research initiatives include primary healthcare, youth suicide, child welfare governance and research ethics.

Eduardo Jovel is currently an Associate Professor and Director of Indigenous Research Partnerships in the Faculty of Land and Food Systems at the University of British Columbia, Canada. His research interests include ethnobotany, Aboriginal health, mycology, and natural product chemistry. He is particularly interested in Indigenous peoples' world-views and their use of ecosystem resources to maintain health and wellness. He has taken an active role in international Aboriginal health research, including Indigenous medicinal systems, food security, research ethics, and Indigenous research methodologies.

Michele Kavanagh is a Consultant Clinical Psychologist who specialises in the area of self-harm with young people and families within the social care system. She is also a trainer on the Clinical Psychology Training Programme for Northern Ireland, based at Queens University Belfast where she has responsibilities for personal and professional development.

Sinead Keeney is Senior Research Fellow in the Institute of Nursing Research and Bamford Centre for Mental Health and Well Being at the University of Ulster, Northern Ireland. Her qualifications include PhD, MRes and her primary degree is in Sociology and Politics. Sinead is currently involved in many research studies in the area of mental health, having recently completed a regional study on male suicide. She is also involved in studies on mental health recovery, research into the effect of social media on suicide and self-harm, and studies on suicide prevention with young people.

Keehan Koorn has an undergraduate degree in Psychology from the University of Waterloo, Canada, and a Master's degree in Family Relations and Human Development from the University of Guelph, Canada. When she is not running Skills for Safer Living groups, she is in training to become a Couple and Family Therapist, with expertise in LGBTQ issues, depression, and anxiety.

Christopher E. Lalonde is currently engaged in research projects that examine the role of culture in the health and well-being of Aboriginal youth. In partnership with the Inter Tribal Health Authority, he is involved in a study of injury rates within First Nations communities on Vancouver Island. In collaboration with the Assembly of Manitoba Chiefs, he has worked on a project in Manitoba that examines culture and healthy youth development. At the University of Victoria, he also helps to direct the LE NONET Project that aims to enhance the success of Aboriginal undergraduate students. He is also the Co-Director of the University of Victoria's Centre for Aboriginal Health Research. His research focuses on cultural influences on identity formation and social-cognitive development.

John Langley is an Assistant Professor in the Department of Psychiatry, University of Toronto, Canada, and he is a staff psychiatrist in the Department of Psychiatry at St Michael's Hospital.

He is the Program Director, Postgraduate Education, Child and Adolescent Psychiatry, University of Toronto. Dr Langley has a strong interest in community and adolescent psychiatry and he has worked with street-involved youth for many years. He provides psychiatric consultation to several inner-city agencies, including Covenant House, the Youth Hostel Outreach Program, Central Toronto Youth Services, and the New Outlook Youth Justice Program. He is also the Medical Director of the STEPS for Youth program at St Michael's Hospital, a program for early intervention in psychosis.

Samuel Law is a Psychiatrist at Mount Sinai Hospital and St Michael's Hospital, Toronto, and Assistant Professor in the Department of Psychiatry at the University of Toronto, Canada.

Alain Lesage is currently Professor, Department of Psychiatry, Faculty of Medicine, University of Montreal, Canada; Adjunct Professor, Department of Psychiatry, Faculty of Medicine, McGill University, Canada; Associate Scientific Director of Fernand-Seguin Research Centre, based at L-H Lafontaine Hospital, since 1987, now known as the Montreal University Mental Health Institute. Since 2009, he has been Associate Scientific Director of the Quebec Suicide Research Network, financed by the Quebec Research Funds. He was an invited research fellow at the Health Systems Research Unit of the Clarke Institute of Psychiatry (Toronto, Canada) in 1994–1995 and Visiting Scientist at the Harvard School of Public Health, 2003–2005. He participated in the development of Best Practice in Reforming Mental Health Services. His work concentrates on the needs of mentally ill persons using evaluative, epidemiological and health services approaches.

Pozi Liu is a Professor and Head of the Department of Psychiatry, Tsinghua University Yuquan Hospital, Beijing, China, and Institute of Mental Health, Peking University, Beijing.

Barry McGale is currently a member of the Northern Ireland Suicide Strategy Implementation Body, which oversees the Northern Ireland suicide prevention strategy, 'Protect Life'. He is also a qualified Cognitive Therapist and the Chairperson of Youthlife, a voluntary organisation that provides services for young people who have experienced loss though separation, divorce or bereavement. Barry was the recipient of the 2012 Florence Nightingale Travel Scholarship where he reviewed postvention services in Australia.

Patrick McGreevy, from Downpatrick in Northern Ireland, is a mental health nurse and has been active in suicide prevention for the past fifteen years. He was twice awarded the Florence Nightingale Travel Scholarship, which enabled him to travel to the United States and Canada to study theories and approaches for application in Ireland and the UK.

John L. McIntosh, PhD, is Interim Executive Vice Chancellor for Academic Affairs and Professor of Psychology at Indiana University South Bend (IUSB). He is the author, co-author, or co-editor of eight published books on suicide including *Suicide and Its Aftermath* (Norton, 1987), *Elder Suicide* (American Psychological Association, 1994), *Grief After Suicide* (Routledge, 2011), and *Devastating Losses* (Springer, 2012). Additionally, he has contributed chapters to several books and articles to many professional journals and has made over 100 professional presentations and many keynote addresses at professional conferences. He serves on the editorial boards of *Suicide & Life-threatening Behavior, Gerontology and Geriatrics Education*, and *Crisis: The Journal of Crisis Intervention and Suicide Prevention*. He is a Past-President of the American Association of Suicidology (AAS) and has been the recipient of AAS's prestigious Edwin Shneidman Award and the Roger Tierney Award for Service. McIntosh has been recognised by Indiana University with the IUSB Distinguished Teaching Award, the Indiana University President's Award for Distinguished Teaching, the IUSB Eldon F. Lundquist Faculty Fellow, and the IUSB Distinguished Research Award.

Hugh McKenna, CBE, PhD, B.Sc(Hons), RMN, RGN, RNT, DipN(Lond), AdvDipEd, FFN RCSI, FEANS, FRCN, FAAN, is a Professor and Pro Vice Chancellor for Research and Innovation at the University of Ulster, UK. His professional background is in general and mental health nursing. He joined the University in 1988 and has held positions as Lecturer, Senior Lecturer, Professor, Research Director, Head of School and Dean. He was Chief Nurse for the Southern Health and Social Care Board responsible for the nursing care of over 300,000 people. He has over 200 publications, including 10 books, and has received over $5 million in grants. He has supervised 16 PhD students to successful completion. He is on the editorial team of the *International Journal of Nursing Studies* and is a Fellow of the Royal College of Nursing (FRCN), Fellow of the European Academy of Nursing (FEAN) and Fellow of the Royal College of Surgeons of Ireland, (FRCSI). In 2008, he was made Commander of the British Empire (CBE) for his work on health and community. In 2009, he obtained the University's Senior Distinguished Research Fellowship and was made an International Fellow of the American Academy of Nursing (FAAN) – only the third person in Europe and the fifteenth worldwide to be given this honour. He also chairs the UK Research Excellence Framework panel for nursing, allied health professions, pharmacy and dentistry, which is tasked with deciding on the allocation of many millions of pounds to UK universities. He has also recently chaired the Hong Kong Accreditation Panel for Health Sciences, and the SWE at the University of Texas, and Trinity College Dublin, and was external examiner for a Master's programme in the Chinese University of Hong Kong.

Kwame McKenzie is a senior scientist within the Health Services and Health Equity Research section, the Medical Director of Access & Transitions as well as a Professor in the Department of Psychiatry at the University of Toronto, Canada. His research focuses on the science of improving mental health services. Key areas of interest include social determinants of health, society and mental health, social capital and mental health, redesigning mental health services for visible minority groups, efficacy of treatment in schizophrenia, psychiatric diagnosis, community engagement, racism, pathways to care, and suicide.

David Miers, PhD is the Counseling and Program Development Manager for Mental Health Services at Bryan Medical Center in Lincoln, Nebraska. Dr Miers holds a BS from Nebraska Wesleyan University, an MS from St. Cloud State University, and a PhD from the University of Nebraska–Lincoln. Dr Miers co-chairs the Nebraska State Suicide Prevention Coalition and helped develop the Lincoln Lancaster County Local Outreach to Suicide Survivors Team in Lincoln. He has published research on family needs following the death of a teenager to suicide.

Melinda M. Moore, PhD, received her doctoral degree in clinical psychology at The Catholic University of America, USA. Since her husband's suicide, she has been involved in a broad range of suicide prevention, research, and advocacy work nationally. Currently, she is a postdoctoral research fellow on the Department of Defense-funded Military Suicide Bereavement Study at the University of Kentucky in Lexington, Kentucky, USA.

Joseph S. Munson is a graduate of the University of Florida, USA, in the Counselor Education doctoral program. His dissertation was on how the impact of suicide affects post-traumatic growth within clinicians who directly experienced a client death by suicide. He has over 13 years specialising in Crisis Intervention, Suicide Prevention, Diagnosis and Assessment of Mental Health disorders, addiction treatment, and Non-Profit Management. He is currently the Vice President for Residential and Related Services at Meridian Behavioral Healthcare in Gainesville, Florida. He is a Licensed Mental Health Counselor in the state of Florida and also a certified trainer in Applied Suicide Intervention Skills Training (ASIST) and in Mental Health First Aid (MHFA).

Eva Neufeld is a Post-Doctoral Fellow in the Department of Psychiatry at Western University in London, Ontario, Canada. Eva's research is primarily in the field of mental health and aging, with particular focus on late-life depression, suicide prevention, risk assessment and mental health in primary care settings. Eva holds an MA in Gerontology from Simon Fraser University and a PhD from the University of Waterloo in Aging, Health and Well-being within the School of Public Health and Health Systems. Her dissertation research was a cross-sectional and longitudinal examination of community-residing older adults who experienced intentional self-harm.

Rosane Nisenbaum is a scientist in the Keenan Research Centre of the Li Ka Shing Knowledge Institute of St Michael's Hospital, Toronto, Canada and an Assistant Professor in the Division of Biostatistics, Dalla Lana School of Public Health, University of Toronto. She has experience of over 20 years as a Senior Biostatistician working in the United States and Canada on projects related to population-based studies of chronic illnesses, neighborhood effects on mental health, homelessness and housing, and suicide studies.

Colleen Pacey earned her Bachelor's degree in business in 1988 and her MSW in 2011. She is a trained instructor in the Roots of Empathy program which she has been facilitating for two years. She has been facilitating Skills and Tools for Emotions Awareness and management (STEAM) groups in elementary schools for four years. Colleen works for the Canadian Mental Health Association – Grand River Branch in Kitchener-Waterloo Ontaria, and is in her third year and fifth group facilitating Skills for Safer Living.

Christopher M. Perlman is an Assistant Professor in the School of Public Health and Health Systems at the University of Waterloo in Waterloo, Ontario, Canada. Christopher holds a BSc. in psychology from Trent University and an MSc and PhD in Health Studies and Gerontology from the University of Waterloo. As a health services researcher, his research incorporates aspects of evaluation, health informatics, and knowledge exchange to better understand and improve the quality of health services for persons with mental health conditions. He is particularly interested in how health information can be organised and presented to improve care decision-making and safety in health care.

Brandon Pierre is a Research Assistant, CAMH, Department of Psychiatry, University of Toronto, Canada.

Joshua A. Rash is a doctorate student in the Psychology Department at the University of Calgary, Canada. His research interests are in suicidal behaviour, behavioural medicine, psychophysiology, stress, pain, mental health in the workplace, and resilience.

Johanne Renaud M.D. M.Sc. FRCPC is a Child Psychiatrist and the Medical Director of the Outpatient Clinic of Depressive and Suicidal Disorders (youth section), at the Douglas Mental Health University Institute, Montreal, Canada. She is also an Associate Professor of Psychiatry, at McGill University. Since 2011, she has been leading the Standard Life Centre for

Breakthroughs in Teen Depression and Suicide Prevention holding both mandates of knowledge transfer and research projects in teen mental health. Since 2003, she has been an active researcher at the McGill Group for Suicide Studies. In New York, she received the 2012 Klerman Prize Honorable Mention, which recognises exceptional clinical research by a National Alliance for Research in Schizophrenia and Depression (NARSAD) Young Investigator grantee, for her research on health care trajectories and youth suicide and suicidal behaviors.

Sophia Rinaldis, MSc is a researcher for the McGill Group for Suicide Studies. She was among the researchers of the Nunavut Suicide Follow Back Study. Her work alongside Rod McCormick was completed in the context of the Network for Aboriginal Mental Health Research summer internship. Her current work focuses on youth suicide and health service trajectories.

Joscelyn Rompogren, BS, is a clinical psychology student at Alliant International University, USA, and editorial manager of several academic journals through the Institute on Violence, Abuse and Treatment. Her current research interests are in emotion regulation and heart-rate variability biofeedback.

Kate Russo is an Assistant Course Director on the Doctorate of Clinical Psychology programme at Queen's University Belfast. She is also an Independent Consultant Clinical Psychologist, specialising in the self-management of chronic and life-limited medical conditions. Dr Russo has a particular interest is using phenomenological research to improve people's lives. She is also an author and eclipse chaser.

Carlos B. Saraiva is Professor of Psychiatry at the University of Coimbra, Portugal, and Director of the Psychiatric Day Hospital of the Department of Psychiatry at the Central University Hospital of Coimbra. He has also been the founder and head of the Suicide Research and Prevention Unit, since 1992. He was the first president of the Portuguese Society of Suicidology (2001–2005). Dr Saraiva received his MD and PhD degrees from the University of Coimbra and trained as a psychiatrist at the Central University Hospital of Coimbra. He also served as scientific advisor to several academic or government institutions. Dr Saraiva is extensively involved in clinical practice, medical education and research, mainly on mood disorders, psychodrama, medical legal issues, and suicidology. He has published more than 100 articles, written two books on suicidology, and several book chapters.

Ayal Schaffer, MD, is Associate Professor, Department of Psychiatry, University of Toronto and Head of the Mood & Anxiety Disorders Program, Sunnybrook Health Sciences Centre, Toronto, Canada.

Monique Séguin, PhD, is a Professor of Psychology at the University of Québec in Outaouais, Canada, and member of the McGill Group on Suicide Studies. She is associated with other research groups including the Fenand-Seguin Research Center and Pierre-Janet Hospital. She spent a year in Toronto with the Arthur Summer Chair in Suicide Studies.

Wes Shera is the Dean Emeritus and Professor, Factor-Inwentash Faculty of Social Work, at the University of Toronto, Canada.

Chris P. Shields is a Clinical Psychologist working in the area of adult mental health in Northern Ireland. Chris's research within the area of suicide was influenced by the death of his nephew by suicide and the impact that this had on the family and wider social circle.

Mark Sinyor, MD, MSc, is Assistant Professor, Department of Psychiatry, University of Toronto, and works at Sunnybrook Health Sciences Centre, Toronto, Canada.

Amresh Srivastava is Associate Professor at the Department of Psychiatry, Western University London, Ontario, Canada.

Paul R. Springer is an Associate Professor in the Department of Child, Youth and Family Studies, and teaches in the Marriage and Family Therapy Program at the University of Nebraska–Lincoln, USA. He received his doctorate degree in Marriage and Family Therapy from Texas Tech University in 2007, a Master's degree in Marriage and Family Therapy from Auburn University in 2003, and his bachelor's degree from Brigham Young University in 2001.

Chris Stevenson, RMN, BA (Hons), MSc, PhD, CPsychol, RPN, has a long career in mental health, including nursing and family therapy which she researched for her PhD. Chris currently conducts psychological assessments for the UK Family Proceedings Courts and works with vulnerable children, young people and adults. Chris has extensive research experience in mental health nursing, psychotherapy and death by suicide. She has published widely both in academic and practice journals. Chris has taught in major UK and Irish universities and also undertaken practice development in mental health services, thereby increasing the impact of her research.

Anne–Grethe Talseth holds a PhD and Master of Science and Bachelor of Science degrees in nursing with a specialty in psychiatric/mental health nursing. She is a member of the Institute Board at the Department of Health and Care Sciences, Faculty of Health Sciences, University of Tromsø, Norway. Her teaching experiences in psychiatric/mental health nursing span more than 30 years. She has served as a consultant to psychiatric/mental health nurses in clinical settings as well as conducted qualitative nursing research. Dr Talseth has authored or co-authored more than 25 publications in various nursing journals. In addition, she has engaged in research collaboration with nursing colleagues in Norway, Sweden and the USA.

Laura Frank Terry is a doctoral candidate at the University of Texas at Arlington School of Social Work. She is a licensed master's level social worker (LMSW) in the state of Texas. She is an Adjunct Professor and her research focus is on the corrections population and mental health.

Darien Thira, PhD, is a Registered Psychologist who serves as a community development/mental health consultant for many Aboriginal communities across Canada and offers training workshops and clinical consultation related to post-colonial community mobilisation/development, trauma, addiction, and suicide. He is an adjunct faculty member at the Adler School of Professional Psychology. His doctoral dissertation related to Aboriginal suicide resilience and social activism and he has been involved in further resilience research at the University of British Columbia. He has previously served as a clinician with suicidal youth at Child and Youth Mental Health, Vancouver, and as the Director of Community Education and Professional Development at the Vancouver Crisis Centre. In relation to suicide prevention, "Through the Pain", a culturally driven community-based program has been used in over 40 Aboriginal communities across the country and as a national program in Australia. His program called "Opening the Circle" is designed to assist communities to develop their own crisis response team. "Choices", his youth suicide awareness education video and seminar was used by more than 250 suicide prevention programs world-wide and he has collaborated on the production of a new version called

"Reaching Out". Darien has presented workshops at many local, provincial, national conferences, and international conferences in Canada, the United States, and Australia.

Sharon Thira is an administrator, facilitator and trainer specialising in knowledge translation for a variety of audiences, but most significantly, Indigenous communities. Believing Indigenous knowledge to be foundational in improving health for Indigenous peoples, her work teleologically centres on holism. She has focused on crisis counselling and suicide prevention and training, residential school trauma and Indigenous health research. She was instrumental in developing the Truth and Reconciliation model negotiated in the Indian Residential School Settlement Agreement, and she developed many residential school response programs including the national Resolution Health Support Worker program. Recently she has developed a community health research training program to build community capacity in research. Her work experience includes 15 years with residential school survivors as the Executive Director of the Indian Residential School Survivors Society; Development Manager for the 15-year-old First Nations House of Healing Residential School Treatment culturally-based program model; and Director of Kloshe Tillicum, the Canadian Institutes of Health Research – Institute of Aboriginal Peoples Health Network Environment for Aboriginal Health Research. She is Lokono, East Indian and Chinese from Guyana and was adopted into the Halalt and Squamish Coast Salish nations.

A Ka Tat Tsang is an Associate Professor, Factor-Inwentash Faculty of Social Work and Factor-Inwentash Chair: Social Work in the Global Community; Expertise in Research, University of Toronto, Canada.

Andrew Tuck is Research Coordinator, Health Systems and Health Equity Research, Centre for Addiction and Mental Health, Toronto, Canada.

Gustavo Turecki, MD, PhD, is a Professor of Psychiatry and Human Genetics at McGill University, Montreal, Canada. He is an award-winning Canadian researcher and clinician who has devoted his career to improving the understanding of the biomedical risk factors and epigenetic mechanisms that lead individuals to commit suicide. Dr Turecki holds a William Dawson Chair and is Director of the McGill Group for Suicide Studies and the Quebec Suicide Brain Bank. In addition, he is the Vice-Chair of Research and Academic Affairs of the Department of Psychiatry at McGill University. His clinical and research interests are focused on the study of biomedical risk factors for suicide and depression. His work has contributed to the understanding of the suicide phenotype through multi-disciplinary studies on suicide completers, as well as molecular studies that inform the understanding of the suicide brain. His recent work has focused on epigenetic mechanisms and he has conducted pioneering research on how early-life adversity impacts the genome and increases long-term risk for suicide. He has authored over 250 publications, including book chapters and research articles in peer-reviewed journals. He has also received numerous grants and distinctions, including several scientific awards, such as the NARSAD Michael Kaplan Investigator Award, the American Foundation for Suicide Prevention Distinguished Investigator Award and the Radio-Canada Researcher of the Year. Dr Turecki is also an engaged clinician and heads the Depressive Disorders Program at the Douglas Mental Health University Institute, Montreal, where he treats patients with refractory major depressive disorder.

Erin F. Ward-Ciesielski, MS, is a doctoral student at the University of Washington, USA. She received her undergraduate degree from Indiana University South Bend and her Master's degree from the University of Washington. Presently, she is a doctoral candidate in the Clinical Psychology program at the University of Washington. She is the principal investigator on an NIMH-funded National Science Research Award to complete her dissertation evaluating the efficacy of a one-time intervention for non-treatment-engaged suicidal adults. She was the recipient of the American Association of Suicidology's Morton M. Silverman Award, in addition to receiving research awards from the American Psychological Association and the American Psychological Foundation.

FOREWORD: A VIEW FROM A SUICIDE SURVIVOR

William T. Feigelman
Professor of Sociology, Nassau Community College,
Garden City, New York

As a relative newcomer to the field of suicidology, with less than ten years research experience to my name, I feel deeply honored to have been chosen to write a foreword for this new, important and path-breaking volume. From my own distinctive vantage point, both as a survivor of my 31-year-old-son's suicide (more than a decade ago), and as a career sociologist, I come to this field with some distinctive perspectives, setting me apart, perhaps, from the many psychologically oriented researchers and practitioners that dominate in this arena. As I glance back, over my shoulder, at the history of this relatively young discipline, I see a very dynamic area of study and practice. It was little more than 50 years ago when Edwin Shneidman coined the term suicidology and founded the American Association of Suicidology, now the oldest professional organization in this field.

For me, there appear to be two distinct streams of intellectual work in this area; one, a wide river of scholarship on the causation of suicide with aims toward applying this knowledge to prevent suicides. This is the relatively well-funded branch of our field, with much support coming from governments and private philanthropic agencies. However, it must be said, that in comparison to the other serious health issues of our times, such as cancer, heart disease, diabetes control, malaria, infant mortality, HIV/AIDS, among other maladies, for suicide and mental health more generally, available research funding here in the U.S. and in most other countries is woefully inadequate to the seriousness and importance of the task. Yet, the work on suicide causation dominates the academic journals of our field.

In the second stream of work in suicidology, commanding a relative trickle of work, compared to the former branch, one finds a much smaller fraction of scholastic activity on postvention research. Here, almost no funding from governmental and philanthropic agencies can be found, though exceptions are observed, most notably in Australia, where an abundance of governmentally funded suicide prevention programs and services for the bereaved are observed. This is indeed a paradoxical outcome considering the large size of the suicide-bereaved population and their empirically demonstrated risks of heightened suicidality. As John McIntosh has demonstrated (in Chapter 12) in his carefully written chapter on the epidemiology of U.S. suicides, there are minimally close to 5,000,000 suicide-bereaved in the U.S. alone. If we apply the bereaved-by-suicide yardstick suggested by Edwin Shneidman—six bereaved for every person completing suicide—to the yearly global totals of suicide of approximately 1,000,000 suicides, we are dealing with a group growing at a rate of 6,000,000 each year. And in the chapter written by Aguirre and Terry (Chapter 22), there is ample documentation to point out that those bereaved-by-suicide stand at greater risk of subsequently taking their own lives.

It is rather remarkable that such a large, risk-prone group has eluded researcher scrutiny. If there is a simple answer for this avoidance of research with the suicide-bereaved, it is perhaps suicide stigma. The bereaved are held at arm's length for fear that any close involvement with them in research will inevitably heighten their suicide risks. Simply asking them about whether they are having suicidal thoughts is believed to induce them into contemplating their own suicides. However, this cautionary precept has usually been taken for granted and has generally not been subjected to any systematic empirical evaluation.

Now, evidence from several recently emerging, careful quantitative researches, cited in Rahel Eynan and her associates' work (Chapter17) and in their own study's findings, show that people with previous evidence of suicidality do not increase their suicidality after participating in a research activity. If anything, they show diminished suicidality at a post-research time point. Studies among the suicide-bereaved completed in Norway (Dyregrov, Dyregrov, & Raundelen, 2000; Dyregrov, 2004) also show great willingness among these survivors to talk about their loss experiences following a suicide who found it cathartic to participate in research and appreciated the caring interests shown by the researchers in their post-loss lives and welfare. Our U.S. survey research, based on a very large sample of 462 suicide-bereaved parents found agreement with the Dyregrovs' findings (Feigelman, Jordan, McIntosh, & Feigelman, 2012). The American bereaved were eager to participate in our research, showing a 72% response rate to our mailed questionnaire survey, comparable to research participation in home interview studies. Few balked at completing our lengthy, 27-page survey and many offered long addendums to their surveys, further explaining their survey answers. Most survivors simply wanted to tell their loss stories to a caring and interested researcher.

A momentum is now growing in the field with the realization that the stigma surrounding suicide must be broken and important neglected at-risk groups such as the bereaved must be studied more closely in future research. Thus, it was a very welcoming sight for me to find that a significant portion of the original articles presented in this anthology were devoted to the suicide-bereaved. This is a feature not found in most previous suicide research anthologies.

If I were assembling my own collection of this field, I don't think I could have arrived at a better and more meaningful synthesis of the materials than the one that John Cutcliffe and his co-editors have chosen. As suicide is an international phenomenon, it makes perfectly good sense to draw the book's contributors from a wide variety of nations, sharing their diverging national viewpoints and reporting on the differing patterns of suicide arising within their home countries. One country, such as Canada, may be likely to have diverging suicide patterns than those found in the USA, Portugal or in the United Kingdom.

It is also vitally important and fitting that the suicide research endeavor be multi-disciplinary in focus, drawn from the many fields that may provide new, original and creative thinking about the causation of suicide and ways of treating those showing suicidal vulnerabilities. It is essential, too, to gather data from the many intersection points where those harboring heightened suicidality can be readily observed and helped: in general and mental hospitals, outpatient mental health clinics, and in the community at large, and from the many other places in society where those with suicidal inclinations may be attracted. The Internet now comprises a new and potentially important resource for studying suicidality and for offering supportive services to those seeking help and information for coping with mental health distress.

Accordingly, besides psychology and psychiatry, anthropology, sociology, social work and nursing all have great potential to add to the knowledge base of the field as long as their practitioners are willing to apply the scientific method of hypothesis testing with observable, empirical data. The editors have created a very meaningful model for future suicidology theory and practice, by including many important previously neglected groups into the enterprise of doing suicide studies and empirically examining the value and benefits from diverging clinical care activities. Psychiatric nurses have a great deal of contact with those distressed by suicidal ideation both in hospital settings and in their home communities. In the many good selections drawn from psychiatric nursing professionals, readers will find much stimulating and provocative content, not found in other suicide research anthologies. For example, they will find great value in the chapter by Cutcliffe and associates (Chapter 3) emphasizing the indispensable importance of close follow-up to formerly hospitalized mental health patients.

Parts II and III on psychiatry and psychology offer many worthy new contributions to the field. To mention one in particular, the selection by Sinyor, Schaffer and Cheung (Chapter 8) which takes a cross-national view of the impact of means restrictions on diminishing suicides shows that a nuanced approach offers an important contribution to our understanding. As a particular means restriction, such as a bridge barrier, may be examined in several different countries, we can more readily observe its value in lessening the numbers of suicides.

The final Part of the book focused on Canadian aboriginal populations and suicides is especially important and valuable. Here the selections highlight the critical role of social marginality as a contributing factor to causing suicide. Today in Australia suicide is the leading death cause above all others among its aboriginal populations, with the youth aboriginal suicide rate far exceeding that of all other groups (Fisher, 2009). When people are held back from full participation in society, unable to get jobs and be respected, when they are looked at with disfavor and disesteem by those in power, they are more likely to have personal problems and to internalize their devalued positions. In turn, they are more likely to become depressed and have low self-esteem. They are also more likely to use drugs and to behave more self-destructively, leading them toward more suicides. Thus, we are led back to Emile Durkheim's important sociological contributions emphasizing the importance of social connectivity to averting suicide.

There is much to like in the many well-written and useful selections in what follows in this richly informative book. Among these carefully chosen selections, readers will find much to extend their knowledge of suicide and how the mentally distressed can be helped to make more meaningful connections with others and ultimately to place more importance and resolve to staying alive.

References

Dyregrov, K. (2004). Bereaved parents' experience of research participation. *Social Science and Medicine*. 58, 391–400.

Dyregrov, K., Dyregrov, A., & Raundelen, M. (2000). Refugee families' experience of research participation. *Journal of Traumatic Stress, 13*, 413–426.

Feigelman, W., Jordan, J.R., McIntosh, J.L., & Feigelman, B. (2012). *Devastating losses: How parents cope with the death of a child to suicide or drugs*. New York: Springer.

Fisher, J. (2009). The stand-by suicide-bereavement response service. Presentation at American Association of Suicidology Conference. San Francisco, CA. April 18, 2009.

FOREWORD: A VIEW FROM A MEMBER OF THE CANADIAN PARLIAMENT

Harold Albrecht
Member of Parliament, Kitchener-Conestoga, Canada

I should begin by noting that I am not an expert in the field of suicide prevention.

I've learned a lot since I began working on my legislation on suicide prevention, Bill C-300, which was signed into law by Governor General David Johnston in December 2012. Even so, all that I've learned has only served to teach me how much I do not know – indeed, how much is entirely unknown – about suicidal ideation and suicide prevention.

In Canada, a multitude of barriers prevent an informed conversation on suicide prevention. We don't even keep accurate numbers. That's why I'm so pleased to see this compendium of cutting-edge research on the subject.

In government, we tend to categorize challenges according to the silo charged with addressing them. Suicide prevention efforts are underway from silos as diverse as Veterans Affairs, the Public Health Agency of Canada, Aboriginal and Northern Affairs, the Canadian Institutes for Health Research, and the Mental Health Commission of Canada. Despite that, efforts on the ground are funded locally at widely varying levels. It is easier to find funding to prove a given program works than to fund the operation of a program proven to work.

But while growing, there still remains a lack of research on the subject. Even experts in one aspect of this field are too often unaware of advances made in other aspects. The *Routledge International Handbook of Clinical Suicide Research* brings together leading research from a variety of fields. My hope is that this will not only result in improved understanding, but that new research will also be inspired. The *Routledge International Handbook of Clinical Suicide Research* will not provide all of the answers. But, hopefully, it will provoke many more questions.

FOREWORD: A VIEW FROM A MEMBER OF THE WORLD HEALTH ORGANIZATION: EUROPE OFFICE

Dr Matt Muijen
Programme Manager, Mental Health and
Neuro-degenerative Disorders, WHO Regional Office for Europe

A book highlighting the many perspectives involved in care of suicidal persons, bringing together the evidence and providing ideas for better actions is very welcome. Any intervention that has the potential to prevent even a single incidence of suicide is worth pursuing. Considering the multi-dimensional causes and consequences of suicide, no single agency, let alone profession, can take, or be held responsible for actions in this field. The multi-disciplinary approach of this book is both welcome and essential.

For the European Region of the WHO, stretching from Iceland in the west to the far eastern parts of the Russian Federation, incorporating all the Central Asian Republics, suicide has always been a major concern and a high priority. Statistics are one reason for this concern. According to WHO data, European countries have consistently been among those with the highest suicide rates, to the extent that around the year 2000 the top nine countries were all in Europe. Lithuania has understandably been very concerned about its position at the top, even though rates have recently decreased somewhat, closely followed by the Russian Federation, Belarus, Kazakhstan and Hungary. Although this suggests an association with previous communist regimes, rates in Western Europe are also above the world average. No doubt the relative position of the European countries is slightly exaggerated due to unreliable data collection elsewhere, but absolute figures are still very high, whatever the rank order of countries.

The high numbers are even more worrying when put in context. In several European countries, suicide is the leading cause of death in young people. Although the rates of men are typically about fivefold higher than women, in some countries rates of completed suicides of young women are rising. Again, Europe appears to be the unfortunate leader in the world of female suicides.

A second reason for concern is how difficult it is proving to reduce suicides in a sustainable way. Many European countries have suicide prevention strategies, and most of these are highly sophisticated, combining universal and targeted primary prevention with follow up of high risk people. Examples of universal prevention are limiting the availability of supply to poisonous substances such as paracetamol and regulating ownership of firearms, uncontroversial in Europe, and safeguarding access to dangerous places such as high buildings and building fences on bridges.

An example of targeted prevention that WHO is actively pursuing is the training of primary care staff in the identification of people with suicide risk. Particularly in many countries of the former Soviet Union, just those with the highest rates of suicide, primary care has no recognised role in diagnosing and treating people with depression. Since we know from research that a high proportion of people with suicidal intent visit family doctors in the weeks preceding an attempt, the ability of properly trained family doctors is crucial. Many inspiring examples of supporting people with a history of suicide attempts are described in the chapters of this book.

It needs to be borne in mind that health care is only one dimension of any effective suicide prevention. Moreover, some of the most effective policy interventions are not directly aimed at suicide prevention, but nevertheless reduce rates very significantly. We know these lessons well, both from past and present experiences. A well known example from the past was the clampdown on alcohol abuse in the Soviet Union during the Gorbachev era by increasing prices and reducing availability. The prime aim was to reduce the mortality rate of men and improve productivity, but a desirable by-product was the reduction of suicides. It is well recognised that the high alcohol consumption in the European Region is correlated to suicide rate. This is true for countries, but even more so if regions within countries are compared. Some rural regions in Eastern Europe that consume high volumes of alcohol also have stunningly high suicide rates. Due to political upheaval, the reforms were not sustained, and both alcohol consumption and suicide rates increased again. But it did demonstrate the feasibility of effective political action.

Unfortunately, the European region is also facing a current crisis that is affecting people's mental health. Many European countries are struggling with the impact of the economic downturn. This is causing an increase in unemployment rates, particularly among the young. Unemployment is associated with depression and alcohol use, both of which increase the risk of suicide. Evidence is accumulating that suicide rates are indeed rising quite significantly. The political question is now how to address economic needs while not negatively affecting the well-being of the population, particularly the most vulnerable groups such as the young and marginalised.

So far, austerity measures have dominated decision making. This can result in a double blow for people at risk of depression. First, unemployment rises, and second, mental health services are cut. This is not inevitable. While Greece has indeed cut investment in mental health care, Ireland has protected its mental health budget. At least equally important as health care spending are measures to protect jobs, income and status, in combination offering 'social inclusion'. As a consequence of the major savings that need to be made, some of the poorest countries have also made cuts to welfare payments, increasing the gap of those with jobs and those without and reducing people's self-esteem. Importantly, we know that suicide rates in countries with the highest social solidarity also are least affected by unemployment. It may be the central policy dilemma of our time, that what is perceived as crucial for the economic condition of a country, austerity measures, is damaging the well-being of the population that governments are aiming to protect.

Some of the chapters in this book address these issues, such as the needs of the most excluded people and the role of agencies to protect them. Each of such agencies will play an essential but separate role in the lives of people at risk of mental health problems and suicide. The challenge, emerging again and again, is how to establish accessible and effective services that people can trust. Such challenges are made even more difficult by the threat of reduced funding for many of these services themselves. Stress and mental health problems of staff are a topic that deserves special attention in its own right.

Many of these points are raised in the new WHO European Mental Health Action Plan. Suicide prevention, mental health promotion, accessible community-based services that are trusted by people with mental health problems and the need for good data are all covered. It also brings to attention the need for multi-disciplinary training and working, and the value of coordinated partnerships between sectors. One example is the agreement of single assessment procedures in order to avoid duplication and delays, so often causing drop outs. Or an opportunity to pool budgets between sectors, creating efficiencies. As is so often exemplified in this book, effective actions do not have to be complex. But all require initiative and trust. This is relevant at both the highest government level and for the person working directly with the man or woman thinking about committing suicide. This book makes this case well, and it deserves to be read widely.

PREFACE

Synergy and serendipity often play a big part in medical and scientific advances.

Julie Bishop

Even the most frustrating of circumstances can give rise to something substantive, meaningful and constructive. On the 14th April, 2010, the Icelandic volcano Eyjafjallajokull began the so-called 'explosive' phase of its eruption which would ultimately lead to the cancellation of thousands of flights, hundreds of thousands of stranded passengers, the loss of millions of dollars for airlines and perhaps (tongue in cheek) – the most important consequence of all – the birth of this book!

One's birthday ought to be a day of celebration but now I had this latest catastrophe to add to the list of historical tragedies that seem to coalesce on the 14th April (for example, President Abraham Lincoln was shot by John Wilkes Booth at Ford's Theatre just before 10.30 p.m. on the 14th April, the *Titanic* struck the iceberg on the 14th at 11.40 p.m., and now this . . .). However, as I continued to watch events in Iceland unfold and develop, it became more and more evident that I was about to be stranded. *There was, however, a 'silver lining' to this ash cloud;* I had the fortune to be stranded with many of the delegates who had been participating in the Horatio European Psychiatric Nursing Congress ('Building Bridges'). One such delegate was my dear friend and colleague Dr José Carlos Santos, from Coimbra, Portugal.

In between calling airlines, checking news reports and listening to the attempts of colleagues as they tried to get home, José and I focused on using the time constructively. We had previously engaged in a number of conversations about suicidology, one of which was an issue that, despite being separated by thousands of miles, he and I had both struggled with. Caring for suicidal people in a formal mental health care system, whether as inpatient or outpatient settings, invariably involves multiple different disciplinary groups. In no order of priority necessarily, these groups include: psychiatrists, psychiatric/mental health nurses, psychologists, social workers and suicide survivors, to name but a few. Formal care for suicidal people is then (and has been for decades) very clearly, a multi-disciplinary endeavour. Moreover, when one starts to widen the conceptual-isation of care to include the prevention of suicide, then even more groups and stakeholders are involved. Yet even a cursory review of the extant literature shows few genuine attempts to bring these groups together and collate their substantive contributions to the body of knowledge in one volume. For José and me, this was a gross oversight and a major gap in the literature.

We wanted a book that combined substantive contributions from the disciplinary groups who are commonly involved in care of the suicidal person. We wanted a book that would 'showcase' the research that these disciplinary groups have been involved in. We wanted a book that included some of the hitherto under-represented groups – specifically suicide survivors and Indigenous/Aboriginal populations. We wanted a book that was not specific to any given discipline. *We wanted a book that brought multi-disciplinarity 'front and centre'.*

Alongside the importance of recognising multi-disciplinarity was the recognition that suicide was (and remains) a global problem. Differences in some cultures, theological positions and beliefs notwithstanding, suicide is ubiquitous. Similarly, while one can acknowledge the variances in suicide rates over time, the history of humankind is 'pockmarked' with suicide. Suicide, the human experience and the human 'condition' appear to be intertwined. Nevertheless, while the global nature of suicide is hardly encouraging, it does create the possibilities for cross-border exchange of ideas, findings and knowledge. It does create opportunities for discovering what may be universally applicable – irrespective of nationality and/or cultural background, while at the same time, highlighting nuanced, idiosyncratic aspects of care of the suicidal person that may exist only in certain countries, certain cultures.

And so as the dust (ash) settled, literally, out of the ashes rose the proposal for this book; an unexpected serendipitous outcome concerned with illustrating and promoting synergy between and among these disciplinary groups. While we had to make very difficult choices about who to invite to edit and/or to contribute, we believe we have brought together a fine collection of scholars who share our understanding and valuing of multi-disciplinarity and internationality. So the next time we are stranded – be it as a result of volcanic eruption or otherwise – we hope it will be once again with like-minded scholars. Who knows what that will lead to?

Dr J. R. Cutcliffe
July 2013, Ontario, Canada

1

INTRODUCTION

Suicide as a significant and growing public health concern: coalescing and building our understanding through interdisciplinary and international scholarship

John R. Cutcliffe

Data collected from a variety of international sources show that suicide continues to be one of the most imposing contemporary public health issues facing many nations of the world today (AGDHA, 2000; Associate Minister of Health, 2006; White, 2003; World Health Organization, 2002). Despite our best efforts, the global rate of suicide has continued to rise since the 1950s. Suicide is expensive in terms of the human cost and associated suffering (Shneidman, 1997, 2004), the economic costs (Institute of Medicine, 2002), the social costs (CASP, 2004; Maris, 1997) and the spiritual costs (Jobes et al., 2000). The international epidemiological picture is equivocal with some countries showing a recent downward trend in suicide rates, such as in the United Kingdom (Department of Health, 2005), Australia (AGDHA, 2000), New Zealand (Associate Minister of Health, 2006) Hungary, Switzerland, Denmark, Belgium and others. Inversely, other countries show alarming upwards trends, such as Ireland, China and former Soviet Bloc countries, such as Lithuania, Russian Federation and the Ukraine.

It is also may be noteworthy that trends in both Canada and the United States[1] also indicate increases in suicide rates; indeed, the Blueprint for a Canadian National Suicide Prevention Strategy (CASP, 2004) indicates that Canada has a higher suicide rate than many other industrialized countries. As a result, though epidemiological evidence should always be treated with a degree of caution (given the epistemological and methodological limitations), the clear trend in this evidence is that suicide remains a significant public health problem and in many parts of the world – is actually on the increase.[2]

What do we know? The significant gaps in the literature

It is reasonable to state that a substantial literature exists that focuses on suicide, nevertheless, it is also accurate to point out that:

1   This literature remains significantly under-developed (see, for examples, Leenaars' 2010 statement that much of the current understanding and research in suicide is at least half-paralyzed).

2   There remain large and highly significant gaps in the literature and our current understanding (see Maris et al., 2000).

3   The literature contains a great deal of repetition (see Rogers and Lester's 2009 comments that recent suicide-focused research has not served to advance our understanding of suicidal behaviour but tends to repeat older research).

4   There is a particular need for inter- (or multi-) disciplinary and international efforts to deepen our understanding of suicide.

The calls for increased inter/multi/trans-disciplinarity and internationality

Several key international calls further indicate the need for evidence-based literature to inform the care of the suicidal person. The American Association of Suicidology (AAS), for example, has urged researchers to produce more 'book-length' manuscripts of research pertaining to care of the suicidal person. Concomitantly, within the substantive area of suicidology, there is a growing requirement for research that gives voice to service users' experiences and thus the associated need for service user involvement in the research process; including the dissemination of research findings (see, for example, Andriessen, 2004). The International Association for Suicide Prevention established a taskforce (as long ago as 1999), to increase awareness of issues concerning suicide survivors and postvention activities. Furthermore, repeated exhortations have been delivered to urge greater international research efforts *vis-à-vis* studying suicide. The National Academy of Sciences (2002) document, for instance, has argued: 'Extending the (increased multi-disciplinary research efforts) into the international arena where cultural differences are large and may provide new information. . .can be fostered.'

Alongside such encouragements, numerous conferences have been held in recent years where the explicit goals of such multi-disciplinary gatherings include the need to unite stakeholders to advance efforts to impact the high suicide rate. In such conferences, researchers, clinicians, bereaved families, and passionate advocates are encouraged to work together to address the critical public health problem of suicide and suicide attempters.

The necessity and benefits of international collaboration

According to Adams et al. (2007), international research collaboration is a rapidly growing component of core research activity for all countries; it is encouraged at a policy level because it provides access to a wider range of facilities and resources. Adams et al., continue that international collaboration enables researchers to formulate and participate in networks of cutting-edge and innovative activity. For researchers, collaboration provides opportunities to move further and faster by working with other leading people in their field; collaborative research is also identified as contributing to some of the highest impact activity. Other gains include access to knowledge and facilities and the establishment of longer-term relationships. It should not be surprising then that the scholarly output from international (and especially multi-disciplinary) teams can provide 'added value'.

Scholarly output from international, multi-disciplinary teams, it can be argued, has more potential impact and utility than uni-disciplinary and/or uni-national scholarly outputs. Internationally focused books such as this text have many times the potential applicability of uni-national focused books; if well written, they reflect the context, culture and experiences of all the contributing authors and editors, thus broadening the appeal of the book. Furthermore, suicide is a global phenomenon; it impacts on people in all nations. And there are both commonalities across individual nations and idiosyncratic elements of the 'problem of suicide' in individual nations. As a result, there is much to be learned from studying the problem in different contexts and cultures, and much to be gained by sharing these findings and insights across international boundaries.

Similar arguments have been made regarding the extra or added value of having multi-disciplinary or inter-disciplinary studies and associated scholarly outputs. It is extremely rare in today's health and social care system(s) that problems exist entirely within the boundaries of one academic/clinical discipline or another. Almost inevitably, these major public health problems transcend and straddle the boundaries of individual disciplines; the range of different disciplinary groups involved in the care of individuals who present with these problems is, again, wide and deep. Suicide and the care of the suicidal person are a case in point. It is well recognized that suicide is influenced by intra- and inter-personal phenomena such as the person's physiology (e.g., biochemistry, genetics); psychology (e.g., personality traits, coping skills); spirituality (e.g., theological views); social connectivity and interactions (e.g., degree of loneliness, degree of connection/engagement); and behaviour (e.g., suicide as an acquired, learned behaviour). Similarly, suicide is also clearly linked to and influenced by extra-personal matters of social policy and economics (e.g., unemployment rates, access to health care). Accordingly, improving the care of suicidal people, creating more efficacious suicide prevention programmes and ultimately preventing deaths by suicide require the input of many disciplinary groups. It is with these very specific issues in mind that the authors have constructed a book that:

1 is clearly international in focus and composition;
2 is clearly multi- or inter-disciplinary in focus and composition;
3 collects contemporary, leading-edge suicide-focused research.

We believe that this is the first book of its kind. This book brings together a collection of eminent suicidology scholars, each of whom has an established track record of publishing in this substantive area or/and engaging in federally funded research that focuses on suicide (or/and issues related to suicide). Our collection of editors includes:

- two former holders of Professorial Endowed Chairs (Dr. Cutcliffe and Dr. Links);
- the former president of the American Association for Suicide Prevention (Dr. Campbell);
- the former president of the Canadian Association for Suicide Prevention (Dr. Links);
- the former president of the Portuguese Association for Suicide Prevention (Dr. Santos);
- two former international representatives to the International Association for Suicide Prevention (Dr. Cutcliffe and Dr. Links);
- several members of numerous journal editorial boards, including suicide-specific journals such as *Crisis* – the journal of the International Association for Suicide Prevention.

The book's editorial team is, for the first time, a purposeful collection of scholars/clinicians from the wide range of disciplines involved in the direct/indirect care of the suicidal person (and/or suicide survivors). Moreover, the editorial team is again intentionally international in composition. These two important design choices were incorporated as an attempt to have the book reflect the global and professional/disciplinary reality of the problem of suicide. Suicide is not restricted to one country or another; it is not restricted to the developing world or the developed world; it is not limited to one ethnic group. All the countries that report data to the World Health Organization show that suicide is a global phenomenon and, moreover, in many places/countries, it is a growing problem. Similarly, the problem of suicide and care of the suicidal person are not restricted to one disciplinary group or another. At the same time, it should be acknowledged that the 'answers' to the problem of suicide are unlikely to exist within the artificial, 'man-made' boundaries of one discipline or another. The logical position is that in order to address the problem of suicide, we ought to draw upon the wisdom, knowledge, experiences, theories and empirical findings from all the groups/disciplines involved (either directly or indirectly) in the care of suicidal people.

The book is divided into six discrete (yet linked) Parts, with each Part focusing on the research work emanating from (and focusing on) the individual disciplines (groups) involved in the care of suicidal people. Not to overstate the unique nature of this book, but no other book that focuses on suicide and suicidology has been written with such a format and clear emphasis on highlighting the multi-disciplinary contributions to the extant knowledge base.

Each Part of the book is a collection of 'cutting-edge' research studies[3] that have focused on suicide and care/management of suicidal people that relates to the particular disciplinary group. Accordingly, by way of an example, Part I, 'Nursing' includes five research reports of studies involving psychiatric/mental health nurses as part of the research teams and/or focusing on psychiatric/mental health nursing care of the suicidal person. Similarly, Part II, 'Psychiatry' includes five research reports of studies involving psychiatrists as part of the research teams and/or focusing on psychiatric care of the suicidal person issues.

Each of these Parts has been edited by key figures from their respective disciplines; they have made previous substantive contributions to the literature in their area and have undertaken research focusing on their particular substantive group. Each Part is buttressed by an introductory editorial and a commentary section where the salient threads and themes that are evident in the research have been highlighted; in some cases, possible future directions for research are highlighted.

Why have we included these issues/parts and not others?

As stated previously, four sections of this book are driven by professionals who belong to the clinical groups (disciplines) who have frequent contact with suicidal people, perhaps most commonly in mental health care settings: psychiatric nurses, psychiatrists, psychologists and social workers (though Part IV also includes contributions from other disciplines). As to which studies/issues to include in the five chapters in each of these Parts, we have deliberately deferred to the expertise of the Editors of these sections in making these choices. In putting together a book that focuses on current and key research activity in suicidology, and operating within word/space limits, the Editors would like to point out that difficult choices had to be made on which studies/issues to include and which to omit. The Editors wish to emphasize that in no way is this list of contemporary research meant to be exhaustive or representative of the only issues that warrant formal study. Understandably, the choice of which studies/issues to include reflects, at least in part, the views, values and to some extent, the interest of the Editors. The idiosyncrasies of the Editors notwithstanding, we believe the studies/issues have currency and meaning for the majority of practitioners involved in the care of suicidal people. They have been selected in part as a result of our communication with the international suicidology community (e.g., the emerging evidence regarding expressed emotion and suicide); as a result of searching the extant literature for recent 'cutting-edge' research (e.g., the encouraging work that uses aspects and ideas of dialectical behavioural therapy to reduce suicide risk); as a result of the introduction of some health care policy and national suicide prevention strategies (e.g., the work with significant others of suicide victims), as a result of empirical responses to recent epidemiological data and trends in suicidology (e.g., recent dramatic rise in rates of suicide in young men) and in part, in an attempt to capture practice and related issues.

The two remaining Parts, those that focus on suicide survivors and Indigenous/Aboriginal people, were included for the following reasons. Even a cursory examination of various countries' national suicide prevention strategies will indicate that they all highlight the need to focus on suicide survivors. Numerous national and international suicide survivor groups are already in existence; their annual meetings are now attached to formal suicidology conferences, and their collective voices are heard by researchers, practitioners and legislators. As a result, the authors believe it would be remiss to produce a book that focuses on cutting-edge research efforts in suicidology without simultaneously giving some attention and focus to those most affected by suicide.

Second, there is an overwhelming body of evidence, when one looks at the international 'picture' that indigenous (Aboriginal) peoples very often have disproportionately high suicide rates (when compared to the general population). See, for example, many First Nation bands in Canada; Aboriginal suicide rates in Australia, indigenous groups living within the circumpolar regions from various countries e.g., Inuit, http://www.itk.ca/Inuit-Approaches-to-Suicide-Prevention, the Inupiat youth in Alaska http://www.ncbi.nlm.nih.gov/pubmed/16952416, the Evenks in China and Russia and the Sami in northern Norway and Finland (though there are some encouraging data relating to the Sami).

There is little doubt, then, that suicide remains one of the most pressing public health concerns in these populations, and despite the fact the indigenous populations can be separated by thousands of miles, there are significant similarities across these groups. Accordingly, for a book that wishes to capture the contemporary and cutting-edge suicidology research, one should logically include work that has focused on one of the highest risk groups. Further, the geographical distribution of these groups perhaps also lends support to the idea that this book will have international appeal and utility, not least because of Part VI that focuses on suicide in indigenous groups.

Finally, as the editors put the 'finishing touches' to this book, the mass media is reporting the spread of suicide to families of military personnel in the United States of America (http://usnews.nbcnews.com/_news/2013/01/16/16540098-like-an-airborne-disease-concern-grows-about-military-suicides-spreading-within-families?lite&ocid=msnhp&pos=3); this follows alarming reports of increasing rates of suicide in the military personnel themselves (http://abcnews.go.com/Health/study-80-percent-army-suicides-start-iraq-war/story?id=15872301). This is despite the existence of a concerted research (the biggest ever) effort to better understand and prevent such suicides (http://www.nimh.nih.gov/science-news/2009/evidence-based-prevention-is-goal-of-largest-ever-study-of-suicide-in-the-military.shtml). Concomitantly, the International Association for Suicide Prevention and the WHO draw attention to how the rate of suicide is increasing; their projections highlight that by 2020 approximately 1.53 million people will die from suicide (each year – on average), this represents a suicide death every 20 seconds and one attempt every 1–2 seconds.

Consequently, there is undeniable evidence that:

1 The problem is on the increase.
2 Previous (no doubt robust and well-meaning) research efforts have not produced widespread, indeed global and permanent reductions in suicide rates.
3 The need to broaden and widen our understanding (and conceptualization) of suicide and what we do as a health care and a social community to help reduce the rate of suicide becomes clear. It is difficult to make the case that our current understanding/conceptualization and approaches to reducing suicide rates have been particularly successful.

For the editors of this book, one such way to broadening our thinking and practice on this matter is to look beyond our historical (artificial, man-made) disciplinary boundaries and beyond international, cultural and ethnic boundaries. It is therefore our hope that this edited volume might be considered one small step in the direction of a truly global, multi-disciplinary body of extant knowledge focused on preventing suicide and we look forward to reading similar contributions from other suicidologists and scholars.

Notes

1   These two countries have been included as examples of the state of affairs in occidental counties and because of the location/associations of the bulk of the editors.
2   This introductory paragraph has been reproduced from Cutcliffe et al. (2006).
3   In a few cases, we have included summaries of research, reviews of literature/existing instruments.

References

Adams, J., Gurney, K., & Marshall, S. (2007). *Patterns of international collaboration for the UK and leading partners.* Leeds: Evidence Ltd.

AGDHA (Australian Government Department of Health and Ageing) Mental Health and Suicide Prevention Branch (2000). Living Is For Everyone (LIFE): A framework for prevention of suicide and self-harm in Australia. National Suicide Prevention Strategy. Available at: http://www.livingisforeveryone.com.au/about_nsps.html (accessed 2013).

Andriessen, K. (2004). Suicide survivor activities: An international perspective. *Suicidologi, 4*(2), 25–27. Available at: http://www.iasp.info/pdf/papers/Andriessen.pdf.

Associate Minister of Health (2006). The New Zealand Suicide Prevention Strategy 2006–2016. Wellington, Ministry of Health. Available at: http://www.moh.govt.nz/moh.nsf/pagesmh/4904/$File/suicide-prevention-strategy-2006-2016.pdf (accessed 2013).

Canadian Mental Health Association (n.d.). Suicide Statistics. Available at: http://www.ontario.cmha.ca/fact_sheets.asp?cID=3965 (accessed 2013).

Canadian Association for Suicide Prevention (2004) *CASP blueprint for a Canadian National Suicide Prevention Strategy.* Edmonton: CASP.

Cutcliffe, J. R., Stevenson, C., Jackson, S., & Smith, P. (2006). A modified grounded theory study of how psychiatric nurses work with suicidal people. *International Journal of Nursing Studies, 43,* 791–802.

Department of Health (2001). *Safety first: Five year report of the national confidential inquiry into suicides and homicides by people with mental health problems.* London: HMSO.

Department of Health (2005). *National suicide prevention strategy for England: 2nd annual report on progress.* London: HMSO.

Institute of Medicine (2002). *Reducing suicide.* Washington, DC: National Academic Press.

Jobes, D. A., Luoma, J. B., Hustead, L. A., & Mann, R. E. (2000). In the wake of suicide: Survivorship and postvention. In R. W. Maris, A. L. Berman, & M. M. Silverman (Eds.), *Comprehensive textbook of suicidology* (pp. 536–560). New York: Guilford Press.

Leenaars, A. (2010). Review of the book, 'Understanding Suicide: Why We Don't and How We Might', J. R. Rogers & D. Lester. Available at: http://www.hogrefe.com/program/understanding-suicide.html (accessed 2013).

Maris, R. (1997). Social suicide. In A. A. Leenaars, R. Maris, & Y. Takahashi (Eds.), *Suicide: Individual, cultural, international perspectives* (pp. 41–49). New York: Guilford Press.

Maris, R. W., Berman, A. L., & Silverman, M. M. (2000). *Comprehensive textbook of suicidology.* New York: Guilford Press.

National Academy of Sciences (2002). *Reducing suicide: A national imperative.* Available at: http://www.nap.edu/openbook/0309083214/html/.

Rogers, J. R., & Lester, D. (2009). *Understanding suicide: Why we don't and how we might.* Cambridge, MA: Hogfree.

Shneidman, E. S. (1997). The suicidal mind. In R. W. Maris, M. M. Silverman, & S. S. Canetto (Eds.), *Review of suicidology* (pp. 22–41). New York: Guilford Press.

Shneidman, E. S. (2004) *Autopsy of a suicidal mind.* Oxford: Oxford University Press.

Suicide in the U.S.: Statistics and Prevention. Available at: http://www.nimh.nih.gov/health/publications/suicide-in-the-us-statistics-and-prevention/index.shtml (accessed 2013).

White, J. (2003). *Report on the workshop on suicide-related research in Canada.* Ottawa: Health Canada/CIHR.

World Health Organization (2002). *Depression/suicide.* Available at: www.int/health_topics/suicide/en/ (accessed 2013).

PART I

Nursing

EDITORIAL INTRODUCTION

For many people, suicide and mental health problems are inextricably linked to the extent that contemporary mental health care, in many parts of the world,[1] is synonymous with providing care and treatment to suicidal people. However, this was not always the case. Prior to the 18th century, the prevailing orthodoxy of and associated discourses about suicide were firmly embedded within theological and philosophical literatures (Cutcliffe & Links, 2008a; 2008b). It was not until the 18th century, however, that 'science' began to offer explanations for suicidal behaviour and 'treatment' (Cutcliffe & Links, 2008a; 2008b). This time period also saw a corresponding and significant rise in the number of suicidal individuals who were admitted (and interned) to so-called 'insane institutions'. Since those days, the association between formal mental health care and suicidal people has strengthened. Admission to formal mental health facilities, which in the main has meant psychiatric inpatient hospitalization, became the mainstay of care and treatment for suicidal people. As a result, psychiatric/mental health (P/MH) nurses now have a long history of working with suicidal people; indeed, of all the different disciplinary groups involved in such care and treatment, P/MH nurses spend more direct contact time with suicidal people than any other. Given this clinical reality, one could be forgiven for expecting that P/MH nurses would have made significant, substantial and frequent contributions to the extant theoretical and empirical suicidology literature; alas, this is not the case.

It has been argued that the discipline of nursing has only recently started to have better scientific evidence to demonstrate the difference nursing makes in health care since the 1990s where studies have been undertaken to bridge the gap in knowledge and identify nursing-sensitive outcomes (Doran, 2011). Despite the fact that nurses are the single largest discipline involved in health care[2] (Benner, Sutphen, Leonard, & Day, 2009), nursing is often absent from health policy decision-making and debates *vis-à-vis* health care, including suicidology. While some literature is available regarding nursing-sensitive outcomes in acute (medical/surgical) care (Yang et al., 1999; Doran et al., 2006; Tourangeau et al., 2006; Blegen et al., 2011), and to a lesser extent in long-term care (Head et al., 2004; Castle et al., 2008), it is limited in the area of psychiatric/mental health nursing. However, although P/MH nursing-originated empirical and theoretical contributions to the suicidology literature remain sparse, especially when compared to some other disciplines, substantive, significant, and meaningful contributions have been made. In focusing on a sample of such substantive contributions, and highlighting the type of research that P/MH nurses are involved in, the editors hope that in some small way, Part I will contribute to rectifying this limitation. It is also noteworthy that the contributions to this section have emanated from different geographical locations, and the editors believe this deserves special attention. Suicidal behaviors are a global problem, P/MH nurses in various different parts of the world encounter the same challenges; the same relative absence of hope, the same experiences of psychache, the same stigma. Accordingly, findings that originate from Ireland, Norway, the USA, Portugal, or the United Kingdom may very well have applicability and transferability to other parts of the world; to other mental health care systems.

Part I begins with Chapter 2 by Gilje and Talseth which reports on a qualitative meta-analysis of how P/MH nurses experienced suicidal patients. They found four major themes: (1) pondering humanistic and mechanistic views of suicide and suicidal patients; (2) contemplating various responses to life and death encounters; (3) discerning complex competencies while relating therapeutically; and (4) needing informal and formal support. Despite the different practices, education and contexts of the studies examined, some commonalities can be identified. According to the authors, adopting a humanistic, person-first perspective enables suicide to be understood in the context of a person's life situation, and this opens up relational possibilities for 'sharing existential despair' and reconnecting with humanity. Inversely, labeling suicidal persons, for example as having a psychiatric diagnosis, conveys a mechanistic perspective. These different options to 'connect' with the patient can help us distinguish the defensive practices of P/MH nurses from more advanced practices, such as engaging with patients. If we consider that suicidal persons need a closer human relationship to reconnect with humanity and re-vision the meaning of life, then such nurses need to have better nursing education, more clinical supervision of practices and more support.

In Chapter 3, Cutcliffe, Links, Harder, Balderson, Bergmans, Eynan, Ambreen and Nisenbaum examine the increased risk of suicide following discharge. They conclude that the risk of suicide remains high in the post-discharge period, with few suicides but more self-injury and suicide attempts within six months of hospital discharge. Some participants even mentioned that their suicidal ideation increased after they were discharged. The authors stress the importance of pre-discharge preparation and post-discharge 'follow-up' care, such as: preparing the person for discharge, involving clients in the decision-making process, post-discharge visits in the community, phone calls, use of social media, and creating a post-discharge plan in collaboration with the patient. Discharge should not be the end of care for the suicidal person, but the beginning of a new approach to caring and supporting in the community, because in many cases suicidal behavior is a chronic condition.

Following this, in Chapter 4, Gordon, Stevenson and Cutcliffe report on a nationally funded, Grounded Theory (GT) (Glaser & Strauss, 1967) study in Ireland, to develop a theoretical understanding of how young men transcend suicidality. They report that the key psychosocial process involved in transcending suicidality was the process of re-vitalizing worthiness and this has two interlinked stages: (1) confronting a crisis of destiny; and (2) earning a life. They underline the importance of including patients in decisions, 'working with them', helping them regain a sense of control over their lives and fostering their sense of self-agency and self-esteem. These actions can be the turning point between life and death. Also important is giving support to practitioners working in this area in order to prevent compassion, fatigue and burnout and enhance job satisfaction.

Chapter 5 by McKenna, Keeney, Cutcliffe and Stevenson reports on a study designed to obtain a comprehensive understanding of the encounters of suicidal men (aged 16–34) with formal mental health services, in order to explicate the specific caring processes that might make 'a difference' to caring for the suicidal person, that is, to inform what health care professionals can do. These authors were concerned with answering the questions: how can mental health care services be most appropriately configured to encourage their use by suicidal men aged 16–34? And: what is the required response of mental health care services for suicidal men, aged 16–34? After analyzing qualitative interviews, they found three major categories: (1) widening access and bolstering pro-active outreach; (2) on becoming a man . . .; and (3) equipping young men for the challenges of 21st-century living. Three main ideas should be underlined: the services should be community-based and open access; they should include the use of 'social media', which have become a regular means of communication among young people; and psychological therapies need to be made available as part of routine care.

And to conclude Part I, in Chapter 6, Santos reports on a qualitative and quantitative study with parasuicidal adolescents who had been admitted to the Emergency Room and their families. He used quantitative tools to characterize the adolescents and qualitative analysis to characterize their families' environment through Expressed Emotion. A follow-up study was conducted during nine months after the parasuicidal behavior. In this study, he concluded that families with high Expressed Emotion had more recurrent parasuicidal behaviors, which remained high after nine months. Patients with recurrent behavior were being followed by a psychiatrist, but none of them had a history of familial intervention. However, the family emerges, in this study, as an important factor in the recurrence of parasuicidal behaviors.

Notes

1   Particularly the occidental world.
2   In terms of numbers of clinicians, and furthermore, this 'picture' is evident when one examines the international and global data on this issue.

References

Benner, P., Sutphen, M., Leonard, V., & Day, L. (2009). *Educating nurses: A call for radical transformation*. San Francisco: Jossey-Bass.

Blegen, M. A., Goode, C. J., Spetz, J., Vaughn, T., & Park, S.H. (2011). Nurse staffing effects on patient outcomes: Safety-net and non-safety-net hospitals. *Medical Care, 49*(4), 406–414.

Castle, N. G. (2008). Nursing home caregiver staffing levels and quality of care: A literature review. *Journal of Applied Gerontology, 27*(4), 375–405.

Cutcliffe, J. R. & Links, P. (2008a) Whose life is it anyway? An exploration of five contemporary ethical issues that pertain to the psychiatric nursing care of the suicidal person: part 1. *International Journal of Mental Health Nursing, 17*, 236–246.

Cutcliffe, J. R. & Links, P. (2008b) Whose life is it anyway? An exploration of five contemporary ethical issues that pertain to the psychiatric nursing care of the suicidal person: part 2. *International Journal of Mental Health Nursing, 17*, 247–255

Doran, D. (2011). *Nursing outcomes: State of the science* (2nd ed.). Toronto, ON: Jones & Bartlett Learning.

Doran, D. M., Harrison, M. B., Laschinger, H. S., Hirdes, J. P., Rukholm, E., Sidani, S., McGillis Hall, L., & Tourangeau, A. E. (2006). Nursing-sensitive outcomes data collecion in acute care and long-term care settings. *Nursing Research, 55* (2S), S75–S81.

Glaser, B. G., & Strauss, A. L. (1967) *The discovery of grounded theory: Strategies for qualitative research*. Chicago: Aldine.

Head, B. J., Lober Aquilino, M., Johnson, M., Reed, D., Maas, M., & Moorhead, S. (2004). Content validity and nursing sensitivity of community-level outcomes from the Nursing Outcomes Classification (NOC). *Journal of Nursing Scholarship, 36*(3), 251–259.

Tourangeau, A. E., Doran, D. M., McGillis Hall, L., O'Brien Pallas, L., Pringle, D., Tu, J. V., & Cranley, L. A. (2006). Impact of hospital nursing care on 30-day mortality for acute medical patients. *Journal of Advanced Nursing, 57*(1), 32–44.

Yang, K. A., Simms, L. M., & Yin, J. T. (1999). Factors influencing nursing-sensitive outcomes in Taiwanese nursing homes. *Online Journal of Issues in Nursing, 4*(2). Available at: ww.nursingworld.org/MainMenu Categories/ANAMarketplace/ANAPeriodicals/OJIN/TableofContents/Volume41999/No2Sep1999/ ArticlePreviousTopic/TaiwaneseNursingHomes.aspx.

2

HOW PSYCHIATRIC NURSES EXPERIENCE SUICIDAL PATIENTS

A qualitative meta-analysis

Fredricka L. Gilje and Anne-Grethe Talseth

Introduction

As psychiatric nurses experience suicidal persons from diverse walks of life, they face pivoting them from a 'death oriented position to a life oriented position' (Cutcliffe et al., 2006, p. 801). This chapter presents a qualitative meta-analysis of how psychiatric nurses experience suicidal patients. Our aim is to summarize and synthesize existing research, revealing understandings that inform nurses in clinical practice and research.

Method

Qualitative meta-analysis, the first component of a meta-study, involves re-analysis of data from published primary studies (Paterson et al., 2001). This study proceeded in three phases: (1) formulating the research question; (2) selecting and appraising primary research; and (3) conducting meta-data analysis.

Formulating the research question

The research question that evolved over time (Timulak, 2009) was 'How do psychiatric nurses experience suicidal patients?' Suicide was defined as physical harm to oneself with the intent of dying (Nock & Kessler, 2006), excluding self-mutilation, euthanasia, parasuicide and assisted suicide.

Selecting and appraising primary research

Eleven selected studies were retrieved from peer-reviewed journals in electronic databases. Inclusion criteria were: at least one nurse author; primary clinical nursing research published in English in peer-reviewed periodicals between 1996 and 2012; qualitative designs or designs where qualitative data were clearly distinguishable; solely psychiatric nurse participants; explicitly focused on suicide or suicide attempts; a clear description of data analyses processes related to findings; and some described ethical considerations and trustworthiness. Exclusion criteria were: research reports; secondary studies; unpublished primary research; non-psychiatric nurse participants;

non-English language publications; and an explicit focus on self-mutilation, euthanasia, para-suicide or assisted suicide. Screening of the studies was based on the above inclusion criteria. Appraisal of quality was based on the criteria of Paterson and associates (2001). The studies were conducted in England (Cutcliffe et al., 2007), Ireland (Bohan & Doyle, 2008; Long & Reid, 1996), Norway (Gilje et al., 2005; Gilje & Talseth, 2007; Talseth et al., 1997; Vråle & Steen, 2005), Sweden (Carlen & Bengtsson, 2007; Larsson et al., 2007), Taiwan (Tzeng et al., 2010) and the USA (Aflague & Ferszt, 2010). Table 2.1 reports a summary of the studies.

Table 2.1 Summary of selected primary studies

Author(s) and year of publication	Participants and context	Methodological orientation	Theoretical orientation
Long & Reid (1996)	N = 45 Psychiatric Ireland	Qualitative Exploratory	Caring for suicidal patients
Talseth, Lindseth, Jacobsen & Norberg (1997)	N = 19 Psychiatric Norway	Qualitative Hermeneutic	Meaning of experiences caring for suicidal patients
Vråle & Steen (2005)	N = 5 Psychiatric Norway	Qualitative Descriptive	Performing constant observation of suicidal patients
Cutcliffe, Stevenson, Jackson & Smith (2007)	N = 20 General health care England	Qualitative Modified Grounded Theory	Meaningful nursing care for suicidal patients
Carlen & Bengtsson (2007)	N = 11 Psychiatric Sweden	Qualitative Exploratory	Experiencing caring for suicidal patients
Gilje & Talseth (2007)	N = 19 Psychiatric Norway	Qualitative Hermeneutic	Responding to suicidal patients
Larsson, Nilsson, Runeson & Gustafsson (2007)	N = 29 General Health Care Sweden	Qualitative Descriptive	Nursing care of suicidal patients
Bohan & Doyle (2008)	N = 9 Emergency Department Ireland	Qualitative Descriptive	Experiencing patient suicide and suicide attempts & support received
Aflague & Ferszt (2010)	N = 6 Psychiatric USA	Qualitative Phenomenography	Assessing suicide
Tzeng, Yang, Tzeng, Ma & Chen (2010)	N = 18 Psychiatric Taiwan	Qualitative Focused Ethnography	Caring dilemmas and responses to suicidal patients

Meta-data analysis

Analytic processes were guided by qualitative content analysis (Graneheim & Lundmann, 2004) and interpretive description (Thorne et al., 2004). These iterative processes were interwoven with disciplined researcher reflexivity and consensual interpretive data analyses. First, the major findings of each study were coded (i.e., Views, Responses, Competencies, Needs) and categorized. Next, subcategories were formulated by both authors until achieving intercoder consensus. From these processes, themes developed. Table 2.2 reports the analyses processes. A summary of the analyses processes is reported in Table 2.3.

Findings

The findings revealed four themes addressing the research question. Psychiatric nurses' experiences with suicidal patients involved: (1) pondering humanistic and mechanistic views of suicide and suicidal patients; (2) contemplating various responses to life and death encounters; (3) discerning complex competencies while relating therapeutically; and (4) needing informal and formal support.

The theme 'Pondering humanistic and mechanistic views of suicide and suicidal patients', was evident in most studies. Findings showed nurses viewed suicide and suicidal patients in positive, humanistic ways (Long & Reid, 1996), as human beings (Bohan & Doyle, 2008; Cutcliffe et al., 2007; Talseth et al., 1997; Vråle & Steen, 2005), and sufferers (Carlen & Bengtsson, 2007; Gilje & Talseth, 2007), needing consolation (Gilje & Talseth, 2007). A mechanistic view described suicidal patients as a label (Carlen & Bengtsson, 2007; Tzeng et al., 2010), a psychiatric diagnosis (Carlen & Bengtsson, 2007), and a diagnosis of depression with accompanying hopelessness (Carlen & Bengtsson, 2007).

The theme, 'Contemplating various responses to life and death encounters', showed nurses maneuvering through moral-ethical, relational and emotional responses to suicidal patients. Moral-ethical responses (Cutcliffe et al., 2007; Gilje & Talseth, 2007; Tzeng et al., 2010) such as respect, and relational responses, such as openness and professional boundaries (Tzeng et al., 2010) were apparent in the studies. Emotional responses (Bohan & Doyle, 2008) included struggling with feelings of despair (Gilje & Talseth, 2007; Long & Reid, 1996), anger (Bohan & Doyle, 2008; Carlen & Bengsteen, 2007; Tzeng et al., 2010), and closeness and distance (Talseth et al., 1997). Lack of distress and anger when encountering suicidal patients were also reported (Long and Reid, 1996).

Professional nursing competencies concerning care for suicidal patients are complex (Aflague & Ferszt, 2010; Carlen and Bengtsson, 2007) and involve 'discerning complex competencies while relating therapeutically', the third theme. The most frequently addressed competency was therapeutic relating (Aflague & Ferszt, 2010; Cutcliffe et al., 2007; Gilje & Talseth, 2007; Long & Reid, 1996; Talseth et al., 1997; Tzeng et al., 2010; Vråle & Steen, 2005). Other competencies included knowledge of risk factors (Aflague & Ferszt, 2010), risk assessment (Aflague & Ferszt, 2010; Vråle & Steen, 2005), close observation (Bolen & Doyle, 2008; Vråle & Steen, 2005), safety (Aflague & Ferszt, 2010), therapeutic milieu (Vråle & Steen, 2005) and collaborating with patients, peers, carers and colleagues (Aflague & Ferszt, 2010).

'Needing informal and formal support' was the fourth theme. Nurses clearly reported needing self-awareness (Larsson et al., 2007; Long & Reid, 1996; Carlen & Bengtsson, 2007), emotional support (Larsson et al., 2007; Talseth et al., 1997) and educational resources (Bohan & Doyle, 2008; Long & Reid, 1997). They also reported an immense sense of helplessness in supporting colleagues while, at the same time, struggling with similar emotions (Bohan & Doyle, 2008).

Table 2.2 Thematic analysis processes: from major findings of selected studies to codes to categories to subthemes and themes

Author year	Major findings of selected studies	Code	Category	Subtheme	Theme
Long & Reid (1996)	Overall nurses had positive attitudes toward working with suicidal patients. Yet some experienced distress while others did not. Length of psychiatric nursing experience did not affect level of satisfaction caring for suicidal patients. Nurses needed further education and practice in interpersonal skills and therapeutic approaches	Views	Humanistic view of suicidal patients	Viewing suicide & suicidal patients in various ways	Pondering humanistic and mechanistic views of suicide and suicidal patients
		Responses	Emotional	Reflecting on various responses	Contemplating various responses to life and death encounters
		Competencies	Therapeutic relating	Judging expertise	Discerning complex competencies while relating therapeutically
		Needs	Self-awareness Education	Needing various kinds of assistance	Needing informal and formal support
Talseth, Lindseth, Jacobsson & Norberg (1997)	Caring meant 'closeness'. 'Distance' placed ethical demands on nurses' interactions with suicidal patients, revealing the importance of reflecting on feelings and needing support	Views	Humanistic view of suicide & suicidal patients	Viewing suicide & suicidal patients in various ways	Pondering humanistic and mechanistic views of suicide and suicidal patients
		Responses	Moral-ethical Emotional	Reflecting on various responses	Contemplating various responses to life and death encounters
		Competencies	Therapeutic – relating	Judging expertise	Discerning complex competencies while relating therapeutically

Study		Needs	Emotional	Needing various kinds of assistance	Needing informal and formal support
Vråle & Steen (2005)	Constant observation involved assessing need for controlling the patient; nurse–patient relationship involved structure-flexibility, control–therapeutic relationship	Competencies	Risk assessment; Constant observation; Therapeutic milieu; Therapeutic relating	Judging expertise	Discerning complex competencies while relating therapeutically
		Views	Humanistic view of suicidal patient	Viewing suicide & suicidal patients in various ways	Pondering humanistic and mechanistic views of suicide and suicidal patients
Cutcliffe, Stevenson, Jackson & Smith (2007)	Reconnecting person with humanity meant reflecting an image of humanity, guiding them back to humanity and learning to live	Views	Humanistic view of suicide & suicidal patients	Viewing suicide & suicidal patients in various ways	Pondering humanistic and mechanistic views of suicide and suicidal patients
		Responses	Moral-ethical	Reflecting on various responses	Contemplating various responses to life and death encounters
		Competencies	Therapeutic relating	Judging expertise	Discerning complex competencies while relating therapeutically
Carlen & Bengtsson (2007)	Caring was experienced as labeling (e.g. psychiatric diagnosis) and suffering (e.g. hopelessness)	Views	Mechanistic & humanistic views of suicide & suicidal patients	Viewing suicide & suicidal patients in various ways	Pondering humanistic and mechanistic views of suicide and suicidal patients
		Needs	Self-awareness	Needing various kinds of assistance	Needing informal and formal support

Table 2.2 Continued

Author year	Major findings of selected studies	Code	Category	Subtheme	Theme
Gilje & Talseth (2007)	Becoming ready to mediate consolation with suicidal patients involved being at-home with self, an ethical way of being	Views	Humanistic view of suicidal patient	Viewing suicide & suicidal patients in various ways	Pondering humanistic and mechanistic views of suicide and suicidal patients
		Responses	Moral–ethical	Reflecting on various responses	Contemplating various responses to life and death encounters
		Competencies	Therapeutic relating	Judging expertise	Discerning complex competencies while relating therapeutically
Larsson, Nilsson, Runeson & Gustafsson (2007)	Nurses mostly used person support; self-support was occasionally used; self-perspective was lacking	Needs	Self-awareness Emotional	Needing various kinds of assistance	Needing informal and formal support
Bohan & Doyle (2008)	Feeling distressed and needing informational support and resources were needed following suicide/suicide attempt	Responses	Emotional	Reflecting on various responses	Contemplating various responses to life and death encounters
		Competencies	Close observation	Judging expertise	Discerning complex competencies while relating therapeutically
		Needs	Educational	Needing various kinds of assistance	Needing informal and formal support

Source					
Aflague & Ferszt (2010)	Structure of suicide assessment was knowledge (e.g. risk factors), method (e.g. listening, significant others) and reference (suicide cases, intuition, collaboration). All skillfully assessed suicidality in various ways without using suicide assessment guidelines or tools, pointing to complexity of suicide assessment	Views	Humanistic view of suicidal patient	Viewing suicide & suicidal patients in various ways	Pondering humanistic and mechanistic views of suicide and suicidal patients
		Competencies	Knowledge of risk factors / Risk assessment / Safety / Therapeutic relating / Collaboration	Judging expertise	Discerning complex competencies while relating therapeutically
Tzeng, Yang, Tzeng, Ma & Chen (2010)	Dilemmas involved opening and closing of figurative 'inner door', a dynamic process. Most effect was when they first opened their own inner door, and then waited outside suicidal patients' inner door to open up. Their response was 'Discouragement', including labeling, using restraints, reflecting on practice, receiving patients' teachings	Views	Humanistic and mechanistic views of suicide & suicidal patients	Viewing suicide & suicidal patients in various ways	Pondering humanistic and mechanistic views of suicidal patients
		Responses	Moral–ethical / Emotional / Relational	Reflecting on various responses	Contemplating various responses to life and death encounters
		Competencies	Therapeutic relating	Judging expertise	Discerning complex competencies while relating therapeutically

Table 2.3 Summary of analysis processes: code to category to subtheme to theme

Code	Category	Sub-theme	Theme
Views	Humanistic Mechanistic	Viewing suicide and suicidal patients in various ways	Pondering humanistic and mechanistic views of suicide and suicidal patients.
Responses	Moral-ethical Relational Emotional	Reflecting on various responses	Contemplating various responses to life and death encounters
Competencies	Knowledge of risk factors Risk assessment Close observation Safety Therapeutic milieu Therapeutic relating Collaboration	Judging expertise	Discerning complex competencies while relating therapeutically
Needs	Self-awareness Emotional Educational	Needing various kinds of assistance	Needing informal and formal support

Reflections and discussion

Findings from this qualitative meta-analysis point to various clinical implications. Nurses' humanistic and mechanistic views of suicide have a bearing on how they experience suicidal persons. A humanistic, person-first perspective sees being suicidal in the context of a person's life situation. This opens up relational possibilities for 'sharing existential despair' (Gilje & Talseth, 2007, p. 549) and reconnecting with humanity (Cutcliffe et al., 2007; Gilje & Talseth, 2007). In contrast, labeling suicidal persons, for example, as a psychiatric diagnosis (Carlen & Bengtsson, 2007; Tzeng et al., 2010), conveys a mechanistic perspective. Of importance is to consider that suicide also occurs in those who do not have a mental health problem (Cutcliffe & Links, 2008b). In the United States, those who die by suicide do not always access the formal mental health system; those who do access it are often diagnosed (Tanney, 2000). Hopelessness poses a significant suicide risk factor, especially when it accompanies depression (Carlen & Bengtsson, 2007; Cutcliffe, 2003). Nurses should realize that diagnostic labels can be dehumanizing and stigmatizing. Stigma often becomes a barrier to caring for suicidal persons (Smoyak, 2001).

Nurses' views of suicide have a bearing on their responses. As nurses contemplate various responses to life and death encounters (Carlen and Bengtsson, 2007; Gilje & Talseth, 2007; Tzeng et al., 2010) and work through value-laden situations concerning their responsibility for another's life and death, they waver (Gilje & Talseth, 2007). This is poignantly exemplified in the following participant's response:

> I feel very heavy each and every time I meet a suicidal patient because I, myself, have to go through my own desire to live or not to live . . . We never do this once and for all. My own attitude about life is activated every time I meet a suicidal patient.
>
> *(Gilje et al., 2005, p. 526)*

Wavering between feeling close and feeling distant occurs in the midst of experiencing difficulty entering into the person's lonely isolation (Talseth et al., 1997). Boundary struggles (Tzeng et al., 2010) likely relate to nurses' humanistic and mechanistic views or Moralist, Libertarian and Relativist perspectives (Cutcliffe & Links, 2008a). (A Moralistic perspective considers suicide sinful; a Libertarian views suicide as rational and reasonable; a Relativistic view is based on situational and contextual variables.)

At a deep level, nurses' responses seem to reveal conflicting and competing moral-ethical dilemmas involving questioning moral justification (Hewitt & Edwards, 2006, p. 667). An example is 'Whose life is it anyway?' (Cutcliffe & Links, 2008a, p. 238). Addressing and responding to this contemporary question is foundational for encountering suicidal persons in meaningful ways. Such encounters demand more than understanding theories and models (Aflague & Ferszt, 2010); they require ethical responses that permeate such encounters.

Contemplating responses prior to and in the midst of encounters with suicidal persons calls for self-understanding. This means understanding one's emotional and mental status and having sufficient time to be available (Tzeng et al., 2010), present (Gilje, 1992) and co-present (Cutcliffe et al., 2007). Through self-reflection, nurses can become present, open up, engage and relate. Engaging, a fundamental process of relating (Cutcliffe & Barker, 2002), involves 'opening an inner door' (Tzeng et al., 2010) and 'being-at-home' (Gilje & Talseth, 2007). 'Opening an inner door' illustrates nurses' open-mindedness to understand both patients and themselves. 'Being-at-home' consoles the nurse's self and fosters readiness for consolation (Gilje & Talseth, 2007). 'Closing the inner door' may be manifest as mood changes and seeking relief from burdensome caregiving (Tzeng et al., 2010). This can happen when nurses do not feel 'at-home' and cannot become ready to either encounter suicidal persons or mediate consolation. It is important for nurses to become aware of their 'inner door' and 'at-homeness' which are dynamic processes. Of importance is for nurses to reflect on their responses (Talseth et al., 1997), which may include their own suffering and need for consolation (Gilje & Talseth, 2007) because a sense of powerlessness can constrain nursing care (Sun et al., 2006). Reflection raises self-understanding and, in turn, affects nurses' readiness to engage in close encounters that reconnect with humanity (Cutcliffe et al., 2007) and preserve human dignity, autonomy and life inviolable (Vatne, 2006).

It makes sense that professional competencies concerning care for suicidal persons are complex (Aflague & Ferszt, 2010; Cutcliffe & Stevenson, 2007; Talseth & Gilje, 2011) and require judging expertise in the midst of relating therapeutically. Therapeutic relating is of utmost importance (Aflague & Ferszt, 2010; Cutcliffe et al., 2007; Gilje & Talseth, 2007; Long & Reid, 1996; Talseth et al., 1997; Tzeng et al., 2010; Vråle & Steen, 2005). A review of the literature on suicide and nursing care (Sun et al., 2005) concluded that competency in therapeutic communication is necessary for the care of suicidal persons. Indeed, 'caring for suicidal people must be an interpersonal endeavor' (Cutcliffe & Stevenson, 2007, p. 950).

Suicidal persons need a close human relationship (Cutcliffe et al., 2006; Vråle & Steen, 2005) to 'reconnect with humanity' (Cutcliffe et al., 2007) and 're-vision the meaning of life' (Gilje & Talseth, 2007). 'Patients are unlikely to explore sensitive issues, distressing thoughts and problems in living unless they are able to experience trusting relationships with mental health professionals' (Hewitt & Edwards, 2006, p. 670). Viewing patients as human beings is important for building trust (Løgstrup, [1956] 1971). Trust can help envelope suffering and turn lives around. Without a relational aspect, suffering that encompasses suicide is not addressed.

Moreover, connecting with others may be an important mediating factor in overcoming suicidal thoughts (Lakeman & Fitzgerald, 2008) and instilling hope. Suicidal persons are imbued with hopelessness; they desire goodness and hope (Gilje & Talseth, 2007). Hope conveyed through the therapeutic relationship is essential for recovery. At a deep level, relational aspects are of utmost importance in inspiring hope (Cutcliffe & Koehn, 2007; Koehn & Cutcliffe, 2007; Talseth et al., 2001). Hope emerges through engagement. Key processes of engagement involve: 'forming a relationship, a human–to–human connection, conveying acceptance and tolerance, and healing and understanding' (Cutcliffe & Barker, 2002, p. 612).

Complex competencies include knowledge of risk factors, risk assessment, close observation, safety, therapeutic milieu and collaboration. Knowledge of risk factors influences assessment; assessment requires knowledge of risk factors. The selected studies showed mixed results about nurses' suicide risk assessments. Some recommended structure to guide suicide assessment (Aflague & Ferszt, 2010; Vråle & Steen, 2005). Others showed no use of guidelines or instruments, asserting that variability in risk assessment furthers understanding of how nurses assess suicide and accentuating the complexity of suicide and suicide assessment (Aflague & Ferszt, 2010). A knowledge gap in suicide assessment and risk factors and a need for comprehensive suicide assessment have been emphasized (Talseth & Gilje, 2011). Comprehensive assessment should include the impact of chronic stress related to an array of social, economic, nutritional and life style factors, neuroendocrine functions and cultural aspects. Cultural variables are important in understanding various views and customs associated with suicide. Of concern is lack of cultural-specific assessment in the selected studies. Approaching assessment in the context of the person's life experiences is important for engaging in meaningful encounters with suicidal persons.

Encounters with suicidal persons often involve close or special observation. An increase in close observation following an attempted suicide often occurs (Bohan & Doyle, 2008). The importance of both a supportive therapeutic relationship as well as concern for safety is emphasized in a few studies (Aflague & Fertz, 2010; Vråle & Steen, 2005) and supported in other literature (e.g., Cleary et al., 1999). The practice of observation can involve a conflict with providing patient safety while regarding patient autonomy (Cutcliffe & Links, 2008b). While it protects physical integrity, too often it serves the organization, averts litigation and does not relieve the despair of suicidal persons (Cutcliffe & Stevenson, 2007). While close observation may uphold non–malfeasance, it may provide only some therapeutic value (Cutcliffe & Barker, 2002). Observation often seems to be 'defensive and custodial' (Cutcliffe & Stevenson, 2007, p. 943), a mechanized way of viewing suicidal persons.

Providing a therapeutic milieu focused on emotional and physical aspects is important for the care of suicidal persons, yet it poses challenges in balancing structure and flexibility (Vråle & Steen, 2005). The complex dynamics, influenced by nurses' views, that comprise the context of the ward environment, impact the therapeutic nurse–patient relationship (Sun et al., 2005) and call for collaboration. Collaboration is a professional responsibility (Alflague & Ferstz, 2010) that provides an opportunity for team members to share expertise, and compile deeper understandings of suicidal situations (Sun et al., 2005).

In light of nurses' pondering diverse views of suicide and suicidal persons, reflecting on their various responses and discerning complex competencies, of importance is for nurses and organizations to advocate for various kinds of support. Support is vital for maneuvering through a myriad of dilemmas encountered with suicidal persons. Nurses need informal and formal support to guide them through the complex labyrinth of encounters with those who live with suicidal intent.

Informal support involves reflecting and engaging with colleagues and peers in a casual way while adhering to confidentiality (Bohan and Doyle, 2008). Engaging in self-awareness is key to addressing nurses' need for support (Carlen & Bengtsson, 2007; Larsson et al., 2007; Long & Reid, 1996; Talseth & Gilje, 2011). Self-awareness is related to self-reflection which is similar to self-assessment, self-determination, self-integration and self-realization (Larsson et al., 2007, p. 224). Reflecting on views of suicide and suicidal persons opens up possibilities for viewing the complexity of professional nursing competencies. Nurses' views of suicidal persons influence discerning professional nursing competencies and have a bearing on their need for support. Meaningful encounters can turn lives around. First-person accounts and stories can evoke provocative insights and emotions about suicidal persons' real-life experiences and what is meaningful to them (Aflague & Ferszt, 2010). Such accounts and stories, shared in informal or formal settings, can stir up dramatic shifts in emotions and views of suicidal persons and aid in discerning nursing competencies. Nurses' self-care needs can also be met in these ways. Self-care is very important to sustain and uphold nurses' resilience (Talseth & Gilje, 2011; Warelow & Edward, 2007) and enables caring for others.

Formal support (Bohen & Doyle, 2008; Long & Reid, 1996) is support offered by an organization. A study of nurses authored by psychiatrists (Takahashi et al., 2011) found nurses needed formal support systems, especially in the aftermath of a patient's suicide death. However, support is not only needed by nurses. Psychiatrists expressed their strong, frightening feelings about mortality, vulnerability and fallibility during interactions with suicidal patients (Talseth & Gilje, 2007). Telling and retelling profound recollections can open up dialogue within and among disciplines (Talseth & Gilje, 2007). Formal support can occur through 'compassionate leave' (Bohan & Doyle, 2008, p. 15), support groups, debriefing sessions, counseling, follow-up phone calls, team building and educational programmes. Ongoing education focused on self-awareness is important (Bohan & Doyle, 2008; Sun et al., 2005). One way to reflect on various responses, moral-ethical issues, challenging questions and relational aspects is clinical supervision. Clinical supervision can provide various kinds of support and reveal poignant understandings about self and others. Similarly, multi-disciplinary teams provide an arena where collaborating with various professionals can provide much-needed support as well as self-awareness about responses to, and understandings of, suicide prevention, intervention and post-discharge follow-up care (Aflague & Ferszt, 2010).

Conclusion

The four themes interpreted from this synthesis of 11 primary clinical nursing studies collectively convey how psychiatric nurses experience suicidal persons. Clinical nursing research focused on this topic is sparse and scattered in a few geographic locations. Major gaps exist in knowledge development related to cultural context. Cultural-sensitive knowledge is needed to shed light on the meaning of suicide in specific contexts.

We acknowledge that the limited diversity and relatively small sample size can be considered a limitation (Timulak, 2009). However, the textual data were sufficient to answer the research question. While the selected studies reported that participants were solely psychiatric nurses, it is unclear if all had specialized education which should affect their experiences with suicidal persons. We acknowledge that educational preparation varies from country to country. Also perspectives on research ethics may differ geographically, influencing the appraisal of quality. The selected studies were conducted in clinical settings, resulting mainly in knowledge about secondary interventions. As we look to the future, resilient practices and education offer ways for nurses to foster patient recovery (Warlow & Edward, 2007). Primary prevention, including protective factors such as resilience (Wagnild & Gantnar, 2011), must be emphasized. Knowledge of neuroscience related to suicide is increasing, so the physiological side of suicide protection, prevention and intervention needs to be addressed.

We consider the findings one of many interpretations (Ricouer, 1976) influenced by our pre-understandings, including our own cultural context. The first author is from the United States; the second is from Norway. Both are psychiatric nurse educators and researchers. Their pre-understandings of nursing and suicidality provided prerequisite understandings of the texts in the selected studies. Throughout the analyses processes, we repeatedly examined the text, posing critical questions to it, engaging in ongoing dialogue concerning it, maintaining a faithful stance to it and reaching consensus of our critical interpretation of the findings shown in the tables. The findings can guide and inform nursing practice and research in psychiatric and, likely, non-psychiatric settings, offering deeper and richer understandings about how nurses experience suicidal persons.

References

Aflague, J. M., & Ferszt, G. G. (2010). Suicide assessment by psychiatric nurses: A phenomenographic study. *Issues in Mental Health Nursing, 31*, 248–256.

Bohan, F., & Doyle, L. (2008). Nurses' experiences of patient suicide and suicide attempts in an acute unit. *Mental Health Practice, 11*,13–16.

Carlen, P., & Bengtsson, A. (2007). Suicidal patients as experienced by psychiatric nurses in inpatient care. *International Journal of Mental Health Nursing, 16*, 257–265.

Cleary, M., Jordan, R., Horsfall, J., Mazoudier, P., & Delaney, J. (1999). Suicidal patients and special observation. *Journal of Psychiatric Mental Health Nursing, 6*, 461–467.

Cutcliffe, J. R. (2003). Research endeavors into suicide: A need to shift the emphasis. *British Journal of Nursing, 12*, 92–99.

Cutcliffe, J. R., & Barker, P. (2002). Considering the care of the suicidal client and the case for 'engagement and inspiring hope' or 'observations'. *Journal of Psychiatric and Mental Health Nursing, 9*, 611–621.

Cutcliffe, J. R., & Koehn, C. V. (2007). Hope and interpersonal psychiatric/mental health nursing: A systematic review of the literature: Part two. *Journal of Psychiatric and Mental Health Nursing, 14*, 141–147.

Cutcliffe, J. R., & Links, P. S. (2008a). Whose life is it anyway? An exploration of five contemporary ethical issues that pertain to the psychiatric nursing care of the person who is suicidal: Part one. *International Journal of Mental Health Nursing, 17*, 236–245.

Cutcliffe, J. R., & Links, P. S. (2008b). Whose life is it anyway? An exploration of five contemporary ethical issues that pertain to the psychiatric nursing care of the person who is suicidal: Part two. *International Journal of Mental Health Nursing, 17*, 246–255.

Cutcliffe, J. R., & Stevenson, C. (2007). Feeling our way in the dark: The psychiatric nursing care of suicidal people – a literature review. *International Journal of Nursing Studies, 45*, 42–53.

Cutcliffe, J. R., Stevenson, C., Jackson, S., & Smith, P. (2006). A modified grounded theory study of how psychiatric nurses work with suicidal people. *International Journal of Nursing Studies, 41*, 791–802.

Cutcliffe, J., Stevenson, C., Jackson, S., & Smith, P. (2007). Reconnecting the person with humanity: How psychiatric nurses work with suicidal people. *Crisis, 28*, 207–210.

Gilje, F. (1992). Being there: A concept analysis of presence. In G. Gaut (Ed.), *The presence of caring in nursing*. New York: National League for Nursing.

Gilje, F., & Talseth, A. G. (2007). Mediating consolation with suicidal patients. *Nursing Ethics, 14*(4), 546–557.

Gilje, F., Talseth, A. G., & Norberg, A. (2005). Psychiatric nurses` response to suicidal psychiatric inpatients: Struggling with self and sufferer. *Journal of Psychiatric and Mental Health Nursing, 12*, 519–526.

Graneheim, U. H., & Lundman, B. (2004). Qualitative content analysis in nursing research: Concepts, procedures and measures to achieve trustworthiness. *Nursing Education Today, 24*, 105–112.

Hewitt, J. L., & Edwards, S. D. (2006). Moral perspectives on the prevention of suicide in mental health settings. *Journal of Psychiatric and Mental Health Nursing, 13*, 665–672.

Koehn, C. V., & Cutcliffe, J. R. (2007). Hope and interpersonal psychiatric/mental health nursing: A systematic review of the literature: Part one. *Journal of Psychiatric and Mental Health Nursing, 14*, 134–140.

Lakeman, R., & FitzGerald, M. (2008). How people live with or get over being suicidal: A review of qualitative studies. *Journal of Advanced Nursing, 64*(2), 114–126.

Larsson, P., Nilsson, S., Runeson, B., & Gustafsson, B. (2007). Psychiatric nursing care of suicidal patients described by the sympathy-acceptance-understanding-competence model for confirming nursing. *Archives of Psychiatric* Nursing, 21, 222–232.

Løgstrup, K. E. ([1956] 1971). *The ethical demand* (Danish original), Philadelphia, PA: Fortress Press.

Long, A., & Reid, W. (1996). An exploration of nurses' attitudes to the nursing care of the suicidal patients. *Journal of Psychiatric and Mental Health Nursing, 3*, 29–37.

Nock, M. K., & Kessler R. C. (2006). Prevalence of and risk factors for suicide attempts versus suicide gestures: Analysis of the national comorbidity survey. *Journal of Abnormal Psychology, 3,* 616–623.

Paterson, B. L., Thorne, S., Canam, C., & Jillings, C. (2001). *Meta-study of qualitative health research: A practical guide to meta analysis and meta synthesis.* Thousand Oaks, CA: Sage.

Ricouer, P. (1976). *Interpretation theory: Discourse and the surplus of meaning.* Fort Worth, TX: Christian University Press.

Smoyak, S. A. (2001). Stigma: Shades of visibility. *Journal of Psychosocial Nursing and Mental Health Services, 39,* 4–5.

Sun, F. K., Long, A., Boore, J., & Tsao, L. I. (2005). Suicide: A literature review and its implications for nursing practice in Taiwan. *Journal of Psychiatric Mental Health Nursing, 12,* 447–455.

Sun, F. K., Long, A., Boore, J., & Tsao, L. I. (2006). Patients and nurses' perceptions of ward environmental factors and support systems in the care of suicidal patients. *Journal of Clinical Nursing, 15,* 83–92.

Takahashi, C., Chida, F., Nakamura, H., Akasaka, H., Yagi, J., Koeda, A., Takusari, E., Otsuka, K., & Sakai, A. (2011). The impact of inpatient suicide on psychiatric nurses and their need for support. *BMC Psychiatry, 11,* 1–8.

Talseth, A. G., & Gilje, F. (2007). Unburdening suffering: Responses of a psychiatrist to a patient's suicide death. *Nursing Ethics, 14,* 620–627.

Talseth, A. G., & Gilje, F. (2011). Nurses' response to suicide and suicidal patients: A critical interpretive synthesis. *Journal of Clinical Nursing, 20,* 1651–1667.

Talseth, A. G., Gilje, F., & Norberg, A. (2001). Being met: A passage way to hope for relatives of patients at risk of committing suicide: a phenomenological hermeneutic study. *Archives of Psychiatric Nursing, 15,* 249–256.

Talseth, A. G., Lindseth, A., Jacobsson, L., & Norberg, A. (1997). Nurses' narrations about suicidal psychiatric inpatients, *Nordic Journal of Psychiatry, 51,* 359–374.

Tanney, B. (2000). Psychiatric diagnosis and suicidal acts. In R. W. Maris, A. L. Berman, & M. M. Silverman (eds.) *Comprehensive textbook of suicidology.* New York: Guilford Press.

Thorne, S., Kirkham, S. R., & O'Flynn-Magee, K. (2004). The analytic challenge in interpretive description. *International Journal of Qualitative Methods, 3,* 1–11.

Timulak, L. (2009). Meta-analysis of qualitative studies: A tool for reviewing qualitative research findings in psychotherapy. *Psychotherapy Research, 19,* 591–600.

Tzeng, W-C., Yang, C-I., Tzeng, N-S., Ma, H-S., & Chen, L. (2010). The inner door: Toward an understanding of suicidal patients. *Journal of Clinical Nursing, 19,* 1396–1404.

Vatne, M. (2006). Psykiatriske sykepleieres forståelse av eget ansvar I arbeid med selvmordsnære pasienter [Psychiatric nurses' understanding of their responsibility working with suicidal patients], *Vård i Norden, 1,* 30–35.

Vråle, G., & Steen, E. (2005). The dynamics between structure and flexibility in constant observation of psychiatric in-patients with suicidal ideation. *Journal of Psychiatric and Mental Health Nursing, 12,* 513–518.

Wagnild, G., & Gantnar, R. (2011) Defeating depression with resilience, *Corporate Wellness.* November 10, available at: http://www.corporatewellnessmagazine.com/article/defeating-depression-with-resilience.html (accessed 26 June 2012).

Warelow, P., & Edward, K-L. (2007). Caring as a resilient practice in mental health nursing. *International Journal of Mental Health Nursing, 16,* 132–135.

3

A MIXED METHODS STUDY OF THE INCREASED RISK OF SUICIDE FOLLOWING DISCHARGE

A long road ahead

John R. Cutcliffe, Paul S. Links, Henry G. Harder, Ken Balderson, Yvonne Bergmans, Rahel Eynan, Munazzah Ambreen and Rosane Nisenbaum

There are no shortcuts to any place worth going.

Beverly Sills

Introduction

There is a significant body of literature which indicates that people whose mental health problems lead them to require psychiatric hospitalization are at a significantly increased risk for suicide (Appleby et al., 1999; Pirkola, Sohlman, & Wahlbeck, 2005; Troister, Links, & Cutcliffe, 2008). However, hospitalization for people at risk of suicide is only 'part of the bigger picture'; the period of time immediately following discharge after such hospitalizations, perhaps rather counter-intuitively,[1] appears to be a particularly high risk time (see Geddes & Juszczak, 1995; Geddes, Juszczak, O'Brien, & Kendrick, 1997; Goldacre, Seagrott, & Hawton, 1993; Ho, 2003; Lawrence, et al., 2001; Troister et al., 2008; Yim et al., 2004). Findings from studies conducted in various parts of the world have highlighted a number of variables which have been shown to be significantly related to suicide after recent discharge such as: previous suicide attempts (Fernando & Storm, 1984; King et al., 2001a; 2001b; King, Baldwin, Sinclair, & Campbell, 2001b; McKenzie & Wurr, 2001; Yim et al., 2004); presence of affective disorder/depressive symptoms, (King, Segal, Kaminski, & Naylor, 1995), unplanned discharge (King et al., 2001a, 2001b), and experience of negative life events following discharge (Pokorny & Kaplan, 1976). Conflicting findings exist regarding the link between duration of hospitalization and increased risk (Qin & Nordentoft, 2005; Ho, 2006).

While there is consensus within the limited literature concerning the existence of this increased period of risk, our comprehension of the phenomenon is in its infancy. Conflicting findings, for example, exist regarding the duration of hospitalization and any positive correlation with increased suicide risk; different studies producing conflicting findings (Ho, 2006; Qin & Nordentoft, 2005). The studies that have been undertaken to explore this phenomenon represent only a 'handful' of mental health facilities and the particular experiences that contribute to this increased risk are far from complete. For instance, the authors could locate no qualitative studies that have systematically examined the post-discharge experiences of former hospitalized suicidal patients. Accordingly, this chapter reports on findings from a federally funded, mixed methods study which sought to do the following:

1 discover whether or not this increased risk of suicide post-discharge was 'present' at an Ontario health facility;
2 better understand the particular experiences associated with the observed increased risk for suicide following discharge from an inpatient psychiatric service(s).

The study combined a pre-test, post-test design ('before and after' design) with an intervention group and a control group with a hermeneutic, phenomenological design, using van Manen's (1997, 2002) internationally established approach to phenomenology. Ultimately, the theoretical understanding of this specific high risk period can help lead to the development of selective prevention strategies that have the potential to assist in decreasing the risk for suicide and suicidal behaviour (Knox, Conwell, & Caine, 2004).

Methodological rationale and background

According to O'Cathain, Murphy and Nicholl (2007), there has been a recent surge of international interest in combining qualitative and quantitative methods in a single study, often called mixed methods research. This interest can be detected in the Canadian Institute for Health Research (CIHR) (http://www.cihr-irsc.gc.ca/e/41382.html, recovered 2012) information and associated positions with specific reference made to mixed method synthesis as an approach subsumed within the 'Knowledge Translation' initiative. Indeed, while a relatively recent development, the United States of America National Institute of Health (NIH) has embraced and endorsed mixed method research designs. The NIH Office of Behavioral and Social Sciences Research was among the first to publish guidelines for qualitative and mixed methods research and included models for combining qualitative and quantitative approaches. Similarly, the National Science Foundation (NSF) held a workshop on the scientific foundations of qualitative research, with five papers devoted to combining qualitative and quantitative methods. Following this, the NIH held their own mixed methods workshop,[2] sponsored by seven NIH institutes and this was followed by various private foundations holding their own workshops. The number of mixed methods studies reported in journal articles continues to increase and this reflects how mixed methods research is being utilized in more and more disciplines and fields of study (Plano Clark, 2005). Indeed, the level of interest has grown substantially to the extent that there now exists a journal which is devoted exclusively to publishing mixed methods studies and discussions about the methodology of mixed methods research;[3] and international conferences dedicated to mixed methods research have been held in various countries since 2005.

The rationale or case for mixed method research designs can be advanced on several methodological and epistemological grounds. The central premise of such designs, it has been argued (Cresswell, 2003), is that the combination of quantitative and qualitative approaches provides a more comprehensive and complete understanding of problems than either approach can alone. Several authors have highlighted how mixed method research designs provide advantages/strengths that offset the limitations/weaknesses of both quantitative and qualitative research (e.g., Cutcliffe & Harder, 2009; Goering & Streiber, 1996; Goldney, 2002, Leenaars, 2002; Lester, 2002). Greene (2007) highlights how mixed method research designs enable questions to be answered that cannot be answered by qualitative or quantitative approaches alone. Mixed methods, according to Cresswell (2003), enable researchers to use all of the tools of data collection available rather than being restricted to the types of data collection typically associated with qualitative research or quantitative research. Further, mixed methods designs encourage the use of multiple world-views or paradigms rather than the typical association of certain paradigms for quantitative researchers and others for qualitative researchers (Cresswell, 2003). This methodological consilience (Wilson, 1998) and the resultant unification of ways of knowing (and associated ways of conducting research) are highly congruent with complex, multi-dimensional health care problems.[4] Professor of Psychiatry Goldney (2002, p. 70) makes this point most clearly: "It is increasingly more difficult for even the most partisan of researchers to ignore the nexus between the qualitative and quantitative approaches."

Despite these methodological and epistemological exhortations, mental health or/and psychiatry, it has been argued, are still somewhat lagging behind other disciplinary/academic groups when it comes to embracing qualitative and mixed methods research designs (see, for example, Bassett, 2010; Whitley, 2009). Mixed methods research is inherently pragmatic; researchers are unrestricted in selecting all methods possible to address a particular research problem. Further, the methodological pragmatism extends to enabling researchers to solve problems using data in the form(s) of numbers and words; to combining inductive and deductive thinking.

Research design and method: the quantitative component

This study was carried out in a large urban general hospital with an active inpatient psychiatric service between May 2007 and December 2009. High-risk patients admitted to the inpatient psychiatric service and a short-stay crisis stabilization unit with a lifetime history of suicidal behavior, accompanied by some level of intent to die and current suicidal ideation based on self-report or chart documentation, were eligible to participate in the study. After receiving permission to approach patients from their treatment team, newly admitted patients were asked for their consent to participate in the investigation. After providing signed informed consent, patients participated in the baseline assessment during their hospital admission. Given the 'vulnerable' nature of the population, and the potentially sensitive nature of the phenomenon of interest, particular attention was devoted to considered ethical issues before commencing the study. Though the research team recognizes that qualitative research interviews do not *ipso facto* re-traumatize interviewees (see Cutcliffe & Ramcharan, 2002; Ramcharan & Cutcliffe, 2001), they were cognisant of the potential risks and so provided a number of 'safety measures' for the participants. All the information collected was treated confidentially and any information provided that could compromise the confidentiality of the person or the programs, was disguised. All electronic data files were protected by a password system and the study computer remained within a locked office. The study received research ethics approval from the hospital Research Ethics Board.

Baseline measures for the quantitative component

While in hospital, the participants were assessed for baseline suicidal ideation measured with the clinician-administered version of the Scale for Suicide Ideation[5] (SSI), (Beck, Kovac, & Weissman, 1979) on the day of the interview and during the preceding week. This scale has demonstrated internal consistency, inter-rater reliability, and concurrent validity (Beck et al., 1979) and adequate predictive validity significantly predicting eventual suicide (Brown, Beck, Steer, & Grisham, 2000). The SSI was administered at 1, 3, and 6 months after hospital discharge. At the sixth month follow-up appointment, participants were asked to report on any self-injury events without intent to die or suicide. A number of other measures and instruments were used in the study and details of these are reported in Links et al. (2012).

Outcomes

For suicidal ideation the authors considered two outcomes: (1) change in SSI scores from baseline to 1 month post-discharge; and (2) SSI scores at 1, 3, and 6 months post-discharge dichotomized as ≥3 (indicating that the patient is positive for suicide ideation) and <3 (negative for suicide ideation). We used these SSI categories due to the high proportion of zero scores at follow-up. For suicide behavior we used the composite of the indicator of self-injury or suicide attempts within 6 months of hospital discharge or death by suicide after discharge.

Research design and method: qualitative component

For the qualitative, phenomenological component, the research team used Van Manen's (1997) interpretation of hermeneutic phenomenology. The researchers obtained a purposive sample of 20 former inpatients, each of whom met the inclusion criteria, (see Box 3.1). Interviews took place at (or close to) the end of the first month following their discharge from the inpatient psychiatric service. Demographic details of the sample are displayed in Table 3.1.

Box 3.1 Participant inclusion criteria

1 Had to be willing to participate and talk about their experiences.
2 Aged 18 years or over.
3 Must have been admitted to hospital with suicidal ideation or/and a lifetime history of suicidal behaviour.
4 Must have subsequently stabilized based on the inpatient psychiatrist's assessment.

Data were collected from the participants as a result of hermeneutic interviews, lasting between 1 and 2 hours; these occurred in a quiet, peaceful environment of the participant's choosing. At the beginning of the interview, the research team was concerned only with attempting to build rapport and helping the participant to feel at ease. While adopting a reflexive technique to qualitative interviewing (Kvale, 1996), the research team were seeking to elicit specific descriptions of the lived-moments of the experience of discharge; therefore certain types of questions needed to be asked to assist the participant in accessing the moment as lived. For example:

• If you could focus on an example of your post-discharge suicidal experience which stands out for its vividness, can you describe your experience of being discharged following your admission for suicidal ideation, as you live(d) through it?

Table 3.1 Socio-demographics of the sample

Socio-demographic	N (%)
Age mean (SD)	36.3 (10.7)
Gender	
Males	10 (50.0)
Females	10 (50.0)
Race/Ethnicity	
Caucasian	13 (65.0)
Black	1 (5.0)
Asian	0
Other	6 (30.0)
Marital status	
Single	14 (70.0)
Married/Common-law	2 (10.0)
Divorced/Separated/Widowed	4 (20.0)
Diagnoses	
Affective disorder	7 (35%)
Affective disorder and borderline personality disorder	8 (40%)
Affective disorder and schizophrenic disorder	1 (5%)
Neither borderline personality disorder nor affective disorder nor schizophrenic disorder	4 (20%)
Education	
Less than high school	1 (5.0)
High school	5 (25.0)
College/University/Graduate school	14 (70.0)[1]
Current place of residence	
Shelter	2 (10.0)
Living with parents/family	1 (5.0)
Rent	14 (70.0)
Own	3 (15.0)
Source of income in the past year	
Disability pension	9 (45.0)
Other	11 (55.0)
Current employment status	
Full-time	6 (30.0)[2]
Part-time	6 (30.0)
Unemployed	2 (10.0)
Disabled	6 (30.0)

Notes: 1 It might be noteworthy that this is a high percentage of participants who have a higher education background. While this may be a nuance or idiosyncrasy of this particular sample, it is also possible that this high number reflects the greater degree of comfort that higher educated individuals feel when participating in research interviews. That is to say that individuals with a higher education background are more likely to be familiar with the research process per se and arguably, less intimated by this.
2 It might be noteworthy that these figures represent higher percentages than are typically associated with the adult population. While sampling for phenomenological studies seek informants who can provide the richest, deepest understanding into the phenomenon and thus deliberately eschew random (representative) samples, it remains possible that different findings may have been discovered from a sample that was representative of the adult population.
Definitions: Affective disorder = bipolar or major depression; Schizophrenic disorder = schizophrenia or schizoaffective.

- Can you try and describe the experience from the inside, as it were? What were your feelings, your mood, your emotions, your thoughts?

And

- Could you describe how your body felt at that time, how things smelled, how they sounded?[6]

Furthermore, given the reflexive nature of hermeneutic interviews, some questions were asked in order to provide clarity in response to initial questions and in response to potential key moments described by the participants. Interviews ceased when the participants felt they had said all they had to say about the experience and when prompts from the interviewer did not elicit any new information.[7]

Following verbatim transcription of the interview(s), the whole research team read the entire transcript. This process has been described as giving the researcher(s) a global sense of the whole (Kleiman, 2004) and/or a feeling for the subject's inherent meanings (see Colaizzi, 1978). The first author then undertook a second reading of the transcript and asked questions of the text such as: What is going on here?, What is this an example of? This enabled the first author to divide the data in meaningful sections and then integrate those that had a similar focus or content. The first author then took each of these sections and formulated meaning in the context of the subject's own words/terms. This was achieved by asking questions of these collated sections such as: What does this passage of text, or more accurately, the collections of passages, say about the essence of the experience of being discharged after receiving inpatient mental health care for the risk of suicide? These meanings, drawn from a number of interviews, are then grouped or clustered (or even reduced) together, as a result of individual meaning units having shared and/or common patterns, content, or trends, into themes. Further, in the repeated examination of the transcripts, themes were supported or exemplified by highlighting and 'lifting' appropriate phrases or capturing singular key statements (thematic statements). Following this, the themes texts were shared with all members of the research team who were encouraged to re-write them as a means

Table 3.2 Initial questions posed during phenomenological interviews

Perhaps if you could focus on an example of your post-discharge suicidal experience which stands out for its vividness, can you describe your experience of being discharged following your admission for suicidal ideation, as you live(d) through it?

Please describe the events leading up to that particular moment. Any events that you feel impacted on and influenced your experience?

Can you try and describe the experience from the inside, as it were? What were your feelings, your mood, your emotions, your thoughts?

Can you describe what your 'world' and those in it, both in a local and wider sense, felt like to you during the moments of dealing with being discharged following your admission for suicidal ideation?

Can you focus on a particular example or incident? Can you describe specific events, particular happenings?

Can you tell me what were you aware of during the experience of feeling suicidal following your discharge?

Could you describe how your body felt at that time, how things smelled, how they sounded?

to enhance the richness and depth of the text. The team then revisited the interview transcripts once more as a means to ensure that their interpretations could be substantiated by reference to the raw data.[8] Consequently, this process of writing and re-writing was used to make aspects of the lived experience reflectively understandable and was guided by van Manen's (2002) recent text on phenomenological writing. Furthermore, the interdisciplinary nature of the research team meant that each member was able to bring his or her particular disciplinary experience and expertise to the data analysis; to the re-writing of the phenomenological text.

Post-discharge elevated risk of suicide: quantitative and qualitative results

At baseline (n = 119), our quantitative measures indicated that discharged clients remained at an elevated risk of suicide; in some cases for many months subsequent to discharge. Further, our qualitative, phenomenological data confirm these quantitative findings whereby, despite the inpatient hospital stay being concluded, (and one could therefore assume that the client was deemed to be 'well' enough to be discharged), a theme of the induced lived experiences indicates that suicide remained an option. For instance, the Scale for Suicide Ideation (SSI) baseline scores ranged from 10 to 31, with a mean of 23.6 and standard deviation of 3.8. Mean (SD) scores post discharge were 7.9 (9.0), 6.6 (7.8), 5.7 (7.8) at 1 month (n = 100), 3 months (n = 96), and 6 months (n = 98), respectively. So while these scores appear to indicate some diminution in suicide ideation between baseline and discharge (and follow-up), the data also clearly indicate that SSI scores remained quite high for some people. It is also important to note that the incidence of death by suicide during the study period was 3.3% (95% confidence interval [CI] = 0.9%–8.3%): 1 participant died (0.8% or 1 in 120) while hospitalized and 3 participants (2.5% or 3 in 120) within 1 month of hospital discharge. Moreover, 41 of 104 (39.4%) (95% CI = 30.0%–49.5%) participants reported self-injury or suicide attempts within 6 months of hospital discharge. Accordingly, our quantitative findings from the prospective cohort design adds to the existing retrospective studies of the risk of suicide in recently discharged patients by confirming the remarkable risk for suicide in recently discharged patients.

When these quantitative results are combined with the phenomenological findings, the post-discharge continuation of elevated suicide risk becomes more difficult to dismiss or refute.

One of the induced sub-themes, 'Suicide remains an option – "But I still feel suicidal"' (see Cutcliffe et al., 2012a, 2012b) describes how for some of the participants in this study, suicide very much remained an option even after they are discharged. Thoughts of ending their lives occurred to some participants on the very day that they were discharged; for others, thoughts of suicide and/or suicide remained in their consciousness as a viable solution to their problems, persisting for many months after discharge and in some cases, years after. These suicidal thoughts/feelings were described by the participants as residing in different (metaphorical) places in their minds. Some referred to how these thoughts/feelings were at the forefront of their minds. Others described a more subconscious location, i.e. at the back of my mind, and yet this location could and did change. Participants referred to how, usually, they became more conscious, more aware of suicide as an option, when times got harder, and/or when they felt more stressed. Others still referred to suicide residing in their unconscious and manifesting itself in their dreams. Perhaps somewhat counter-intuitively, some participants described their suicidal thoughts/feelings as being worse after they were discharged. Participants described, again perhaps somewhat paradoxically, that having suicide as an option for them post-discharge actually served as a 'security blanket'. There was a sense of participants being willing to try and resolve their issues but if they couldn't, if they couldn't cope . . . then they still had a way out in the form of suicide. Participants were very clear that, for the most part, the act and experience of being discharged in no way prevented them from still feeling suicidal. Just because the formal mental health care system (services) had decided that it would be safe to discharge someone, did not necessarily mean that the person's suicidality had been resolved; that the suicidal 'episode' was now concluded. It may well have been the case that the crisis point or highest point of risk had elapsed, but participants were adamant that they left the hospital still feeling suicidal. Some participants described their experiences as the system letting them down; they described not getting their issues resolved or that their 'recovery' was incomplete. For some, the experience of being discharged before they felt that they had resolved their suicidal issues actually served to potentially increase their risk. Some participants referred to the increased sense of hopelessness that resulted from going to a place/organization where they were expecting things to improve, and yet they didn't improve. There was a sense of "Where can I get help? If I can't get help from these guys, the formal mental health services, then where can I get help?" Some participants' experiences appeared to indicate that it takes a great deal longer to resolve these complex issues and that at times, their experience of the health care system was one characterized as a 'Band-Aid' approach. Evidence of the continued elevated risk of suicide post-discharge was captured by the research participants in their quotes:

> I'm probably going to still be depressed and, you know, suicide will be on the table, um, you know, kind of as one of the options.
>
> *Interview 4*

> What was going through your head on the day of discharge? I'm going to end my life.
>
> *Interview 13*

> Yeah, yeah, and, ah, basically, you know, before being admitted and after being admitted I pretty much just think about like suicide all the time, you know, it's, um, you know, I know people sit there and just say change your attitude or go for a walk or blah, blah, blah . . . and when I got home, for the first week, it's actually, it's actually getting a little worse.
>
> *Interview 20*

> I was still suicidal when they let me go but they did what they were supposed to do. They upped my drugs, they gave me some sleeping medication and they were all kosher like everything was cop esthetic, and it doesn't matter where you're at, and so I'm still struggling with it.
>
> *Interview 9*

> Well, Thursday, when I had told the nurse that I was having suicidal thoughts, she told me that my, the psychiatrist wanted, said that I would be discharged Friday, that was the first I had heard anything of it. I just knew by Friday morning that if I had told them I was still having suicidal thoughts, I'd still be in restraints, so I lied, and I was taken out of restraints, two hours later, I was discharged and then two days, two or three days later I ended up at (mental health facility name).
>
> *Interview 7*

> I think the burden part is kind of not never ending, cause even, now I, I, very rarely tell my parents, um, more than they really need to know, um, but in terms of the fear

and, um, you know, the thoughts of suicide and things like that, that's still in hospital and right after getting out of hospital.

Interview 4

When my doctor told me I was being discharged, I was very, very sad because I was, like, I don't understand what I did . . . I don't understand what I am supposed to do. I felt much more lost and so much more worried.

Interview 16

Like, I immediately want my safety blanket of suicide and for me that's a safety blanket, that's where I want to be. It's hard, like, day-to-day is a struggle and you're always in fluctuation with your emotions. You can't control them. You can't trust your relationships. You're always trying to figure things out. It's very tiring.

Interview 9

It came, it just came to that, to that mind space that it's like, okay, I can't deal with this, you know, and it's like I have a way out and, um, you know it, there's just like so much anxiety around it and I just felt like, okay, you're sending me home, I understand that I need to go home but it's like I don't feel like I'm ready to go home, you know, it's like because all the problems are still there.

Interview 20

Not really, because when they discharged me I was still suicidal, and even more so because of the fact that, you know, that I was hopeless in a way and they were happy. You know, like, the mental health system was happy because they decided to discharge me and it didn't matter where I was.

Interview 9

No, I think it's the same. It hasn't changed with me. I'm on very high antidepressants, like the maximum you could take and, um, no I still want to kill myself, I'm still there.

Interview 11

It remains but you get better at hiding it. It's a matter of hiding it and trying not to feed it, um, I try to distract myself from it and I try to get on board with trying to connect with my boyfriend although I can pretend and I can mimic, um, but it doesn't go deeper than superficial and I know that's a problem. But I'm getting good at mimicking and pretending but I guess that's why I stay suicidal. You know it seems like I never know when it's going to hit and yet the outside factors are detonators for action.

Interview 9

Um, that's the mind space was just, like, the only thing that I really remember was the fact that it's like I'm not ready, and I can't deal with this, and that I was just going to go home and, and like overdose and then everything would be okay.

Interview 20

Discussion

Combining the quantitative and qualitative findings in this study results in robust evidence to suggest that the risk of suicide continues long after the client has been discharged. Given these findings the need for a range of post-discharge support orientated 'interventions' is indicated such as: scheduled visits in the community from a mental health clinician, follow-up phone calls, text messages, emails, and/or postcards. If the client is willing to give his/her consent, the discharge process might also be adapted to include notification sent to family, friends and formal carers (e.g. managers of homeless centres). There is some corroboration within the, albeit limited, empirical literature[9] that supports such amendments to practice. Driscoll (2001), for example, found that carers who were present with their patients when they received information concerning post-discharge care experienced a decrease in anxiety during their patients' convalescence at home, greater satisfaction with the information they received, and their patients experienced fewer medical problems post-discharge. More specific to follow-up care for suicidal people, the novel studies by Motto and Bostrom (2001) and Carter and colleagues (2005; 2007) show that simply utilizing letters or postcards as an intervention following discharge suggests that social connectedness, feeling that somebody still cares, may be a crucial component of post-discharge support. Other qualitative findings in this study indicated that there were a range of experiences (and variables) which contributed to this ongoing, elevated risk of suicide post discharge including: participants feeling scared, anxious, fearful and/or stressed; the degree of preparedness felt by the participants; participants' sense of leaving the place of safety; their sense of feeling like they were a burden; participants' ongoing need for post-discharge support; participants' sense of feeling lost, uncertain, disorientated, and feeling alone and/or isolated.

The reported sense(s) of fear, dread and anguish about leaving their 'place of safety' and being sent 'back into the lion's den' was lessened when the participant felt more prepared; felt that he/she had a degree of control over when and how this happened. While mindful of the many factors that influence (if not drive) decisions regarding discharge, relatively slight alterations in current practice appear to have potential and significant utility in helping to alleviate this post-discharge problem. Involving patients in the decision-making process, encouraging expression and 'ventilation' of fears/anxieties; acknowledging that such fear is to be expected; seeking and taking account of the patient's views *vis-à-vis* readiness for discharge; where possible, addressing specific concerns and exploring what can be put in place to help patients feel more supported, and, wherever possible, not forcing the discharge on patients who do not feel ready and/or prepared, would appear not only to be indicative of good practice but simultaneously would potentially reduce the risk of further suicide attempts post-discharge. Similar calls for involving patients (and their family carers) in discharge decision-making have been advocated in the United Kingdom (see Social Care Institute for Excellence Research Brief 12, accessed 2010) and are common in policy documents (see, for example, Department of Health, accessed 2010). However, the norm is that people are not usually consulted about the planning of their discharge or care (SCIE, accessed 2010). Indeed, the limited literature shows that a 'top-down' or 'paternalistic' approach is the norm for discharge planning (Bull, Hanson, & Gross, 2000; Cornes and Clough, 2001; Mountain and Pighills, 2003). And yet the empirical findings, such as they are, indicate that patients who perceived that the time of discharge was consistent with the stage of their illness experienced significantly higher recovery (Schröder, Larsson, & Ahlström, 2007).

Further practice implications arising out of these findings include the need to commence the discharge process as soon as possible after admission, and in this way, being discharged can then be experienced as a gradual process, one where the patient has time to prepare and plan. If possible, and the authors are mindful of the possible logistical difficulties, it would be prudent to introduce the patient to his/her post-discharge support staff before the discharge occurs (and thus enhance the continuity of care). The findings also indicated that a variable (or dynamic) that appeared to be contributing to the post-discharge continued elevated risk of suicide was that of the major disconnect between the expectations of admitted patients and what realistically could be offered by the formal mental health care services. For example, some participants referred to the expectation of getting fixed or cured; they expected[10] that being admitted to inpatient care would result in the cure/solution to their problem. The difficulties associated with misconceptions/unrealistic expectations about formal psychiatric care have been documented previously (see, for example, Douglas, Noble, & Newman, 1999). Such disconnections are linked with drop-out rates (Bunn et al., 1997) and levels of satisfaction (Balogh et al., 1995). Interventions to enhance the congruence between patients' expectations and what the mental health care services can realistically offer have resulted in improved attendance/satisfaction and decreased anxiety (Webster, 1992). Accordingly, the authors assert that early exploration of and reconciling patients' expectations regarding inpatient care for their suicidality might be an intervention that could diminish the post-discharge risk for further suicide attempts; though this hypothesized intervention requires further empirical testing.

A further variable (or dynamic) that appeared to be contribute to the post-discharge continued elevated risk of suicide was that of participants reporting how when they arrived home, they did not know what to do next; they were uncertain about so many aspects of their lives. Accordingly, there appears to be significant utility in creating a post-discharge plan, working in collaboration with the client; which can subsequently explore pragmatic issues such as: What to do now/next? What needs to be addressed first and what can wait? How to begin re-engaging in life? How to pick up the threads of one's life again? Where can the client go for additional help/support? Providing information of post-suicide support groups, be they physical 'face-to-face' groups and/or 'virtual' online groups, might also be useful. This ongoing, post-discharge support can be offered from both the mental health services and the voluntary sectors (including peer support) and should logically include some work on helping the client become more comfortable with this sense of uncertainty, helping the client understand that this sense of being 'dazed' is normal, is to be expected and that this too shall pass. Mental health services might similarly think about augmenting their discharge process by producing some post-discharge literature and/or pamphlets. Perhaps analogous to current best practice in some medical/surgical situations, for example, patients about to be discharged following a new diagnosis for diabetes, or the patients about to be discharged following a myocardial infarction, are inevitably provided with pamphlets and literature regarding their ongoing, post-discharge recovery and how to reduce the risk of post-discharge complications.

While there is little evidence in the extant suicidology literature regarding post-discharge interventions, valuable lessons can be learned by drawing on related practices in other areas of health care. For example, in their thorough meta-analysis, Phillips et al. (2004) found that comprehensive discharge planning plus post-discharge support for older patients with congestive heart failure (CHF) significantly reduced readmission rates and may improve health outcomes such as survival and Quality of Life without increasing costs. The ongoing suicide risk, particularly in recently discharged patients admitted for suicidal behaviour, with high levels of depression, hopelessness or impulsivity must be monitored at discharge and in the early weeks and months following discharge (Links et al., 2012). In conjunction with ongoing risk, monitoring clinicians should help clients to understand that, even after discharge, there remains much work to be done; that the recovery from suicide can take a considerable length of time; that the short inpatient stay for the suicidal crisis can be just the beginning of their holistic recovery. In conjunction with this is the need for the suicidology community to perhaps re-visit what we consider to be an appropriate time frame for dealing with suicidality. There is a need to reflect how, for many suicidal patients, (see, for example, Maris, 1981; Beautrais, 2013), a more useful and accurate perception of the formal mental health care response to high risk suicidal clients would be to regard the inpatient care as the acute, crisis stabilization necessary as a preface to a longer-term, community-based recovery period. In such a model, the suicidology community would then acknowledge that the majority of the recovery work is likely to be undertaken post-discharge.

Some support for such a conceptualizations can be found in the relevant theoretical and empirical literature. While acknowledging its vintage yet significant status, the work of Maris (1981), *Pathways to Suicide*, drew attention to the notion of suicidal careers. The central premise of his thesis was that individuals who took their own lives had long suicidal careers involving complex mixes of biological, social and psychological factors. More recently, Joiner's (2005) illuminating book contains three central premises: (1) that people who make a serious attempt to end their own lives feel real disconnection from others; (2) they feel that they are a burden on others; and (3) the ability to enact the lethal self-injury is acquired. Relatedly, Beautrais' important work on looking at the trends and outcomes of all admissions for suicide attempts to a New Zealand hospital over ten years, reports similar findings. Beautrais (2013) argues that her results clearly show that suicidal behaviour, for many, is a chronic condition, not just a single, impulsive event and rather worryingly, for many the situation does not change much following a suicide attempt, because people do not get the help they need. Beautrais concludes that suicide is a complex response by vulnerable people who need extensive long-term treatment, care and support.

Acknowledgements

Some sections of this chapter book have been adapted or reproduced from original papers authored by the research team; which is not uncommon with mixed methods research designs. While we have included specific reference details in the chapter where this is the case, we wish once more to offer our most profound and heartfelt thanks to the following publishing houses:

Churchill Livingstone/Elsevier Ltd., for allowing the use of the paper published in *General Hospital Psychiatry*:
Links, P. S., Nisenbaum, M., Ambreen, M., Balderson, K., Bergmans, Y., Eynan, R., Harder, H., & Cutcliffe, J. R. (2012). Prospective study of risk factors for increased suicide ideation and behavior following recent discharge. *General Hospital Psychiatry, 34*(1): 88–97. Available online. DOI:10.1016/ j.physletb.2003.10.071.
Hogfree Publishing Ltd., for allowing the use of papers published in *Crisis: The Journal of Crisis Intervention and Suicide Prevention*:
Cutcliffe, J. R., Links, P. S., Ahern, R., Ambreen, M., Balderson, K., Bergmans, Y., Harder, H., & Nisenbaum, R. (2012). Understanding the risks of recent discharge: The phenomenological lived-experiences – 'existential angst at the prospect of discharge'. *Crisis: The Journal of Crisis Intervention and Suicide Prevention, 33*(1): 21–29.
Cutcliffe, J. R., Links, P. S., Ahern, R., Ambreen, M., Balderson, K., Bergmans, Y., Harder, H., & Nisenbaum, R. (2012) Understanding the risks of recent discharge: The phenomenological lived-experiences – 'Trying to survive while living under the proverbial "Sword of Damocles"', *Crisis: The Journal of Crisis Intervention and Suicide Prevention*. Available online = DOI: 10.1027/0227-5910/a000132.

The authors also wish to acknowledge the research team who undertook this research: John Cutcliffe, Paul Links, Henry G. Harder, Ken Balderson, Yvonne Bergmans, Rahel Eynan, Munazzah Ambreen, and Rosane Nisenbaum.

Rosane Nisenbaum gratefully acknowledges the support of the Ontario Ministry of Health and Long-Term Care. The views expressed in this publication are the views of the authors and do not necessarily reflect the views of the Ontario Ministry of Health and Long-Term Care.

Notes

1 One would expect that hospitalization ought logically to improve (or in some cases even 'cure') the situation.
2 Which was entitled, 'Design and Conduct of Qualitative and Mixed-Method Research in Social Work and Other Health Professions', and ran in 1994.
3 *Journal of Mixed Methods Research*, editors J. W. Creswell, A. Tashakkori, & V. L. Plano-Clark, published by Sage.
4 And here the authors will not belabor the obvious utility of undertaking mixed-methods studies in suicidology given that the multi-dimensionality and complexity of suicide have been very well documented, perhaps even to the extent that the multi-dimensionality and complexity of suicide are now regarded as axiomatic.
5 This is a 21-item, interviewer-administered rating scale that measures the current intensity of the participants' specific attitudes, behaviours, and plans to die by suicide.
6 A full list of our initial interview questions is provided in Table 3.2.
7 For hermeneutic phenomenology, the act of writing is not something that occurs ex-post-facto; writing is closely fused into the research activity. However, for ease of understanding, here the authors describe their approach to data analysis in a linear rather than cyclic (or iterative) fashion.
8 Please see the direct quotes from the interviews that substantiate the induced themes.
9 In terms of quantity and scope.
10 Analogous to their experiences of receiving care for physical/medical problems.

References

Appleby, L., Shaw, J., Amos, T., et al. (1999). Suicide within 12 months of contact with mental health services: National clinical survey. *British Medical Journal, 318,* 1235–1239.
Balogh, R., Simpson, A., & Bond, S. (1995). Involving clients in clinical audits of mental health services. *International Journal of Quality in Health Care, 7,* 343–353.
Bassett, R. (2010).Time to catch up . . . qualitative research in child and adolescent psychiatry. *Journal of Canadian Academic Child & Adolescent Psychiatry, 19*(1), 2.
Beautrais, A. (2013). Suicidal behavior needs long-term follow-up. Available at: http://www.thefreelibrary.com/Suicidal+behavior+needs+long-term+follow-up.-a0149058950 (accessed May 28, 2013).
Beck, A. T., Kovac, M., & Weissman, A. (1979). Assessment of suicidal ideation: The Scale for Suicide Ideation. *Journal of Consulting and Clinical Psychology, 47,* 343–352.
Brown, G. K., Beck, A. T., Steer, R. A., & Grisham, J. R. (2000). Risk factors for suicide in psychiatric outpatients: A 20-year prospective study. *Journal of Consulting and Clinical Psychology, 68,* 371–377.
Bull, M. J., Hanson, H. E., & Gross, C. R. (2000). A professional-patient partnership model of discharge planning with elders hospitalized with heart failure. *Applied Nursing Research, 13* (1), 19–28.
Bunn, M. H., O'Connor, A. M., Tansey, M. S., et al. (1997). Characteristics of clients with schizophrenia who express uncertainty about continuing treatment with depot neuroleptic medication. *Archives of Psychiatric Nursing, 11,* 238–248.
Canadian Institutes of Health Research (2012). A Guide to Knowledge Synthesis. Available at: http://www.cihr-irsc.gc.ca/e/41382.html.
Carter, G. L., Clover, K., Whyte. I. M., Dawson, A. H., & D'Este, C. (2005). Postcards from the Edge project: Randomized controlled trial of an intervention using postcards to reduce repetition of hospital-treated deliberate self-poisoning. *British Medical Journal, 331,* 805–810.
Carter, G. L., Clover, K., Whyte. I. M., Dawson, A. H., & D'Este, C. (2007). Postcards from the Edge: 24-month outcomes of a randomized controlled trial of hospital-treated self-poisoning. *British Journal of Psychiatry, 191,* 548–553.
Colaizzi, P. (1978). Psychological research as the phenomenologist views it. In R. Valle, & M. King (Eds.), *Existential phenomenological alternatives for psychologists.* New York: Oxford University Press.
Cornes, M., & Clough, R. (2001). The continuum of care: Older people's experiences of intermediate care. *Education and Ageing, 16*(2), 179–202.
Cresswell, J. W. (2003). *Research design: Qualitative, quantitative and mixed methods approaches* (2nd ed.). Thousand Oaks, CA: Sage.
Cutcliffe, J. R., & Harder, H. (2009). The perpetual search for parsimony: Enhancing the epistemological and practical utility of qualitative research findings. *International Journal of Nursing Studies, 46,* 1401–1410.

Cutcliffe, J. R., Links, P. S., Ahern, R., Ambreen, M., Balderson, K., Bergmans, Y., Harder, H., & Nisenbaum, R. (2012a). Understanding the risks of recent discharge: The phenomenological lived-experiences – 'existential angst at the prospect of discharge'. *Crisis: The Journal of Crisis Intervention and Suicide Prevention, 33*(1), 21–29.

Cutcliffe, J. R., Links, P. S., Ahern, R., Ambreen, M., Balderson, K., Bergmans, Y., Harder, H., & Nisenbaum, R. (2012b). Understanding the risks of recent discharge: the phenomenological lived-experiences – 'Trying to survive while living under the proverbial "Sword of Damocles"'. *Crisis: The Journal of Crisis Intervention and Suicide Prevention.* Available online: DOI: 10.1027/0227-5910/a000132.

Cutcliffe, J. R., & Ramcharan, P. (2002) Levelling the playing field: Considering the 'ethics as process' approach for judging qualitative research proposals. *Qualitative Health Research, 12*(7), 1000–1010.

Douglas, B. C., Noble, L. M., & Newman, S. P. (1999). Improving the accuracy of patients' expectations of the psychiatric out-patient consultation. *Psychiatric Bulletin, 23*, 425–427.

Driscoll, A. (2001). Managing post-discharge care at home: An analysis of patients' and their carers' perceptions of information received during their stay in hospital. *Journal of Advanced Nursing, 31*(5), 1165–1173.

Fernando, S., & Storm, V. (1984). Suicide among psychiatric patients of a district hospital. *Psychological Medicine, 14*, 661–672.

Geddes, J. R., & Juszczak, E. (1995). Period trends in rate of suicide in first 28 days after discharge from psychiatric hospital in Scotland, 1968–92. *British Medical Journal, 311*, 357–360.

Geddes, J. R., Juszczak. E., O'Brien, F., & Kendrick, S. (1997). Suicide in the 12 months after discharge from psychiatric inpatient care, Scotland, 1968–92. *Journal of Epidemiological Community Health, 51*, 430–434.

Goering, P. N., & Streiber, D. L. (1996). Reconcilable differences: The marriage of qualitative and quantitative methods. *Canadian Journal of Psychiatry, 41*(8), 491–497.

Goldacre, M., Seagrott, V., & Hawton, K. (1993). Suicide after discharge from psychiatric inpatient care. *Lancet, 342*, 283–286.

Goldney, R. D. (2002). Qualitative and quantitative approaches in suicidology: Commentary. *Archives of Suicide Research, 6*(1), 69–73.

Greene, J. (2007). *Mixed methods in social inquiry.* London: Sage.

Ho, T. P. (2003). The suicide risk of discharged psychiatric patients. *Journal of Clinical Psychiatry, 64*, 702–707.

Ho, T. P. (2006). Duration of hospitalization and post discharge suicide. *Suicide and Life-threatening Behavior, 36*(6), 682–686.

Joiner, T. (2005). *Why people die by suicide.* Cambridge, MA: Harvard University Press.

King, C. A., Segal, H., Kaminski, K., & Naylor, M. W. (1995). A prospective study of adolescent suicidal behavior following hospitalization. *Suicide Life-Threatening Behavior, 25*(3), 327.

King, E. A., Baldwin, D. S., Sinclair, J. M. A., et al. (2001a). The Wessex recent in-patient suicide study, 1. Case-control study of 234 recently discharged psychiatric patient suicides. *British Journal of Psychiatry, 178*, 531–536.

King, E. A., Baldwin, D. S., Sinclair, J. M. A., & Campbell, M. J. (2001b). The Wessex recent in-patient suicide study, 2. Case-control study of 59 in-patient suicides. *British Journal of Psychiatry, 17*, 537–542.

Kleiman, S. (2004). Phenomenology: To wonder and search for meanings. *Nurse Researcher, 11*(4): 7–19.

Knox, K. L., Conwell, Y., & Caine, E. D. (2004). If suicide is a public health problem, what are we doing to prevent it? *American Journal of Public Health, 94*, 37–45.

Kvale, S. (1996). *Interviews: An introduction to qualitative research interviewing.* Thousand Oaks, CA: Sage.

Lawrence, D., Holman, C. D. J., Jablensky, A. V., et al. (2001). Increasing rates of suicide in Western Australian psychiatric patients: A record linkage study. *Acta Psychiatrica Scandinavica, 104*, 443–451.

Leenaars, A. (2002). Qualitative and quantitative approaches in suicidology: Commentary. *Archives of Suicidology Research, 6*(1), 69–73.

Lester, D. (2002). Qualitative versus quantitative studies in psychiatry: Two examples of cooperation from suicidology. *Archives of Suicide Research, 6*(1), 15–18.

Links, P. S., Nisenbaum, M., Ambreen, M., Balderson, K., Bergmans, Y., Eynan, R., Harder, H., & Cutcliffe, J. R. (2012). Prospective study of risk factors for increased suicide ideation and behavior following recent discharge. *General Hospital Psychiatry, 34*(1): 88–97 Available online: DOI:10.1016/j.physletb.2003.10.071.

Maris, R. W. (1981). *Pathways to suicide.* Baltimore, MD: Johns Hopkins University Press.

McKenzie I., & Wurr C (2001). Early suicide following discharge from psychiatric hospital. *Suicide and Life-Threatening Behavior, 31*(3), 358–363.

Motto, J. A., & Bostrom, A. G. (2001). A randomized controlled trial of post-crisis suicide prevention. *Psychiatric Services, 52,* 828–833.

Mountain, G., & Pighills, A. (2003). Pre-discharge home visits with older people: Time to review practice. *Health and Social Care in the Community, 11*(2), 146–154.

O'Cathain, A., Murphy, E., & Nicholl, J. (2007). Why, and how, mixed methods research is undertaken in health services research in England: A mixed methods study. *BMC Health Services Research, 7,* 85. DOI:10.1186/1472-6963-7-85.

Phillips, C. O., Wright, S. M., Kern, D. E., Singa, R. M., Shepperd, S., & Rubin, H. R. (2004). Comprehensive discharge planning with post-discharge support for older patients with congestive heart failure: A meta-analysis. *JAMA, 17,* 291(11): 1358–1367.

Pirkola, S., Sohlman, B., & Wahlbeck, K. (2005). The characteristics of suicides within a week of discharge after psychiatric hospitalization: A nationwide register study. *BMC Psychiatry, 5,* 32.

Plano Clark, V. (2005). *Cross-disciplinary analysis of the use of mixed methods in physics education research, counseling psychology, and primary care ETD collection for University of Nebraska-Lincoln.* Paper AAI3163998. University of Nebraska-Lincoln.

Pokorny, A. D., & Kaplan, H. B. (1976). Suicide following psychiatric hospitalization. *Journal of Nervous and Mental Disorders, 162*(2), 119–125.

Qin, P., & Nordentoft, M. (2005). Suicide risk in relation to psychiatric hospitalization: Evidence based on longitudinal registers. *Archives of General Psychiatry, 62,* 427–432.

Ramcharan, P., & Cutcliffe, J. R. (2001). Judging the ethics of qualitative research: Considering the 'ethics as process' model. *Health and Social Care, 9*(6), 358–367.

Schröder, A., Larsson, B. W., & Ahlström, G. (2007). Quality in psychiatric care: An instrument evaluating patients' expectations and experiences. *International Journal of Health Care Quality Assurance, 20*(2), 141–160.

Social Care Institute for Excellence (accessed 2010). SCIE Research Brief 12: Involving individual older patients and their carers in the discharge process from acute to community care: Implications for intermediate care. Available at: http://www.scie.org.uk/publications/briefings/briefing12/index.asp.

Troister, T., Links, P., & Cutcliffe, J. R. (2008). Review of predictors of suicide within 1 year of discharge from a psychiatric hospital. *Current Psychiatry Reports, 10,* 60–65.

United States of America Department of Health and Human Services: Office of Behavioral and Social Sciences Research (2011). *Best practices for mixed methods research in the health sciences.* Available at: http://obssr.od.nih.gov/scientific_areas/methodology/mixed_methods_research/section4.aspx.

Van Manen, M. (1997). *Researching lived experience: Human science for action-sensitive pedagogy.* Albany, NY: State University of New York Press.

Van Manen, M. (2002). *Writing in the dark: Phenomenological studies in interpretive inquiry.* London, Ontario: Althouse Press.

Webster, A. (1992). The effect of pre-assessment information on clients' satisfaction, expectations and attendance at a mental health day centre. *British Journal of Medical Psychology, 65,* 89–93.

Whitley, R. (2009). Introducing psychiatrists to qualitative research: A guide for instructors. *Academic Psychiatry, 33,* 252–255.

Wilson, E. O. (1998). *Consilience: The unity of knowledge.* London: Little Brown & Co.

Yim, P. H. W., Yip, P. S. F., Li, R. H. Y. et al. (2004). Suicide after discharge from psychiatric inpatient care: A case-control study in Hong Kong. *Australian New Zealand Journal Medicine, 38*(1–2), 65–72.

4

TRANSCENDING SUICIDALITY
Facilitating re-vitalizing worthiness

Evelyn Gordon, Chris Stevenson and John R. Cutcliffe

Introduction

In recent years there has been a notable increase in suicide rates in many countries, including Ireland, where this trend has been particularly evident among young men (NOSP, 2005), giving rise to concern about how best to understand and respond to this group. Ironically, despite their prominent role in providing care to the suicidal person, many mental health professionals are ill-prepared to work with this population due to lack of training. As a means to help remedy this situation, the authors undertook a government-funded Grounded Theory (GT) (Glaser & Strauss, 1967) study in Ireland, to develop a theoretical understanding of how young men transcend suicidality. The theory that emerged from this study entitled, "Re-vitalizing Worthiness", refers to how the study participants regained a sense of value as individuals who were deserving of life (Gordon, Cutcliffe, & Stevenson, 2011). The study also highlighted key social and treatment practices that facilitated and hindered their movement from a death orientation to a life orientation, drawing attention to the important role of the mental health practitioner in this process.

Background: the picture in Ireland and beyond

Within the vast and growing suicidology literature much has come to be known about suicide and self-injury rates and trends, risk and protective factors and the efficacy and effectiveness of a number of prevention, intervention and postvention strategies (Maris, Berman, & Silverman, 2000; Hawton, 2005). One consistent and troubling trend has been an increase in prevalence rates in suicide and suicidality in many countries, including Ireland (NOSP, 2010; WHO, 2010). It is estimated that around one million people die by suicide each year worldwide and suicide rates are significantly higher among men, while there are higher rates of attempted suicide and self-injury among women (Guo & Harstall, 2004). In Ireland, over 500 people die by suicide and more than 12,000 people attend Emergency Departments each year following acts of self-injury (NSRF, 2012). Rates of completed suicide are notably higher among young men aged 16–34 years, who accounted for almost 40% of suicides in 2003 (NOSP, 2005). While there has been a downward trend in the period 2003–2010, numbers remain concerning and are envisaged to increase again with stresses related to the economic downturn (NOSP, 2010). This has given rise to social and professional concerns about how best to understand and respond to this group, particularly in view of their well-documented restrictive and disabling attitudes and behaviours towards help-seeking. For example, men are less likely than women to recognize, acknowledge and seek help for psychological problems (Burke, Kerr, & McKeown, 2008). In addition to gender- and age-related factors, a number of other risk factors have been identified such as social isolation, trauma including exposure to suicide and self-injury, substance misuse, and mental health problems.

There is much debate regarding the efficacy and effectiveness of treatment responses, with psychiatric and psychological treatments being most prominent in Western cultures. The emphasis on such approaches has been critiqued as restrictive, failing to account for other aspects of the person and his/her life, such as his/her existential/spiritual self (Webb, 2002). Emerging evidence suggests that working with suicidality requires an integrated and flexible approach as it is a complex, multidimensional and multifaceted phenomenon (Maris et al., 2000; Shneidman, 2001; Hawton, 2005). Despite the vast literature in the area it has also been argued that due to an emphasis on quantitative methodology, a focus on causation, and the ethical and practical challenges associated with conducting suicide research (Gibbons, Stirman, Brown, & Beck, 2010), understanding of the suicidal process and suicidal person is limited (Aldridge, 1998; Shneidman, 2001; Webb, 2002).

The social, psychological and economic burden associated with suicide and suicidality is well documented, incorporating individual suffering and disability, family stress and grief, community unease and fear of issues such as contagion, and the cost of health and social service provision (Maltsberger & Goldblatt, 1996; Maris et al., 2000; Hawton, 2005). While there is a strong focus on suicide prevention in government policy and strategy prevention, intervention and postvention can be viewed as interlinked as those exposed to suicidality are more likely to develop suicidal impulses (Grad, 2005). Emerging literature has also highlighted the negative consequences of failure to recognize the complexity and demands of practice in this area for professionals. For example, it has been noted that professionals experience feelings of professional inadequacy and personal loss in the aftermath of suicide (Links, 2001; Ting, Sanders, Jacobson, & Power, 2006). Indeed, Hawton (1994) suggests that it is in the best interests of all concerned to acknowledge the inevitability of death by suicide in order to allay unwarranted guilt and distress across personal and professional systems.

It is ironic that while mental health professionals have a prominent role in responding to the suicidal person, with encountering suicide described as an occupational hazard, many individuals, from a variety of disciplines, are ill-prepared for this work due to lack of training in this specific area (Maltsberger & Goldblatt, 1996; Ting et al., 2006; Cutcliffe & Stevenson, 2007). This may reflect the profound fear (Becker, 1973), social and moral stigma (Sommer-Rothenberg, 1998) and professional discomfort (Gibbs, 1990) associated with the topic of suicide. For example, while the meaning of suicide has evolved over time, reflecting changing social and cultural discourses that have promoted a more tolerant and less pathologizing understanding of suicide (Shneidman, 2001), some predominantly negative views and myths prevail in the Western world that directly influence professional response (Gibbs, 1990; Gordon, 2010; Joiner, 2010). One such myth is that talking about suicide can make the person feel worse; another that those who attempt suicide but do not die do not intend ending their lives. Indeed, it could be argued that such social and professional beliefs fuel practices that focus primarily on the physical safety of the person overshadowing the need for emotional safety and holistic care.

The cited study addressed these theoretical and practice gaps by drawing directly upon the views and experiences of young men who had been highly suicidal, and had been involved with the mental health services, to inform practice in this area. The emergent theory, re-vitalizing worthiness, describes and explains how participants resolved their painful pull between life and death by confronting their ambivalence about living and dying and incorporating "death awareness" (Deci & Ryan, 2004), or awareness of the inevitability and unpredictability of death, into their new sense of self. Hence, the term "transcending" is used to depict a sense of evolution and transformation. The study also highlighted key social and treatment practices that facilitated and hindered this process, for example, acknowledgement of their struggles with life was deemed helpful while responses that minimized their subjective experiences were viewed as unhelpful.

The study

In-depth face-to-face interviews were conducted with 17 men, with an average age of 25 years, who had contact with the mental health services. They came from diverse socio-economic and educational backgrounds and had a range of suicidality profiles, typical of those who present to mental health services, see Figure 4.1.

ID No.	Age	Marital Status	No. of Children	Educational Level	Work	No. of Suicide Attempts	MH Service Contact
1	27	S	1	Pre. L Cert	U/E	2	6 months
2	25	S	0	Pre. L Cert	Manual	1	6 weeks
3	26	S	0	3rd Level	Prof.	1	6 months
4	26	CoH	2	Pre. L Cert	Manual	3	6 weeks
5	20	S	0	3rd Level	Student	1	6 years
6	30	S	0	3rd Level	Student	1	6 years
7	32	S	1	Jnr. Cert	U/E	1	1 year
8	26	S	0	L Cert	Semi-prof	2	8 years
9	21	S	0	Primary	Manual	6	4 years
10	26	S	0	3rd Level	Skilled	0	6 weeks
11	30	S	0	Pre. Jnr. Cert	D/P	20	17 years
12	32	S	0	3rd Level	D/P	12	2 years
13	21	S	0	3rd Level	Student	5	4 years
14	19	S	0	3rd Level	Student	1	4 weeks
15	21	Separated	0	L Cert	Prof.	1	6 weeks
16	34	S	0	3rd Level	Prof.	0	6 years
17	22	S	1	3rd Level	Student	1	6 weeks

Figure 4.1 Participant profile

Key: Marital status: S – Single, CoH – cohabiting, Separated – separated following marriage.
Educational level: Primary – did not progress to secondary level, Jnr. Cert – mid-secondary level, L Cert – completed secondary level, 3rd Level – university.
Work: Prof – professional, Semi-prof – semi-professional, Skilled – tradesperson, Manual – unskilled labour, U/E – unemployed, D/P – disability pension.

Methodology and methods

A Grounded Theory (GT) methodology was employed for this study. A GT study generates a substantive theory in a particular area. First, it identifies the core concern or the issues that preoccupy those involved in the substantive area and then goes on to explore and theorize how this concern is resolved, which is captured in the theory. The theory emerges from the data as opposed to being predetermined by existing assumptions (Glaser & Strauss, 1967; Glaser, 1998). Thus, while an initial literature review can inform researcher sensitivity and provide a sound rationale for a study, a thorough literature review is conducted at the later stages of theory-building which serves as further data (Glaser, 1998). A GT study incorporates a number of interlinked processes as outlined in Figure 4.2.

To counter the challenges associated with studying men in general, and intimate life transitions in particular (Begley, Chambers, Corcoran, & Gallagher, 2004), one-to-one in-depth interviewing was used as the main source of data collection. This also provided scope to unpack participants' unique stories (Kvale, 1996), providing rich data for analysis across participant accounts.

Ethical considerations

Suicide research involves a number of ethical considerations as the topic is deemed sensitive and the population may be viewed as vulnerable and are frequently transient, which contributes to recruitment, engagement and follow-up challenges (Grad, 2005; Gibbons et al., 2010). In this study it was important that participants had adequate information and time to be able to make an informed choice about participation. To counter coercion, they were made fully aware that their decision would not influence their existing relationship with the services from which they

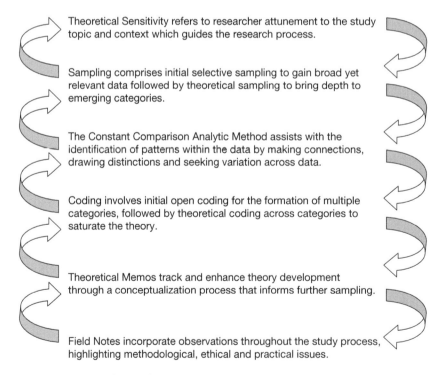

Theoretical Sensitivity refers to researcher attunement to the study topic and context which guides the research process.

Sampling comprises initial selective sampling to gain broad yet relevant data followed by theoretical sampling to bring depth to emerging categories.

The Constant Comparison Analytic Method assists with the identification of patterns within the data by making connections, drawing distinctions and seeking variation across data.

Coding involves initial open coding for the formation of multiple categories, followed by theoretical coding across categories to saturate the theory.

Theoretical Memos track and enhance theory development through a conceptualization process that informs further sampling.

Field Notes incorporate observations throughout the study process, highlighting methodological, ethical and practical issues.

Figure 4.2 GT procedures and processes

were recruited. Interviews were arranged in a quiet, comfortable and convenient location and de-briefing time was incorporated following interview to provide space to reflect on the interview process. Additionally participants were directed to sources of further information and support when this emerged as an issue for the interviewee. Hence, recruitment from well-established services provided a safeguard for participants as support could easily be accessed. It was also important to consider researcher safety and to provide adequate preparation and ongoing support to prevent psychological overload and responsibility anxiety as the first author engaged directly with those disclosing distressing information (Downey, Hamilton, & Catterall, 2007).

The theory

The main concern, *negotiating a dialectic of destiny,* describes two opposing pulls felt by the participants, one that yearned for death and the other that yearned for life. They attempted to conceal this inner battle in order to protect themselves and others from their deep pain. They experienced profound ambivalence and were caught between their desire for life and their drive toward death, while because of perceived social and moral stigma they feared recrimination if this were revealed. This concern occupied their daily living and being, as they tried to work out if and how they should be in the world.

The study identified that re-vitalizing worthiness, which means regaining a sense of value as an individual who is deserving of life, was central to resolving this concern of being. This was a complex process unique to each individual, nevertheless, common patterns were identified as the participants renegotiated the nature and meaning of their relationships with living and dying. The process describes how the young men faced their worst fears about themselves and their lives and transformed their identities in the move from a preoccupation with death to a focus on life, thereby transcending suicidality. The transition was influenced by interpersonal encounters with others in their social and treatment networks, thus the study also identified practices that enhanced and impeded their recovery process. Helpful practices were those that were validating of the participants and their lives, such as acknowledging their struggles and fears, while unhelpful responses involved those that perpetuated their sense of difference and powerlessness, such as exclusionary and controlling actions. Re-vitalizing worthiness has two interlinked stages, *confronting a crisis of destiny* and *earning a life*, described in detail elsewhere (Gordon et al., 2011), and depicted in Figure 4.3.

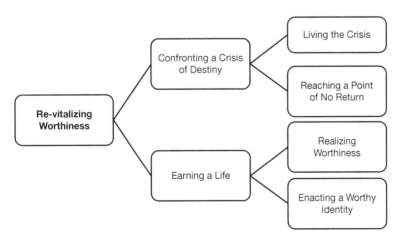

Figure 4.3 The core category and sub–categories

Briefly, confronting a crisis of destiny refers to how participants faced and resolved their torturous pull between life and death, which they had endured for some considerable time as they lived through a period of intense crisis. Finding themselves devoid of value as human beings due to their profound sense of failure and lack of belongingness, they tried to protect themselves and others from their inner pain by cutting themselves off from the world. They became increasingly isolated and alone and frequently masked this by giving the impression that they were content, however, maintaining this false exterior further fuelled their aloneness and experience of living a superficial life.

> Like you don't know who you are and it's horrible to feel like that . . . and a lot of people don't understand when you say that.

They believed that they had nothing to offer to the world, describing themselves in derogatory terms such as a freak or a failure. They were also not sure that life had anything to offer them and sometimes experienced living as more painful than dying. Hence, it made sense to think that they did not belong and were not deserving of life. They behaved in ways that reflected their ambivalence about life and death and their anger and frustration with themselves and the world, such as engaging in self and other directed aggression.

> I was so pissed off with people around me and so pissed off with myself because there was nothing I could do to change it [life].

Eventually their lives and their uncontrollable state of being became intolerable and, having reached a point of no return, they were forced to decide whether to live or die. The participants in this study chose life, which may have reflected the extent of their ambivalence and/or their courage and resilience. It is interesting to note that this shift frequently followed a suicide attempt which resulted in a close encounter with death, such as those described by the "Golden Gate suicide attempt survivors". Therefore, such episodes may have served as an impetus for change or a "turning point", which is said to change one's way of being in the world (Strauss, 1969).

> If I wanted to stay alive I had to change my life, I knew I had to change the situation.

The second stage, earning a life, refers to how the participants re-established themselves in the world as people of value who were deserving of life, thereby realizing their own worthiness. They began to develop a sense of importance as individuals who mattered to themselves and others and had something to contribute in their lives. They opened their ears, eyes and selves and began to see positive aspects of themselves and others. They reconsidered their negative self, other and world perceptions and began to appreciate the simple yet rewarding aspects of their lives.

> I'm starting to see the finer things in life, for example, my car, and holidays and things like that. But for all this to happen, I have to work for it and that's the bottom line.

They disconnected from those who had a negative influence on them despite how difficult this was and reconnected with people who were validating toward them. They also became involved in activities that demonstrated to themselves and others that they had purpose and meaning in their lives. They thereby created and enacted a new worthy identity and a life of which they could be proud rather than ashamed, which reflected their learning from their near death experience and how they had incorporated this into their being.

> I started to think about the future . . . "I might have a place in this world . . . What do I want from my life?"

Re-vitalizing worthiness captures the process which the young men in this study underwent to address their profound existential questions about the meaning and nature of their relationship with living and dying. They confronted and overcame their deep fears about their selves, their lives and their fates, repairing their sense of fragmentation and emerging as stronger and more integrated people. They reclaimed their place as people deserving of life, thereby transcending their suicidality and resolving their crises of destiny.

Enhancing worthiness: what helped and hindered?

The study highlighted that mental health professionals, among others, through their encounters with these young men both enhanced and reduced opportunities for re-vitalizing worthiness. Such encounters occurred at different points on the participants' suicide trajectory and in different contexts, from initial consultations with a general practitioner (GP) to in-patient psychiatric treatment. Thus, examples of helpful and unhelpful interactions across treatment domains and practices are provided.

In general, interactions that were experienced as invalidating, such as controlling, coercive, objectifying and stigmatizing actions further alienated them and confirmed their sense of unworthiness and aloneness. For example, when the professional worked *on* rather *with* them, focused on their suicidal behaviour rather than on them as a person and excluded them from decision-making about their own care and treatment.

> At the time the powerlessness, the injustice, the lack of being heard, was excruciating. It was absolutely horrific . . . Still when I think back to it, and talk about it now, I feel quite upset. I still feel angry about that.

On the contrary, interactions identified as contributing positively to their recovery process incorporated those that openly acknowledged their ambivalence about living and their struggles with life tasks and roles. Despite their shame about their suicidal thoughts and feelings, acknowledgement of their pain, concerns and suicidal desire was experienced as helpful. This facilitated them in confronting and resolving their fears. They also valued a collaborative approach that involved them in their own care and treatment decisions which supported them in re-engaging with living on their terms and at their pace. This was important in helping them to regain a sense of control in their lives and fostering their sense of self-agency and self-esteem.

> I just thought that this transparency, this openness . . . whereby not only do I have a voice but this person is even willing to say, "Well, this is how I work, and if it is something you are interested in. I will share even the mode of work I do with you and see if that is interesting for you, or see if it might inform how we work together."
> Extraordinary.

The study drew attention to how the person in suicidal distress can be highly sensitive to their environment, particularly criticism, and that apparently minor exchanges can make a big difference in their lives. Thus, the mental health practitioner can influence the person's suicide trajectory significantly through his/her daily interactions with the person, for example, greeting the person with genuine interest. This highlights the importance of making and taking opportunities for engaging in validating encounters with the suicidal person, giving the message that the person is someone of value.

Worthiness was also facilitated more formally through therapeutic engagement that sought to establish a safe context for reflection and disclosure of inner turmoil and demonstrate belief in their potential to recover and renew their life. Participants recognized and sought out practitioners who were able to work in this way with them and this allowed them to be more open and willing to face their worst fears about themselves and their lives.

Discussion: what can you do?

The study highlighted that there are a number of ways that the health practitioner can influence the suicidal desire through formal and informal responses to the suicidal person. At an informal level, daily interactions provide opportunities for recognizing the person as someone of value, such as how the person is greeted when they present for treatment. Study participants confirmed that their sense of being valueless and unworthy of consideration was sometimes confirmed by practitioners who did not signal interest in them, or indeed gave the explicit message that they were not deserving of help. This is a crucial issue as early experiences with health professionals determine the help-seeking pathway of the patient. Hence, it can be helpful to acknowledge the suicidal person's decision to seek help following a suicide attempt or self-injury episode as this increases their chances of seeking and receiving appropriate follow-up help. While the precise outcome of such encounters cannot be predetermined and they may not directly impact the person's mental pain, they may interrupt their suicidal urge momentarily. This pause can create temporary space for reflection, which can reorientate them toward life and challenge self-destructive patterns (Orbach, 2001), ultimately serving as a deterrent against suicide (Shneidman, 2001).

It is important to note that the mental health practitioner may be influenced by social myths and stigma and can sometimes act out of negative values and beliefs that are outside of awareness (Joyce et al., 2007). For example, the suicidal person has reported being treated as if they were undeserving of treatment and wasting valuable staff time raising questions about their perceived care value (Gordon, 2010). Therefore, opportunities to reflect upon and challenge one's own views and practices can be useful, which can be done informally with colleagues or formally through clinical supervision. Indeed it has been suggested that the latter provides an important source of support for practitioners working in this demanding area (Cutcliffe & Stevenson, 2007).

Risk assessment is deemed to be a crucial aspect of mental health assessment for the suicidal person and there seems to be a prevailing emphasis on the provision of physical safety. However, it is important to remember that assessment provides a snapshot of the person's suicidal status at a moment in time rather than a static picture of this (Anderson, 1999). Therefore, it is temporarily valid in guiding response and needs to be reviewed as the person's situation evolves. This means focusing on the whole person rather than solely on his/her suicidal status and considering his/her psychological and spiritual safety and well-being in addition to physical safety. Therefore, developing a care/treatment plan that takes account of challenging aspects of the person's life and how these areas might be managed while also identifying intrapersonal and interpersonal resources is important, such as personal resilience, spiritual beliefs and supportive family members and friends. Of course, it is also useful to identify activities and people who may be exacerbating the person's state of suicidal crisis so that these can be addressed in due course, which may mean disengaging from significant people and changing unhealthy coping strategies.

Intervention with each person is unique and requires tailoring to meet his/her needs rather than relying on convenient and conventional methods. An individualized approach facilitates the person to begin to view themselves as important, thereby challenging their sense of unworthiness. This requires the practitioner to be flexible, patient and tolerant as it means engaging with the person's "dark side", sustaining a supportive role throughout their unpredictable journey of self-discovery and respecting their expertise on their own life. This facilitates the person in gaining a sense of agency and control in their lives and learning from and integrating their experiences, however difficult these might have been. Ironically, remembering some of their pain and negativity can serve as an impetus for sustaining change. Furthermore, assessment and intervention can usefully be viewed as interconnected rather than distinctly separate processes (Gordon & Stevenson, 2009). Thus, they can inform each other in dynamic ways that evolve with the person's changing personal and social circumstances.

The suicidal person is frequently treated in isolation from family and friends who are not involved with the professional system except to provide collateral information on the patient. This can further a sense of being disconnected, being a burden and not belonging, which are common concerns of the suicidal person (Joiner, 2005), inadvertently perpetuating their suicidality. This is an important issue as it is well documented that one's social network and resources impact recovery (Barker et al., 1999; Barker, 2009), and that reconnecting with life and living is a crucial part of this process (Cutcliffe & Stevenson, 2007). At times, however, this means distancing from those who have a negative influence on one, which can be difficult if this involves close family members, for example, exiting abusive relationships. Furthermore, those who are exposed to the suicide or attempted suicide of a family member can experience extreme distress which negatively influences relationships (Magne-Ingvar & Ojehagen, 1999). The mental health practitioner is ideally situated to connect with the significant other to both reduce their stress and to engage in dialogue about how they can best assist the suicidal person. This can promote helpful communication and reduce tensions between the patient and the family and between the family and the treatment system, making the person's care more co-ordinated. This is important in terms of planning after-care following in-patient treatment which is a time of particular high risk (Cutcliffe & Stevenson, 2007).

Thus, it is clear that there are multiple opportunities for the health practitioner to consider the therapeutic usefulness of their response to the suicidal person. However, this work is emotionally and ethically challenging and physically demanding and can place conflicting demands on the practitioner, which may give rise to him/her questioning their professional competence. In order to counter negative consequences such as compassion fatigue and burnout, and enhance job satisfaction and practitioner morale, the practitioner needs support and opportunities for personal and professional reflection and integration. Ongoing professional and personal development also serves to sustain emotional tolerance and psychological awareness and promotes an ethos of critical enquiry which ultimately nurtures holistic care, safety-enhancing practices and therapeutic engagement. This enables one to embrace a prevention approach while also focusing on care rather than cure and connection rather than control.

Implications for practice education, policy and research

There is ongoing debate as to whether mental health professionals are born or created (Barker, 2004). What is clear from the above discussion is that working with people in suicidal crisis requires being comfortable with others' tangible distress. It is likely that being able to accommodate that distress without being overwhelmed requires a practitioner who does not have low self-esteem or poor self-worth. Working with people in life and death ambivalence and their associated distress may be easier for those who have a level of security in their internal model of relationships such that they do not try to meet their own needs through helping others. Otherwise, the professional may not be able to take the necessary risk to allow the person to express and manage his/her suicidality. For example, a practitioner who fears that a death by suicide will reflect badly on his/her career may attune to physical rather than emotional risk, leaving the suicidal person physically safe but emotionally insecure.

Undoubtedly, some people who train in mental health professions will do so because of a high level of emotional openness and a belief that they can provide a context in which people can begin to heal themselves. However, others may need intensive training in order to reach a point where they do not close off from others but seek to appreciate the inner worlds of those with suicidal desire and intent, a quality which resonates with the idea of emotional intelligence in nursing (Akerjordet & Severinsson, 2004) and empathy in counselling/psychotherapy (Rogers, 1961). The ability to function reflectively in relation to the emotional states of self and others is achievable through training in mentalization, which refers to the ability of humans to make sense of their social world by imagining the mental states (e.g. beliefs, motives, emotions, desires, and needs) that underpin their own and others' behaviours in interpersonal interactions.

It is important to also consider the value of the person with expertise by experience (EBE). While peer support has frequently been cited as helpful in overcoming stigma and a sense of being alone in one's distress, the EBE is frequently an untapped resource in mental health settings. It is highly likely that a person who has survived the ambivalence and darkness of a close encounter with death is able to imagine the beliefs, motives, emotions and needs of the person living on the edge of suicide. Such attunement can be reassuring for the distressed person contemplating suicide both as an emotional connection and proof that life after suicidality is possible. Clearly, the "wounded helper" would have to achieve a place of peace with his/her own relationship to suicide and be able to maintain that place in a caring exchange. Consideration of curricula and service structures may be required to address such issues.

In respect of policy, help for the suicidal person can occur any time and anywhere, hence the importance of stressing shared ownership for suicidality and emphasizing that social exchanges can enhance or reduce one's sense of worthiness. A striking finding in the study was that the young men were often a long time travelling to their point of utter despair, and could detail important trials and disappointments going back into childhood that influenced their route. Thus, any policy must take account of the broadest range of points of intervention that might assist finding a better road to travel. For example, documented risk factors which aid suicidality to thrive such as family instability and violence, educational challenges and school bullying, sexual orientation conflict, social isolation and exclusion, and poor health and living conditions require active attention.

From this discussion it is clear that there is scope for much future research regarding the relationships between the various factors that can influence the suicide trajectory. For example, it would be worthwhile exploring the relationship between suicidality and adult attachment patterns and between the witnessing of violence (e.g. domestic violence) and being hurtful to oneself. Furthermore, given the tendency of young men to conceal their suicidality, it would be important to explore how to recognize the unobvious distress in a range of settings such as a school environment.

Conclusion

This chapter suggests that overcoming suicidality is influenced by contextual factors, intrapersonal resources and interpersonal encounters. Therefore, others including the mental health practitioner can have a vital role to play in the dynamic re-vitalizing worthiness process, which facilitates the suicidal person to transcend suicidality. It is important to note that any interaction with the suicidal person can present a potential opportunity to influence his/her suicide trajectory and life journey. In addition to specifically designed therapeutic interventions, this can also take the form of simple humane acts of kindness which reinforce his/her worthiness as a person of value who is deserving of life. Such acts may be intuitive or rely on an expansion of the emotional abilities of mental health professionals.

In general, validating interactions include a collaborative, respectful and individualized approach, belief in the value of the person, and genuine care and concern on the part of the practitioner. In contrast, actions that reinforce the patient–professional hierarchy perpetuate feelings of difference, abnormality and unworthiness, and overshadow opportunities for a caring connection.

This work is challenging and the mental health practitioner needs support and space to reflect upon his/her values and biases in addition to opportunities to enhance knowledge and skills, which may require curricular reform, education and training. This can counter the negativity and fears that influence his/her response to the suicidal person, restrict his/her creativity and lead to low morale.

References

Akerjordet, K., & Severinsson, E. (2004). Emotional intelligence in mental health nurses talking about practice. *International Journal of Mental Health Nursing, 13*(3), 164–170.

Aldridge, D. (1998). *Suicide: The tragedy of hopelessness.* London: Jessica Kingsley Publishers.

Anderson, M. (1999). Waiting for harm: Deliberate self-harm and suicide in young people: A review of the literature. *Journal of Psychiatric and Mental Health Nursing, 6,* 91–100.

Barker, P. (2004). *Assessment in psychiatric and mental health nursing: In search of the person* (2nd ed.). Cheltenham: Nelson Thornes Ltd.

Barker, P. (Ed.). (2009). *Psychiatric and mental health nursing: The craft of caring* (2nd ed.). London: Hodder Arnold.

Barker, P., Campbell, P., & Davidson, B. (Eds.). (1999). *From the ashes of experience: Reflections on madness, survival and growth*. London: Whurr.

Becker, E. (1973). *The denial of death*. New York: Free Press Paperbacks.

Begley, M., Chambers, D., Corcoran, P., & Gallagher, J. (2004). *The male perspective: Young men's outlook on life*. Cork: University College Cork Press.

Burke, S., Kerr, R., & McKeown, P. (2008). Male secondary school students' attitudes towards using mental health services. *Irish Journal of Psychological Medicine, 25*(2), 52–56.

Cutcliffe, J. R., & Stevenson, C. (2007). *Care of the suicidal person*. Philadelphia, PA: Elsevier.

Deci, R. M., & Ryan, E. L. (2004). Avoiding death or engaging life as accounts of meaning and culture: Comment on Pyszczynski et al. (2004). *Psychological Bulletin, 130*(3), 473–477.

Downey, H., Hamilton, K., & Catterall, M. (2007). Researching vulnerability: What about the researcher? *European Journal of Marketing, 41*(7), 734–739.

Gibbons, C. J., Stirman, S. W., Brown, G. K., & Beck, A. T. (2010). Engagement and retention of suicide attempters in clinical research. *Crisis, 31*(2), 62–68.

Gibbs, A. (1990). Aspects of communication with people who have attempted suicide. *Journal of Advanced Nursing, 15*, 1245–1249.

Glaser, B. G. (1998). *Doing grounded theory: Issues and discussions*. Palo Alto, CA: Sociology Press.

Glaser, B. G., & Strauss, A. (1967). *The discovery of grounded theory: Strategies for qualitative research*. Chicago: Aldine Publishers.

Gordon, E. (2010). Discourses on suicide: Consideration for therapeutic practice. *Feedback: Special Issue on Suicide, 12*(2), 3–15.

Gordon, E., Cutcliffe, J. R., & Stevenson, C. (2011). Re-vitalizing worthiness: A theory of overcoming suicidality among young men in Ireland, *The Grounded Theory Review, 10*(2), 21–44.

Gordon, E., & Stevenson, S. (2009). The context of assessment: Connecting assessment & intervention. In P. Barker, *Psychiatric and mental health nursing: The craft of caring* (2nd ed.). London: Hodder Arnold.

Grad, O. (2005). Suicide survivorship: An unknown journey from loss to gain – from individual to global perspective. In K. Hawton (Ed.), *Prevention and treatment of suicidal behaviour: From science to practice*. Oxford: Oxford University Press.

Guo, B., & Harstall, C. (2004). *For which strategies of suicide prevention is there evidence of effectiveness?* Copenhagen: WHO Regional Office for Europe (Health Evidence Networka report). Available at: http://www.euro.who.int/__data/ assets/ pdf_file/0010/74692/E83583.pdf (accessed 24 January 2007).

Hawton, K. (1994). Suicide. In E. S. Paykel, & R. D. Jenkins (Eds.), *Prevention in psychiatry*. London: Gaskell.

Hawton, K. (2005). *Prevention and treatment of suicidal behaviour: From suicide to practice*. Oxford: Oxford University Press.

Joiner, T. E. (2005). *Why people die by suicide*. Cambridge, MA: Harvard University Press.

Joiner, T. E. (2010). *Myths about suicide*. Cambridge, MA: Harvard University Press.

Joyce, T., Hazelton, M., & McMillan, M. (2007). Nurses with mental illness: Their workplace experience. *International Journal of Mental Health Nursing, 16*, 373–380.

Kvale, S. (1996). *Inter-views: An introduction to qualitative research interviewing*. Thousand Oaks, CA: Sage.

Links, P. S. (2001). Therapists of patients who committed suicide reported a wide range of emotional responses. *Evidence Based Mental Health, 4*(96), 412–420.

Magne-Ingvar, V., & Ojehagen, A. (1999). Significant others of suicide attempters: Their views at the time of the acute psychiatric consultation. *Social Psychiatry and Psychiatric Epidemiology, 34*, 470–476.

Maltsberger, J. T., & Goldblatt, M. J. (Eds.). (1996). *Essential papers on suicide*. Albany, New York: New York University Press.

Maris, R. W., Berman, A. L., & Silverman, M. M. (2000). *Comprehensive textbook of suicidology*. New York: Guilford Press.

National Office for Suicide Prevention (NOSP). (2005). *Reach out: National strategy for action on suicide prevention 2005–2014*. Dublin: Health Service Executive.

National Office for Suicide Prevention (NOSP). (2010). *Annual report 2009*. Dublin: Health Service Executive.

National Suicide Research Foundation (NSRF). (2012). *National Registry of Deliberate Self Harm Ireland: Annual Report 2011*. Cork: UCC.

Orbach, I. (2001). Therapeutic empathy with the suicidal wish: Principles of therapy with suicidal individuals. *American Journal of Psychotherapy, 55*(2), 166–184.

Rogers, C. A. (1961). *On becoming a person: A therapist's view of psychotherapy.* London: Constable.

Shneidman, E. S. (2001). *Comprehending suicide: Landmarks in 20th-century suicidology.* Washington, DC: American Psychological Association.

Sommer-Rothenberg, D. (1998). Suicide and language. *CMAJ, 159*, 239–240.

Strauss, A. L. (1969). *Mirrors and masks: The search for identity.* Palo Alto, CA: Sociology Press.

Ting, L., Sanders, S., Jacobson, J. M., & Power, J. R. (2006). Dealing with the aftermath: A qualitative analysis of mental health social workers' reactions after a client suicide. *Social Work, 51*(4), 329–341.

Webb, D. (2002). The many languages of suicide. Paper presented at Suicide Prevention Australia (SPA) Conference, Australia.

World Health Organization (WHO) (2010). *World Health Statistics.* Available at: htpp://www.who/int/topics/suicide/en/ (accessed 28 August 2012).

5

PROVIDING MEANINGFUL CARE

Using the experiences of young suicidal men to inform mental health care services

Hugh McKenna, Sinead Keeney, John Cutcliffe and Chris Stevenson

Introduction

Suicide is the act of deliberately ending one's own life and is among the top 20 leading causes of death globally for all ages. Every year, almost one million people die by suicide. This translates to a 'global' mortality rate of 16 per 100, 000 or one death every 40 seconds. Before 1950, suicides were more common in people over 45 years of age. In the latter half of the 20th century, this pattern changed significantly, so that the majority of suicides were within the 15–45 age range. One of the most important factors underpinning this shift in age-related trends was the epidemic rise in suicide among young men in most industrialised nations. And while the most recent epidemiological data from certain parts of the world perhaps indicate an encouraging decline in suicide rates in this age group, notable exceptions exist. For instance, the well-documented rise in suicide in Northern Ireland in general, as well as in relation to young men, is a disturbing trend.

Background

A recent paper in the journal, *New Scientist*, estimated that suicide accounts for approximately 1.5% of all deaths worldwide, following a 60% increase in global suicide since 1965 (Pool, 2009). Trend data show that it is now among the three leading causes of death among those aged 15–44 years in several countries and the second leading cause of death in the 10–24 age group (WHO, 2009). However, the successful suicide statistics hide a deeper problem with twenty uncompleted suicide attempts for every successful one (Pool, 2009).

The worldwide trend in suicide continues upward with eastern European countries displaying some of the highest recorded rates. Belarus reportedly has 63.3 suicides per 100,000 males and 10.3 per 100,000 females, followed closely by Lithuania with rates per 100,000 of 53.9 and 9.8 respectively. Caribbean countries have some of the lowest rates in the world (e.g. Barbados, 1.4 suicides per 100,000 males). Current UK figures are 10.1 per 100,000 males and 2.8 per 100,000 females and those of Ireland are 17.4 per 100,000 males and 3.8 per 100,000 females. These statistics are informative and useful but it must be stressed that because of the stigma surrounding suicide, often related to prevailing religious beliefs, it is possible that suicide remains under-reported; this may account, for example, for the low rates recorded for the Philippines and Iran (WHO, 2009; OECD, 2010).[1]

Since the late 1990s, rates of suicide in young men across the industrialised West have declined (Levi et al., 2003). After a sustained increase in Australian young male suicide rates over the previous 30 years, there has been a dramatic reduction among the 20–34 age group, declining from approximately 40 per 100,000 in 1997/1998 to approximately 20 per 100,000 in 2003 (Morrell, Page, & Taylor, 2007). By 2005, suicide rates were at their lowest level in England and Wales for approximately 30 years; rates in men aged 15–24 fell to almost half the peak rate and those in men aged 25–34 had decreased by almost one-third (Biddle, Brock, Brookes, & Gunnell, 2008). In Scotland, a marked reduction occurred in the 15–29 age group, from 42.5 per 100,000 in 2000 to 24.5 per 100,000, representing a 42% decrease (Stark, Stockton, & Henderson, 2008). While the figures for the USA are unclear, recent evidence suggests a reduction in adolescent male suicide in the recent past (Bridge, Barbe, & Brent, 2005).

In comparison to the trends identified above, the rise in suicide in Northern Ireland in general, as well as in relation to young men, is a more recent phenomenon, beginning in the late 1990s and still ongoing. Thus, after remaining relatively static throughout the latter half of the 20th century, between 1999 and 2008, there was a 64% increase in suicide in Northern Ireland (Samaritans, 2009). Northern Ireland now has more suicides per 100,000 persons than England and Wales, but less than our close neighbours, Scotland and the Republic of Ireland (DHSSPS, 2006). In large part, the dramatic increase has been fuelled by a rise in male suicide, particularly marked in the 15–34 year age group. The sustained nature of this increase in young male suicide is demonstrated by the following figures: in 2002, almost 76% of all suicides were male, with 60% of these occurring in the 15–34 age group; by 2008, 77% of all suicides were by males but the percentage occurring in the 15–34 age group had increased to 72% (Samaritans, 2009). Other sources confirm this dramatic increase in young male suicide. According to the Department of Health in Northern Ireland, in 2010, the number of suicides in Northern Ireland was 315, reflecting the continuing rise across recent years. This is despite £6 million per year being allocated to suicide prevention by the Department of Health for the 1.8 million population of Northern Ireland.

Figures from the 'Protect Life' Document (DHSSPS, 2006) show that in the Belfast Trust area there were 16 deaths by suicide among young men aged 15–34 years in 1998. This increased to 30 deaths in 2008. The average across these years was 17 deaths per year for this age range. This alarming rise in suicide, particularly among young men in Northern Ireland, prompted the Department of Health to produce the first ever local-level Northern Ireland Suicide Prevention Strategy, 'Protect Life: A Shared Vision' (DHSSPS, 2006). Included in this strategy is an acknowledgement of the need for research to inform the development of policy as well as local-level service provision. The study reported here was one such research initiative funded by the Health and Social Care Research & Development Division of the Public Health Agency. It was an investigation undertaken by the University of Ulster and Queens University, Belfast, in collaboration with colleagues at University College Dublin and the University of Maine. It focused on those areas of Northern Ireland evidencing some of the highest rates of suicide among the male population in the 16–34 age group.

Aims of the study

The overarching aim of the study was to obtain a comprehensive understanding of the encounters of suicidal men aged 16–34 to underpin the provision of accessible, acceptable and appropriate mental health services. In line with this aim, study objectives were to do the following:

- elicit the encounters of men (aged 16–34) of being suicidal and their understandings of what would constitute meaningful caring;

- explicate the specific caring processes that might make 'a difference' to caring for the suicidal person, that is, to inform what health care professionals can do.

The above aims and objectives were developed in order to answer two research questions:

- How can mental health care services be most appropriately configured to encourage their use by suicidal men aged 16–34?
- What is the required response of mental health care services for suicidal men, aged 16–34?

Method

An underpinning conceptualization of suicide as a multidimensional, complex phenomenon was reflected in the choice of a qualitative research design for this study. The fact that relatively little is known about young men's encounters and incidents of suicide further validated this approach. Consequently, in-depth interviews were chosen as the means of data collection. A purposive sample of young men was obtained according to: (1) age range; and (2) contact/lack of contact with statutory and non-statutory mental health services. The final sampling frame targeted four 'categories' of young suicidal men, defined primarily in relation to their (non-)engagement with services. These were:

- *Men aged 16–34 currently engaged with statutory mental health services*: access was obtained through both the Belfast HSC Trust and Southern HSC Trust.
- *Men aged 16–34 previously engaged with statutory mental health services*: access was obtained through both the Belfast HSC Trust and Southern HSC Trust.
- *Men aged 16–34 currently using a range of non-statutory counselling organisations*: access was obtained through a wide range of local-level community sector counselling organisations that dealt with suicidal young men in both the Belfast HSC Trust and Southern HSC Trust areas.
- *Men aged 16–34 who had not had any contact with statutory or non-statutory mental health services*: access was obtained through a comprehensive advertising campaign across a range of media.

A total of 36 young men were subsequently recruited. Data were collected by means of semi-structured interviews. All interviews were audio-recorded, with permission. Although questions were determined primarily by the unfolding discussion between the interviewer and participant, a limited number of pre-specified issues were introduced. These included a question addressing the support, including both formal and/or informal (mental) health care services, which a participant had sought, and a question addressing the factors that had helped and continued to help maintain his wish to stay alive.

Data analysis

The aim was to provide an analysis with *explanatory* value in terms of understanding suicidal behaviour among young men. That is, we were aiming to identify patterns and relationships within the data that would offer suggestions concerning how care and services could be developed appropriately. Consequently, we wanted to move beyond the mere description of recurrent or common 'themes' observable in the interview data to offer an analysis that explored the context of and relationships between these themes (and their constituent 'properties' and associated concepts). This offered a means of thinking about a range of relevant issues to do with the provision of care to young suicidal men.

After initial verbatim transcription, Glaser and Strauss's (1967) process of open coding was applied to each interview transcript. That is, the text was examined line by line in order to identify and subsequently 'code' processes in the data. Such a process of 'substantive coding' codified the substance of the data, frequently using the participant's own words. Following this initial coding, individual labels (that is, codes) were compared with each other in order to develop clusters or categories of codes according to obvious fit. This allowed a tentative conceptual framework to be developed, comprising a number of categories (with associated labels). This latter process was accomplished by examining common themes and/or concepts evident in each of the categories or, alternatively, by identifying if there was a process or theme underpinning several of the categories that would allow them to be grouped together. This framework was subsequently confirmed by further, conceptually led reduction of the data. Here, the tentative categories were gradually grouped together under 'umbrella terms' by examining all the categories to identify how they clustered or connected. Each of these umbrella terms thus encompassed several initial tentative categories. This extended process gradually enabled the development of a number of core categories (see Figures 5.1, 5.2 and 5.3 below), which encompassed the entire dataset and captured the essential processes evident in the data.

The following procedures and processes were followed in order to enhance the validity and reliability of data analysis (Silverman, 2006). In terms of reliability: (1) all interviewers were trained with a view to establishing consistency in the conduct of interviews; (2) all digital recordings were transcribed verbatim; and (3) transcripts were distributed among the research team for individual analyses, which were then shared in order to promote the full possibilities for analytical insight. In terms of validity: (1) comprehensive data treatment meant that all data were analysed and accounted for; and (2) constant comparison ensured that the final analytical framework was incrementally built up through comparison both within and across interview datasets.

Ethics/research governance

The study adhered to all relevant research governance requirements. It received full Office of Research Ethics Committee, Northern Ireland (ORECNI) approval (REC Reference: 06/NIR02/149). In addition, it complied with the research governance requirements of the Health and Social Care Trusts in Northern Ireland.

Findings

Three 'core categories' were developed: (1) *Widening access and bolstering pro-active outreach*; (2) *On becoming a man. . .*; and (3) *Equipping young men for the challenges of 21st-century living*. Collectively, these categories answered the two research questions.

Widening access and bolstering pro-active outreach

Essentially, this category is concerned with current formal mental health services (see Figure 5.1). Findings indicated that the type, nature, and geographical location of these services offered only limited help to address young men's suicidal thoughts and behaviours. Importantly, there was a clear need for more 'pro-active', 'outreach', suicide prevention services in addition to/distinct from responsive or reactive suicide services. In keeping with such a development was the parallel need for increasing awareness in the community, including among young men, of the existence of such services. Further, the data highlighted how any media-based outreach attempts could

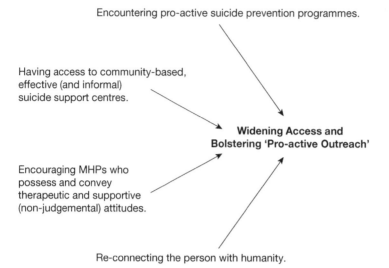

Encountering pro-active suicide prevention programmes.

Having access to community-based, effective (and informal) suicide support centres.

Widening Access and Bolstering 'Pro-active Outreach'

Encouraging MHPs who possess and convey therapeutic and supportive (non-judgemental) attitudes.

Re-connecting the person with humanity.

Figure 5.1 Core category and Phase One: Widening access and bolstering pro-active outreach

profitably make use of technology more appropriate to the younger age group (for example, social media, 'text messaging', email). In addition, findings confirmed the value in creating (more) community-based and relatively informal 'drop-in' suicide centres in line with young men's preferred contexts of (social) interaction.

The category also addresses the particular qualities and skills that young suicidal men found helpful in people with whom they worked. Especially in relation to the initial stage of the process of recovery, young suicidal men placed immense emphasis on such qualities and skills which emerged as the principal 'interventions' of which the mental health practitioners (MHPs) made use. A firm interpersonal connection not only served as the platform upon which all future interventions were built but was made possible because of the practitioner possessing and, importantly, communicating certain attitudes. Finally, this category is concerned with initial attempts to combat the pervasive sense of disconnection referred to by the young men in the study. Their accounts indicated that having a sense that they mattered, that someone else was concerned about and interested in them, was immensely important and had a specific countering effect on their suicidal ideation and perspectives.

On becoming a man . . .

Participants described a range of issues, problems and perceptions that were significantly contributing to their initial and ongoing increased risk for suicide. Accordingly, this category is concerned with the interventions and services that could be provided to young men as a means of alleviating this risk. Participants made reference to possessing certain perceptions of what it was to be a 'successful' man in 21st-century Northern Ireland. These perceptions were, by and large, unhelpful and unrealistic and served to contribute to their low self-esteem, level of personal stress and ultimately, to their increased risk of suicide. Accordingly, one role of MHPs was to gently challenge these constructs and perceptions and replace them with more realistic, helpful and attainable views of being a successful man (see Figure 5.2).

Further, study data suggested the relevance of being able to access a 'peer group' in which young men can find support and hope from mixing with survivors of suicide. Being among others

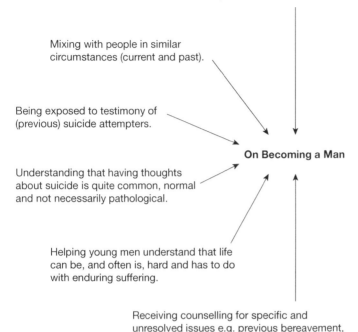

Gently challenging unhelpful and unrealistic perceptions of what it is to be a (successful) man in 21st-century Northern Ireland.

Mixing with people in similar circumstances (current and past).

Being exposed to testimony of (previous) suicide attempters.

On Becoming a Man

Understanding that having thoughts about suicide is quite common, normal and not necessarily pathological.

Helping young men understand that life can be, and often is, hard and has to do with enduring suffering.

Receiving counselling for specific and unresolved issues e.g. previous bereavement, childhood abuse, addiction.

Figure 5.2 Core category and Phase Two: 'On becoming a man . . .'

who were 'the same' created an opportunity for the young men to vocalise their feelings and behaviours in what was perceived as a 'safe' forum. In addition, hearing the testimonies of other (formerly suicidal) young men highlighted the possibility of recovery and provided some form of conceptual understanding of the likely processes involved. Additionally, being exposed to these testimonies served as a protective factor, in that learning of the 'pain' of suicide from (multiple) others directly ushered the suicidal young men towards an understanding of suicide as unacceptable.

Finally, this category addresses suicidal young men's requirement for counselling (therapy) to address specific, unresolved issues. Participants referred to a wide variety of problems and issues, each of which, to a greater or lesser extent, was contributing to their risk for suicide. Accordingly, a wide variety of forms or types of counselling services were required (for example, for abusive childhood, relationship/marriage problems, addictions and dependency, loss and bereavement and family dysfunctionality). Evidently, where suicidal young men had received such specific forms of counselling help, they found it useful.

Equipping young men for the challenges of 21st-century living

This category is concerned with the processes and activities with which the young men engaged on their path to recovery from suicidality. It captures how this 'journey' was seldom completed quickly or easily and that recovery involved a process of establishing meaning in the young men's lives. Individual ways through which this (new) meaning was generated varied, but there were distinct commonalities across participants. In the context of their increasing sense of dissatisfaction with a 'meaningless life', MHPs could play an important role in helping the young men (re)discover personally meaningful phenomena and experiences. As a result of finding this (new) meaning and purpose, the elevated risk of suicide appeared to diminish. Furthermore and importantly, participants found meaning in 'doing for other people', particularly other people who were experiencing similar challenges. Accordingly, there appears to be particular utility and value (as a suicide deterrent) to be involved in helping other people overcome their own challenges with suicidal thinking and actions (see Figure 5.3).

The category is also concerned with providing suicidal young men with a range of opportunities to engage in pragmatic life skills, social skills, educational programmes and other meaningful activities. All of these, to a greater or lesser extent, provide them with a wide range of skills required to navigate their way successfully through the contemporary challenges of modern life in Northern Ireland. Further, such opportunities play an important role in keeping the young men occupied, thereby avoiding exposure to excessive isolation and rumination. Additionally, the category reflects suicidal young men's (growing) awareness of the powerful protective factor that having close, loving, concerned 'significant others' (most especially, family) can provide. Moreover, participants needed to be aware that their suicidal behaviour had been accepted by these others; such acceptance affected their outlook, making them feel more hopeful about the future.

Finally, the category highlights the suicidal young men's acknowledgement of 'recovery' from their suicidality as an ongoing and long-term process and that within this extended time frame, 'hard work' on their part would be required. There is also a strong sense that while they were willing to engage in this long-term work, they would require ongoing support from mental health services and others who have endured a similar situation. To a lesser extent, this category

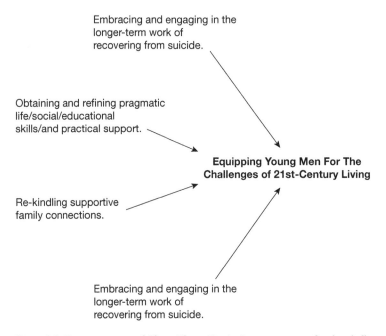

Figure 5.3 Core category and Phase Three: Equipping young men for the challenges of 21st-century living

is also concerned with the participants, in essence, 'learning to live' again. This included the important process of 'making sense' of their suicidality; interestingly, none of the young men referred to this process of 'sense making' in the past tense or as something they had completed. Additionally, it was evident that a number of inter- and intra-personal processes were involved, not least the continued support from and involvement of (in this instance) the MHPs and fellow 'travellers' on the 'recovery' path.

Discussion and conclusions

The findings of this study corroborate some of the core principles enshrined in national suicide prevention strategies of many Western countries. These include: the United States (USDHHS, 2001), England (DoH, 2002), Scotland (Scottish Executive, 2002), Ireland (HSE, 2005), New Zealand (Associate Minister of Health, 2006) and Australia (AGDHA, 2000). All have been developed in direct response to a significant global increase in the rate of suicide. Examination of these documents shows much conceptual and strategic overlap and corresponding similarities in emphases in relation to priorities set for the prevention of suicide (Cutcliffe & Stevenson, 2008). One such emphasis is that of interventions to help combat the stigma associated with suicide. Our research shows this to be particularly pertinent to the uptake and utilisation of mental health services among young men in Northern Ireland.

Encouragingly, there is evidence that national suicide prevention strategies can be effective in helping to reduce the rate of suicide in young males. For example, Morrell et al. (2007) traced a reduction in suicide in young men in Australia to the National Youth Suicide Prevention Strategy (NYSPS). This strategy ensured that health and social care providers were resourced to implement a wide range of national and local-level interventions across primary prevention programmes, capacity-building services and treatment support. Further, Stark et al. (2008) suggested that the recent priority given to promoting mental health and well-being in Scotland, as part of the national suicide prevention strategy work, may have had an impact on reducing young male suicide. Specific interventions which mirror the policy and practice recommendations outlined in respect of this study include the 'See Me' anti-stigma programme, the 'Breathing Space' confidential telephone helpline targeted at young men, the development of a recovery-oriented mental health programme (the Scottish Recovery Network), as well as a large investment in media publicity about the nature and prevalence of suicidal behaviour.

Underpinning the development of the *range* of programmes and related measures included in national suicide strategies has been the ongoing debate concerning the most appropriate approach to suicide prevention. While a public health approach within suicide prevention is necessary in that it permits a broad range of social, economic, health, mental health, cultural and other risk factors to be integrated and targeted (Jenkins & Singh, 2000; Jenkins, 2002), the need remains for more targeted interventions (Beautrais et al., 2005), including and particularly in relation to identified high-risk populations such as young men.

Recommendations

In the following, the two original research questions are used to structure study findings in terms of what they suggest as relevant to the provision of care for young suicidal men:

1. How can mental health care services be most appropriately configured to encourage their use by suicidal men aged 16–34?

The recommendations in reply are:

- Suicide-related services need to reach out to young men *pro-actively*. These services should be community based and open access.
- Part of this pro-active, community-level service provision should be embedded in manifestly non-'mental health' contexts. These include sports clubs, schools, the workplace and community interest/self-help groups.
- Services, particularly those based in the community, need to be advertised more widely and in ways which reach out to young men. A range of media should be used to promote access and provide culturally relevant care, including media which have become a regular means of communication among young people.
- Services should be premised on an acknowledgement of the need for support to be provided to young men over the long term so that they are to be enabled to move forward with their lives in a positive manner once the initial risk of suicide has been removed.
- Novel forms of suicide prevention outreach work should include those media that have become a regular means of communication among young people. This includes social networking systems, the Internet, text messaging and/or email.
- Services must continue to address the concerns of young men about issues of stigma and confidentiality regarding the care and treatment of suicidality. Some issues around signposting and labelling of suicide prevention services should be addressed immediately.
- Care should be based on a broad recovery approach. The need to skill and support young men operates at both an individual and societal level and a fundamental part of this must involve creating an appropriate environment to promote participation and social inclusion of young suicidal men generally.
- Irrespective of the particular form of care/service provision, help and support needs to be delivered by those appropriately skilled and resourced.

2 What is the required response of mental health care services for suicidal men, aged 16–34?

The recommended responses are:

- It is essential that health care professionals care for young suicidal men in ways which respond to their basic emotional and interpersonal needs. It should be ensured that health professionals possess and convey therapeutic and supportive (non-judgemental) attitudes and realise the important bonding role they have in enabling young men to *reconnect with humanity*.
- Health care professionals should appreciate that their demeanour and attitude are crucial to a young man's sense of meaningful therapeutic engagement. Effective care is as much about how a young man perceives the relationship between himself and his professional carer as it is about the 'technical' components of care.
- Care should be premised on an explicit acknowledgement of a young man as a human being with a unique personal biography.
- It should be ensured that treatment and care are relevant to recovery and onward trajectory through life, if it is to be perceived as effective by young men. As part of this sense of 'moving forward', care should include help and support to develop a realistic appreciation of the (personal) possibilities that life offers as well as the skills to pursue these possibilities once envisaged.
- People with experience of suicide should be involved in care delivery and support. Hearing *first-hand* about these experiences serves as a powerful disincentive to suicide, and learning

about lives built successfully thereafter can act as an incentive for/basis of personal growth and development.

- Psychological therapies need to be made available as part of routine care, particularly those that equip young men with fundamental cognitive resources, including coping strategies (e.g. for dealing with stress, anxiety and disappointment) as well as other dimensions of mental/emotional well-being such as, for example, self-esteem.
- Maximising access must include taking steps to address the major challenges posed by stigma and discrimination, including comprehensive, population-level advertising and awareness-raising campaigns as well as more targeted educational and workplace initiatives.
- Care should be premised on a recovery rather than a 'risk reduction' approach.
- Additional education/training needs to be provided to health care professionals in order to support the provision of relevant care to young suicidal men.

Coda

The evidence from this study highlights the importance of implementing a 'package' of measures. These include Northern Ireland-wide, population-level public health measures directed at reducing the stigma and discrimination associated with suicidal behaviour and related help-seeking. In addition, measures should be targeted specifically at the 'at risk' population of young men themselves (for example, care which is specifically configured around the help-seeking preferences of young men). These measures are inextricably linked; put basically, young men have to 'turn up' for care in order for that care to have a chance of being effective. They will continue not to attend services they perceive as both stigmatised and stigmatising, irrespective of the quality of care these services may provide. However, as outlined above, there is growing evidence that, once implemented, such measures can be effective in reducing young male suicide.

Note

1   Editors' note: Or other countries that hold deeply held or devout religious beliefs wherein suicide is regarded as a 'sin'.

References

AGDHA (2000). *The national suicide prevention strategy*. Canberra: AGDHA.

Associate Ministry of Health (2006). *The New Zealand suicide prevention strategy, 2006–2016*. Wellington: Associate Ministry of Health.

Beautrais, A. L., Collings, S. C. D., Ehrhardt, P. et al. (2005). *Suicide prevention: A review of evidence of risk and protective factors and points of effective intervention*. Wellington: Ministry of Health.

Biddle, L., Brock, A., Brookes, S. T., & Gunnell, S. (2008). Suicide rates in young men in England and Wales in the 21st century: Time trend study. *British Medical Journal, 336*, 539–542.

Bridge, J. A., Barbe, R. P., & Brent, D. A. (2005). Recent trends in suicide among US adolescent males, 1992–2001. *Psychiatric Services, 56*(5), 222.

Cutcliffe, J. R., & Stevenson, C. (2008). Never the twain? Reconciling national suicide prevention strategies with the practice, educational and policy needs of Psychiatric/Mental Health Nurses: part one. *International Journal of Mental Health Nursing, 17*, 341–350.

Department of Health (DoH) (2002). *National suicide prevention strategy for England*. London: Department of Health.

DHSSPS (2006). *Protect life: a shared vision: The Northern Ireland suicide prevention strategy and action plan, 2006–2011*. Belfast: DHSSPS.

Glaser, B. G., & Strauss, A. L. (1967). *The discovery of grounded theory: Strategies for qualitative research*. New York: Aldine de Gruyter.

Health Services Executive (HSE) (2005). *National suicide prevention strategy in Ireland.* Dublin: HSE.

Jenkins, R. (2002). Addressing suicide as a public-health problem. *Lancet, 359* (9309), 810–814.

Jenkins, R., & Singh, B. (2000). General population strategies of suicide prevention. In K. Hawton, & K. van Heeringen (Eds.) *The international handbook of suicide and attempted suicide* (pp. 597–615). New York: John Wiley and Sons Ltd.

Levi, F., La Vacchia, C., Lucchini, F., Negri, E., Saxena, S., Maulik, P. K., & Saraceno, B. (2003). Trends in mortality from suicide, 1965–1999. *Acta Psychiatrica Scandinavica, 108*(5), 341–349.

Morrell, S., Page, A. N., & Taylor, R. J. (2007) .The decline in Australian young male suicide. *Social Science and Medicine, 64,* 747–754.

Organisation for Economic Co-operation and Development (2010). *Statistics on suicide.* Available at: http://www.oecd.org/home/0,3305,en_2649_201185_1_1_1_1_1,00.html (accessed 25 August 2010).

Pool, R. (2009). Why do people die that way? *New Scientist, 28* February, pp. 37–39.

Samaritans (2009). *Suicide in the UK and Republic of Ireland, 1999–2008.* London: Samaritans.

Scottish Executive (2002). *Choose life: A national strategy and action plan to prevent suicide in Scotland.* Edinburgh: The Stationery Office.

Silverman, D. (2006). *Interpreting qualitative data* (3rd ed.). London: Sage.

Stark, C., Stockton, D., & Henderson, R. (2008). Reduction in young male suicide in Scotland. *BMC Public Health, 8,* 80.

United States Department of Health and Human Services (USDHHS) (2001). *National strategy for suicide prevention.* Washington, DC: USDHHS.

World Health Organisation (2009). Suicide rates per 100,000 by country, year and sex. Available at: http://www.who.int/mental_health/prevention/suicide_rates/en/index.html (accessed 25 June 2010).

6

EXPRESSED EMOTION AND SUICIDAL BEHAVIORS

José Carlos Santos

Introduction

Suicidal behaviors have been examined and addressed from different perspectives: anthropological, philosophical, sociological, bio-medical and theological, to name a few, but they still remain one of the most mysterious phenomena known to man (Cobb, 1801, cited in Saraiva, 1999). There has been a growing interest in suicidal behaviors in recent years; one of the reasons for this interest is the increase in the number of suicides worldwide. While some nations appear to produce more suicide-focused research than others, there are still potentially valuable lessons and insights to be learned from research that is undertaken in less prominent countries.

For instance, in a previous study conducted in Portugal, Santos (2000) performed a retrospective study in a hospital emergency room in the Central Region. He concluded that 58% of adolescent parasuicides went home without any indication of follow-up in the psychiatric hospital or community care; 32% were sent to psychiatric consultation; and 10% stayed in the hospital. This study considered it important to study these families because many of them have to deal with these suicidal behaviors once the adolescent returned home, and this often produced a significant sense of fear, insecurity and guilt. Suicide and suicidal behaviors are not easy phenomena to understand or to have to cope with. Even for mental health professionals who have formal training in this area, these behaviors can evoke powerful and sometimes negative emotions and reactions (Cutcliffe & Santos, 2012). It may not be entirely surprising then to expect difficulties in coping with parasuicides in families. This line of thinking led the author to think about the concept of expressed emotion (EE); and an interest in applying the concept to the families of parasuicides, particularly given that very few studies have been conducted in this area (Santos, Saraiva, & Sousa, 2009). Accordingly the remainder of this chapter focuses on the theoretical, clinical and empirical background of EE, and then reports on further recent research in this area.

A brief overview of expressed emotion (EE)

EE is a multidimensional theoretical construct based on research in the area of Social Psychiatrics conducted in the 1950s and 1960s (Wearden, Tarrier, Barrowclough, Zastowny, & Rahill, 2000) in the United Kingdom. Brown and colleagues (Brown, 1958; Brown, Carstairs, & Topping,

1958; Brown, Monck, Carstairs, & Wing, 1962) raised the issue of different outcomes depending on patient destination after discharge and showed that relapses are less common in patients who do not live with their parents. They identified five factors mentioned by relatives as being correlated with patients' relapse, such as hostility and dominant or directive behaviors. These domains are clearly distinguished from patients' emotions towards their relatives. Later on, Brown and Rutter (1966) considered the interview to be the best option to collect information which should then be recorded and classified. This interview should address the current crisis, the psychiatric background and the patient's participation in the family dynamics, and identified three dimensions of EE: (1) critical comments; (2) hostility; and (3) emotional over-involvement of the family towards the patient. EE is considered high when there are seven or more critical comments, hostility or a high over-involvement evidenced during a 3-hour individual interview. It is sufficient for one of the relatives to reach this score. In a joint interview with the patient, EE is considered high if there are at least two or more critical comments. Brown designed a script for an interview with patients' relatives, the Camberwell Family Interview (CFI) (Brown, Birley, & Wing, 1972). According to Vaughn and Leff (1976a), instead of the seven comments previously considered necessary, EE is considered high if there are at least six critical comments.

Dimensions of expressed emotion

The critical comments refer to any statement which, referring to the manner in which it is expressed, constitutes an unfavorable comment upon the behavior or personality of the person to whom it refers. The assessment should take into account the critical content, in which there is a clear statement of the relative saying that he/she dislikes, disapproves or resents any behavior or characteristic. There can also be a clear sign of rejection. The vocal aspects should also be considered, namely, variations in voice tone when the relative states something which is potentially neutral, positive or negative.

If an individual is referred to by what he/she is and not for what he/she does, if negative feelings are generalized and expressed against the individual and not against specific behaviors or attitudes, then criticism is generalized, "he's a failure in everything he does." The signs of rejection imply a generalized negative feeling which involves a clear antipathy. Hostile comments, i.e. an attitude of rejection or negative comments towards someone, are always considered critical comments. However, critical comments are not necessarily hostile. Hostility, like over-involvement, is generally analyzed based on the interview as a whole to obtain a final score.

Together with the critical comments, hostile comments can also be classified in terms of content. These comments may not be comments of clear criticism of specific traits or behaviors, but suggest an attitude of overall rejection of the individual. The context, the content and the voice tone are important aspects to define a comment as being critical. However, to define a comment as being hostile, there must be some evidence of its content. In case of doubt, the definition of hostility is removed.

Emotional over-involvement was developed for interviews of parents of over-18-year-olds, but it has also been successfully applied to other age groups (Leff & Vaughn, 1985). It is based on both the report on the behavior towards the individual and the individual's behavior during the interview. The behavioral report is based on three aspects: (1) an exaggerated emotional response (in the past or resulting from a demonstration of over-identification between the relative and the patient); (2) a relationship characterized by an exaggerated self-sacrifice; and/or (3) an exaggerated devotion. Emotional over-involvement can also be assessed based on what the patient has demonstrated and verbalized during the interview: statements about the relative's attitude towards the patient or the impact of the disease, intrusion phenomena, or over-protection.

Dramatization can be carried out through the description of trivial events or small problems, through voice tone and intonation, and through the complete and detailed description being given. It must be associated with an excessively high anxiety towards a minor aspect of the individual's behavior or way of living to be considered.

The assessment of the environment of over-involvement is based on the interview as a whole. During the interview, the interviewer registers some non-verbal evidence and, later on, the relevant material is transcribed from an audiotape. The final score should be given based on the detailed notes of the interview. Warmth is rated on a 6-point scale (0–5), according to Table 6.1. Warmth is assessed based on several aspects. The tone of voice is perhaps the most important one, and so the interviewer should be alert to the enthusiasm with which the relative speaks about the patient. In the same way, a monotonous or cold tone of voice should also be taken into account in the final assessment of warmth. The spontaneity of the expressions which show warmth (if they are not direct responses to questions) should also be considered. On the other hand, the lack of expressions of warmth in crucial moments of the interview should also be registered. Sympathy, concern and empathy are usually present when relatives talk about the individual's behavior or problems. It is also important to demonstrate interest for the person by showing enthusiasm for the individual, his/her activities and accomplishments.

There are other aspects which should not be considered as being relevant: deductions about the real affective warmth; the warm-hearted personality of the interviewee; comparisons regarding warmth towards others; interviewee's depression; criticism or hostility; stereotyped affection and positive comments. Positive remarks are statements in which the interviewee praises, approves or appreciates the behavior or personality of the patient. This should be considered whenever it is a response to an interviewer's question. The positive remark is primarily characterized for its content, although the tone of voice itself cannot determine a positive remark.

Table 6.1 Characteristics of family attitudes according to their expressed emotion

Dimensions	Low EE	High EE
Cognitive	Accept the illness as genuine Decrease in the expectations, according to the situation of the individual	Doubt the legitimacy of the illness, believing that the individual may control the symptomatology Expectations maintained, not accepting the decrease in the functioning levels
Emotional	Attention centered on the individual, sensitive towards his/her needs Empathy, with an effort to understand the vision of the individual Calm/Greater balancing Objectivity Greater adjustment to the emotions	Attention centered on themselves Intense anger and/or stress
Behavioral	Adaptation, flexibility Attempt to solve the problems Non-intrusive Non-conflictual	Little flexibility Inadequate and strict strategies used in the management of difficulties Intrusive Conflictual

Source: Adapted from Leff and Vaughn (1985) and Vaughn (2003b).

Assessment of expressed emotion

Despite the difficulty in measuring, quantifying and replicating social factors (Kuipers, 1994), EE can be rated and play an independent and causal role in the relapse process (Hooley & Gotlib, 2000). Among interviews and surveys, there are many instruments to measure EE. The most important ones are: CFI (Brown et al., 1972; Vaughn & Leff, 1976b); Five Minutes Speech Sample (Gottschalk & Gleser, 1969; Magana, Goldstein, Karno, Miklowitz, & Falloon, 1985); Level of Expressed Emotion (Cole & Kazarian, 1988); Influential Relationships Questionnaire (Baker, Helmes, & Kazarian, 1984); Perceived Criticism (Hooley & Teasdle, 1989); Family Emotional Involvement and Criticism Scale (Shields, Franks, Harp, McDaniel, & Campbell,1992); Patient Rejection Scale (Kreisman, Simmes, & Joy, 1979); Questionnaire Assessment of Expressed Emotion (Docherty, Serper, & Harvey, 1990); Family Attitude Scale (Kavanagh et al., 1997).

In a literature review, Van Humbeeck, Van Audenhove, De Hert, Pieters, and Storms (2002) compared the CFI with 11 alternative EE measures (among them, those previously mentioned). The authors concluded that the CFI remains the best tool for assessing the quality of the relationship, and the most reliable predictor of the relapse rate because it has a higher sensitivity to assess the climate with high EE. Hooley and Holly (2006), after analyzing several EE measures, concluded that the CFI is also the only form of EE assessment that provides data on all five EE variables (criticism, hostility, emotional over-involvement (EOI), warmth, and positive remarks). Another major advantage of the CFI is that, when it is conducted by a skilled clinical researcher, it can be a remarkably positive experience for the relative being interviewed, and, finally, another major advantage of the CFI is that it provides a great deal of information beyond that needed to make EE ratings.

Perceived criticism ratings are in no way a substitute for the CFI. However, in circumstances that call for a fast estimate of the affective climate in the family, the minimal time cost of a Perceived Criticism assessment appears to be greatly outweighed by its possible benefits as negative prognostic indicator. Although they can be more appealing for their briefness, Vaughn (2003b) calls attention to the importance of the quality of the instruments to the research findings, underlining the power of the CFI to address, explore and reveal facts to rate EE. We can conclude that the CFI is the most complete EE measure and that it provides an extremely good return on the time investment that it demands (Van Humbeeck et al., 2002; Hooley & Holly, 2006).

The objectives of the CFI are: to gather information on the individual's psychiatric background, behavior symptoms, and the role played by the individual in the six months prior to hospital admission. The interviewer also tries to collect data on the relatives' subjective attitudes and feelings towards the patient and the disease. During the session, the interviewer shows interest in every detail shared by the relatives, but he/she should never comment or criticize attitudes or behaviors.

Cultural validity of expressed emotion

Over the last 50 years, the study of EE has become an international concern worldwide and in different clinical populations. Cultural validity has been under discussion since the study on EE expanded beyond the United Kingdom. Kuipers (1992) mentioned a study on the research on EE in Europe, which is not culturally specific and can be used in different situations and in different countries, stating that EE can be a new way to assess the impact of severe conditions in different cultures.

Moreover, Butzlaff and Hooley (1998), in an analysis of studies previously conducted in different geographic areas, concluded that the scores obtained in Eastern Europe were higher than in the other groups: the United Kingdom, Northern Europe, Southern Europe, North America, Australia and Asia, with the lowest score in Australia. They also concluded that the studies from Eastern Europe accounted for much of the heterogeneity. However, they stated that the correlation between the geographic location and EE findings was not sufficiently relevant and that further research was needed, particularly in Eastern Europe and Asia. Previously, Bebbington and Kuipers (1994) found no significant differences when they analyzed the geographic location, thus concluding that there was no variation between EE and the location of research. Based on this finding, Kuipers (1994) stated that the capacity of EE to cross cultural and linguistic barriers was perhaps unique for a social measurement tool. However, Bhugra and Mckenzie (2003) argue that critical comments, emotional over-involvement and hostility should be embedded in the specific cultural context and family relationships and, most importantly, that they should also be analyzed based on warmth and positive remarks. They also mention that EE is not a single directional concept and that it should not be seen in isolation from intermediary factors, such as the role of kinship, attitudes of the family to mental illness, and cultural dynamics. The same authors also mention that the interaction between expressed emotion and patient outcomes is complex, so it is best measured by a person from the same cultural group because that person is familiar with the nuances of language and cultural expression to rate any of the components of EE.

Implications and areas of study

A high EE has proven to be an important predictor of relapse in different pathologies (schizophrenia, depression, bipolar disease, borderline personality, eating disorders, dementia, epilepsy, behavior disorders, alcoholism, anxiety disorders, diabetes mellitus, abdominal pain, post-traumatic distress, asthma, rheumatoid arthritis), although, according to Hooley and Gotlib (2000), high EE levels are usually common in long-term diseases. There was also a correlation between the individual's level of functioning and the professionals' perception of the individual's role during the disease, which is important to rate EE. Based on an analysis of the relatives' characteristics, we found differences of relationship among the families according to their EE.

Expressed emotion and suicidal behavior

Michelson and Bhugra (2012) said that it is surprising that only a few studies published have specifically considered EE and its relationship to self-harm in youth populations (Table 6.2).

Further research is needed on this issue. As we have seen, because of the wide range of tools to assess EE and different samples under analysis, it has been difficult to draw any conclusions. However, the influence of the parenting relationship in parasuicidal behaviors is considered important in all of these studies. Hence the interest in understanding the role of expressed emotion in parasuicidal behaviors. Innovative and pioneering, the study conducted in Hong Kong (Hong Kong Jockey Club Centre for Suicide Research and Prevention, 2005) adds a new area of research in a postvention situation. This study contributed to better understanding of the role played by EE in completed suicides. However, the fact that it did not use a full version of an instrument (only 16 items of EE were used) makes it impossible to draw any conclusions on the role of EE in completed suicides. Nonetheless, given its role in non-fatal suicidal behaviors, further studies are needed to analyze its importance in completed suicides.

Table 6.2 Studies assessing EE and suicidal behaviors

Authors / Date	Study	Method	Instruments to assess EE	Conclusions	Suggestions
Pollard, USA, 1996	20 adolescents who attempted suicide, plus 19 in the control group	Follow-up (0–6–12 months)	FMSS	A correlation was found between hostility and criticism as predictors of suicide attempt.	Larger sample size; Use of CFI; Use of a control group without psychopathology; assess relatives' psychopathology; assess the stability of hostility and criticism during the study.
Wedig & Nock, UK, 2007	36 adolescents with self-injurious thoughts and behaviors	Cohort study	FMSS	EE was associated with each type of SITB assessed: suicide ideation, suicide plans, suicide attempts, and nonsuicidal self-injury. Analyses also revealed that one specific component of EE (parental criticism) was strongly associated with SITB, whereas the other (emotional overinvolvement) was not and that the relationship between EE and SITB was not explained by the presence of mental disorders. Finally, a moderation model was supported in which the relationship between parental criticism and SITB was especially strong among adolescents with a self-critical cognitive style.	Future work should examine whether treatments that aim to lower criticism in the family and/or adolescent decrease such criticism and ultimately whether they also decrease the likelihood of self-injurious thoughts and behaviors.

Hong Kong Jockey Club Centre for Suicide Research and Prevention, 2005	150 suicides among 15–19 years and 150 control group	Psychological autopsy. The interviews were carried out on average 7.4 months after the suicide	LEE. 16 items to measure the informants' perception about the intrusiveness, emotional response, attitude towards the subjects and tolerance or expectations on the subjects by their influential family members at home	Compared to the live controls in the general population, those who committed suicide were more likely to be single, less educated, unemployed or underemployed, indebted, had experienced physical abuse at home (either as the recipient or the perpetrator), earned less monthly income, lived alone, had experienced negative expressed emotions at home.	Strategic interventions in Hong Kong should be adopted with public health approach which emphasizes both raising public awareness of psychiatric illnesses (depression in particular); providing timely, accessible, and individualized follow up services for attempters; developing extensive networks and social support for the unemployed and people who are in debt; and educating the public on the importance of integrated familial and interpersonal support for healthy mental well-being.

The Santos (2007) study: method and ethics

Our study was approved by the ethics committees of the three hospitals where we interviewed the adolescents and contacted the parents or the significant persons. The aims of the study were explained to all participants who agreed with the study. In case of under-age adolescents, parents agreed to the adolescent's inclusion in the study. Our sample was composed of 67 individuals divided into two groups. One group (N = 34) consisted of individuals (aged 15–24 years old) with parasuicidal behaviors living in the city of Coimbra (the central region of Portugal) or in the surrounding areas who had been admitted to the Emergency Room. The second group (N = 33) was a control group with individuals with no parasuicidal behaviors but with similar characteristics (age, gender, and residence) to the first group.

Measurement instruments

The adapted version of the Interview for Suicidal Behavior Assessment (EACOS) is a measurement tool created by and used at the Coimbra University Hospital's Suicide Research and Prevention Unit. Thirty-three items were selected following the objectives mentioned above, and taking into account social-demographic characteristics, family interaction, personal background, circumstantial factors, and suicidal behavior:

- The Clinical Self-Concept Inventory (ICAC) is a 20-question self-report inventory aimed to measure self-concept (Vaz-Serra, 1986).
- The Problem-Solving Inventory (IRP) is a self-report inventory aimed at evaluating coping strategies (Vaz-Serra, 1988).
- The Clinical Depression Assessment Inventory (IACLIDE) is a self-report inventory aimed at measuring the intensity of the frame of reference in clinically depressed patients (Vaz-Serra, 1994).
- The IPC is a self-report inventory aimed at measuring the locus of control (Levenson, 1972; Relvas, Vaz-Serra, Saraiva, & Coelho, 1984).
- The SSQ6 is a self-report inventory aimed at measuring social support (Sarason, Sarason, Shearin, & Pierce, 1987; Pinheiro & Ferreira, 2002).
- The Camberwell Family Interview (CFI) was used to measure EE.

Results and discussion

The mean age of parasuicides was 19.31 (SD = 2.97), most of them were female (82.3%), and single (91.7%). Students represented 60% of the sample, and 31.4% of these were enrolled in higher education. The control group had similar characteristics of age, gender, and residence, with no statistically significant differences. Most (77.1%) parasuicides mentioned affective problems (mainly marital or family conflicts/quarrels) but did not have financial difficulties (82.9%). The majority did not mention the grieving process (82.9%), denying cases of suicide of friends (74.3%), in the family (68.6%) or in the community (68.6%). Most parasuicidal patients had attempted suicide only once (54.3%) and indicated an affective conflict as the reason for the suicide attempt (77.1%). The most common method to commit suicide was drug intoxication (88.6%). This parasuicidal behavior did not occur on any specific day of the week but took place more often between 4 p.m. and 12 p.m. (48.6%).

In this sample, individuals with parasuicidal behaviors had a higher number of depressive symptoms, higher difficulties in problem solving, mostly external locus of control, higher levels of neurotic personality, a smaller social support network, and a lower self-concept than the control group. Hence this profile of the parasuicidal patient coincides with those outlined by Sampaio (1994), Saraiva (1999; 2006) and Santos (2007) for the Portuguese population, as well as other authors such as Webb (2002), Beautrais (2003), and Fox and Hawton (2004).

In terms of expressed emotion and in relation to reference people, parents are mentioned more often, although there were also other relatives and friends mentioned by parasuicides. Most interviews were conducted at the homes of the parasuicides. The context of these interviews was very important to better understand the parasuicides' daily environment and to get away from the "power relation" specific to hospital settings. The average interview length in our study was about 50 minutes.

These interviews showed that most family environments had a high EE. The factor EOI was found more often, followed by critical comments and hostility. A high EOI was common among the mothers, which can be explained by a higher proximity and a higher level of control of the mothers compared to the fathers.

A high EE (73.5%) was found in relatives of parasuicides, whereas in the control group, it was only 6.1%. The dimensions which account for a high EE in this sample were emotional over-involvement (23), critical comments (18), and hostility (7). In some situations, more than one dimension was high. In the control group, all the dimensions were significantly different, with the exception of positive remarks. This situation is explained by the over-protective type of mother, which was mentioned in most interviews, and by the authoritarian type of father. These three scales are usually co-predictors of a relapse. The high levels of EE found do not support in Pollard's (1996) and Wedig and Nock's (2007) conclusions. In their studies they found only a small percentage, 33% and 25%, respectively, of relatives with high EE. These differences may be explained by the use of FMSS by these authors, which is less sensitive in detecting a high EE than the CFI (Van Humbeeck et al., 2002; Vaughn, 2003a; Hooley & Holly, 2006). Moreover, Pollard (1996) did not measure EOI.

The scores in the "protection" scales (warmth and positive remarks) were lower than in the control group, which contradicts the perception of parasuicides who mentioned having a good relationship. We can speculate about the individuals' expectations concerning a good family relationship, or assume they answered according to socially desirable behaviors. Emotional over-involvement was mainly translated into excessive self-sacrifice and becoming over-emotional during the interview (Table 6.3). Critical comments (CC) (Table 6.4) and hostility (H) (Table 6.5) were related to personal characteristics, general behavior or parasuicidal behavior.

At the 9-month evaluation, the sample registered a slight decrease in high EE (70.6%), while the level in the control group remained 6.1%. Once again, EOI was the dimension with highest scores, but significant differences were registered in all dimensions, with the exception of H.

In order to understand EE stability over the 9-month period, we compared the scores obtained at the beginning of the study and those obtained at the 9-month evaluation period. In relation to EE stability, we verified that, even if the majority of the interviewees had a high EE, all dimensions decreased with significant differences at the 9-month evaluation period, with the exception of H and warmth. Nevertheless, this decrease was not enough to be considered a low EE. The situation remained the same 9 months after the crisis that had influenced the parasuicidal behavior. Families made no structural changes in their involvement. Most families did not understand parasuicidal behavior as a "cry for help" but as a sign of bad behavior which needed to be controlled and punished.

Eight individuals repeated parasuicide during these 9 months. Seven individuals came from families with high EE and one came from a family with low EE. The number of individuals with repeated parasuicidal behavior and whose family environment had a high EE is significantly higher

Table 6.3 Examples of EOI of families in which adolescents had recurrent parasuicidal behaviors

Type	EOI
Over-identification	She's exactly like me, she's as nervous as I was (AMM01) She eats very little, but I was also like this . . . I'm sad and she's sad too, if I'm sad she's also sad (AMT05) I never thought this could happen to me (child's parasuicidal behavior), I wish this had never happened to me (AMM36)
Over-protection	Every day I take her to school and then I pick her up, sometimes it is very cold and late (she studies at night), it is very painful, you can't imagine what I do (AMI19) At home I cook different types of dishes to please her, she likes the food in a certain way and I do it for her to eat (AMM26) I need to solve all my son's problems here (at home), in the city, with his friends (AMM28 He gave me money and I take care of everything for my son, it is always like this, I do everything (AMM36)
Dramatization	It's a desperate situation, I can't communicate with her, I'm helpless . . . when she cries I feel sad, powerless, desperate (AMP01)
Exaggerated emotional response	I panicked, I could no longer press my cellphone buttons (AMC03) I can't talk about it (parasuicidal behavior), I ask people not to talk about it . . . I don't even want to think it really happened (AMM36)
Assertions of attitude	I'm everything for S. . . . she lives for me and I live for her (AMT05) I feel desperate, scared, unsafe . . . it's horrible . . . that's the right word, sometimes I want to run away, I'm afraid I won't do things well, afraid to fail even more, because I should have soon realized that J. was like this, that this could happen (parasuicidal behavior) [...[I'm tormented, it's hard to explain, it's very hard to endure because I suffer a lot (AMM08) I can't live without him and he can't live without me . . . I'm everything to him (AMM28) He doesn't help me do anything, anything, but I am the one to blame because I didn't raise him right (AMM36)
Excessive self-sacrifice	I'm getting to like her more and more, if she tells me to stop talking to someone, I stop talking with that person from the moment she tells me so . . . when I argue with her, she beats me but I've never beaten her (AMT05) I often give him things that I need, I often give him everything I earned in the whole day (AMM28) I make everything I can not to get into his nerves, everything has to be as he pleases, as he wants, as he thinks and that's it, it must be that way . . . I can't say anything . . . I let him do what he wants, even if it's very hard for me (AMM36)
Intrusiveness	I call her many times a day to see if everything is ok, whom she's with . . . I don't know what else to do, I'm always checking up on her, I often stop by the school with my husband just to see where she is [...] I call her friends . . . I let her fall asleep and then I check her bag to see if I can find anything, letters, cigarettes . . . (AMM26) I slept in his room and then he slept in mine . . . he didn't want it but this way I felt more tranquil (AMM36)

Table 6.4 Examples of CC of families in which adolescents had recurrent parasuicidal behaviors

Type	CC
Regarding personal characteristics	She lies a lot, because she wants to create a certain image and so she lies . . . she is always lying . . . she is a liar (AMM01; AMM19)
	She is very irritable, very unstable, very tearful . . . she is still a child (AMP01)
	She feels like everything and everyone is against her, that we are only here to bother her, it is not even good to talk about it because it's hard . . . she always plays the victim (AMI19)
	with this behavior, we've been going through hell with her (AMM19)
	He calls me names and I don't tolerate it, and he is a pig, he doesn't want to shower (AMM28)
	He is aggressive, he kicks me, he yells at me, I can't stand him (AMM28)
	He is a quitter, he backs out of everything (AMI34)
Regarding parasuicidal behavior	She began to interiorize it and then did this foolish thing (parasuicidal behavior) (AMP01)
	She could have had more control over her disease (parasuicidal behavior) (AMM05; AMM08; AMM26; AMP36)
	I never thought she would do this (parasuicidal behavior), she had no reasons to do it (AMM11)
	She does it (parasuicidal behavior) but she doesn't even think about it, because the poison must taste bad (AMI34)
	Such a thing (parasuicidal behavior) is not for a boy like him to do . . . I don't know why he did such a foolish thing (AMM36)
Regarding general behavior	One moment she is affectionate, and then she starts screaming and yelling . . . at everyone (AMP01)
	Sometimes she makes stupid comments and then I lose control . . . I scream . . . I get angry (AMP01)
	She stays up late and then she is all sleepy, but it's what she wants, she isn't in her right mind (AMP01)
	She was very aggressive, especially to me, and I felt desperate . . . she's been trying me (AMM08)
	The music is always so loud . . . there's no peace and quiet (AMM08)
	She does nothing other than being in bed. She can spend all day in bed, even in sunny days . . . always in bed . . . always in bed (AMM19)
	She is rude, disobedient (AMM19)
	With this behavior, we've been going through hell with her (AMM19)
	She does nothing . . . nothing, she doesn't want to do anything (AMM19)
	She only says silly or stupid things (AMI19)
	She puts on her pajama and goes to bed, and after 10 minutes, she already wants to go out in the streets, she is very unstable (AMM28)
	When he is irritated it is very difficult, things have to be done his own way (AMP36)

Table 6.5 Examples of H of families in which adolescents had recurrent parasuicidal behaviors

Type	Examples
Rejection	I have even hated my daughter . . . I couldn't even see her. . . she wouldn't collaborate (AMP09)
	Will I have to live all my life with my daughter despising me? (AMM09)
	I told her, from now on I will pretend you're not at home . . . because she says she hates me (AMM10)
Generalization	She seems to do that on purpose for me to hurt her. Everything that is bad for her, she has a tendency for that, to mess with my head (AMI30)

than the individuals whose family environment had a low EE. EE did not decrease during this period.

The eight cases of repeated parasuicidal behaviors used the same methods that had been previously used (six cases of drug intoxication, one by household chemicals and one by phlebotomy). Patients with recurrent behaviors were being followed by a psychiatrist, but none of them had a history of family intervention.

Clinical implications

This study underlined the need to evaluate the familiar environment to better understand suicidal behaviors. EE proved to be a good concept to characterize, understand and evaluate the familiar climate and also to identify the needs of the families who require intervention. Based on this research, we can develop a familiar intervention program to prevent recurrent suicidal behaviors through psycho-education interventions on mental health, adolescence and suicidal behaviors. In the program, it is important to deal with parents' feelings of guilt, shame and insecurity and also improve family communication strategies and problem-solving strategies. This study reinforced the role played by the family in suicidal behaviors and promoted the systemic approach.

Research implications

Further research should be carried out in a well-controlled prospective study, and should use the CFI because it is more sensitive and comprehensive in detecting EE. A larger sample should be used and EE should be assessed in other regions to increase knowledge in this field. Another step ahead is to test models of family intervention to reduce EE.

Conclusion

A high EE emerges as an important family factor for parasuicidal behavior, and, therefore, we would like to draw attention to this fact due to its impact on dealing with the families of parasuicides. The EE of parasuicides' relatives is mainly characterized by EOI (marked by feelings of excessive self-sacrifice and assertions of attitude), followed by criticism and hostility. EE is considered a predictor of repeated parasuicidal behaviors. Seven out of eight individuals with repeated parasuicidal behaviors had a family environment with high EE. Overall, EE remained stable during the 9-month period, decreasing in dimensions after the parasuicidal behavior (though still remaining high).

Acknowledgements

The author wishes to acknowledge the cooperation of the research team which supervised the research in this chapter: Carlos Saraiva, Professor of Psychiatry at the University of Coimbra and Coimbra University Hospital, and Liliana de Sousa, Professor at the Abel Salazar Institute for Biomedical Sciences (ICBAS), Oporto University.

Thanks also to the Taylor & Francis Group, for allowing us to reproduce parts of a paper published in *Archives of Suicide Research*, "The role of Expressed Emotion, Self-concept, coping, and depression in parasuicidal behavior: A follow-up study" (Santos et al., 2009).

References

Baker, B., Helmes, E., & Kazarian, S. (1984). Past and present perceived attitudes of schizophrenics in relation to rehospitalization, *British Journal of Psychiatry, 144*, 263–269.

Beautrais, A. (2003). Life course factors associated with suicidal behaviors in young people. *American Behavioral Scientist, 46*(9): 1137–1156.

Bebbington, P., & Kuipers, E. (1994). The predictive utility of Expressed Emotion in schizophrenia: An aggregate analysis. *Psychological Medicine, 24*, 707–718.

Bhugra, D., & Mckenzie, K. (2003). Expressed Emotion across cultures. *Advances in Psychiatric Treatment, 9*, 342–348.

Brown, G. (1958). Experiences of discharged chronic schizophrenic mental hospital patients in various types of living groups. *Millbank Memorial Fund Quarterly, 37*, 105–131.

Brown, G., Birley, J., & Wing, J. (1972). Influence of family life on the course of schizophrenic disorders: A replication. *British Journal of Psychiatry, 121*, 241–258.

Brown, G., Carstairs, G., & Topping, G. (1958). Post hospital adjustment of chronic patients. *The Lancet*, 685–689.

Brown, G., Monck, E., Carstairs, G., & Wing, J. (1962). Influence of family life on the course of schizophrenic illness, *British Journal of Preventive Social Medicine, 16*, 55–68.

Brown, G., & Rutter, M. (1966). The measurement of family activities and relationships: A methodological study. *Human Relations, 19*(3), 241–263.

Butzlaff, R., & Hooley, J. (1998). Expressed emotion and psychiatric relapse. *Archives General of Psychiatry, 55*, 547–552.

Cole, J., & Kazarian, S. (1988). The level of expressed emotion scale: A new measure of expressed emotion. *Journal of Clinical Psychology, 44*(3), 392–397.

Cutcliffe, J., & Santos, J. (2012). *Suicide and self-harm: an evidence-informed approach*. London: Quay Books.

Docherty, N., Serper, M., & Harvey, P. (1990). Development and preliminary validation of a questionnaire assessment of expressed emotion. *Psychological Reports, 67*, 565–578.

Fox, C., & Hawton, K. (2004). *Deliberate self-harm in adolescence*. London: Jessica Kingsley.

Gottschalk, L., & Gleser, C. (1969). *The measurement of psychological states through analysis of verbal behavior*. Berkeley: University of California Press.

Hong Kong Jockey Club Centre for Suicide Research and Prevention (2005). *The Psychological Autopsy Study of Suicides in Hong Kong*. Hong Kong: Hong Kong Jockey Club Centre for Suicide Research and Prevention, The University of Hong Kong.

Hooley, J., & Gotlib, I. (2000). A diathesis-stress conceptualization of expressed emotion and clinical outcome. *Applied & Preventive Psychology, 9*, 135–151.

Hooley, J., & Holly A. (2006). Measuring expressed emotion: An evaluation of the shortcuts. *Journal of Family Psychology, 20*(3), 386–396.

Hooley, J., & Teadsle, J. (1989). Predictors of relapse in unipolar depressives: Expressed emotion, marital distress, and perceived criticism. *Journal of Abnormal Psychology, 98*(3), 229–235.

Kavanagh, D., O'Halloran, P., Manicavasagar, V., Clark, D., Piatkowska, O., Tennant, C., & Rosen, A. (1997). The Family Attitude Scale: Reliability and validity of a new scale for measuring the emotional climate of families. *Psychiatry Research, 70*, 185–195.

Kreisman, D., Simmens, S., & Joy, D. (1979). Rejecting the patient: Preliminary validation of a self-report scale. *Schizophrenia Bulletin, 5*(2), 220–222.

Kuipers, L. (1992). Expressed Emotion research in Europe. *British Journal of Clinical Psychology, 31*, 429–443.

Kuipers, L. (1994). The measurement of expressed emotion: Its influence on research and clinical practice. *International Review of Psychiatry, 6,* 187–199.

Leff, J., & Vaughn, C. (1985). *Expressed emotion in families.* New York: Guilford Press.

Levenson, H. (1972). Distinctions within the concept of internal-external control: Development. *Proceedings of the Annual Convention of the American Psychological Association, 10,* 261–262.

Magana, A., Goldstein, M., Karno, M., Miklowitz, J., & Falloon, I. (1985). A brief method for assessing expressed emotion in relatives of psychiatric patients. *Psychiatry Research, 17,* 203–212.

Michelson, D., & Bhugra, D. (2012). Family environment, expressed emotion and adolescent self-harm: A review of conceptual, empirical, cross-cultural and clinical perspectives. *International Review of Psychiatry, 24*(2): 106–114.

Pinheiro, M., & Ferreira, J. (2002). O Questionário de Suporte Social: Adaptação e validação da versão portuguesa do Social Support Questionnaire (SSQ6). *Psychologica, 30,* 315–333.

Pollard, C. (1996). Attempted adolescent suicide and expressed emotion. PhD dissertation, The Catholic University of America, Washington, DC.

Relvas, J., Vaz-Serra, A., Saraiva, C., & Coelho, I. (1984). Resultados da aplicação da Escala IPC (Internal, Powerful and Others) de Levenson a estudantes universitários. *Psiquiatria Clínica, 5*(3), 119–124.

Rutter, M., & Brown, G. (1966). The reliability and validity of measures of family life and relationships in families containing a psychiatric patient. *Social Psychiatry, 1*(1), 38– 53.

Sampaio, D. (1994). *Ninguém morre sozinho. Os adolescentes e o suicídio* (5th ed.). Lisbon: Caminho.

Santos, J. (2000). O para-suicídio no Concelho de Coimbra: Contributos para o seu estudo. *Revista Sinais Vitais, 28,* 15–19.

Santos, J. (2007). *Para-suicídio, o que dizem as famílias. A Emoção Expressa.* Coimbra: Formasau.

Santos, J., Saraiva, C., & Sousa, L.(2009). The role of Expressed Emotion, Self-concept, coping, and depression in parasuicidal behaviour: A follow-up study. *Archives of Suicide Research, 13,* 358–367.

Saraiva, C. (1999). *Para-suicídio. Contributos para uma compreensão clínica dos comportamentos para-suicidários recorrentes.* Coimbra: Quarteto Editora.

Saraiva, C. (2006). *Estudos sobre o para-suicídio. O que leva os jovens a espreitar a morte.* Coimbra: Redhorse.

Sarason, I. G., Sarason, B. R., Shearin, E. N., & Pierce, G. R. (1987). A brief measure of social support: Practical and theoretical implications. *Journal of Social and Personal Relationships, 4,* 497–510.

Shields, C., Franks, P., Harp, J., McDaniel, S., & Campbell, T. (1992). Development of the Family Emotional Involvement and Criticism Scale (FEICS): A self-report scale to measure expressed emotion. *Journal of Marital and Family Therapy, 18* (4): 395–407.

Van Humbeeck, G., Van Audenhove, C., De Hert, M., Pieters, G., & Storms, G. (2002). Expressed emotion: A review of assessment instruments. *Clinical Psychology Review, 22*(3), 321–341.

Van Humbeeck, G., Van Audenhove, C., Pieters, G., Storms, G., Vertommen, H., Peuskens, J., & Heyrman, J. (2004). Expressed Emotion in the client-professional caregiver dyad: A comparison of three expressed emotion instruments. *European Journal of Psychological Assessment, 20*(4), 237–246.

Vaughn, C. (2003a). What became a EE? Apresentado numa reunião de homenagem a Julian Leff. Unpublished paper, Institute of Psychiatry, London.

Vaughn, C. (2003b). Apontamentos fornecidos no decorrer do Expressed Emotion Course (unpublished).

Vaughan, C., & Leff, J. (1976a). The influence of family and social factors on the course of psychiatric illness. A comparison of schizophrenic and depressed neurotic patients. *British Journal of Psychiatry, 129,* 125–137.

Vaughn, C., & Leff, J. (1976b). The measurement of expressed emotion in the families of psychiatric patients. *British Journal of Social and Clinical Psychology, 15*(2), 157–165.

Vaz-Serra, A. (1986). O inventário clínico de auto-conceito. *Psiquiatria Clínica, 7* (2), 67–84.

Vaz-Serra, A. (1988). Um estudo sobre coping: O Inventário de Resolução de Problemas. *Psiquiatria Clínica, 9*(4), 303–315.

Vaz-Serra, A. (1994). *IACLIDE, Inventário de Avaliação Clinica da Depressão* (1st ed.). Lisbon: Edição Psiquiatria Clínica.

Vaz-Serra, A., Ponciano, E., & Freitas, F. (1980). Resultados da aplicação do EPI Eysenck Personality Inventory a uma amostra da população portuguesa. *Psiquiatria Clínica, 1*(2), 127–132.

Wearden, A, Tarrier, N., Barrowclough, C., Zastowny, T., & Rahill, A. (2000). A review of expressed emotion research in health care. *Clinical Psychology Review, 20*(5), 633–666.

Webb, C. (2002). Deliberate self-harm in adolescence: A systematic review of psychological and psychosocial factors. *Journal of Advanced Nursing, 38*(3): 235–244.

Wedig, M., & Nock, M. (2007). Parental expressed emotion and adolescent self-injury. *Journal of Academic Child Adolescence Psychiatry, 46*(9): 1171–1178.

EDITORIAL COMMENTARY

Each of the chapters in Part I – on their own – makes a substantive and valuable contribution to the extant literature. P/MH nurses and other associated mental health professionals are greatly in need of contemporary evidence, particularly evidence that helps guide their practice day-by-day, hour-by-hour and minute-by-minute (Cutcliffe & Santos, 2012). As valuable as these contributions are individually, when they are examined for themes, commonalities or shared, congruent findings and implications, then arguably their significance becomes more clear. Accordingly, the editors of this section will focus on a number of such themes, namely:

1 Moving practice forward: the key roles of psychiatric and mental health nurses in care of suicidal people 1. – talking as the centre piece.
2 Moving education forward: specialized training for caregivers to suicidal people.

Moving practice forward

Despite the aforementioned long history of P/MH nurses working with suicidal people, an honest appraisal of the 'state of the science' indicates that the P/MH nursing care of the suicidal person is not an area of care that can claim to be grounded on an abundance of empirical literature, thus, as a result, P/MH nurses have to 'feel their way in the dark' so to speak (Cutcliffe & Stevenson, 2008). However, as the findings in four of the five chapters in Part I indicate, there is an emerging body of evidence which highlights what suicidal people want/need and find helpful from their P/MH nurses; that is: practice that is an interpersonal endeavour – concerned with fostering engagement, connectivity and increased hopefulness; one personified by talking and listening; one that eschews defensive, custodial and containment-orientated interventions, It is important to note that these findings echo the views (and findings) of the founder of suicidology as a discrete area of science and clinical practice: Professor Ed Shneidman. And while much of contemporary care for suicidal people can be described as moving away from this interpersonal, engagement-driven focus, for P/MH nurses who wish to practise in this way, there is great reassurance in knowing that such emphasis was the original founding focus of suicidology. Shneidman eloquently captures the essence of this message when he states:

> There is a basic rule to keep in mind: We can reduce the lethality if we lessen the anguish, the perturbation. Suicidal individuals who are asked, "Where do you hurt?"

intuitively know that this is a question about their emotions and their lives, and they answer appropriately, not in biological terms but with some literary or humanistic sophistication, in psychological terms. What I mean by this is to ask about the person's feelings, worries and pain.

(1997, p. 29)

This view is supported by Maris, Berman and Silverman, who state:

As important as the biological treatment of hopelessness is, any treatment of a suicidal patient that relies solely on impersonal therapies (e.g. psychoactive medication, seclusion, restraint, and 15 minute checks (observations) may be second rate . . . Many psychiatrists argue that the heart of the treatment of suicidal individuals is the relationship of the therapists and the patient.

(2000, p. 13)

Accordingly, we encourage other P/MH suicidologists to pursue this area of research and add to the accumulating body of evidence that focuses on these ways of working with suicidal people, secure in the knowledge that in so doing, they would be 'standing on the shoulders' of suicidology pioneers and luminaries.

Alongside the need to move towards and embrace an 'engagement'-focused approach to care of the suicidal person, is the corresponding need for mental health care of the suicidal person to move away from defensive, surveillance and containment-orientated practices, which are perhaps best epitomized by the over-zealous use of close observations (Cutcliffe & Santos, 2012). In our earlier and recent publication (see Cutcliffe & Santos, 2012), we included a review of the extant literature pertaining to close observations and the key findings that emerge from this literature review are:

1 The evidence pertaining to the effectiveness of close observations as a means of providing safe and therapeutic care to suicidal people is equivocal. The scientific and clinical community really does not know if placing people under observation reduces suicidality or makes them feel less suicidal. *We do know that placing people under observation does not guarantee their physical safety.*
2 Unfortunately, major ethical and methodological problems are associated with undertaking the studies that would help to answer these questions.
3 The findings pertaining to the experience of being observed are equivocal, with data showing that clients experience observations as non-therapeutic, though some data do show the opposite.
4 Some tentative evidence suggests that the client's experience of being observed, and the associated therapeutic value of close observations, depend upon who performs them.
5 Some tentative evidence suggests that the client's experience of being observed, and the associated therapeutic value of close observations, depend upon both the collective unit and the individual practitioner's views and attitudes toward close observations.
6 Some tentative evidence suggests that it may *be certain micro-skills or micro-interventions that appear related to the therapeutic effectiveness of close observations rather than the experience of being observed per se.*
7 *Inversely, some evidence suggests that certain ways of enacting close observations are experienced as non-therapeutic and may exacerbate suicidality.*

8   The innovative use of mixed methods will provide a more comprehensive and translational understanding of the usefulness of, and alternatives to, close observation in treating suicidal individuals.

Moving education forward

Despite the long history of P/MH nurses caring for (and with) suicidal people, only sparse attention and time have been dedicated to suicide in nursing curricula. For generic nursing programmes, where mental health issues have to 'compete' with more popular nursing content (such as adult medical-surgical nursing; child and mother nursing; midwifery), suicide-focused curriculum content is even less evident. Where content is included, common elements include: an introduction to the principal theories of suicide; perhaps some material on risk and risk assessment and – if the curriculum is 'progressive', an introduction to some suicide risk-assessment instruments (Cutcliffe & Stevenson, 2007). Reference to treatment, much to the chagrin of the editors – if it is included at all – usually focuses on pharmacology and containment measures (see above).

Given the space restrictions in such curriculum and nursing programmes, it is likely that judicious and thoughtful choices will have to be made about which suicide-focused educational elements are the most important to include, such as: listening, communication skills to convey empathy, engagement skills, personal awareness raising, and the beginnings of the development of the required 'humanistic' qualities.

So, while even a cursory increase in suicide-focused material in nursing curricula would be most welcome, the authors would advance the argument that this may still be insufficient to produce nurses who are confident and skilled when faced with working with suicidal people. It may well be that additional specialist, and/or post-graduate, advanced education and training is required for those nurses who wish to focus on or specialize with working with suicidal people (Cutcliffe & Stevenson, 2007). Just as one would not expect newly graduated nurses to take on a caseload of people requiring specialist psychotherapy, the editors suggest it would be clinically prudent not to expect newly graduated nurses to take on a caseload 'heavy' with highly suicidal people. This appears to be particularly logical and sensible, given the previously mentioned complexity of suicide and the emotional requirements such clients demand of their nurses (Cutcliffe & Stevenson, 2007). In the light of these foci, one might conclude that the current preparation of nurses to work with suicidal people is deficient in providing them with the skills, attitudes and knowledge necessary for delivering adequate, therapeutic, transformative care for suicidal people (see Cutcliffe & Stevenson, 2007). Hence, there is a clear need to provide additional education/training to address this matter. As a result, we propose the following outline for a post-graduate course/module in caring for suicidal people (Box I.1).

Box I.1 Minimum educational components to be included in a post-basic programme in equipping nurses to provide effective, meaningful caring responses to suicidal people

- self-awareness training – specifically dealing with one's own mortality;
- cognitive re-framing techniques and skills;
- experiential work around being comfortable with stillness;

- monitoring one's self – particularly one's own level of hope;
- experiential work around hearing about death, dying and suicide;
- techniques and qualities associated with inspiring hope;
- techniques and qualities associated with presencing;
- listening (without prejudice or discomfort);
- recognizing limiting personal constructs, cognitive distortions (such as catastrophizing, over-generalizing, selective abstraction, arbitrary interference, magnification and minimizing, emotional reasoning, use of 'shoulds and oughts'; labelling and mislabelling, for instance, the use of gentle, implicit challenges;
- giving and receiving clinical supervision;
- a basic understanding of and ability to detect transference and counter-transference;
- familiarity with and comfort using empathy-promoting interpersonal techniques: simple reflection, selective reflection, empathic building, paraphrasing, summarizing, clarifying, open questions, closed questions, appropriate self-disclosure;
- creating a calming, peaceful external (physical) environment;
- experiential work on becoming comfortable with not having erudite answers;
- interventions and attitudes to build trust;
- interventions geared to explore and facilitate understanding of the meanings attached to the suicidal act (e.g., catalytic interventions, empathic building, selective reflection);
- role modelling and the use of simulators.

References

Cutcliffe, J. R., & Stevenson, C. (2007). *Care of the suicidal person*. Edinburgh: Churchill Livingstone/Elsevier.

Cutcliffe. J. R., & Stevenson, C. (2008). Feeling our way in the dark: The psychiatric nursing care of suicidal people. *International Journal of Nursing Studies 45*, 942–953.

Cutcliffe, J. R., & Santos, J. C. (2012). *Suicide and self-harm: An evidence-based approach*. London: Quay Books.

Maris, R. W., Berman, A. L., & Silverman, M. M. (2000). *Comprehensive textbook of suicidology*. New York: Guilford Press.

Shneidman, E. S. (1997). The suicidal mind . In R. W. Maris, M. M. Silverman, & S. S. Canetto. (Eds.), *Review of suicidology* (pp. 22–41). New York: Guilford Press.

Shneidman, E. S. (2001). *Comprehending suicide: Landmarks in 20th-century suicidology*. Washington, DC: American Psychological Association.

PART II

Psychiatry

EDITORIAL INTRODUCTION

Moving beyond diagnosis: Expanding the psychiatrist's role in suicide prevention

In Part II, we will provide five unique chapters that highlight the depth and breadth of psychiatric research in suicide prevention. These five chapters illustrate the contribution psychiatrists can make in understanding the biological, psychological, social and cultural factors that shape suicidal behaviour. They also emphasize the importance of multi-disciplinary approaches and the roles psychiatrists can play in the development and evaluation of suicide prevention strategies and shaping of health policy.

Brandon Pierre and Vincenzo De Luca's Chapter 7 on genetics and suicide speaks to the psychiatrist's role as a clinician-scientist, using cutting-edge expertise in biologically based research to better understand who is at risk for suicide and to guide interventions targeting the illnesses that are risk factors for suicide.

Chapter 8 by Mark Sinyor, Ayal Schaffer and Amy Cheung reviews means restriction as a strategy for suicide prevention and illustrates the contribution psychiatrists can make in shaping policies to prevent suicide. These policies can include advocating for barriers for bridges and public transportation as well as safer prescribing practices to prevent overdose. Sinyor, Schaffer and Cheung stress the importance of evidence-based approaches to evaluate the efficacy of these strategies and describe two innovative studies whose findings can guide future research and inform policy decisions.

Chapter 9 by Kwame McKenzie, Andrew Tuck and Samanthika Ekanayake adds another important layer by highlighting the need to address cultural and ethnic diversity in suicide prevention. Although suicide prevention strategies address mental illness and means restriction, factors discussed in Chapters 7 and 8, suicide must also be viewed through a cultural lens. By discussing epidemiological data on suicide in the Southeast Asian population in the United Kingdom, they make a persuasive case for addressing the needs of diverse populations in a Canadian suicide prevention strategy.

Chapter 10 by Juveria Zaheer, Paul Links, Samuel Law, Wes Shera, Tat Tsang, Catherine Cheng, Alan Fung and Pozi Liu builds on McKenzie et al.'s work to discuss the role of culture and gender in understanding suicide with a focus on Chinese women and women of Chinese descent living in North America. This chapter discusses the benefits of qualitative and cross-cultural approaches in suicide prevention by describing a novel study aimed at better understanding the experiences of these women in order to develop culturally appropriate suicide prevention strategies.

Finally, Paul Links, Juveria Zaheer, Rahel Eynan and Amresh Srivastava tie the threads of the previous chapters in Part II together by describing a model for rural suicide prevention as it applies to Canada and India. The model incorporates the identification and management of mental illness, means restriction, culturally appropriate interventions and rigorous mixed methods procedures to evaluate the interventions. They also underscore the benefits of collaborating across international boundaries. These benefits include the clarification of the impact of culture as a causal factor for suicide, improved understanding of other cultures as well as our own with respect to needs, strengths and challenges related to suicide prevention, and addressing the needs of minority groups, including Indian-born Canadians and Canadians of Indian descent.

7

GENETICS OF THE SEROTONERGIC SYSTEM AND IMPLICATIONS FOR SUICIDE RESEARCH

Brandon Pierre and Vincenzo De Luca

Introduction

Over the past 45 years, suicide rates have increased by 60% worldwide with a global mortality rate of one death every 40 seconds (WHO, 2012). Identified risk factors include comorbid psychiatric illness, impulsive behaviour and aggression, substance abuse, and stress; however, the exact aetiology of suicidal behaviour remains unclear.

While suicide is generally understood to be an amalgamation of complex social, psychological, and biological interactions, genetics research may elucidate the underlying biological mechanisms of suicidality. Preliminary evidence from twin and adoption studies suggests a genetic basis of suicidal behaviour. Monozygotic (MZ) twins have a higher suicide concordance rate than dizygotic (DZ) twins (Roy, Rylander, & Sarchiapone, 1997). Furthermore, when one twin commits suicide, a living MZ co-twin has a higher suicide concordance rate than a DZ co-twin (MZ: 18.45% > DZ: 0.68%; Roy & Segal, 2001). Adoption studies further substantiate a genetic component of suicide while seemingly ruling out environmental factors (Von Borczyskowski, Lindblad, Vinnerljung, Reintjes, & Hjern, 2011).

Anomalies in the dopaminergic, noradrenergic, and serotonergic systems may increase vulnerability to suicidal behaviour; however, the serotonin (5HT) system is of particular interest due to its role in mood regulation. Suicide victims have low cerebrospinal (CSF) concentrations of 5-HT metabolite 5-hydroxyindoleacetic acid (5-HIAA), an indicator of 5-HT metabolism in the cerebral cortex (Åsberg, 1997). Moreover, low CSF 5-HIAA may indicate trait-impulsivity and aggression (Higley & Linnoila, 1997), may be hereditary (Rogers et al., 2004), and may signal suicide risk (Mann et al., 2006). A better understanding of the genetics of the 5-HT system may, therefore, deepen our knowledge of the suicide phenotype (i.e., ideation, attempt, and completion).

This chapter will review the genetic studies on the role of the serotonergic system in the pathophysiology of suicidal behaviour with an overview of their implications for clinical suicide research. Candidate gene studies investigate genetic variants and their association with suicidal behaviour. Current suicide research involving the 5-HT system examines single nucleotide polymorphisms (SNPs) in genes that encode proteins involved in 5-HT synthesis, binding, and reuptake. Given the complexity of neurobiology, no unique gene should be held wholly responsible for creating a 5-HT diathesis to suicidality. The continuum of suicidal behaviours remains the consequence of complex social, psychological, and biological interactions and thus a comprehensive stress–diathesis model is proposed.

The proposed stress–diathesis model incorporates various genetic and environmental risk correlates for suicidal behaviour to create a unified theory of suicidal pathogenesis. First, genetic factors represent additive or intergenic effects modifying the 5-HT system. These genetic variants may alter 5-HT synthesis (TPH1, TPH2), receptor binding (HTR1A, HTR1B, HTR2A), and reuptake (SLC6A4). Second, environmental factors include stressors such as psychiatric diagnosis and adverse life experiences. Together, these components produce both the suicide phenotype (i.e., ideation, attempt, and completion) and intermediate endophenotypes (i.e., markers of emotional, behavioural, and cognitive dysregulation). For our purposes, intermediate endophenotypes will be discussed and assessed in relation to their genetic susceptibility.

Tryptophan hydroxylase (TPH) polymorphisms and suicidal behaviour

Dysregulation of TPH, the rate-limiting enzyme of 5-HT biosynthesis, was initially thought to increase vulnerability for suicidal behaviour. Early studies associated the A779 allele in the TPH gene, with lower CSF 5-HIAA levels (Jönsson et al., 1997), trait aggression (Rujescu et al., 2002), and deliberate self-harm (Pooley, Houston, Hawton, & Harrison, 2003).

However, TPH (now TPH1) was found to be primarily expressed in the peripheral nervous system, with minimal expression in the central nervous system (CNS), while TPH2 is expressed exclusively in the CNS (Walther et al., 2003). Hence, many studies fail to demonstrate a link between suicidal behaviour and either A779C genotypes (Bellivier, Chaste, & Malafosse, 2004) or A218C genotypes (Rujescu et al., 2002; Viana, De Marco, Boson, Romano-Silva, & Corrêa, 2006).

The highest TPH2 expression is in the brain stem, specifically the raphe nuclei, which control the release of 5-HT in the CNS. The dorsal raphe nucleus (DRN) has ascending projections to the forebrain and amygdala, which conjointly regulate limbic systems that modulate emotionally influenced behaviour (McDevitt & Neumaier, 2011). Reduced TPH2 expression in the DRN may indicate violent suicide risk in depressed patients (Gos et al., 2008). A risk TPH2 haplotype may also signal aggressive-impulsive and suicidal tendencies (Perez-Rodriguez et al., 2010).

Animal models further illustrate the functional relationship between TPH2, impulsivity, and aggression. TPH2-deficient mice demonstrate increased impulsive-aggressive behaviours (Waider, Araragi, Gutknecht, & Lesch, 2011) whereas injecting TPH2's precursor immediately attenuates these behaviours (Angoa-Pérez et al., 2012). Furthermore, adverse early life experiences may potentiate a gene–environment interaction in which individuals with increased TPH2 expression are vulnerable to stress-induced change in the 5-HT system (Hale, Shekhar, & Lowry, 2011).

To summarize, 5-HT hypofunction could be the consequence of reduced TPH2 enzyme activity due to allelic variation. The highest TPH2 expression is in the DRN, which has ascending projections to brain regions implemented in executive function and emotionally regulated behaviours. Reduced TPH2 may explain impulsive-aggressive behaviours in mice (Angoa-Pérez et al., 2012) and violent suicides in humans (Gos et al., 2008). Nonetheless, it is unlikely that single TPH2 polymorphisms are wholly responsible for suicidal behaviour. Findings from association studies, post-mortem samples, and animal models all indicate complex intergenic and gene–environment interactions.

5-HT receptor genes and suicidal behaviour

5-HT receptors are separated into seven families, modifying various biological and neurological processes such as aggression, cognition, learning, memory, and mood. Molecular studies of suicidal behaviour generally focus on genes encoding 5-HT receptor subtypes 5-HT$_{1A}$, 5-HT$_{1B}$, and 5-HT$_{2A}$ (HTR1A, HTR1B, and HTR2A, respectively).

5-HT$_{1A}$

The HTR1A gene codes proteins for 5-HT$_{1A}$ receptors that are found particularly in the septum, hippocampus, and amygdala – regions believed to control mood and stress reactivity (McDevitt & Neumaier, 2011). The raphe nucleus features somato-dendritic 5-HT$_{1A}$ autoreceptors, regulating the 5-HT system by inhibiting neural firing. 5-HT$_{1A}$ receptor dysregulation can be envisaged as two processes: reduced post-synaptic receptor binding, resulting in blunted 5-HT response (Arango et al., 2001); and over-expression of autoreceptors, reducing 5-HT neuro-transmission (Lemonde et al., 2003).

Further research indicates that these mechanisms are not mutually exclusive. The G-allele of the C1019G promoter polymorphism may alter transcription of factors that reduce the expression of 5-HT$_{1A}$ autoreceptors in the raphe nucleus (Parsey et al., 2010). 5-HT$_{1A}$ receptor dysregulation thus consists of an allelic variant inhibiting transcription factors that normally reduce the expression of 5-HT$_{1A}$ receptors. Subsequently, 5-HT$_{1A}$ autoreceptor over-expression signals the 5-HT system to reduce post-synaptic receptors, thereby decreasing 5-HT neurotransmission.

Extensive molecular genetics studies reveal the role of the HTR1A gene C1019G polymorphism in 5-HT diathesis for major depression and suicide. The G allele is twice as prevalent in major depression cases and four times as prevalent in post-mortem samples of suicide completers (Lemonde et al., 2003). Other research indicates a risk G allele for suicide attempt (Sawiniec, Borkowski, Ginalska, & Lewandowska-Stanek, 2007), impulsivity (Benko et al., 2009), and suicide completion (Lemonde et al., 2003; Rad et al., 2012) – but not replicated in other studies (Murphy et al., 2011).

Interestingly, the 1019G variant is also associated with higher 5-HT$_{1A}$ binding potential (Lemonde et al., 2003; Lemonde et al., 2004; Miller et al., 2009; Parsey et al., 2010). Increased 5-HT$_{1A}$ receptor binding potential in major depression may also predict blunted response to antidepressants (Parsey et al., 2006).

5-HT$_{1B}$

The HTR1B gene encodes the protein for 5-HT$_{1B}$ receptors, which are concentrated in the striatum, basal ganglia, and frontal cortex – areas implemented in motivation and executive function. Animal models suggest some involvement of 5-HT$_{1B}$ receptors in human pathology. Notably, mice lacking HTR1B (Zhuang, Gross, Santarelli, Compan, Trillat, & Hen, 1999) and non-human primates with low 5-HT levels (Higley & Linnoila, 1997) exhibit enhanced aggressive behaviour. Moreover, suicide completers have reduced HTR1B expression in the orbito-frontal cortex, hippocampus, and amygdala (Anisman et al., 2008). Dysregulation of the orbito-frontal cortex is implemented in impulse control disorders (Winstanley, Theobald, Dalley, Cardinal, & Robbins, 2006) and impulsive aggressive disorders (Best, Williams, & Coccaro, 2002). These neurobiological correlates are interesting because impulsivity and aggression are known to be suicide risk factors.

Some researchers investigate impulsive-aggressive behaviours (IABs) as an intermediate endophenotype between the phenotype of suicidality and its genetic origin. From an evolutionary standpoint, suicidality detracts from reproductive fitness and so it may be genetically transmitted through aggression. Reduced HTR1B expression creates aggressive behaviour in animals (Higley & Linnoila, 1997; Zhuang et al., 1999) and therefore may generate trait-aggression exhibited in some suicidal individuals.

HTR1B gene polymorphism A161T has been associated with substance abuse (Cao et al., 2011), major depression (Huang et al., 2003), and IABs (Zouk et al., 2007; Stoltenberg, Christ, & Highland, 2012).

Regarding suicide, HTR1B gene polymorphisms seem to interact with NTRK2 and SLC1A2/3 (Murphy et al., 2011), as well as other 5-HT-related genes (Stoltenberg et al., 2012). Nonetheless, several studies fail to associate the G861C polymorphism with deliberate self-harm (Pooley et al., 2003) and suicide completion (Videtic et al., 2006; Zupanc, Pregelj, Tomori, Komel, & Paska, 2010). Although the link between HTR1B and aggression in animals is possible, its exact role in creating a vulnerability to suicidal behaviour remains unclear.

Therefore, the HTR1B gene may be related to aggression, but presents minimal suicide risk. Complex gene–gene interactions may account for inconsistent findings. A weak direct association between HTR1B and suicide may be further explained by a gene–environment interaction in which aggressive tendencies are triggered by adverse life events before being internalized. This hypothesis concurs with the evolutionary standpoint and the stress–diathesis model; however, current genetic research did not investigate HTR1B variants related to the hypothesized shift from internalized aggression to suicidal behaviour.

5-HT$_{2A}$

Analysis of post-mortem samples reveals greater 5-HT$_{2A}$ receptor binding in the prefrontal cortex of suicide completers than non-suicide controls (Turecki et al., 1999). The T102C and A1438G polymorphisms were found to mediate HTR2A expression where the 102T/-1438A haplotype is mainly associated with violent suicides. The T102C polymorphism has been associated with impulsivity, aggression and suicide attempts (Zalsman et al., 2011) as well as suicide completion (Videtic et al., 2006).

Nonetheless, subsequent meta-analysis failed to associate HTR2A gene polymorphism and suicidality (Serretti, Drago, & De Ronchi, 2007). Differences could not be found between suicidal, non-suicidal depressed patients, and healthy controls in 5-HT$_{2A}$ binding (Roggenbach et al. 2007). These inconsistencies warrant more gene–environment interaction studies.

For example, Brezo et al. (2010) investigated the interaction with childhood physical or sexual abuse in the onset of mood disorders and suicide attempts. Among their findings, the HTR2A gene mediated mood disorders and suicide attempts by different mechanisms. Genotype (AA) carriers had 2.4 times the risk of G carriers for mood disorders through a recessive main effect of the SNP rs9316235. Contrarily, the T-allele genotypes (rs7997012) provided protection from suicide risk in the presence of childhood sexual abuse. Childhood anxiousness and disruptiveness, relating to adult impulsivity and aggression, did not mediate the effects of mood disorder.

Recent data from a family study suggests a gene–environment interaction with the HTR2A rs6313 gene and stressful life events. Ben-Efraim et al. (2012) report a risk (CT) genotype for suicide attempts in individuals exposed to stressful life events and a protective (TT) genotype among the unexposed.

SLC6A4 and suicidal behaviour

The SLC6A4 gene encodes the protein for 5-HT transporter (5HTT), which regulates synaptic 5-HT levels through reuptake. The 5-HT transporter-linked polymorphic region (5HTTLPR) of the SLC6A4 gene is a functionally triallelic insertion/deletion polymorphism and consists of a long (L_A, L_G) and short (S) allele.

One meta-analysis identifies the L and S alleles as protective and risk variants, respectively (Li & He, 2007). The S allele of the 5HTT gene has been associated with anxiety-related personality traits (Munafò et al., 2009), depression (Karg, Burmeister, Shedden, & Sen, 2011), and suicidality in response to adverse life experiences (Zalsman et al., 2006). Despite the overlap, some authors argue a distinct biology of suicidality (for a review, see Gonda et al., 2011).

Methodological limitations of candidate gene studies

Candidate gene and association studies present several methodological limitations. First, many association studies compare patients with suicidal tendencies with and without varying comorbidity (e.g., schizophrenia, major depression). Degree of suicidality may vary in different psychiatric disorders. In the case of post-mortem studies, the neurobiological effects of psychiatric illness, pharmaceutical treatment, and suicidality often cannot be separated. For example, one alternative design might evaluate a theoretical biological marker in suicidal depressed patients, non-suicidal depressed patients, and matched controls.

Second, the definition of the suicidal phenotype varies greatly, ranging from suicidal ideation to suicide attempt to completed suicide. Some studies erroneously correlate genotypes with self-report measures instead of clinical diagnosis. Comorbidity and sex may mediate the lethality and frequency of suicidal behaviour. This becomes problematic for meta-analytic and interpretative purposes.

Lastly, many candidate gene and case-controlled association studies have poor sample stratification, i.e., individuals are drawn from different ethnic subpopulations that may not share the same allelic variants. Misrepresentation of one subpopulation increases the risk for Type II errors. One alternative is to limit the study to one ethnic population; however, ethnically homogenous samples limit the generalizability of the study as candidate SNPs may confer a specific risk only in certain population. These methodological limitations impede the detection of small genetic variants that could be relevant in the genetic aetiology of suicide.

Recent findings from genome-wide association studies (GWAS)

Curiously, no GWAS to date have found the SNPs of 5-HT genes associated with suicide-related phenotypes. At present, few GWAS target suicidality and most use psychiatric populations featuring Axis I disorders. Despite the high suicide rates in schizophrenic patients, no GWAS to date have addressed suicidality in this population.

Perlis et al. (2010) identified 11 loci with suggestive association with suicidality (6 in depressed subjects, 5 in bipolar subjects); however, none of the initial significant findings could be replicated. Schosser et al. (2011) evaluated genetics of suicidal ideation and behaviour in depressed subjects; however, the identified SNPs failed to achieve genome-wide significance and could not be replicated. Small effect sizes of multiple genetic variants are one hypothesized source of this result. Conversely, Galfalvy et al. (2011) identified seven genes and 58 SNPs independently associated with suicidality.

Willour et al. (2012) compared bipolar subjects with and without a history of attempted suicide to produce 2507 SNPs associated with suicide attempt history. Results could not be replicated;

however, combining the samples produced marginally significant data for the chromosomal region 2p25 (associated with the ACP1 gene). ACP hydrolyzes tyrosine phosphate to tyrosine, the substrate for tyrosine hydroxylase, which is the synthesizing enzyme of L-DOPA. Other GWAS on suicidality have linked chromosome 2p12 and suicidality. Willour et al. (2007) provided suggestive evidence for chromosome-wide linkage of chromosome 2p12 and attempted suicide in bipolar subjects. None of the markers surpassed the genome-wide significance threshold; however, subsequent research on mood disorders and suicidality provided suggestive evidence for linkage to 2p12 (Butler et al., 2010).

Conclusion

Several lines of research propose 5-HT dysregulation as a major component of suicide pathophysiology. Candidate 5-HT genes such as TPH2, HTR1A, HTR1B, HTR2A, and SLC6A4 seem to interact as components of the same neurotransmission that, in turn, can create widespread 5-HT disruption. Although allelic variations in these genes may be risk factors for suicidality, gene–environment interaction studies suggest an underlying genetic diathesis instigated by stressors such as psychiatric diagnosis and adverse life events. Hence, the stress–diathesis model incorporates the genetic and environmental factors that conjointly produce the phenotype of suicide and intermediate endophenotypes.

IABs and 5-HT binding are promising intermediate endophenotypes primarily due to their association with suicide risk and 5-HT neurotransmission. The functional relationship between 5-HT genes and IABs in animals is fascinating, given the relationship between impulsivity/ aggression and suicide in humans. Similarly, antidepressant-induced suicidal behaviour provides more clues as to the underlying mechanisms of 5-HT dysregulation in suicidality. Future research must clarify the precise mechanism by which altered 5-HT neurotransmission generates these intermediate endophenotypes.

Identifying other intermediate endophenotypes of suicidal tendencies would have tremendous implications for the treatment and care of at-risk individuals. Studying genetic variants in the 5-HT system is essential to providing personalized health care and prevent adverse reactions to pharmacological treatment (e.g., antidepressant-induced suicidal behaviour). As IABs are a known suicide risk factor, extensive study on the relationship between 5-HT dysregulation, IABs, and suicide will provide additional insight into the underlying mechanisms of suicidal behaviour. Understanding the genetics and neurobiology of suicide will subsequently aid in the production of reliable biological tests to screen for a combination of risk genetic variants.

Lastly, negative or inconsistent GWAS results are produced by a number of methodological hurdles. Conservative significance thresholds and multiple testing of hundreds of thousands of SNPs render genome-wide significance for single SNPs difficult. Additive or interactive effects between small genetic variants may collectively be responsible for the genetic diathesis of suicide. In keeping with the stress–diathesis model, environmental factors such as psychiatric diagnosis and adverse life experiences may differentially act upon these genetic variants, thereby creating the suicidal phenotype.

Future GWAS and candidate gene research must therefore address environmental factors (e.g., childhood trauma) and 5-HT-specific genetic interactions. These findings could be combined with imaging data for a better understanding of suicide neurobiology. Future GWAS research must also clarify the relationship between 5-HT dysregulation and intermediate endophenotype(s) such as IABs and 5-HT receptor binding potential.

References

Angoa-Pérez, M., Kane, M. J., Briggs, D. I., Sykes, C. E., Shah, M. M., Francescutti, D. M., Rosenberg, D. R., et al. (2012). Genetic depletion of brain 5HT reveals a common molecular pathway mediating compulsivity and impulsivity. *Journal of Neurochemistry, 121*(6), 974–984.

Anisman, H., Du, L., Palkovits, M., Faludi, G., Kovacs, G. G., Szontagh-Kishazi, P., Merali, Z., & Poulter, M. O. (2008). Serotonin receptor subtype and p11 mRNA expression in stress-relevant brain regions of suicide and control subjects. *Journal of Psychiatry and Neuroscience, 33*(2), 131–141.

Arango, V., Underwood, M. D., Boldrini, M., Tamir, H., Kassir, S., Chen, J. J., et al. (2001). Serotonin 1A receptors, serotonin transporter binding and serotonin transporter mRNA expression in the brainstem of depressed suicide victims. *Neuropsychopharmacology, 25*(6), 892–903.

Åsberg, M. (1997). Neurotransmitters and suicidal behavior: The evidence from cerebrospinal fluid studies. *Annals of the New York Academy of Sciences, 836,* 158–181.

Bellivier, F., Chaste, P., & Malafosse, A. (2004). Association between the TPH gene A218C polymorphism and suicidal behavior: A meta-analysis. *American Journal of Medical Genetics, Part B Neuropsychiatric Genetics, 124B*(1), 87–91.

Ben-Efraim, Y. J., Wasserman, D., Wasserman, J., & Sokolowski, M. (2012). Family-based study of HTR2A in suicide attempts: Observed gene, gene x environment and parent-of-origin associations. *Molecular Psychiatry,* 1–9. doi:10.1038/mp.2012.86.

Benko, A., Lazary, J., Molnar, E., Gonda, X., Tothfalusi, L., Pap, D., Mirnics, Z., et al. (2009). Significant association between the C(-1019)G functional polymorphism of the HTR1A gene and impulsivity. *American Journal of Medical Genetics, Part B Neuropsychiatric Genetics, 153B*(2), 592–599.

Best, M., Williams, J. M., & Coccaro, E. F. (2002). Evidence for a dysfunctional prefrontal circuit in patients with an impulsive aggressive disorder. *Proceedings of the National Academy of Sciences USA, 99*(12), 8448–8453.

Brezo, J., Bureau, A., Mérette, C., Jomphe, V., Barker, E. D., Vitaro, F., Hébert, M., et al. (2010). Differences and similarities in the serotonergic diathesis for suicide attempts and mood disorders: A 22-year longitudinal gene–environment study. *Molecular Psychiatry, 15*(8), 831–843.

Butler, A. W., Breen, G., Tozzi, F., Craddock, N., Gill, M., Korszun, A., Maier, W., et al. (2010). A genome-wide linkage study on suicidality in major depressive disorder confirms evidence for linkage to 2p12. *American Journal of Medical Genetics Part B, 153B*(8), 1465–1473.

Cao, J.-X., Hu, J., Ye, X.-M., Xia, Y., Haile, C. A., et al. (2011). Association between the 5-HTR1B gene polymorphisms and alcohol dependence in a Han Chinese population. *Brain Research, 1376,* 1–9.

Galfalvy, H., Zalsman, G., Huang, Y.-Y., Murphy, L., Rosoklija, G., Dwork, A. J., Haghighi, F., et al. (2011). A pilot genome-wide association and gene expression array study of suicide with and without major depression. *World Journal of Biological Psychiatry,* 1–9. doi:10.3109/15622975.2011.597875.

Gonda, X., Fountoulakis, K. N., Harro, J., Pompili, M., Akiskal, H. S., Bagdy, G., & Rihmer, Z. (2011). The possible contributory role of the S allele of 5-HTTLPR in the emergence of suicidality. *Journal of Psychopharmacology, 25*(7), 857–866.

Gos, T., Krell, D., Brisch, R., Bielau, H., Trübner, K., Steiner, J., Bernstein, H. G., & Bogerts, B. (2008). Demonstration of decreased activity of dorsal raphe nucleus neurons in depressed suicidal patients by the AgNOR staining method. *Journal of Affective Disorders, 111*(2), 251–256.

Hale, M. W., Shekhar, A., & Lowry, C. A. (2011). Development by environment interactions controlling tryptophan hydroxylase expression. *Journal of Chemical Neuroanatomy, 41*(4), 219–226.

Higley, J. D., & Linnoila, M. (1997). Low central nervous system serotonergic activity is traitlike and correlates with impulsive behaviour: A nonhuman primate model investigating genetic and environmental influences on neurotransmission. *Annals of the New York Academy of Sciences, 836,* 39–56.

Huang, Y.-Y., Oquendo, M. A., Friedman, J. M. H., Greenhill, L. L., Brodsky, B., et al. (2003). Substance abuse disorder and major depression are associated with the human 5-HT1B receptor (HTR1B) G861C polymorphism. *Neuropsychopharmacology, 28*(1), 163–169.

Jönsson, E. G., Goldman, D., Spurlock, G., Gustavsson, J. P., Nielsen, D. A., Linnoila, M., et al. (1997). Tryptophan hydroxylase and catechol-O-methyltransferase gene polymorphisms: Relationships to monoamine metabolite concentrations in CSF of healthy volunteers. *European Archives of Psychiatry and Clinical Neurosciences, 247*(6), 297–302.

Karg, K., Burmeister, M., Shedden, K., & Sen, S. (2011). The serotonin transporter promoter variant (5-HTTLPR), stress, and depression meta-analysis revisited: Evidence of genetic moderation. *Archives of General Psychiatry, 68*(5), 444–454.

Lemonde, S., Du, L., Bakish, D., Hrdina, P., & Albert, P. (2004). Association of the C(-1019)G 5-HT1A functional promoter polymorphism with antidepressant response. *International Journal of Neuropsychopharmacology, 7*(4), 501–506.

Lemonde, S., Turecki, G., Bakish, D., Du, L., Hrdina, P. D., Bown, C. D., Sequiera, A., et al. (2003). Impaired repression at a 5-Hyroxytryptamine 1A receptor gene polymorphism associated with major depression and suicide. *The Journal of Neuroscience, 23*(25), 8788–8799.

Li, D., & He, L. (2007). Meta-analysis supports association between serotonin transporter (5-HTT) and suicidal behavior. *Molecular Psychiatry, 12*(1), 47–54.

Mann, J. J., Currier, D., Stanley, B., Oquendo, M. A., Amsel, L. V., & Ellis, S. P. (2006). Can biological tests assist prediction of suicide in mood disorders? *International Journal of Neuropsychopharmacology, 9*(4), 465–474.

McDevitt, R. A., & Neumaier, J. F. (2011). Regulation of dorsal raphe nucleus function by serotonin autoreceptors: A behavioral perspective. *Journal of Chemical Neuroanatomy, 41*(4), 234–246.

Miller, J. M., Brennan, K. G., Ogden, T. R., Oquendo, M. A., Sullivan, G. M., Mann, J. J., & Parsey, R. V. (2009). Elevated serotonin 1A binding in remitted major depressive disorder: Evidence for a trait biological abnormality. *Neuropsychopharmacology, 34*(10), 2275–2284.

Munafò, M. R., Freimer, N. B., Ng, W., Ophoff, R., Veijola, J., Miettunen, J., Järvelin, M-R., et al. (2009). 5-HTTLPR genotype and anxiety-related personality traits: A meta-analysis and new data. *American Journal of Medical Genetics, Part B Neuropsychiatric Genetics, 150B*, 271–281.

Murphy, T. M., Ryan, M., Foster, T., Kelly, C., McClelland, R., O'Grady, J., Corcoran, E., et al. (2011). Risk and protective genetic variants in suicidal behaviour: Association with SLC1A2, SLC1A3, 5-HTR1B & NTRK2 polymorphisms. *Behavioral and Brain Functions, 7*(1), 22.

Parsey, R. V., Ogden, R. T., Miller, J. M., Tin, A., Hesselgrave, N., Goldstein, E., Mikhno, A., et al. (2010). Higher serotonin 1A binding in a second major depression cohort: Modeling and reference region considerations. *Biological Psychiatry, 68*(2), 170–178.

Parsey, R. V., Olvet, D. M., Oquendo, M. A., Huang, Y-Y., Ogden, R. T., & Mann J. J. (2006). Higher 5-HT1A receptor binding potential during a major depressive episode predicts poor treatment response: Preliminary data from a naturalistic study. *Neuropsychopharmacology, 31*(8), 1745–1749.

Perez-Rodriguez, M. M., Weinstein, S., New, S. A., Bevilacqua, L., Yuan, Q., Zhou, Z., Hodgkinson, C., et al. (2010). Tryptophan-hydroxylase 2 haplotype association with borderline personality disorder and aggression in a sample of patients with personality disorders and healthy controls. *Journal of Psychiatric Research, 44*(15), 1075–1081.

Perlis, R. H., Huang, J., Purcell, S., Fava, M., Rush, J., Sullivan, P. F., Hamilton S.P. et al. (2010). Genome-wide association study of suicide attempts in mood disorder patients. *American Journal of Psychiatry, 167*(12), 1499–1507.

Pooley, E. C., Houston, K., Hawton, K., & Harrison, P. J. (2003). Deliberate self-harm is associated with allelic variation in the tryptophan hydroxylase gene (TPH A779C), but not with polymorphisms in five other serotonergic genes. *Psychological Medicine, 33*(5), 775–783.

Rad, B. S., Ghasemi, A., Seifi, M., Samadikuchaksaraei, A., Baybordi, F., & Danaei, N. (2012). Serotonin 1A receptor genetic variations, suicide, and life events in the Iranian population. *Psychiatry and Clinical Neurosciences, 66*(4), 337–343.

Rogers, J., Martin, L. J., Comuzzie, A. G., Mann, J. J., Manuck, S. B., Leland, M., & Kaplan, J. R. (2004). Genetics of monoamine metabolites in baboons: Overlapping sets of genes influence levels of 5-hydroxyindolacetic acid, 3-hydroxy-4-methoxyphenylglycol, and homovanillic acid. *Biological Psychiatry, 55*(7), 739–744.

Roggenbach, J., Müller-Oerlinghausen, B., Franke, L., Uebelhack, R., Blank, J., & Ahrens, B. (2007). Peripheral serotonergic markers in acutely suicidal patients. 1. Comparison of serotonergic platelet measures between suicidal individuals, nonsuicidal patients with major depression and healthy subjects. *Journal of Neural Transmission, 114*(4), 479–487.

Roy, A., Rylander, G., & Sarchiapone, M. (1997). Genetics of suicide: Family studies and molecular genetics. *Annals of the New York Academy of Sciences, 836*, 135–157.

Roy, A., & Segal, N. L. (2001). Suicidal behavior in twins: A replication. *Journal of Affective Disorders, 66*(1), 71–74.

Rujescu, D., Giegling, I., Bondy, B., Gietl, A., Zill, P., & Möller, H-J. (2002). Association of anger-related traits with SNPs in the TPH gene. *Molecular Psychiatry, 7*(9), 1023–1029.

Sawiniec, J., Borkowski, K., Ginalska, G., & Lewandowska-Stanek, H. (2007). Association between 5-hydroxytryptamine 1A receptor gene polymorphism and suicidal behavior. *Przegl Lek, 64*(4–5), 208–211.

Schosser, A., Butler, A. W., Ising, M., Perroud, N., Uher, R., Ng, M. Y., Cohen-Woods, S., et al. (2011). Genome-wide association scan of suicidal thoughts and behaviour in major depression. *PLoS ONE, 6*(7): e20690. doi:10.1371/journal.pone.0020690.

Serretti, A., Drago, A., & De Ronchi, D. (2007). HTR2A gene variants and psychiatric disorders: A review of current literature and selection of SNPs for future studies. *Current Medicinal Chemistry, 14*(19), 2053–2069.

Staner, L., Uyanik, G., Corrêa, H., Trémeau, F., Monreal, J., Crocq, M., Stefos, G., Morris-Rosendahl, D. J., & Macher, J. (2002). A dimensional impulsive-aggressive phenotype is associated with the A218C polymorphisms of tryptophan hydoxylase gene: A pilot study in well-characterized impulsive inpatients. *American Journal of Medical Genetics, 114*(5), 553–557.

Stoltenberg, S. F., Christ, C. C., & Highland, K. B. (2012). Serotonin system gene polymorphisms are associated with impulsivity in a context dependent manner. *Progress in Neuropsychopharmacology & Biological Psychiatry, 39*(1), 182–191.

Turecki, G., Brière, R., Dewar, K., Antonetti, T., Lesage, A. D., Séguin, M., Chawky, N., et al. (1999). Prediction of level of serotonin 2A receptor binding by serotonin receptor 2A genetic variation in postmortem brain samples from subjects who did or did not commit suicide. *American Journal of Psychiatry, 156*(9), 1456–1458.

Viana, M. M., De Marco, L. A., Boson, W. L., Romano-Silva, M. A., & Corrêa, H. (2006). Investigation of A218C tryptophan hydroxylase polymorphism: Association with familial suicide behaviour and proband's suicide attempt characteristics. *Genes, Brain and Behavior, 5*(4), 340–345.

Videtic, A., Pungercic, G., Pajnic, I. Z., Zupanc, T., Balazic, J., Tomori, M., & Komel, R. (2006). Association study of seven polymorphisms in four serotonin receptor genes on suicide victims. *American Journal of Medical Genetics, Part B Neuropsychiatric Genetics, 141B*(6), 669–672.

Von Borczyskowski, A., Lindblad, F., Vinnerljung, B., Reintjes, R., & Hjern, A. (2011). Familial factors and suicide: An adoption study in a Swedish National Cohort. *Psychological Medicine, 41*(4), 749–758.

Waider, J., Araragi, N., Gutknecht, L., & Lesch, K-P. (2011). Tryptophan hyodroxylase-2 (TPH2) in disorders of cognitive control and emotion regulation: A perspective. *Psychoneuroendocrinology, 36*(3), 393–405.

Walther, D. J., Peter, J. U., Bashammakh, S., Hortnagl, H., Voits, M., Fink, H., & Bader, M. (2003). Synthesis of serotonin by a second tryptophan hydroxylase isoform. *Science, 229*(5603), 73.

Willour, V. L., Seifuddin, F., Mahon, P. B., Jancic, D., Pirooznia, M., Steele, J., Schweizer, B., et al. (2012). A genome-wide association study of attempted suicide. *Molecular Psychiatry, 17*(4), 433–444.

Willour, V. L., Zandi, P. P., Badner, J. A., Steele, J., Miao, K., Lopez, V., MacKinnon, D. F., et al. (2007). Attempted suicide in bipolar disorder pedigrees: Evidence for linkage to 2p12. *Biological Psychiatry, 61*(5), 725–727.

Winstanley, C. A., Theobald, D. E. H., Dalley, J. W., Cardinal, R. N., & Robbins, T. W. (2006). Double dissociation between serotonergic and dopaminergic modulation of medial prefrontal and orbitofrontal cortex during a test of impulsive choice. *Cerebral Cortex, 16*(1), 106–114.

World Health Organization (2012). *Suicide prevention (SURPRE)*. Available at: http://www.who.int/mental_health/prevention/suicide/suicideprevent/en/.

Zalsman, G., Huang, Y-Y., Oquendo, M. A., Burke, A. K., Hu, X-X., Brent, D. A., Ellis, S. P., et al. (2006). Association of a triallelic serotonin transporter gene promoter region (5-HTTLPR) polymorphism with stressful life events and severity of depression. *American Journal of Psychiatry, 163*(9), 1588–1593.

Zalsman, G., Patya, M., Frisch, A., Ofek, H., Schapir, L., Blum, I., Harell, D., et al. (2011). Association of polymorphisms of the serotonergic pathways with clinical traits of impulsive-aggression and suicidality in adolescents: A multi-center study. *World Journal of Biological Psychiatry, 12*(1–2), 33–41.

Zhuang, X., Gross, C., Santarelli, L., Compan, V., Trillat, A-C., & Hen, R. (1999). Altered emotional states in knockout mice lacking 5-HT1A or 5-HT1B receptors. *Neuropsychopharmacology, 21*(2), 52S–60S.

Zouk, H., McGirr, A., Lebel, V., Benkelfat, C., Rouleau, G., & Turecki, G. (2007). The effect of genetic variation of the serotonin 1B receptor gene on impulsive aggressive behaviour and suicide. *American Journal of Medical Genetics, Part B Neuropsychiatric Genetics, 144*(8), 996–1002.

Zupanc, T., Pregelj, P., Tomori, M., Komel, R., & Paska, A. V. (2010). No association between polymorphisms on four serotonin receptor genes, serotonin transporter gene and alcohol-related suicide. *Psychiatria Danubina, 22*(4), 522–527.

8

MEANS RESTRICTION AS A SUICIDE PREVENTION STRATEGY

Lessons learned and future directions

Mark Sinyor, Ayal Schaffer and Amy H. Cheung

Introduction

It has become widely accepted that restricting access to the means of suicide not only prevents suicide by that means but can prevent suicide deaths entirely (Cantor & Baume, 1998; Daigle, 2005; Mann et al., 2005; Yip et al., 2012). Commonly held rationales for this assertion are: (1) that people often express a preference for a specific method of suicide; (2) that suicidal crises may often be fleeting; and (3) that suicidal behaviours are frequently impulsive (Daigle, 2005; Hawton, 2007). It follows therefore that when immediately or easily available methods of suicide are removed, people will not invariably seek out other methods. In certain instances, this is almost certainly true; however, important counter-examples can also be seen. Researchers and policy-makers must be mindful of this complexity as they develop comprehensive suicide prevention programs. In this chapter, we will use two of the research studies we have conducted to illustrate the relative merits and limitations of means restriction as a suicide prevention strategy. We will argue that restricting access to the means of suicide is an important consideration for any large program targeting suicide. However, given that means restriction is a downstream intervention that does not address the fundamental antecedents of suicide, we will also argue for the importance of not overstating the power of means restriction for suicide prevention especially where more nuanced and/or targeted approaches may be called for.

Before proceeding, it is important to clearly define what we are talking about when we use the term "suicide prevention," as it relates to means restriction strategies. Every reasonably conceived effort to restrict access to a particular method of suicide has resulted in fewer suicides by that method. This finding is not under debate. To truly "prevent" suicides, however, such efforts also need to be accompanied by a decrease in suicides overall. In other words, there cannot be a parallel increase in suicides by other methods that abolishes the effect of the means restriction program. In this chapter, we will examine what happens to both method-specific and overall suicide rates when such programs are implemented, while keeping in mind an important limitation: every study examining suicide prevention by means restriction is an uncontrolled, natural experiment. There are numerous factors that influence suicide rates such as changes in average income as well as unemployment and divorce rates (Gunnell, Middleton, Whitley, Dorling, & Frankel, 2003; Ceccherini-Nelli & Priebe, 2011). These factors contribute to the plasticity of suicide rates and may help to either mask or magnify the effects of suicide prevention initiatives. This limitation notwithstanding, we hope to invite the reader to draw some educated conclusions from the literature that exists, imperfect as it is.

Inadvertent suicide prevention by means restriction

Over the past half-century, numerous programs have been undertaken to restrict access to the means of suicide. In some cases, the intent from the beginning has been to prevent suicides while in others new technology, such as cleaner energy, or new public policies unrelated to suicide prevention, such as restrictions on access to pesticides, have inadvertently resulted in significant changes in suicide rates. Some of the earliest examples of successful suicide prevention by means restriction involve the latter: inadvertent suicide prevention programs that were neither intended to prevent suicides nor advertised as such to the public. In the seminal 1976 article "The Coal Gas Story", Norman Kreitman explains how between 1955 and 1975, coal-based gas with a 10–20% carbon monoxide (CO) concentration was gradually phased out in the United Kingdom in favor of natural gas which had a negligible carbon monoxide concentration (Kreitman, 1976). As a result, suicides by CO poisoning which were 4–6/100,000/year for males in the U.K. and 3–4/100,000/year for females in 1956 dropped to below 1/100,000/year in both groups by 1971. This was accompanied by a clear and persistent drop in overall suicide rates in England and Wales over that period by 4 suicides/100,000/year for men and by 2 suicides/100,000/year for women. These were extraordinary findings with far-reaching implications although reductions in suicide rates were not found to be as robust in Scotland. What happened to suicides by methods other than CO poisoning? Recent reviews have tended to discount or minimize the problem of method substitution in the coal gas story (Cantor & Baume, 1998; Daigle, 2005), however, Kreitman (1976) himself wrote: "Far from any improvement the non-CO suicide rate has been shown to be increasing, especially in Scotland, among women in [England and Wales as well as Scotland], and among the young and middle-aged." The conversion of household gas in the UK was associated with lasting changes in overall suicide rates but not uniformly across age and gender. It is notable that the effect was most pronounced for older males. We know that suicide methods are often influenced by culture and that certain subgroups within a population may be more likely to use specific means of suicide death. It is possible, for example, that older males may have been more attached to the "traditional" method of suicide by CO poisoning than were younger males or females and that this may explain why they were most influenced by the lack of access to CO.

As one might expect, other countries in Europe and elsewhere also converted to cleaner household gas. Each of them saw a dramatic drop in suicides by CO poisoning. However, only Switzerland saw the same significant overall decrease in suicides observed in the UK (Lester, 1990a). The drop in suicides by household gas observed in other countries was accompanied by parallel increases in suicide deaths by other means such as inhalation of car exhaust in the United States (Lester, 1990b), by ingestion of other poisons in Germany (Wiedenmann & Weyerer, 1993) and by various methods in the Netherlands (Lester, 1991). The overall rate of suicides in each of those countries was unchanged.

Household gas was not the only dangerous gas detoxified in the latter part of the 20th century. The use of catalytic converters significantly diminished the lethality of inhaling car exhaust. In the United Kingdom, the use of catalytic converters was associated with a reduction in overall suicide rates in both men and women (McClure, 2000). Suicides by motor vehicle exhaust also dropped dramatically after catalytic converters were introduced in the United States (Mott et al., 2002) although no study has examined the impact on overall rates of suicide.

The literature on firearm restriction strategies is also somewhat ambiguous. Overall suicide rates as well as suicide rates by firearms decreased in Canada after legislation restricting access to firearms was enacted, with only a small increase in suicides by other means (Bridges & Kunselman, 2004). When suicides specifically in adolescents aged 15–19 were examined, there was a reduction in suicides by firearms but this coincided with an increase in suicides by hanging/suffocation leaving the suicide rate in this age group unchanged (Cheung & Dewa, 2005). An Australian study found that while firearm restriction reduced suicides in provincial city areas, these restrictions were not associated with any reduction in rates in rural or large metropolitan areas (Cantor & Slater, 1995). In the United States, firearm restrictions resulted in fewer suicides overall in only males over the age of 55 (Ludwig & Cook, 2000). Notably, this reduction was most pronounced in areas which also required background checks and longer waiting periods.

Finally, when the pesticide parathion was restricted in Finland, suicide by that method decreased but suicides by other methods increased, leaving overall rates unchanged. The authors concluded: "Restriction of a method reduces its use for suicide, but other methods tend to replace it. Restrictive measures should focus on some specific situations" (Ohberg, Lonnqvist, Sarna, Vuori, & Penttila, 1995).

Clearly, some societal advances that unintentionally result in restricting access to the means of suicide are often associated with lasting reductions in suicide rates. However, just as often, they seem to have little impact. Unfortunately, a specific pattern does not appear to be associated with the success or failure of these strategies. Suicide rates are known to differ in terms of demographics and across regions even within the same country (Masocco et al., 2010). Therefore, the explanation for why some means restriction efforts reduce suicides and others do not is likely complex and specific to each culture, region, population and method.

Intentional efforts to prevent suicide by means restriction

Suicide prevention barriers on bridges

The first study our own group conducted examined the effect of a suicide prevention barrier at the Bloor Street Viaduct in Toronto, which had been the bridge with the second highest yearly suicide rate in the world, next to the Golden Gate Bridge in San Francisco (Sinyor & Levitt, 2010). Our study, and the debate about the effectiveness of suicide prevention barriers on bridges in general, suitably demonstrate the ambiguity of the literature as a whole on targeted means restriction strategies.

The idea of placing suicide barriers on specific bridges stems from early studies of people who jumped or threatened to jump from the Golden Gate Bridge. In 1975, David Rosen published interviews with six survivors of suicide attempts by jumping from the Golden Gate (Rosen, 1975). The suicide plans of all six involved only the Golden Gate Bridge. Four of the six said they would not have attempted suicide had the Golden Gate Bridge been unavailable and all favored a suicide prevention barrier at that location. This study was followed up by two articles by Richard Seiden. One showed that a substantial proportion of those dying by suicide at the Golden Gate Bridge actually drove over the Oakland Bay Bridge to get there (Seiden & Spence, 1983). The other followed people who had been brought to the emergency department after a suicide threat or attempt at the Golden Gate Bridge and found that after a median follow-up of more than 26 years, only 5% of those people had gone on to die from suicide (Seiden, 1978). This was persuasive evidence that barriers on bridges might prevent suicides, although it ought to have been accompanied by three important caveats. First, the Golden Gate Bridge is a cultural icon and it was unclear whether evidence from that bridge was applicable to other, less iconic bridges. Second, it is unclear what proportion of those people taken to the emergency department after a suicidal gesture were actually intent on dying from suicide, which complicates the interpretation of Seiden's 1978 study. Third, being taken to hospital after a threat or, in the case of Rosen's six subjects, an actual jump off the bridge is a potentially life-changing event where people would have received psychiatric treatment. A physical barrier might theoretically deter a suicidal person in the moment and therefore increase the likelihood of that person receiving professional help but barriers by themselves do not specifically facilitate that outcome.

The first study looking at the impact of an actual suicide prevention barrier on a bridge examined the barrier on the Duke Ellington Memorial Bridge in Washington, DC (O'Carroll & Silverman, 1994). It found that the barrier prevented nearly all suicides at that location with virtually no increase in suicides at the nearby Taft Bridge. However, it did not analyze the impact on suicide rates as a whole in Washington. Similarly, Pelletier (2007) looked at suicides at the Memorial Bridge in Maine before and after a suicide prevention barrier was installed. That study found no further suicides at that bridge and no increase in suicides at other bridges in Maine. However, it did not examine overall rates and with a low baseline suicide rate of 0.6 suicides/year from the bridge, it would likely have been impossible to demonstrate any difference. A study of the barrier on the Clifton Suspension Bridge in Bristol, England, was the first to examine the impact of a barrier on overall rates in an area (Bennewith, Nowers, & Gunnell, 2007). Interestingly, despite the fact that for architectural reasons the barrier did not span the entire length of the bridge, suicides were still halved from 8 per year before the barrier to 4 per year after the barrier. This was accompanied by a non-significant rise in suicides by jumping from other nearby locations from 6 to 8. In other words, suicides by jumping decreased overall by 2 per year. The overall rate of suicide was noted to be statistically unchanged at 10.5/100,000/year compared to 11.2/100,000/year though it should be noted that this non-significant reduction is roughly what one would expect for an overall drop in suicides by jumping of 2 per year without any method substitution. In their more recent follow-up to that initial study, Bennewith and colleagues (2011) note on the success of the barrier that: "The number of incidents on the bridge did not decrease after barriers were installed but Bridge staff reported that the barriers 'bought time', making intervention possible."

The last study we would like to call attention to before discussing our own does not involve a suicide barrier being erected. It involves the *removal* of a barrier from the Grafton Bridge in Auckland, New Zealand, in 1996. When this was studied, it was found that in the two years prior to the barrier's removal, there were two suicides at the bridge and 12 suicides by jumping from other sites in the area (Beautrais, 2001). In the two years after the barrier was removed, suicides at the Grafton Bridge increased by seven but suicides from other locations dropped to seven leaving the total number of suicides by jumping exactly unchanged at 14. A follow-up study found that suicides at the Grafton Bridge subsequently decreased again when the barrier was reintroduced a few years later (Beautrais, Gibb, Fergusson, Horwood, & Larkin, 2009).

Our own study examined the Bloor Street Viaduct in Toronto, Canada, which had seen nearly 10 suicide deaths by jumping per year in the decade prior to a suicide barrier being erected (Sinyor & Levitt, 2010). Toronto had an annual rate of approximately 250 suicide deaths before the barrier and that rate decreased by about 28 suicides in the four years after the barrier. However, this was accounted for by a decrease in suicides by means other than jumping of almost exactly 28 suicides per year. Suicide rates by jumping were nearly identical in the two periods. This was the result of a statistically significant increase in suicides by jumping from other bridges in the city from 8.7 per year before the barrier to 14.7 per year after the barrier, as well as a non-significant but numerical increase in suicides by jumping from buildings over that time period. To date, this is the best powered study to detect changes in suicide rates by jumping and, unfortunately, the first to show a statistically significant increase in suicides by location substitution.

One important issue when interpreting this and other studies of bridge barriers is whether people may have traveled large distances to an iconic bridge. If so, prevented suicides may be obscured in studies that examine only local data. Our study found that, of 23 people who died from suicide at the Bloor Street Viaduct in the three years prior to the suicide barrier, only two lived outside the city of Toronto and one of those lived in a close suburb. Data examining 225 people who died from suicide at the Golden Gate Bridge found that 87% of them lived in San Francisco and surrounding counties (Blaustein & Fleming, 2009). Therefore, while the issue of travel is an important consideration in interpreting studies of suicide barriers, it appears the majority of people who die from iconic bridges live relatively close by.

While not exactly analogous, a related topic concerns suicide barriers on subways. One study was recently conducted examining the impact of the implementation of such barriers on one subway line (the "MTR" line) in Hong Kong but not on an adjacent line (the "KCR" line) (Law et al., 2009). The barriers decreased suicides on the MTR line from 38 in the 5 years before they were in place to only 7 in the five years afterwards, with suicides on the adjacent KCR line essentially unchanged. During the same time period, however, suicides in Hong Kong increased from 4,444 to 5,104. While it is clear that the barriers prevented suicides on the MTR subway line, it seems almost impossible to interpret a drop of about 30 suicides in the context of a city-wide increase of nearly 700.

All of the above studies are fraught with confounders and if we only emphasize the impact of bridge barriers on suicide rates, we neglect other important reasons to have them. These include, for example, the importance of sending a message that society cares about suicide prevention. Especially when coupled with efforts to assist in accessing treatment services such as distress phones on bridges, these barriers have the potential to be powerful symbols for hope to people contemplating suicide. Unfortunately, the opposite can sometimes occur. There were several reports in the news media that expressed skepticism about the barrier at the Bloor Street Viaduct around the time of its creation which may have undermined the impact of the barrier's intended message of hope. In the future, one important consideration would be the possibility of coupling such barriers with media campaigns aimed at greater awareness about mental illness and how to access treatment for suicidality.

Barriers may also be important for public safety reasons. The Bloor Street Viaduct spans two major freeways and the tragedy of people dying from suicide at that location was augmented by the safety risk to those driving on the roads below. There may also be specific cases in which barriers may have an increased likelihood of making an impact on overall rates as has been argued about the Golden Gate Bridge (Blaustein & Fleming, 2009), which dwarfs other locations in terms of its place in the public consciousness. However, it is also important to be aware of the real limitations of suicide prevention barriers. The tenor of conclusions reached regarding these barriers is often overly positive with respect to suicide rates. Take the authors of the study at the Grafton Bridge which shifted suicides but did not affect overall rates. They conclude: "This natural experiment . . . shows that safety barriers are effective in preventing suicide: their removal increases suicides; their reinstatement prevents suicides" (Beautrais et al., 2009). The evidence is in fact much murkier than this statement and other similar ones in the literature imply.

Suicide prevention by restricting access to lethal substances and moving beyond means restriction

There have been several recent efforts to restrict access to both prescription and over-the-counter medications that could be used in suicide. These interventions build on evidence suggesting that the diminishing use of more lethal medications such as barbiturates has been associated with a significant drop in suicides by overdose (Crome, 1993; Ohberg et al., 1995) although over the long term, suicides using other newer medications have increased (Carlsten et al., 1996).

In 1998, the UK introduced legislation that limited the size of over-the-counter packages of paracetamol (acetaminophen) and salicylates. This meant that people contemplating suicide by overdose would have to purchase multiple packages of these medications in order to obtain a lethal dose. Keith Hawton and his group at Oxford studied the effect of this intervention and found that there was a 22% decrease in intentional deaths from ingestion of these medications as well as a decrease in morbidity in people attempting suicide (Hawton et al., 2004). This research interested our group. After the somewhat disappointing results observed with the Bloor Street Viaduct suicide barrier, we were looking for other more targeted means restriction strategies that might be worth implementing in Toronto. We decided to characterize all suicides by overdose in the city in order to determine whether there were certain over-the-counter or prescription medications that would be amenable to this sort of restriction strategy. While we were completing that work, a reanalysis of the UK data was released. It persuasively argues that rates of suicide by paracetamol and salicylates followed the same pattern as multiple other medications that were unaffected by the legislation, meaning that the observed reductions were part of a broader trend of reduction in suicide by all ingestions rather than as a result of package size limitation (Bateman, 2009).

We completed our study which had a variety of interesting results including the fact that diphenhydramine, the active ingredient in new over-the-counter sleep aids, is used more often in completed suicide than acetaminophen and salicylates combined (Sinyor, Howlett, Cheung, & Schaffer, 2012). However, we chose not to recommend that the sale of any of these medications be limited. Rather we decided to argue for suicide prevention initiatives that were more targeted. For example, opioids were a cause of death in one-third of all suicides, and cardiac medications, particularly diltiazem, were used for suicide in a number of cases. We therefore called for increased awareness and screening for depression and suicidal ideation at pain, cancer and heart clinics. In another example, we found 10 cases of suicide where the only drug(s) causing death were newer antidepressants and in seven of those cases, venlafaxine, mirtazapine and citalopram were involved. This is in keeping with Professor Hawton's work showing that these are the three most toxic non-TCA antidepressants when taken in overdose (Hawton et al., 2010). We therefore recommended that clinicians take this into account when prescribing antidepressants to people at high risk for overdose and consider avoiding these specific antidepressants.

In short, we did not conclude that means restriction was pointless, quite the contrary. However, we have taken a more nuanced view of this approach. More work clearly needs to be done to propose, implement and then study suicide prevention initiatives to determine which ones are truly effective. In the meantime, we can try to make some educated guesses about the kinds of interventions we should be considering. We can speculate that it may be helpful to separate "population-based" means restriction strategies from more targeted "patient-based" means restriction. As we have seen, evidence for the former is mixed and the few cases with clear reductions in suicide rates, such as the coal gas story, involve programs that were not specifically designed for suicide prevention that eliminated access to a method of suicide that was both entrenched in the culture and available in all homes across the country. It is our contention that means restriction may be better placed in the clinician's office and targeted at high risk patients and/or high risk times. The interventions may include judicious prescription practices, having family members dispense medications, and efforts to secure firearms. While psychiatrists already routinely do these things, they need better information, such as our findings about specific antidepressants and over-the-counter hypnotics, so that their means restriction practices can be most effective. Furthermore, we would argue that these practices need to be better disseminated to family physicians and other medical specialists treating patients with elevated suicide risk. While there may be a place for means restriction in broader public policy, we think that governments are better poised for other strategies for suicide prevention. These include public and media education programs, programs to both improve detection and eliminate the stigma of mental illness as well as efforts to optimize access to mental health care. In our view, governments ought to spend most of their energy creating a society where mental health is an emphasis, whereas clinicians should be the ones to implement specific treatment which may include restricting access to lethal means where indicated. It should be noted that many of the strategies we are proposing here suffer from the same paucity of evidence for reducing suicide rates as means restriction. But while we now have a relatively rich literature on means restriction, rigorous studies examining the interventions listed above are lacking. We hope that in the near future research will be undertaken in an effort to clarify whether any of these approaches may truly prevent deaths from suicide.

Conclusion

We still do not fully understand the role of population-based means restriction strategies for suicide prevention. No doubt, many research projects that continue to investigate this issue are underway at the moment. To truly inform us, these studies must provide context for their findings. That means that they need to examine changes in suicide rates overall, not just by a specific method. Preferably, they should also try to account for broader trends by making comparisons to rates in nearby regions where the intervention has not occurred.

Regardless of the outcomes of these studies, there will be always be societal efforts to limit access to potentially fatal materials and methods such as guns, poisons and carbon monoxide, either for the explicit purpose of suicide prevention or for other reasons. In some cases these efforts will result in fewer deaths from suicide and, it should be noted, accidental deaths and homicides as well. There is also likely a role for means restriction efforts targeting suicide "hot spots" such as the Golden Gate Bridge, especially since such programs, if carefully designed, may help to create a meaningful public dialogue about suicide, work to destigmatize mental illness and send a message of hope to people contemplating suicide. These latter points are crucial. Although they are difficult to quantify, means restriction efforts may have very important outcomes even if there is no immediate impact on overall rates of suicide. However, to view means restriction programs as a panacea is reductionist. We cannot bubble-wrap our society. Means restriction will never, for example, tackle hanging, the most common method of suicide worldwide. Ultimately our emphasis has to be on the fundamental antecedents of suicide such as mental and physical illness, despair, hopelessness and maladaptive coping strategies. We are finally beginning to have a public conversation about how to address these underlying problems and we should be aware that the topic of means restriction will always be somewhat lateral to that conversation. Of course, the mental health community needs to continue to combat the popular but misguided notion that suicide is inevitable. At the same time we must embrace our responsibility to find nuanced solutions for a highly complex problem.

Acknowledgements

This chapter is, in part, based on articles published in the *BMJ* (Sinyor & Levitt, 2010) and the *Canadian Journal of Psychiatry* (Sinyor, Howlett, Cheung, & Schaffer, 2012) as well as a presentation at the 2011 Ontario Psychiatric Association Annual Conference (Sinyor & Howlett, 2011).

The authors wish to thank Dr. Anthony Levitt and Dr. Andrew Howlett for their work on the projects on which this chapter is based as well as Marcus Allen for his assistance with the literature review.

References

Bateman, D. N. (2009). Limiting paracetamol pack size: Has it worked in the UK? *Clinical Toxicology, 47,* 536–541.

Beautrais, A. L. (2001). Effectiveness of barriers at suicide jumping sites: A case study. *Australian and New Zealand Journal of Psychiatry, 35,* 557–562.

Beautrais, A. L., Gibb, S. J., Fergusson, D. M., Horwood, L. J., & Larkin, G. L. (2009). Removing bridge barriers stimulates suicides: An unfortunate natural experiment. *Australian and New Zealand Journal of Psychiatry, 43*(6), 495–497.

Bennewith, O., Nowers, M., & Gunnell, D. (2011). Suicidal behaviour and suicide from the Clifton Suspension Bridge, Bristol, and surrounding area in the UK, 1994–2003. *European Journal of Public Health, 21*(2), 204–208.

Bennewith, O., Nowers, M., & Gunnell, D. (2007). Effect of barriers on the Clifton Suspension Bridge, England, on local patterns of suicide: Implications for prevention. *British Journal of Psychiatry, 190,* 266–267.

Blaustei, M., & Fleming, A. (2009). Suicide from the Golden Gate Bridge. *American Journal of Psychiatry, 166*(10): 1111–1116.

Bridge, F. S., Kunselman, J. C. (2004). Gun availability and use of guns for suicide, homicide, and murder in Canada. *Perceptual & Motor Skills, 98,* 594–598.

Carlsten, A., Allebeck, P., & Brandt, L. (1996). Are suicide rates in Sweden associated with changes in the prescribing of medicines? *Acta Psychiatrica Scandinavica, 94,* 94–100.

Cantor, C. H., & Baume, P. J. (1998). Access to methods of suicide: What impact? *Australian and New Zealand Journal of Psychiatry, 32,* 8–14.

Cantor, C. H., & Slater, P. J. (1995). The impact of firearm control legislation on suicide in Queensland: Preliminary findings. *Medical Journal of Australia, 162,* 583–585.

Ceccherini-Nelli, A., & Priebe, S. (2011). Economic factors and suicide rates: Associations over time in four countries. *Social Psychiatry and Psychiatric Epidemiology, 46*(10): 975–982.

Cheung, A. H., & Dewa, C. S. (2005). Current trends in youth suicide and firearms regulations. *Canadian Journal of Public Health, 96*(2): 131–135.

Crome, P. (1993). The toxicity of drugs used for suicide. *Acta Psychiatrica Scandinavica Suppl, 37,* 133–137.

Daigle, M. S. (2005). Suicide prevention through means restriction: Assessing the risk of substitution. A critical review and synthesis. *Accident Analysis and Prevention, 37,* 625–632.

Glasgow, G. (2011). Do local landmark bridges increase the suicide rate? An alternative test of the likely effect of means restriction at suicide-jumping sites. *Social Science and Medicine, 72*(6): 884–889.

Gunnell, D., Middleton, N., Whitley, E., Dorling, D., & Frankel, S. (2003). Why are suicide rates rising in young men but falling in the elderly? A time-series analysis of trends in England and Wales 1950–1998. *Social Science and Medicine, 57*(4): 595–611.

Hawton, K. (2007). Restricting access to methods of suicide: Rationale and evaluation of this approach to suicide prevention. *Crisis, 28*(suppl. 1): 4–9.

Hawton, K., Bergen, H., Simkin, S., Cooper, J., Waters, K., Gunnell, D., & Kapur, N. (2010). Toxicity of antidepressants: Rates of suicide relative to prescribing and non-fatal overdose. *British Journal of Psychiatry, 196*(5): 354–358.

Hawton, K., Simkin, S., Deeks, J., Johnston, A., Waters, K., Arundel, M., Bernal, W., Gunson, B., Hudson, M., Suri, D., & Simpson, K. (2004). UK legislation on analgesic packs: Before and after study of long-term effect on poisonings. *BMJ, 329*: 1076.

Kreitman, N. (1976). The coal gas story: United Kingdom suicide rates, 1960– 971. *British Journal of Preventive and Social Medicine, 30*: 86–93.

Law, C. K., Yip, P. S. F., Chan, W. S., Fu, K. W., Wong, P. W., & Law, Y. W. (2009). Evaluating the effectiveness of barrier installation for preventing railway suicides in Hong Kong. *Journal of Affective Disorders, 114*: 254–262.

Lester, D. (1990a). The effect of the detoxification of domestic gas in Switzerland on the suicide rate. *Acta Psychiatrica Scandinavica, 82,* 383–384.

Lester, D. (1990b) The effects of detoxification of domestic gas on suicide in the United States. *American Journal of Public Health, 80*, 80–81.

Lester, D. (1991). Effects of detoxification of domestic gas on suicide in the Netherlands. *Psychological Reports, 68*, 202.

Ludwig, J., & Cook, P. J. (2000). Homicide and suicide rates associated with implementation of the Brady Handgun Violence Prevention Act. *JAMA, 284*, 585–591.

Mann, J. J., Apter, A., Bertolote, J., et al. (2005). Suicide prevention strategies: A systematic review. *JAMA, 294*, 2064–2074.

Masocco, M., Pompili, M., Vanacore, N., Innamorati, M., Lester, D., Girardi, P., Tatarelli, R., & Vichi, M. (2010). Completed suicide and marital status according to the Italian region of origin. *Psychiatric Quarterly, 81*(1), 57–71.

McClure, G. M. (2000). Changes in suicide in England and Wales, 1960–1997. *British Journal of Psychiatry, 17*, 664–667.

Mott, J. A., Wolfe, M. I., Alverson, C. J., Macdonald, S. C., Bailey, C. R., Ball, L. B., Moorman, J. E., Somers, J. H., Mannino, D. M., & Redd, S. C. (2002). National vehicle emissions policies and practices and declining US carbon monoxide-related mortality. *JAMA, 288*, 988–995.

O'Carroll, P. W., & Silverman, M. M. (1994). Community suicide prevention: the effectiveness of bridge barriers. *Suicide and Life-threatening Behavior, 24*(1), 89–99.

Ohberg, A., Lonnqvist, J., Sarna, S., Vuori, E., & Penttila, A. (1995). Trends and availability of suicide methods in Finland: Proposals for restrictive measures. *British Journal of Psychiatry, 166*(1), 35–43.

Pelletier, A. R. (2007). Preventing suicide by jumping: The effect of a bridge safety fence. *Injury Prevention, 13*, 57–59.

Rosen, D. H. (1975). Suicide survivors: A follow-up study of persons who survived jumping from the Golden Gate and San Francisco-Oakland Bay Bridges. *Western Journal of Medicine, 122*, 289–294.

Seiden, R. H. (1978). Where are they now? A follow-up study of suicide attempters from the Golden Gate Bridge. *Suicide and Life-threatening Behavior, 8*, 203–216.

Seiden, R. H., & Spence, M. (1983). A tale of two bridges: Comparative suicide incidence on the Golden Gate and San Francisco-Oakland Bay Bridges. *Omega, 14*: 201–209.

Sinyor, M., & Howlett, A. (Presenters). (2011). A debate: Do suicide prevention strategies lower suicide rates? Ontario Psychiatric Association Annual Meeting. April. Toronto, Ontario, Canada.

Sinyor, M., Howlett, A., Cheung, A. H., & Schaffer, A. (2012). Substances used in completed suicide by overdose in Toronto: An observational study of coroner's data. *Canadian Journal of Psychiatry, 57*(3), 184–191.

Sinyor, M., & Levitt, A. J. (2010). Effect of a barrier at Bloor Street Viaduct on suicide rates in Toronto: Natural experiment. *BMJ, 341*, c2884.

Wiedenmann, A., & Weyerer, S. (1993). The impact of availability, attraction and lethality of suicide methods on suicide rates in Germany. *Acta Psychiatrica Scandinavica, 88*, 364–368.

Yip, P. S., Caine, E., Yousuf, S., Chang, S. S., Wu, K. C., & Chen, Y. Y. (2012). Means restriction for suicide prevention. *Lancet, 23*, 379(9834), 2393–2399.

9

SUICIDE IN DIVERSE POPULATIONS

Implications for Canada's suicide strategies

Kwame McKenzie, Andrew Tuck and Samanthika Ekanayake

Introduction

Developing services and interventions that meet the needs of diverse populations is a common challenge for health services in high income countries. Globalization is leading to rapid urbanization and international migration which are increasing our already diverse populations. Suicide prevention strategies need to consider the possible differential effectiveness of interventions on diverse populations but often this is not taken into account. For instance, though health equity is one of the cornerstones of the Mental Health Strategy for Canada, launched in May 2012 (Mental Health Commission of Canada, 2012a), it is not clear that health equity is similarly enshrined in the work that is developing a national suicide strategy (Canadian Association for Suicide Prevention, 2010; Mental Health Commission of Canada, 2012b) or in provincial strategies.

Nationally, groups have come together including the Mental Health Commission, the Canadian Association of Suicide Prevention and the Canadian Institutes of Health Research to increase the capacity for effective suicide prevention by connecting people, ideas, and resources on a pan-Canadian level. This national collaborative on suicide prevention aims to enhance capacity building for suicide prevention in Canada, promote knowledge exchange and mobilization on suicide prevention across Canada, and inform suicide prevention policy development at the local, provincial, territorial, and national levels (Mental Health Commission of Canada, 2012c).

The members are to include researchers, practitioners, decision-makers, family caregivers and people with lived experience with a vested interest in and commitment to suicide prevention. The work will be based on principles of collaboration; independence and interdependence; diversity (meaning they will embrace many perspectives and expertise that they call research, practice, policy, and including caregivers and people with lived experiences); community; results; leverage; and, transparency.

Many national suicide prevention strategies attempt to address issues of health equity by bringing attention to a public health concern that is often stigmatized and marginalized. Those suffering from mental health concerns or having thoughts of suicide often have difficulty accessing support services. Further, because the rate of suicide on some Aboriginal reserves in Canada ranks among the highest in the world, Canada will include specific work on this group in their plans (Kirmayer et al., 2007a). However, a considered approach must also be taken to address the needs of ethnic minorities at risk for suicide. Canada is a diverse population of immigrants. Visible minority groups significantly outnumber Aboriginal populations and may need their own place in any strategy.

Ethnic diversity and suicide

There is a significant literature documenting differences in the rates of suicide between ethnic groups within countries (McKenzie, Serfaty, & Crawford, 2003). For example, higher suicide rates have been reported in some migrant populations of the South Asian diaspora and those from Eastern Europe around the world when compared to the host populations. Evidence may also suggest that rates of suicide in Chinese origin female immigrants may be higher than those seen in their male counterparts (McKenzie et al., 2003; 2008). Rates in non-migrant minority populations may also differ; suicide rates among African Americans are half that of White Americans (US Department of Health and Human Services, 2001).

Early work on relative rates of suicide in different ethnic groups reported that in the USA the rank order of suicide rates in immigrant groups was similar to the rank order of suicide rates for their countries of origin (Sainsbury & Barraclough, 1968). Immigrants who came from countries with high suicide rates had higher rates in the USA than immigrants who came from countries with medium or low rates of suicide. However, there was some convergence towards the rate of the host population. One potential explanation suggested that some aspects of the culture of their home country that are linked to suicide risk stay with immigrants despite the fact that they have moved to a new country. These aspects are modified by the host culture but may dissipate over time, so that immigrant groups will acquire the rates of suicide of the host population as they acculturate and change their patterns of risk and resilience (McKenzie et al., 2003). However, the evidence for this explanation is mixed. For instance, in Sweden, the rates of suicide in migrants from areas with traditionally higher suicide rates is increased, rather than decreased, in their Swedish-born children (Hjern, 2002).

The theory that migrants continue to keep some of the culture of their countries of origin and this is linked to their suicide rate in part relies on the assumption that people who migrate are typical, or at least carry the same liability to suicide, as those left in a country. However, people who migrate may be different to those who stay. They may be more resilient, may be leaving because of persecution, because of their social position or because they lack opportunity. Minorities within a country may be more likely to migrate than majority populations. In the United Kingdom, for example, 28% of the Indian population is Sikh, although they make up only 2% of the Indian population (Office for National Statistics, 2013).

The theory that suicide rates for minority ethnic populations always move towards the suicide rates of the majority or economically dominant population is also not supported. For instance, rather than diminishing or being equal, there have been persistently low rates of suicide in some groups such as African Americans and consistently higher rates in other ethnic minority populations such as the native populations of Canada, the USA and Australia (US Department of Health and Human Services, 2001; McKenzie et al., 2003; Kirmayer et al., 2007a). The rate of suicide in any group is a result of complex and inter-related environmental and psychological factors. Contrary to previous theories, there is no simple single trajectory of suicide rates in a minority ethnic group (McKenzie et al., 2003). This is because of their unique and differential exposures to factors that have an impact on suicide risk.

Four dimensions of social aetiology and suicide

A simplified model for understanding multi-level aetiology of mental health problems has been published (Shah, Mizrahi, & McKenzie, 2011). Using this may offer an outline for considering the factors that are important in changing suicide risk for a particular group. Understanding the reasons for differences in risk may help to develop or target suicide prevention strategies (US Department of Health and Human Services, 2001). A four-dimensional model of aetiology posits that the causes of an illness can be individual, ecological, an interaction between the individual and ecological factors, and, linked to time (Shah et al., 2011).

A non-exhaustive list of the possible risk factors for suicide at an individual level could include education, mental health, social circumstances, spiritual and religious views, exposure to risk factors and response to stress. At an ecological level, the list could include the amount of risk factors in the environment, a group's acceptance of suicide as a way of dealing with problems, the level of social cohesion or social efficacy and the availability of social support (National Institutes for Mental Health, 2003). An example of the interaction between individual risk and ecological risk would be the processes through which the amount of risk factors in the environment fosters individual resilience or produces health problems or behaviours which increase the risk of suicide.

Lastly, time could include issues such as the latent impacts of exposure to risk factors for suicidal behaviour or differences in exposure to risk factors linked to the social history and trajectory of a group in a country (Shah et al., 2011). The factors that are acting on a particular ethnic group may change over time and this may mean that rates of suicide may change over time. Also because risks interact, even if exposure to risk factors stays the same the impact of risk factors may change over time.

Because different sub-groups, such as age groups, may have different exposures to risk factors, have dissimilar social contexts and do not have the same histories, the rates of suicide in different age groups may differ and may change at different rates in different directions. One size, therefore, does not fit all. People from the same cultural group in different places, at different chronologies in their time in a new country, may have different rates of suicide. This finding is influenced not only by culture but by interaction between who they are, where they are and how they and their host populations interact.

Diversity in Canada

Such complexity poses a challenge to countries developing suicide prevention strategies and particularly to Canada. Canada is one of the most diverse countries in the world. Statistics Canada classifies 16% of the population as a visible minority (Statistics Canada, 2008) which is defined by the Employment Equity Act as "persons other than aboriginal peoples, who are non-Caucasian in race or non-white in colour" (Statistics Canada, 2011). The visible minority population in Canada is rapidly increasing and is projected to reach 22% by 2017 (Bélanger & Molenfant, 2005) and 31% by 2031 (Statistics Canada, 2010). The majority of recent Canadian immigrants are from South or East Asia. The 2006 census reported that the South Asian origin population had surpassed the East Asian population and was the biggest visible minority group (Statistics Canada, 2008).

The improvement in health services, access to care, and health outcomes for ethnic minority populations have been recognized as national and provincial priorities (Health Canada, 2011). Equity in access and outcomes for Canada's diverse population is one of the aims of the national mental health strategy (Mental Health Commission of Canada, 2009) and provincial strategies (Ministry of Health and Long Term Care, 2010). Variability in the rates of specific illnesses between groups, generations, classes of immigrant, refugee and visible minority groups as well as differences in use of services offer a complex challenge to policy-makers. A recent Mental Health Commission of Canada publication concluded that the development of equitable services for immigrant, refugee, ethno-cultural and racialized groups should be based on an understanding of the needs of specific groups rather than on general assumptions about visible minority groups (Hansson et al., 2010). Due to the large diversity within Canada we have focused on people of South Asian origin, the largest visible minority ethnic grouping in Canada, as an example to indicate issues that may be experienced when looking at different groups. We will use the national and some of the international literature to consider what Canada may want to consider when developing an equitable suicide prevention strategy.

The South Asian population of Canada

The South Asian origin group makes up 4% of the Canadian population (1,262,865). The majority of South Asian newcomers settle in Ontario (Statistics Canada, 2008). Projections suggest that the South Asian population in Canada will grow to 1.8 million by 2017 (Bélanger & Molenfant, 2005). The South Asian origin population in Canada is a diverse group with significant ethnic, religious, and linguistic differences. For instance, South Asian origin immigrants in Ontario are from India (443,690), Pakistan (133,285), Sri Lanka (105,670), Bangladesh (33, 230), with smaller numbers from other countries such as Nepal (3,645), Bhutan (130) and the Maldives (30) (Statistics Canada, 2008). People from India are mainly Hindu and Sikh, whereas the majority of individuals from Pakistan are Muslim. Most are economic migrants but many from Sri Lanka are refugees. There are also significant differences between those born abroad and those born in Canada (Samuel, 2010). It has been argued that there are commonalities in social networks, family interactions, and preservation of customs and traditions (Tran, Kaddatz, & Allard, 2005; Lai & Surood, 2008), but the use of the catch-all term South Asian may hide significant cultural differences that are important for exposure to risk factors and use of services.

Mental health status and service utilization of the South Asian diaspora in Canada and internationally

Mental health is one of the most important risk factors for suicide. Internationally, there has been significant research on mental health, mental illness, social determinants of mental illness and service utilization, and barriers to care in the South Asian diaspora. The UK has perhaps the best developed literature (Fenton & Sadiq-Sangster, 1996; Jacob et al., 1998; Bhui, Bhugra, & Goldberg, 2002; McCabe & Priebe, 2004; Lawrence et al., 2006a; 2006b; McKenzie et al., 2008). Australia (Ghuman, 2000; Somasundaram, 2010) and the USA (Mehta, 1998; Diwan, Jonnalagadda, & Gupta, 2004; Karasz, 2005) have also investigated this group. These studies indicate that differences may exist in rates of mental illness between South Asian origin groups and host populations, lower levels of service usage, changing patterns of service usage between generations and changing rates of suicide with women specifically at higher risk. Research results vary considerably and there has been no systematic synthesis of the international literature. Moreover, because of the impact on health and service use of the reasons for migration and the social situation that South Asian origin populations find themselves in – including differences in the availability and access to health services – the international literature may be a guide but local studies are needed to inform service changes (Rodney & Copeland, 2009).

In Canada, research based on national-level data reports lower rates of mental health problems among immigrants (Ali, 2002; Wu et al., 2003), including those of South Asian origin. However, longer-term studies of well-being indicate that the healthy immigrant effect may be temporary (Beiser, 1988). After five years, immigrants have the same level of ill-health as those who are Canadian-born and longer-term immigrants have worse general health and well-being (Beiser, 1988; Xu & McDonald, 2010). Small-scale studies report increased rates of specific mental health problems in particular South Asian immigrant groups (Lai & Surood, 2008; Jibeen & Khalid, 2010).

Studies show that new immigrants and the Canadian-born population have similar rates of access to general medical care (Kirmayer et al., 2007b), however, both new and longer-term immigrants are less likely to receive mental health care even though they suffer from mental health problems (Whitley, Kirmayer, & Groleau, 2006). This may be similar in the South Asian origin group (Tiwari & Wang, 2008; Lai & Surood, 2008; Surood & Lai, 2010). There is evidence of systematic inequalities in the mental health service provision for the ethnic minorities in Canada which may be a result of a lack of culturally adapted services (Kirmayer & Minas, 2000). There are significant differences in the risk of illness and service use in refugee populations compared to immigrant populations (Beiser, 1988). Within the immigrant population, new immigrants are less likely to use services if they have a mental illness than longer-term immigrants (Whitley et al., 2006). There may also be differences in health status and service use for rural or low concentration South Asian groups not in high populous cities (Sadavoy, Meier, & Ong, 2004). There is significant information available but this has not been synthesized or considered through the lens of people interested in suicide prevention.

Suicide in diverse populations in the South Asian population in Canada

There is little published work on suicide in the South Asian population in Canada. We could not identify national studies of suicide in the South Asian population in Canada. Data from the Canadian Vital Statistics Data Base and the World Health Statistics Annual of the WHO (Malenfant, 2004) have been used to produce a comparison suicide in immigrant and Canadian-born people of all ages. The study calculated death rates between the years 1990–1992 and 1995–1997. The rate of suicides per 100,000 for 1990–1992 was Canadian-born 13.0, Immigrant 8.3, and between 1995–1997 Canadian-born 13.3 and Immigrant 7.9. The results were not broken down further by country of origin or whether the immigrants were from visible minorities.

Some information may be gleaned from trends in suicidal ideation and attempts. Though this should be done with caution because there may be different risk factors involved, the trends may be informative. Data from the CCHS Cycle 1 looked at 61,673 people over the age of 18 from September 2000 and February 2001 (Clarke et al., 2008). Respondents were asked to report suicidal ideation and or non-fatal suicide attempts in the previous 12 months. Similar to actual suicides, the minority populations were less likely than Canadian White populations to have suicidal ideation or attempts. Some 2.3% answered yes in the Anglophone White population, 1.3% in the Foreign-born White population and 1.5% in the visible minority population (Clarke et al., 2008).

The only specific data on suicidal ideation and attempts in the South Asian populations of Canada comes from a study of 1135 first-, second- and third-generation immigrant students in British Columbia (Kennedy et al., 2005). There were 459 European, 574 Chinese and 102 Indo-Asian respondents. The study investigated the lifetime prevalence of suicidal thoughts, plans or attempts. It reported differing rates and trajectories of suicidal thoughts for the different ethnic groupings. European origin immigrant groups had increasing rates of suicidal ideation between first and third generations whereas both Indian and Chinese origin students had decreasing rates of suicidal thoughts across the generations. Some 52% of first-generation Indian students had thought about suicide, as had 49% of second-generation and 44% of third-generation Indian students. All groups had increasing rates of plans for suicide between first and third generations. However, 0% of first-generation Indian origin students had planned a suicide, though 10% of second-generation and 22% of third-generation Indian origin students had. Though suicide attempts were lower in the third compared to the first generation in European and Chinese students, in Indian students the percentage of suicide attempts jumped from 0% in the first generation to nearly 7% in the second generation to 11% in the third generation (Kennedy et al., 2005).

The research so far in Canada seems to indicate that there are variations in suicidal ideation and suicide attempts between groups. There are also differences in completed suicide. Though it could be argued that the low rates of suicide in immigrant groups means there is little reason to focus on them for suicide prevention, it is likely that simple comparisons between immigrants and non-immigrants may mask underlying differences between ethnic groups. There may be sub-populations at high risk of suicide that are missed. Moreover, the 4-D aetiological model would predict that rates may change over time. Research into perhaps the best investigated part of the South Asian diaspora, the population in the UK, demonstrates how such complexities may play out.

Suicide in the South Asian diaspora in the UK

According to the 2001 UK Census, there were approximately 2,331,000 South Asians, constituting 4.0% of the population of the UK (Office for National Statistics, 2007). This proportion is similar to the proportion of South Asian origin people in Canada. Those of Indian origin numbered 1,053,411 (1.8% of the population), 747,285 people were of Pakistani origin (1.3%), 283,063 were of Bangladeshi origin (0.5%), and 247,664 were other Asian (0.4%). South Asians make up 50.3% of the UK's non-European population (Office for National Statistics, 2007). The consistent findings over the years in the UK are that South Asian women, particularly young women, have higher rates of suicide and South Asian men have lower rates. Those of South Asian origin are for historical cultural reasons more likely to use suicide by fire as a method than other groups and are more likely to use lethal methods (Raleigh et al., 1990; Raleigh & Balarajan, 1992a; 1992b; Patel & Gaw, 1996; Raleigh, 1996; Neeleman et al., 1997; McKenzie et al., 2003; Gunnell & Lewis, 2005; Tuck et al., 2012).

Recent studies have demonstrated the importance of contemporary information and the use of best scientific methods available as risks and rates may change over time and rates may differ depending on the methodology used. A recent study investigated suicide in the South Asian diaspora in the UK to try to confirm the low rates in older men and high rates in young women. Previous studies had mainly used place of birth to identify people of South Asian origin. Calculating suicide rates for ethnic minorities in any other way in the UK is difficult because only the place of birth is recorded on death certificates. Though place of birth was a reasonable proxy measure when the South Asian origin population of the UK were mainly first generation, now that 50% are born in the UK, its utility has waned. A new method with good validity, sensitivity and specificity is to use computer-based names algorithms. Suicide rates were calculated between 1993 and 2003 using the South Asian Name and Group Recognition Algorithm (SANGRA) computer software. The age-standardized suicide rate for men of South Asian origin was lower than for other men in England and Wales, and the rate for women of South Asian origin was only marginally raised. Contrary to previous studies, the suicide rate in young women of South Asian origin was lower than that for women in England and Wales but the suicide rate in those over 65 years was double that of England and Wales. Older, rather than younger, women of South Asian origin seem to be an at-risk group. Over the 11 years of the study the suicide rate in women of South Asian origin had decreased (McKenzie et al., 2008).

The reasons for the changes in suicide rates may follow the 4-D model. At an individual level, suicide is complex and a number of factors across a life course influence risk. Increasing educational achievement and changing socio-economic situations may have had an influence (Gunnell & Lewis, 2005). At an ecological level, the UK South Asian origin group is composed of people of Bangladeshi, Pakistani, Indian and mixed origins. The findings could reflect differences in the composition of the South Asian origin population over time. The Pakistani and Bangladeshi origin populations are younger than the Indian population. Their proportion in the younger population at risk increased over the study period while the proportion of Indian South Asians decreased from 59% to 41%.

The interaction between the individual risk and the ecological risk in the overall suicide rate may come in part because risks vary between sub-groups (Office for National Statistics, n.d., 2002; Weich & McManus, 2002; McKenzie et al., 2003). And it is not clear that traditional risk factors have the same impact on all groups (Raleigh, Bulusu, & Balarajan, 1990). In addition, different religious groups also have different rates of suicide. The Pakistani and Bangladeshi groups are over 90% Muslim, a religion which generally prohibits suicide, while the Indian group is 75% Hindu or Sikh (Commission for Racial Equality, n.d.). Because of religious, socio-economic and socio-cultural factors, different South Asian origin subgroups may have different risk factors for suicide. As the composition of the South Asian origin population varies, so may the rates of suicide.

Time may also be important. All previous studies report rates of suicide for older women of South Asian origin that are similar to or lower than England and Wales, or White comparison groups (Raleigh et al., 1990; Raleigh & Balarajan, 1992a; Raleigh, 1996; Neeleman, Mak, & Wessely, 1997). However, this study reported a marked increase in suicide rates particularly in people aged over 65 years. Older groups remain predominantly of Indian origin so changes are unlikely to reflect changes in the composition of the South Asian origin population. The long-term impact of social risk factors, migration and acculturation may be important but it may also be that bereavement and long-term illness are an issue. The life expectancy of men of South Asian origin is lower than that for England and Wales, leaving an increasing number of bereaved older women of South Asian origin. Older women of South Asian origin are also more likely to suffer from a limiting long-term illness (Evandrou, 2005). Both bereavement and long-term illness are known risk factors for depression and suicide. However, though it may be that the possible differential rate of suicide is due to known risk factors, it is perhaps useful to note that there is little evidence that these risk factors are cross-culturally applicable in the UK.

Another recent study undertook a descriptive analysis of suicide by burning in this group. A population study of all those who died by suicide in England and Wales between 1993 and 2003 inclusive found that 1.77% of suicides in the general population and 8.45% of suicides in the South Asian origin population were by burning (Tuck et al., 2012). The suicide rate by burning was 0.8/100000 person-years for England and Wales and 2.9/100000 person-years for the South Asian origin population. The odds of suicide by burning were increased in the South Asian group as a whole (OR 3.06, 95% CI 2.30 to 4.08). Those born in Asia and Africa were at higher risk than those born in the UK (OR 2.69, 95% CI 2.01 to 3.60 and OR 2.10, 95% CI 1.46 to 3.01, respectively). The increased risk was for those aged 25–64 years. Rather than decreasing with time in the UK, the rate of suicide by burning was still a significant cause of death in the South Asian population in the UK (Tuck et al., 2012). The study found that the suicide rate per 100,000 for all South Asians, in 2001 was 5.50 compared to 9.32 for the population of England and Wales.

When the South Asian group was categorized into religious groups, the suicide rates ranged from a low of 4.39 for Muslims to a high of 8.25 for Hindus. The SMR were 0.88 (0.83–0.95) Hindu, 0.47 (0.42–0.52) Muslim and 0.85 (0.64–1.05) Sikh (Tuck et al., unpublished).

Perhaps the easiest groups to reach for suicide prevention are those in mental health services because they are potentially accessible for targeted interventions. A recent study in the UK found that people of South Asian origin are less likely to be in contact with mental health services; the standardized suicide ratio for those in contact with mental health services in the last year is lower for both South Asian men and women than it is for White men and women; for those who have been admitted to hospital in the last year, the suicide rate is lower for South Asian women but is no different than White for South Asian men. However, there were some differences in risk by age group. In 25–39-year-old women, the standardized suicide ratio was nearly three times higher in the South Asian group if this is coupled with the lack of difference in population rates of suicide from the SANGRA analysis detailed above, thus, it is reasonable to conclude that people of South Asian origin in this age group who commit suicide are three times more likely to have been in contact with services in the previous year.

Taken together, these studies indicate that, on a population level, those of South Asian origin with higher comparative risks are South Asian older women, with men and Muslims at lower risk. Suicide by burning is an important issue. And for those in contact with services, women in the 25–39 age group are particularly at risk, though, in general, risk in South Asian groups is either the same or lower than the White population. Given the differences in rates of suicide, different age groups that are at risk and different methods of suicide, generic suicide prevention strategies may have differential impacts on the South Asian origin population compared to the ethnic majority population in England and Wales. So in the UK if the aim was to ensure equitable outcomes from the national suicide prevention strategy, there would need to be a mitigation strategy to ensure that the initiatives are equally effective. Clearly as things change, there would also need to be a data and research strategy to ensure that timely and up-to-date information on trends is available.

Suicide prevention in Canada

The situation in Canada is even more complex than in the UK but the research effort with regards to ethnic minority groups would seem to be a long way behind. After the development of the UK suicide prevention strategy, a black and minority ethnic groups suicide prevention project was commissioned (Department of Health, 2002; 2005; National Institutes for Mental Health in England, 2003). It succeeded in summarizing the literature, developing the evidence base, identifying possible avenues for future research and outlining suggestions for targeted initiatives. The overwhelming message was that there was a need for more information and better information so that they could be confident that services are equitable, and that black and minority ethnic groups are benefiting from the success of the suicide prevention strategy. Specific initiatives to improve public awareness, staff skills as well as research and development were proposed by stakeholders.

The research reports from the UK on the South Asian origin population, plus the Canadian research, demonstrate a trend towards higher suicide attempts in the Indian origin population and different trends in the Chinese origin population. This points to the need for a deeper investigation of suicide in Canada. In order to develop equitable suicide prevention strategies both at the provincial and national levels, more research on the rates, risks and social processes acting on diverse populations and associated with suicide are needed. The 4-D model may help in organizing thoughts and considering what interventions and at what level may be useful.

Canada can learn a lot from the UK. Rather than including a stream that investigates Canada's diversity after strategies are launched, national and provincial leads could do it from the beginning. As the most diverse country on the planet, it is possible for Canada to lead the way in developing state-of-the-art suicide prevention strategies for all of its people.

References

Ali, J. (2002). Mental health of Canada's immigrants. Supplement to Health Reports, *Statistics Canada Catalogue, 13,* 82-003.

Beiser, M. (1988). Influence of time, ethnicity and attachment on depression in Southeast Asian refugees. *American Journal of Psychiatry, 145,* 46–51.

Bélanger, A., & Molenfant, E. C. (2005). Ethno cultural diversity in Canada: Prospects for 2017. *Canadian Social Trends,* Statistics Canada Catalogue No 11– 008, 18–21.

Bhui, K., Bhugra, D., & Goldberg, D. (2002). Causal explanations of distress and general practitioners' assessments of common mental disorder among Punjabi and English attendees, *Social Psychiatry and Psychiatric Epidemiology, 37,* 37–45.

Canadian Association for Suicide Prevention (CASP) (2010). *The CASP National Suicide Prevention Strategy* (2nd ed.). Winnipeg, Manitoba: CASP. Available at: www.casp.acps.ca (accessed 30 July 2012).

Clarke, D. E., Colantonio, A., Rhodes, A. E., et al. (2008). Pathways to suicidality across ethnic groups in Canadian adults: The possible role of social stress. *Psychological Medicine, 38,* 419–431.

Commission for Racial Equality (n.d.). *A guide to ethnic groups in Britain.* London: Commission for Racial Equality. Available at: http://83.137.212.42/sitearchive/cre/diversity/ethnicity/index.html.

Department of Health (2002). *National suicide prevention strategy for England.* London: Department of Health.

Department of Health (2005). *Delivering race equality and action plan.* London: Department of Health.

Diwan, S., Jonnalagadda, S. S., & Gupta, R. (2004). Differences in the structure of depression among older Asian Indian immigrants in the United States. *Journal of Applied Gerontology, 23,* 370.

Evandrou, N. (2005). Health and well being. In A. Soule, P. Babb, N. Evandrou, S. Balchin, & L. Zealey (Eds.), *Focus on older people* (pp. 39–49). London: Office for National Statistics.

Fenton, S., & Sadiq-Sangster, A. (1996). Culture, relativism and the expression of mental distress: South Asian women in Britain. *Sociology of Health and Illness, 18,* 66–85.

Ghuman, P. A. S. (2000). Acculturation of South Asian adolescents in Australia. *British Journal of Educational Psychology, 70*(3), 305–316.

Gunnell, D., & Lewis, G. (2005). Studying suicide from the life course perspective: Implications for prevention. *British Journal of Psychiatry, 187,* 206–208.

Hansson, E., Tuck, A., Lurie, S., et al. (2010). *Issues and options for improving services for immigrants, ethno-cultural and refugee groups in Canada.* Mental Health Commission of Canada, Calgary. Available at: http://www.mentalhealthcommission.ca/SiteCollectionDocuments/Key_Documents/en/2010/Issues_Options_FINAL_English%2012Nov09.pdf.

Health Canada (2011). *Health Canadians: A federal report on comparable health indicators 2010.* Ottawa, Ontario. Available at: http://www.hc-sc.gc.ca/hcs-sss/pubs/system-regime/index-eng.php.

Hjern, A. (2002). Suicide in first and second generation immigrants in Sweden: A comparative study. *Social Psychiatry and Psychiatric Epidemiology, 37,* 423–429.

Jacob, K. S., Bhugra, D., Lloyd, K. R., et al. (1998). Common mental disorders, explanatory models and consultation behaviour among Indian women living in the UK. *Journal of the Royal Society of Medicine, 91,* 66–71.

Jibeen, T., & Khalid, R. (2010) Predictors of psychological well-being of Pakistani immigrants in Toronto, Canada. *International Journal of Intercultural Relations, 34*(5), 452–464**.**

Karasz, A. (2005). Cultural differences in conceptual models of depression. *Social Science and Medicine, 60,* 1625–1635.

Kennedy, M. A., Parhar, K. K., Samra, J., et al (2005). Suicide ideation in different generations of immigrants. *Canadian Journal of Psychiatry, 50,* 353–356.

Kirmayer, L., Brass, G., Holton, T., et al. (2007a). *Suicide among Aboriginal people in Canada.* The Aboriginal Healing Foundation, Ottawa, Canada. Available at www.ahf.ca/downloads/suicide.pdf (accessed 15 January 2012).

Kirmayer, L. J., & Minas, I. H. (2000). The future of cultural psychiatry: An international perspective. *Canadian Journal of Psychiatry, 45,* 438–446.

Kirmayer, L. J., Weinfeld, M., Burgos, G., et al. (2007b). Use of health care service for psychological distress by immigrants in an urban multicultural milieu. *Canadian Journal of Psychiatry, 52*(5), 295–304.

Lai, D. W. L., & Surood, S. (2008). Predictors of depression in aging South Asian Canadians. *Journal of Cross-Cultural Gerontology, 23*, 57–75.

Lawrence, V., Banerjee, S., Bhugra, D., et al. (2006a). Coping with depression in later life: A qualitative study of help-seeking in three ethnic groups. *Psychological Medicine, 36*, 1375–1383.

Lawrence, V., Murray, J., Banerjee, S., et al. (2006b). Concepts and causation of depression: A cross-cultural study of the beliefs of older adults. *The Gerontologist, 46*(1), 3–32.

Malenfant, E. C. (2004). Suicide in Canada's immigrant population. *Health Reports, 15*, 9–17.

McCabe, R., & Priebe, S. (2004). Explanatory models of illness in schizophrenia: Comparison of four ethnic groups. *British Journal of Psychiatry, 185*, 25–30.

McKenzie, K., Bhui, K., Nanchahal, K., et al. (2008). Suicide rates in people of South Asian origin in England and Wales: 1993–2003. *British Journal of Psychiatry, 193*, 406–409.

McKenzie, K., Serfaty, M., & Crawford, M. (2003). Suicide in minority ethnic groups. *British Journal of Psychiatry, 183*, 100–101.

Mehta, S. (1998). Relationship between acculturation and mental health for Asian Indian immigrants in the United States. *Genetic, Social, and General Psychology Monographs, 124*(1), 61–78.

Mental Health Commission of Canada (2009). Toward recovery & well-being: A framework for the Mental Health Strategy for Canada. Available at: http://www.mentalhealthcommission.ca/SiteCollection Documents/boarddocs/15507_MHCC_EN_final.pdf (accessed 21 July 2011).

Mental Health Commission of Canada (2012a). *Changing directions, changing lives: The mental health strategy for Canada.* Calgary: AB.

Mental Health Commission of Canada (2012b). Catalyzing action around suicide prevention. Available at: http://www.mentalhealthcommission.ca/English/Pages/Catalyzing_Action_Suicide_Prevention_ENG. aspx (accessed 30 July 2012).

Mental Health Commission of Canada (2012c). National collaborative for suicide prevention. Mental Health Commission of Canada Knowledge Exchange Centre Available at: https://kec.mentalhealth commission.ca/communities_initiatives/ncsp (accessed 30 July 2012).

Ministry of Health and Long Term Care (2010). Respect, recovery and resilience: Recommendations for Ontario's mental health and addiction strategy. The Minister's Advisory Group on the 10 year mental health and addictions strategy. Available at: http://www.health.gov.on.ca/en/public/publications/ ministry_reports/mental_health/mentalhealth_rep.pdf.

Nanchahal, K., Mangtani, P., Alston, M., et al. (2001). Development and validation of a computerized South Asian Names and Group Recognition Algorithm (SANGRA) for use in British health-related studies. *Journal of Public Health Medicine, 23*, 278–285.

National Institutes for Mental Health in England (2003). *National Suicide Prevention Strategy for England: Annual report on progress.* London: Department of Health.

Neeleman, J., Mak, V., & Wessely, S. (1997). Suicide by age, ethnic group, coroners' verdicts and country of birth: A three-year survey in inner London. *British Journal of Psychiatry, 171*, 463–467.

Office for National Statistics (n.d.). Ethnicity: education. Available at: http:/www.statistics.gov.uk/ CCI/nugget.asp?ID=268&Pos=3&ColRank=2&-Rank=1000 (accessed May 2007).

Office for National Statistics (2002). *Ethnicity: Labour market.* London: The Stationery Office. Available at: http://www.statistics.gov.uk/CCI/nugget.asp?ID=271&Pos=4&ColRank=2&Rank=1000.

Office for National Statistics (2007). *Population estimates by ethnic group, 2001–2005 (experimental).* London: The Stationery Office. Available at: http://www.statistics.gov.uk/statbase/Product.asp?vlnk=14238.

Office for National Statistics (2013). *2011 Census: Detailed characteristics for local authorities in England and Wales.* Available at: http://www.ons.gov.uk/ons/publications/re-reference-tables.html?edition=tcm% 3A77-306085.

Patel, S. P., & Gaw, A. C. (1996). Suicide among immigrants from the Indian subcontinent: A review. *Psychiatric Services, 47*, 517–521.

Raleigh, V. S. (1996). Suicide patterns and trends in people in Indian subcontinent and Caribbean origin in England and Wales. *Ethnicity & Health, 1*, 55–63.

Raleigh, V. S., & Balarajan, R. (1992a). Suicide levels and trends among immigrants in England and Wales. *Health Trends, 24*, 91–94.

Raleigh, V. S., & Balarajan, R. (1992b). Suicide and self-burning among Indians and West Indians in England and Wales. *British Journal of Psychiatry, 161* 365–368.

Raleigh, V. S., Bulusu, L., & Balarajan, R. (1990). Suicides among immigrants from the Indian subcontinent. *British Journal of Psychiatry, 156*, 46–50.

Rodney, P., & Copeland, E. (2009). The health status of Black Canadians: Do aggregated racial and ethnic variables hide health disparities? *Journal of Health Care for the Poor and Underserved, 20*(3), 817–823.

Sadavoy, J., Meier, R., & Ong, A. Y. M. (2004). Barriers to access to mental health services for ethnic seniors: The Toronto study. *Canadian Journal of Psychiatry, 49*(3), 192–199.

Sainsbury, P., & Barraclough, B. (1968). Differences between suicide rates. *Nature, 220*, 1252.

Samuel, S. (2010). Mating, dating and marriage: Intergenerational cultural retention and the construction of diasporic identities among South Asian immigrants in Canada. *Journal of Intercultural Studies, 31*(1), 95–110.

Shah, J., Mizrahi, R., & McKenzie, K. (2011). The four dimensions: A model for the social aetiology of psychosis. *British Journal of Psychiatry, 199*, 11–14.

Singh-Carlson, S., Neufeld, A., & Olson, J. (2010). South Asian immigrant women's experiences of being respected within cancer treatment settings. *Canadian Oncology Nursing Journal, 20*, 188–189.

Somasundaram, D. (2010). Using cultural relaxation methods in post-trauma care among refugees in Australia. *International Journal of Culture and Mental Health, 3*(1), 16–24.

Statistics Canada (2008). *Ethnic origin and visible minorities, Release no. 7.* Available at: http://www12.statcan.gc.ca/census-recensement/2006/rt-td/eth-eng.cfm.

Statistics Canada (2010). *Population projections for Canada, provinces and territories 2009 to 2036.* Available at: http://www.statcan.gc.ca/pub/91-520-x/91-520-x2010001-eng.htm.

Statistics Canada (2011). *Proportion of foreign-born and visible minority populations by census metropolitan area, 2006 and 2031.* Available at: http://www.statcan.gc.ca/daily-quotidien/100309/t100309a1-eng.htm.

Surood, S., & Lai, D. W. L. (2010). Impact of culture on use of western health services by older South Asian Canadians. *Canadian Journal of Public Health, 101*(2), 176–180.

Tiwari, S. K., & Wang, J. L. (2008). Ethnic differences in mental health service use among White, Chinese, South Asian and South East Asian populations living in Canada. *Social Psychiatry and Psychiatric Epidemiology, 43*(11), 866–871.

Tuck, A., Bhui, K., Nanchahal, K., et al. (2012). Suicide by burning in the South Asian origin population in England and Wales: A secondary analysis of a national data set. *BMJ Open 2011*, 1, e000326. doi:10.1136/bmjopen-2011-000326.

Tuck, A., Bhui, K., Nanchahal, K., et al. (unpublished). Religion and suicide in the South Asian origin population in England and Wales.

Tran, K., Kaddatz, J., & Allard, P. (2005). South Asians in Canada: Unity through diversity. *Canadian Social Trends: Statistics Canada Catalogue No. 11-008*, 20–25.

US Department of Health and Human Services (2001). *Mental health: Culture, race and ethnicity. A supplement to mental health: A report of the Surgeon General.* Rockville, MD: US Department of Health and Human Services, Substance Abuse and Mental Health Services Administration, Center for Mental Health Services.

Weich, S., & McManus, S. (2002). Common mental disorders. In K. Sproston, & J. Nazroo (Eds.), *Ethnic minority psychiatric rates in the community.* London: The Stationery Office.

Whitley, R., Kirmayer, L. J., & Groleau, D. (2006). Understanding immigrants' reluctance to use mental health services: A qualitative study from Montreal. *Canadian Journal of Psychiatry, 51*(4), 205–209.

Wu, Z., Noh, S., Kaspar, V., et al. (2003). Race, ethnicity, and depression in Canadian society. *Journal of Health and Social Behavior,* Special Issue: Race, Ethnicity, and Mental Health, *44*(3), 426–441.

Xu, M. A., & McDonald, J. T. (2010). The mental health of immigrants and minorities in Canada: The social and economic effects. *Canadian Issues, Summer*, 29–32.

10

SUICIDE-RELATED BEHAVIOUR IN CHINESE WOMEN

Illustrating the role of cultural conceptions of gender in understanding and preventing suicide

Juveria Zaheer, Paul S. Links, Samuel Law, Wes Shera, A Ka Tat Tsang, Catherine Cheng, Alan Fung and Pozi Liu

Introduction

Suicide is a major international public health concern. Each year, approximately one million people die of suicide worldwide; this number may even represent an underestimate due to variability on reporting practices across countries, shame and stigma, and religious, cultural and legal traditions (Hendin et al., 2008). In almost every country in the world, women have higher rates of suicidal ideation and behaviour, but lower rates of death by suicide than men. Canetto and Sakinofsky (1998) labeled this phenomenon the "gender paradox" of suicidal behaviour, and it is most striking in industrialized nations, specifically English-language countries such as Canada, the United States, Great Britain, Canada and Australia (S. Canetto, 2008). Studies have also shown that more than 90% of suicides meet criteria for a *Diagnostic and Statistical Manual of Mental Disorders*, Fourth Edition (DSM-IV) psychiatric illness, and mood disorders have been associated with about 60% of suicides (Mann et al., 2005). Along with mental illness and male sex, established risk factors for suicide also address the availability of lethal means, alcohol and drug abuse, access to psychiatric treatment, attitudes to suicide, help-seeking behaviour, physical illness, marital status, and age.

The "gender paradox" of suicidal behaviour identifies males as being at higher risk of death by suicide than women, and women as having higher risk for non-fatal suicidal behaviour (S. Canetto & Sakinofsky, 1998). Suicide prevention strategies have focused on addressing risk factors in high risk groups, with a strong focus on the identification and treatment of mental illness, specifically depression. While research in suicide prevention has considered the importance of cultural diversity, it has focused largely on developing programs that are of potential use for any population in any part of the world (Mishara, 2006). It is crucial to consider the important role that cultural factors may play in the etiology and prevention of suicide. As Mishara suggests, we assume commonalities, guidelines, methods of prevention and clinical practices would need only language translation and minor adaptation to a region's culture and mental health delivery system. However, universality does not explain the wide variability of suicide rates, demographics, attitudes and methods seen cross-culturally.

This chapter will discuss gender and cultural factors related to suicidal behaviour by exploring the limitations of the "gender paradox" of suicidal behaviour. By accepting this belief as a manifestation of basic differences in the nature of men and women, we do not appreciate that this finding is not constant across cultures and ignore our own cultural biases. The chapter will consist of four parts: (1) a review of the demographics of gender and suicide worldwide; (2) a review of the prevailing cultural discourses of gender and suicide; (3) an illustration of gender and cultural factors and suicide in Chinese women; and (4) a discussion describing how knowledge of gender and cultural factors can be applied to suicide prevention. We will focus on ways to examine these differences and apply the findings in practice, with a description of a novel study as an example of qualitative work in this field.

In this chapter, we will conceptualize "sex" as the physiological characteristics related to reproduction, and "gender" as the phenomena and issues related to social and cultural influences (S. Canetto, 2008). "Culture" will be defined as "a product of people living together and creating traditions, patterns norms and values that manifest as a pattern in a specific group of people", as per Joe et al.'s (2008) article focusing on the advancement of culturally focused research on suicide prevention. Suicide-related behaviour will refer to self-inflicted, potentially injurious behaviour for which there is evidence (either explicit or implicit) either that (1) the person wished to use the appearance of attending to kill him or herself in order to attain some end; or (2) the person intended at some undetermined or some known degree to kill him or herself (Silverman, Berman, Sanddal, O'Carroll, & Joiner, 2007). Suicide-related behaviours comprise self-harm, undetermined suicide-related behaviours, and suicide attempts (Silverman et al., 2007).

Demographics of suicide by sex

Although suicide rates vary widely from country to country, in almost every country in the world, males have higher rates of death by suicide, while women have higher rates of non-fatal suicide-related behaviour. In general, suicide rates are highest in Eastern Europe and lowest in Central and South America; rates seen in the United States, Western Europe and Asia tend to fall in the middle (Nock et al., 2008) . Although the ratio of male to female suicide rates tends to be quite high (3.1–7.5 to 1) in North America and Europe, the difference is less pronounced in other parts of the world, specifically Asia (S. Canetto, 2008; Nock et al., 2008). As we will discuss, China is the only country in the world where women die by suicide more than men do. In this section, we present a brief review on the differences in suicide rates by sex in several countries worldwide.

In the United States, suicide represents the eleventh leading cause of death for all ages at a rate of 11/100,000 (Centers for Disease Control (CDC), 2007). According to CDC data, males die by suicide at nearly four times the rate of females and represent 79.0% of all US suicides, while women engage in suicide-related behaviour with intent to die about 2 to 3 times more often than men (Centers for Disease Control (CDC), 2009). No group differences are seen in suicide rates until mid-adolescence; at this time the rate among males rises significantly (Nock et al., 2008). Firearms are the most commonly used method of suicide among males and poisoning is the most common method seen in female deaths by suicide (Centers for Disease Control (CDC), 2009). Suicide rates are the highest for males aged 75 or older (35.7/100,000) (Centers for Disease Control (CDC), 2007). Certain cultural groups are at higher risk for death by suicide, such as American Indian and Alaskan Native adolescents, who have a suicide rate 1.8 times higher than the national average for that group (Centers for Disease Control (CDC), 2009).

Elsewhere in North America, almost 4000 Canadians die by suicide each year and many more deliberately harm themselves. While significantly more men die by suicide than women at a rate of 3.2:1, women are at significantly greater risk than men for non-fatal suicide attempts (Langlois & Morrison, 2002). In Mexico, the age-standardized suicide rate from 1980–2006 is lower than those observed in the US and Canada (4.9/100,000 for males, 0.9/100,000 for females), but a significant male to female ratio of 5:1 is seen (Milner, McClure, & De Leo, 2012). This pattern (lower absolute rates of suicide than those seen in North America or Europe but significant differences in male and female rates) rates are in keeping with those seen in Central and South America (Milner et al., 2012).

European countries consistently show higher rates of death by suicide in males and higher rates of suicide-related behaviour in females. According to World Health Organization data, the average suicide rates in Europe are 13.9/100,000, with the highest rates seen in Russia and other former Soviet Republics (Marusic & Farmer, 2001). With respect to suicide-related behaviours, the World Health Organization/Euro Multicentre Project on Parasuicide used data from 16 centres in 13 European countries to assess trends on the epidemiology of suicide attempts (Schmidtke et al., 1996). Suicide attempts were defined as a deliberate act of self-harm or ingestion of a substance in excess of what is therapeutic in order to realize change via the actual or expected physical consequences. Average age-standardized rates of suicide attempts were 136/100,000 for males and 186/100,000 for females. In 15 of 16 centres, the suicide attempt rates were higher among women, ranging from 69/100,000 in Guipuzcoa, Spain, to 462/100,000 in Cergy-Pontoise, France (Schmidtke et al., 1996)

Although significant variability is seen in suicide rates across Asia, most countries do show significantly higher rates of male suicide. The Republic of Korea has a high suicide rate 28.4 per 100,000 (Cheong et al., 2012). A large-scale study using cause of death source data indicated that males have a suicide rate of 33.2/100,000 compared with 15.8/100,000 for women, a ratio of approximately 2:1 (Cheong et al., 2012). In Japan, data show a male to female ratio of 2.7 (Kim, Kim, Kawachi, & Cho, 2011). These ratios are lower than those typically seen in North and South America and Europe.

In India, the suicide rate can be difficult to quantify; many researchers believe the rates in the literature are artificially low due to vast underreporting of deaths by suicide (Manoranjitham, Jayakaran, & Jacob, 2006). As per World Health Organization data, the overall suicide rate in India is 13/100,000 for men and 7.8/100,000 for women, a ratio of 1.7:1 (WHO, 2012). In Steen and Meyer's (2004) review of modernization and the male–female suicide ratio in India from 1967 to 1997, the male to female suicide ratio ranged from 1.27:1 to 1.51:1. They found that male and female suicide rates co-varied over the time period relative to each other, and commented on the difficulty in finding trends in suicide ratio data in a developing country that has major social and regional disparities (Steen & Meyer, 2004). Patel et al.'s (2012) study used a nationally representative mortality survey of deaths between 2001 and 2003 to quantify suicide mortality in India in 2010. They estimated age-standardized suicide rates for those ages 15 or older to be 26.3/100,000 for men and 17.5/100,000 for women, a ratio of 1.5:1 (Patel et al., 2012). This ratio is lower than the more typical over 3:1 ratio seen in most countries in the world.

Based on recent estimates, China's suicide rate is estimated to be approximately 23/100,000, which is approximately 2 to 3 times the global average (Ma et al., 2009). In percentages, China has 21% of the world's population, but 44% of world's total suicides, and 56% of the world's female suicides (Phillips, Li, & Zhang, 2002). This translates to close to 300,000 suicide deaths in China each year (Phillips et al., 2002). China has a unique problem with suicide as the Chinese national reports on suicide have shown a strong reversal of the international trend: in those who are under age 60, female rates exceed male rates by an average of 26%, with rural female rates exceeding rural male rates by 66% (Murray & Lopez, 1996; Ji, Kleinman, & Becker, 2001). While male sex has consistently been considered a risk factor for suicide and female sex has been considered a risk factor for non-fatal suicide-related behaviour, this is not consistent worldwide. Two countries, India and China, do not show a significantly higher rate of male suicide; however, these two countries contain more than one-third of the world's population and cannot be discounted simply as having an "atypical" pattern (Nock et al., 2008). A further exploration of gender and suicide is required to identify at-risk groups and to understand the ways in which gender and culture influence suicide-related behaviour and can be targeted in prevention strategies.

Exploring the relationship between cultural conceptions of gender and suicide

Although it is taken for granted in suicide research that women engage in higher levels of suicide-related behaviour while men are more likely to die by suicide, this "gender paradox" is not constant within or across countries, and cultural factors must be considered (Canetto, 2008). Rather than only being seen as an outcome in males with mental illness, suicide should also be viewed as a cultural and gender-bound phenomenon. Cultural and social determinants of suicide may sanction behaviour among males and females, and social construction of gender plays a crucial role in the way individuals perceive their options and communicate distress (Chung, 2004; Cleary, 2012). It is important to note that gender is only one social construction of human experience and other factors including psychiatric illness, ethnicity, social class, and sexual orientation also are important to consider in suicide research (Canetto & Lester, 1998).

The cultural diversity in gender patterns and interpretations of suicide-related behaviour cannot be explained by epidemiology or oppressive life circumstances, and cultural meanings of gender and suicide-related behaviours have been studied in order to better understand this diversity. Sylvia Canetto (2008) proposed a cultural script theory of suicide-related behaviour, suggesting that the "collective implicit beliefs about the meaning of suicidal behavior – including when it is a possibility and what form it takes – determine the ways in which behaviors are given significance and legitimacy and guide responses to suicidal behavior". This section will explore the relationship between cultural conceptions of gender and patterns of suicide and suicide-related behaviour in countries where the "gender paradox" of suicide-related behaviour is seen and examine the cultural scripts of suicide-related behaviour in men and women. We will also discuss the ways in which subscribing to gender-based assumptions of suicide-related behaviour can be problematic in understanding and preventing suicide.

In most countries in the world, men die of suicide approximately three to seven times more often than women, while women are more likely to experience non-fatal suicidal ideation and behaviour (Nock et al., 2008). As Anne Cleary (2012) describes, explanations for this finding have ranged from essentialist and biological arguments to simply accounting for men's preference for using more lethal methods. However, in countries where the gender paradox of suicidal behaviour is documented, non-fatal and fatal suicidal behaviours are often considered "naturally" gendered – killing oneself is perceived as masculine while non-fatal suicide-related behaviour is considered feminine (Canetto, 2008). Cultural and sociological explanations of this finding have often betrayed gender bias. Emile Durkheim hypothesized that suicide requires a degree of energy, courage and intelligence found only in men, implying that women were too unsophisticated and timid to die by suicide (Canetto, 2008). Although this perspective is not widely held today, it does speak to a way of understanding men and women in binary, oppositional terms (Cleary, 2012).

Based on these binary notions, suicide in males has often been portrayed as rational, with causation related to work or economic spheres (Cleary, 2012). With respect to older men, the masculine protector and provider role can be lost through unemployment, retirement and illness (Oliffe, Han, Ogrodniczuk, Phillips, & Roy, 2011). Braswell and Kushner (2012) hypothesized that high rates of male suicide in the US military may be linked to fatalistic aspects of military masculinity. In Mensah Adinkrah's (2012) qualitative research with suicide experience-related men in Ghana, subjects connected the pursuit of masculine ideals in shaping suicide-related behaviour. They described shame in not meeting economic responsibilities and associated the expression of distress and help-seeking as feminine (Adinkrah, 2012).

Although it is reasonable to assume that both men and women are suffering from some kind of distress prior to engaging in suicide-related behaviour, the ways in which emotions are expressed are highly gendered. Emotional expression has been seen as a feminine trait, and men may be less likely to express negative emotions (Cleary, 2012). Men who subscribe to traditional male gender roles may be also be less likely to seek help (Houle, Mishara, & Chagnon, 2008). The adverse impacts of the traditional male gender role as well as male reluctance to seek help have been posited as factors that increase their risk of suicide. These hypotheses were tested by Houle et al. (2008), who compared two groups of men who had experienced comparable severely stressful life events during the past 12 months with and without a history of suicide-related behaviour. A strongly held belief in the traditional male gender role appeared to increase the risk of suicide-related behaviour by undermining their mental state and by inhibiting protective facets of help seeking and social support (Houle, Mishara, & Chagnon, 2008). In Desaulniers and Daigle's (2008) study, men at higher risk for suicide were found to have lower education but higher income, tended to associate emotional reticence with virility, and were less comfortable with non-fatal suicidal acts. Studies have also described male sex-role stereotyping and the ideology of self-reliance as risk factors for suicide in rural Australian males (Robertson & Fitzgerald, 1992). High-risk men may also be less open about their suicide intentions and men who present to the emergency department intoxicated and suicidal face many barriers to getting proper mental health assessments and care (Links et al., 2007). In a study of men with recurrent suicide-related behaviour in the emergency department, one-half scored high and another quarter scored moderate on alexithymia testing, and frustration was felt by both patients and staff regarding difficult communication, especially during an acute crisis (Strike, Rhodes, Bergmans, & Links, 2006). Heisel (2006) identified social isolation as well as white race, mental illness, personality vulnerability, medical illness and social isolation as risk factors for suicide-related behaviour in older men. Men at risk for suicide may be less likely to seek help from their female partners in order to protect them and for fear of appearing un-masculine (Cleary, 2012). Stigma and reluctance to seek help may lead to self-medicating depression and suicidal ideation with substance use as a by-product of stigma, which may contribute to lower rates of clinically diagnosed depression and higher rates of suicide (Oliffe, Han, Ogrodniczuk, Phillips, & Roy, 2011).

While dying by suicide has traditionally been associated as masculine, non-fatal suicide-related behaviour has often been characterized as feminine (Canetto, 2008). Feminist theorists highlight the problematic language used to describe suicide-related behaviour as an example of gender inequality (Range & Leach, 1998). Suicidal acts that do not result in death, seen more often in women, are often described as "attempted suicide", while dying by suicide, seen more often in men, is often called completed suicide, implying that women are unsuccessful even when they survive (Range & Leach, 1998). As Dahlen and Canetto (2002) discuss, in the United States, suicide tends to be viewed more negatively if the person who died is female, as killing oneself is seen as a masculine act. On the other hand, Dahlen and Canetto point out that non-fatal suicide-related behaviour is often perceived as feminine, youthful behaviour; for example, young women receive more sympathy for suicidal behaviour than men or older women (Stillion, White, Edwards, & McDowell, 1989).

Accepting gendered explanations of suicide-related behaviour without examining these assumptions can have deleterious consequences for men and women at risk for suicide. While male suicide is receiving attention as a focus for prevention, little research attempts to understand their individual experiences. By researching suicide by using only a macro-level, quantitative framework, we rely on gender assumptions that tend to adopt unitary notions of men, as well as binary, oppositional concepts of masculinity and femininity (Cleary, 2012). Anne Cleary's (2012) work of in-depth interviews with 52 young Irish men who made a suicide attempt examines suicidal behaviour and found that these men experienced high levels of emotional pain but had problems identifying symptoms and disclosing distress. By examining and challenging gender-based assumptions of suicidal behaviour, new opportunities for suicide prevention strategies can emerge, for example, establishing and evaluating interventions focused on identifying at-risk men, supporting emotional expression of distress, and working to reduce stigma.

Widely held gender assumptions can lead to inappropriate generalizations about suicide across populations. For example, Mac An Ghaill and Haywood (2012) suggest caution in identifying and explaining pre-adolescent suicide-related behaviour. They suggest that the media accounts reporting a rise in pre-adolescent suicidal behaviour tend to explore suicide through simplistic dyadic categories of male and female, suggesting that boys and men appear to share the same lifestyle challenges. However, their work suggests that existing models of masculinities may not be able to capture the generational specificities of boys – boys can get caught in these narratives and do not account for other important social and cultural codes (Mac An Ghaill & Haywood, 2012).

Gender assumptions can also have negative effects with respect to suicide prevention in women. Researchers have hypothesized that changing gender roles for women, including education, employment, and independence would put them at higher risk for suicide, although this has not been borne out in research studies (Platt & Hawton, 2000). Accepting gender assumptions may lead to potentially ignoring improved education and employment as potential interventions for decreasing the risk of suicide in women.

Gender assumptions can also be problematic cross-culturally. Cultural insensitivity has also been seen in sociological discussions of suicide; suicide was seen an act of civilized men, and primitive and simple people (including women and non-Western societies) were incapable of doing so (Canetto, 2008). In other cultures with higher than expected rates of women's suicide, we may see ideologies that call for a woman's suicide under certain conditions, and suicide can be explicitly defined as a feminine behaviour or sign of weakness (Canetto, 2008). Further, certain minority groups may be at higher risk for suicide based on discourses of suicide-related behaviour. For example, data from the Netherlands shows that minority women from Turkey, Morocco and South Asia have rates of non-fatal suicide-related behaviour 2–4 times higher than the women comprising the cultural majority (van Bergen, van Balkom, Smit, & Saharso, 2012). Higher rates of suicide-related behaviour in ethnic minority women have also been seen in other countries. Bhugra and Desai's (2002) research on the high rate of suicide-related behaviour in South Asian women in the UK could not be explained by increased rates of depression and they suggested culture conflict as a potential explanation. In van Bergen's work, participants described gender-role related themes of self-sacrifice and lack of autonomy and described the cultural value of female endurance. They also described suicidal behaviour as a way of managing to survive and protesting their victimization (van Bergen et al., 2012).

As Sylvia Canetto's (1997) work on gender and suicide states, "Gender is whatever a culture defines and prescribes as masculine and feminine – culturally specific and transient – can only be understood contextually." She posited that the cultural diversity in gender patterns and interpretations of suicide-related behaviour challenges essentialist perspectives on gender and suicide-related behaviour and she points to the pitfalls of theorizing about clinical phenomena as if they were culture-free, and calls for culturally grounded theory, research and practice.

Cultural conceptions of gender and suicide in Chinese women

Suicide-related behaviour is complex and multifactorial, and culture, social and sociopolitical stress and stigma must be considered. These factors can shape the ways in which suicide-related behaviour is understood in the context of gender role and shapes the cultural scripts of suicide. The next section of this chapter will discuss these cultural and gender factors to better understand the high rates of death by suicide in Chinese women, both in China and in North America.

Cultural factors

Suicide is rarely depicted as a mental health issue in China. Suicide-related behaviour is rarely found in medical or psychiatric textbooks, and has been conceptualized as a response to social stress and act of free will rather than as part of a mental illness (Ji, Kleinman, & Becker, 2001). "Diu mianzi", or loss of face, is a powerful cultural construct that has cultural relevance in suicide-related behaviour (Pritchard, 1996). The fear of shame is very powerful and suicide may be a culturally sanctioned means for resolving interpersonal conflict or as a morally sanctioned act (Pritchard, 1996). Religious beliefs have been considered protective against suicide-related behaviour. However, this may not be the case in rural China, as individuals who die by suicide have been found to be more likely than controls to be religious and believe in the afterlife (Zhang, Conwell, Zhou, & Jiang, 2004). Suicide may be seen as morally acceptable under particular circumstances as Confucian doctrine allows suicide as expression of high moral or emotional protest (Zhang & Xu, 2007). Fei (2005) discusses the relationship between cultural beliefs and family structure, describing the important role of family conflict and the importance of "Qi", which was translated as "the origin and essence of the universe . . . a vital fluid in the human body, encompassing air, breath and vigor". Its psychological meaning implies "both dignity and anger". Fei theorizes suicide is often a result of power dynamics in the family and a result of impulsive anger, closely tied with the significance of moral capital and the concept of saving face. Impulsive suicide-related behaviour is conceptualized as a "trump card"; it is an unimpeachable defence of one's dignity in these complex power games (Fei, 2005).

Social factors that may impact suicide include disintegration of traditional supports for the elderly and various economic changes and stressors accompanying economic reforms; suicide cases tend to be likely to be poor, less educated and unemployed, and rural suicides are more likely to occur during the summer months and in daytime, secondary to pesticide availability in farming communities (Zhang et al., 2004).

Social change in China may explain some trends in suicide rates in urban and rural China. Elderly suicide has decreased significantly in urban areas, perhaps influenced by improvement in long-term care systems, and a general improvement in living conditions and educational opportunities in rural China may have led to decreasing rates of suicide in rural areas (Yip, Liu, Hu, & Song, 2005). Further measures such as reducing taxes on farmers were also suggested (Yip et al., 2005).

Gender factors

Chinese women have higher rates of suicide-related behaviour and suicide than men, and significant differences in cultural patterns and interpretations of suicide. As we have described, in Western countries, suicide is seen as a masculine act and "failing at suicide" is feminine. For Chinese women, however, suicide can be considered to be a feminine "act of the powerless" and males exhibiting suicide-related behaviour are seen as effeminate or weak (Canetto, 2008).

Rural suicides largely account for the unusually high female suicide rates in China. Yip et al. (2001) examined years of life lost (YLL) from 1990–2000 using data from the Ministry of Health in China. Some 90% of YLL resulted from rural suicide with rural women aged 25–39 contributing the largest share of YLL. Pearson, Phillips, He, and Ji (2002) found that suicide-related behaviour in young rural women was characterized by high levels of impulsivity, little effort to seclude themselves and low rates of mental illness, including depression. Some 29% of women reported taking the poison in front of someone else and 65% were found within five minutes of the attempt. Common interpersonal stressors included an unhappy marriage (65%), financial problems (43%), spousal abuse (38%), changed routines (33%), conflict with mother-in-law (32%), and a large loan (24%) (Pearson et al., 2002). Traditional Chinese cultural values may put women at a disadvantage because in family disputes or crisis, women are typically blamed (Zhang & Xu, 2007). A study of men and women admitted for suicide-related behaviour to six hospital emergency departments in a rural area of North-eastern China found family and love crises occur in 61% of females compared to 40% of males; females also showed significantly higher levels of metempsychosis (a culturally bound desire to transform to the opposite gender) than males and non-suicidal female controls, perhaps indicative of this gender inequality (Zhang & Xu, 2007). China's one-child policy, instituted in 1979, must also be considered in a discussion of gender. In rural areas, a second child is generally allowed after five years, but this may only apply if the first child is female, highlighting the traditional preference for male children; gender ratios in rural areas is 1.17:1, significantly higher than before the policy was instituted (Hesketh, Lu, & Xing, 2005). In one study, 60% of Chinese fathers respond coldly to the birth of a female child (Aubert, Daigle, & Daigle, 2004). Women may also face considerable emotional and financial stress from family planning workers with respect to contraception, abortion and sterilization (Hesketh et al., 2005).

A common presentation of suicide in rural China involves a young woman who lives in a highly conflicted family environment and has openly voiced that she feels her life is worthless; subsequently, the young woman impulsively ingests pesticides after an acute family conflict (Zaheer et al., 2011). Rural women have low status, restricted economic options, and significant gender role conflict with kin, for example, being forbidden to go to high school, limiting their choice of marriage partner, or sexual assault; married women can be isolated from their family of origin and often experience conflict with mothers-in-law (Zaheer et al., 2011). He and Lester (1998) suggest that for women in rural China, suicide is not considered a mental health issue but rather a strategy available to powerless people to influence the behaviour of others, or for a powerless individual to exact revenge upon those who have made their lives intolerable. The act of suicide can bring tension to a community and shame to the victim's family, who are seen to have caused this extreme action by relentless persecution of the victim (Canetto, 2008). Rural men have a wider arsenal to fight social problems due to possessing more status and power; they often live in the same area of their families and do not have to manage in-law stress and social isolation, seek formal legal recourse, or move to a different community; a man who attempts suicide would be using a traditionally female coping strategy and may be perceived as weak or effeminate (Canetto, 2008).

Women of Chinese descent in North America

In the US, Asian American women aged 15–24 and over 65 have the highest rate of female suicide across all racial/ethnic groups (Noh, 2007). These statistics highlight the importance of cultural background and gender on rates of suicide. Recent studies have highlighted themes of gender role stress of Asian-born women and women of Asian descent residing in North America who have experienced suicidal ideation and behaviour, including conflict between traditional and Western female roles (Chung, 2004). Eliza Noh's (2007) examination of the narratives of Asian American women who have attempted suicide suggested that over-reliance on Western psychotherapeutic philosophy and the systematic minimization of racial and sexual subjugation result in a lack of understanding of the issues that these women face. Irene Chung (2004) posited that Asian American women resort to suicide-related behaviour to express their emotional distress rather than engaging in externalizing behaviour such as substance use, and that their distress did not manifest in functional decline or seeking help from family, friends or mental health services. Alternatively, Aubert et al. (2004) hypothesize that a narrowing in rates of suicidal ideation in male and female Chinese Canadian students compared to their Chinese counterparts can be explained by a reduction in gender role stress, as gender equality is established by law and evident in daily life. They suggested that while Chinese women were clearly identified as second-class citizens, with a lower social status than men, women who immigrate to Canada enjoy better social status and greater control of lives, while Chinese men may lose some social status and control (Aubert et al., 2004).

Several studies of suicide-related behaviour in Asian American women have described stressors related to the "Model Minority" myth. Irene Chung (2004) describes this myth as ascribing a gender role to women that is compliant, hard-working, disciplined, and leading a stable and promising life. A perceived failure of women to live up to the expectations of family and culture, as well as the ways in which they are perceived by the dominant culture, can lead to stress within the family, psychological distress, and impact help seeking behaviour, and can cause internal and external conflict in terms of the ways in which this identity is rejected or accepted.

Familial obligations and stresses related to gender have been described in the accounts of Chinese women with suicide-related behaviour as well as women of Chinese background living in North America. For example, Canetto and Lester (1998) describe the ways in which childlessness or failure to produce a son may trigger abuse and eventual suicide-related behaviour in Chinese women. In a study of Asian American female college students with a history of suicide-related behaviour, the expectation that women should take care of parents, succeed academically and sacrifice their own interests to show love was noted as a significant stressor (Chung, 2004).

Suicide prevention informed by research on cultural conceptions of gender

Suicide studies research has stressed the importance of individual-level suicide prevention strategies based on modifying universal risk factors over population-level culturally informed suicide prevention strategies. Certainly, individual-based interventions hold value in suicide prevention. In Mann's (2005) systematic review of suicide prevention strategies, physician education in depression recognition and treatment and restricting access to lethal methods did reduce suicide rates. However, by utilizing only universal, quantitative frameworks, we cannot appreciate the variability and impact of cultural scripts in suicide prevention. Earlier in this chapter, we outlined the importance of qualitative studies geared to challenging the binary concepts of masculinity and femininity to better understand the individual experiences of those at risk for suicide and suicide-related behaviours. This knowledge can help inform culturally appropriate suicide prevention strategies. We also discussed gender and cultural factors that shape suicide and suicide-related behaviours in Chinese women in China and North America. In this section, we will describe a novel qualitative study aiming to explore the relationship between gender, culture and suicide-related behaviour that is being undertaken jointly between the University of Toronto in Toronto, Canada, and Tsinghua University in Beijing, China.

In this study, 30 women from Beijing, China, and 30 women of Chinese descent from the Greater Toronto Area in Canada with a history of suicide-related behaviour will be interviewed in order to explore their experiences. We are interested in examining the impact of gender as a social and cultural construction on their lives, including self-image, relationships, ways of coping, and the communication of distress. We will explore narratives of suicide-related behaviour presented by the informants, with respect to the chosen course of action, the impressions of suicide-related behaviour by the community, and the "typical actors", conflicts, and emotions attributed as causes in order to better understand cultural scripts of suicide-related behaviour in this group of women (Canetto, 1998).

A qualitative analysis of the impact of social and cultural conceptions of gender on the meanings and experiences of suicidal behaviour in Chinese-Canadian women is needed for several reasons. While the impact of gender role stress has been postulated as a risk factor for suicide, the need for further evidence, specifically an understanding and appreciation of their experiences, has been stressed in the literature. As Noh (2007) points out, while studies of suicide in women of Asian descent in North America often recognize "psychosocial stressors" as a risk factor, empirical studies, specifically from the perspectives of the women themselves, are scarce. Pearson and Liu (2002) suggest that further studies are needed to address the impact of social stress and inequality on Chinese women, specifically those in rural areas, and the lack of social and economic support to manage this stress.

Joe et al. (2008) have recommended qualitative ethnographic studies in order to appreciate the complex experiences of ethnic minorities. Qualitative methods may be more culturally congruent with the preferred modes of communication compared with more structured, Western diagnostic interviews, and can be adapted to different ethnic groups. Integrating cross-cultural research with well-known risk and protective factors can increase the understanding of how ethnicity, culture and social factors mediate the risk of suicide. Prevention researchers must consider the relevance of cultural values, customs and strengths to determine the preferred way for community members to manage crisis situations. Stigma regarding mental illness and suicidal behaviour in communities can have significant clinical and prevention implications and can exert considerable influence on the perception, implementation, delivery and outcome of interventions (Joe, Canetto, & Romer, 2008). An accurate depiction of community perspectives, in this case, an understanding of the experiences of Chinese and Chinese-Canadian women with suicidal behaviour, is crucial in the development of appropriate and effective screening and service provision (Hicks & Bhugra, 2003). Furthermore, if gender-related stress is identified as a specific risk factor for suicidal behaviour, new possibilities for prevention, treatment and intervention can be developed and studied (Hicks & Bhugra, 2003).

Conclusion

Suicide and suicide-related behaviours constitute a major public health concern worldwide. While men generally have higher rates of death by suicide and women have higher rates of non-fatal suicide-related behaviours, these differences are related to complex factors and are not consistent across all cultures. Research in suicide prevention must consider the importance of cultural conceptions of gender in order to better understand the experiences of those who are at risk for suicide and suicide-related behaviours. Cultural and gender factors can shape the ways in which suicide and suicide-related behaviours are understood and carried out. Preventative intervention research design should consider and adapt to cultural and social context, as culture is a reflection of values, history and patterns of behaviour in a group of people, and can exert considerable influence on the perception, implementation, delivery and outcome of interventions.

A specific discussion of the impact of cultural conceptions of gender on suicidal behaviour in Chinese women and women of Chinese descent in North America underscores the importance of qualitative research strategies in suicide prevention.

Acknowledgements

Parts of this chapter have been adapted from:

Zaheer, J., Links, P. S., Law, S., Shera, W., Hodges, B., Tsang, A. K. T., et al. (2011). Developing a matrix model of rural suicide prevention. *International Journal of Mental Health*, *40*(4), 28–49. doi:10.2753/IMH0020-7411400403.

References

Adinkrah, M. (2012). Better dead than dishonored: Masculinity and male suicidal behavior in contemporary Ghana. *Social Science & Medicine (1982)*, *74*(4), 474–481. doi:10.1016/j.socscimed.2010.10.011.

Aubert, P., Daigle, M. S., & Daigle, J.-G. (2004). Cultural traits and immigration: Hostility and suicidality in Chinese Canadian students. *Transcultural Psychiatry*, *41*(4), 514–532. doi:10.1177/1363461504045647.

Bhugra, D., & Desai, M. (2002). Attempted suicide in South Asian women. *Advances in Psychiatric Treatment*, *8*(6), 418–423. doi:10.1192/apt.8.6.418.

Braswell, H., & Kushner, H. I. (2012). Suicide, social integration, and masculinity in the U.S. military. *Social Science & Medicine (1982)*, *74*(4), 530–6. doi:10.1016/j.socscimed.2010.07.031.

Canetto, S. (2008). Women and suicidal behavior: A cultural analysis. *The American Journal of Orthopsychiatry*, *78*(2), 259–66. doi:10.1037/a0013973.

Canetto, S., & Sakinofsky, I. (1998). The gender paradox in suicide. *Suicide & Life-threatening Behavior*, *28*(1), 1–23. Available at: http://www.ncbi.nlm.nih.gov/pubmed/9560163.

Canetto, S. S. (1997). Meanings of gender and suicidal behavior during adolescence. *Suicide & Life-threatening Behavior*, *27*(4), 339–51. Available at: http://www.ncbi.nlm.nih.gov/pubmed/9444729.

Canetto, S. S., & Lester, D. (1998). Gender, culture, and suicidal behavior. *Transcultural Psychiatry*, *35*(2), 163–190. doi:10.1177/136346159803500201.

Centers for Disease Control (CDC) (2007). WISQARS (Web-based Injury Statistics Query and Reporting System). Available at: http://www.cdc.gov/injury/wisqars/index.html (accessed September 30, 2012).

Centers for Disease Control (CDC). (2009). Suicide facts at a glance. Available at: http://www.cdc.gov/ViolencePrevention/pdf/Suicide-DataSheet-a.pdf (accessed September 30, 2012).

Cheong, K.-S., Choi, M.-H., Cho, B.-M., Yoon, T.-H., Kim, C.-H., Kim, Y.-M., & Hwang, I.-K. (2012). Suicide rate differences by sex, age, and urbanicity, and related regional factors in Korea. *Journal of Preventive Medicine and Public Health*, *45*(2), 70–7. doi:10.3961/jpmph.2012.45.2.70.

Chung, I. (2004). Examining suicidal behavior of Asian American female college students. *Journal of College Student Psychotherapy*, *18*(2), 31–47. Retrieved from http://www.tandfonline.com/doi/abs/10.1300/J035v18n02_04.

Cleary, A. (2012). Suicidal action, emotional expression, and the performance of masculinities. *Social Science & Medicine (1982)*, *74*(4), 498–505. doi:10.1016/j.socscimed.2011.08.002.

Dahlen, E., & Canetto, S. (2002). The role of gender and suicide precipitant in attitudes toward nonfatal suicidal behavior. *Death Studies*, *26*(2), 99–116. Available at: http://www.tandfonline.com/doi/abs/10.1080/074811802753455235.

Desaulniers, J., & Daigle, M. S. (2008). Inter-regional variations in men's attitudes, suicide rates and sociodemographics in Quebec (Canada). *Social Psychiatry and Psychiatric Epidemiology*, *43*(6), 445–453. doi:10.1007/s00127-008-0340-2.

Fei, W. (2005). "Gambling for Qi": Suicide and family politics in a rural North China county. *The China Journal*, *54*(July), 7–27. Available at: http://www.jstor.org/stable/10.2307/20066064.

He, Z. X., & Lester, D. (1998). Methods for suicide in mainland China. *Death Studies*, *22*(6), 571–579. doi:10.1080/074811898201407.

Heisel, M. J. (2006). Suicide and its prevention among older adults. *Canadian Journal of Psychiatry/Revue canadienne de psychiatrie*, *51*(3), 143–154. Available at: http://www.ncbi.nlm.nih.gov/pubmed/16618005.

Hendin, H., Phillips, M. R., Vijaykumar, L., Pirkis, J., Wang, H., Yip, P., et al. (2008). *Suicide and Suicide Prevention in Asia.* Available at: http://wwwlive.who.int/entity/mental_health/resources/suicide_prevention_asia_firstpages.pdf.

Hesketh, T., Lu, L., & Xing, Z. W. (2005). The effect of China's one-child family policy after 25 years. *The New England Journal of Medicine, 353*(11), 1171–1176. doi:10.1056/NEJMhpr051833.

Hicks, M. H.-R., & Bhugra, D. (2003). Perceived causes of suicide attempts by U.K. South Asian women. *The American Journal of Orthopsychiatry, 73*(4), 455–462. doi:10.1037/0002-9432.73.4.455.

Houle, J., Mishara, B. L., & Chagnon, F. (2008). An empirical test of a mediation model of the impact of the traditional male gender role on suicidal behavior in men. *Journal of Affective Disorders, 107*(April), 37–43.

Ji, J., Kleinman, A., & Becker, A. E. (2001). Suicide in contemporary China: A review of China's distinctive suicide demographics in their sociocultural context. *Harvard Review of Psychiatry, 9*(1), 1–12. Available at: http://www.ncbi.nlm.nih.gov/pubmed/11159928.

Joe, S., Canetto, S. S., & Romer, D. (2008). Advancing prevention research on the role of culture in suicide prevention. *Suicide & Life-threatening Behavior, 38*(3), 354–362. doi:10.1521/suli.2008.38.3.354.

Kim, S. Y., Kim, M.-H., Kawachi, I., & Cho, Y. (2011). Comparative epidemiology of suicide in South Korea and Japan: Effects of age, gender and suicide methods. *Crisis, 32*(1), 5–14. doi:10.1027/0227-5910/a000046.

Langlois, S., & Morrison, P. (2002). Suicide deaths and suicide attempts. *Health Reports, 13*(2), 9–19. Available at: http://sites.google.com/site/victimass2/statCanLangloisMorrisonSuicideCanada.pdf.

Links, P., Strike, C., Ball, J., Bergmans, Y., Rhodes, A. E., Spence, J. M., et al. (2007). The experience of suicidal, substance-abusing men with severe personality disorders in the emergency department. *Personality and Mental Health, 1*(1), 51–61. doi:10.1002/pmh.

Ma, X., Xiang, Y.-T., Cai, Z.-J., Li, S.-R., Xiang, Y.-Q., Guo, H.-L., et al. (2009). Lifetime prevalence of suicidal ideation, suicide plans and attempts in rural and urban regions of Beijing, China. *The Australian and New Zealand Journal of Psychiatry, 43*(2), 158–166. doi:10.1080/00048670802607170.

Mac An Ghaill, M., & Haywood, C. (2012). Understanding boys' thinking through boys, masculinity and suicide. *Social Science & Medicine (1982), 74*(4), 482–429. doi:10.1016/j.socscimed.2010.07.036.

Mann, J. J., Apter, A., Bertolote, J., Beautrais, A., Currier, D., Haas, A., et al. (2005). Suicide prevention strategies: A systematic review. *JAMA: The Journal of the American Medical Association, 294*(16), 2064–2074. doi:10.1001/jama.294.16.2064.

Manoranjitham, S. D., Jayakaran, R., & Jacob, K. S. (2006). Suicide in India. *The British Journal of Psychiatry: The Journal of Mental Science, 188*, 86. doi:10.1192/bjp.188.1.86.

Marusic, A., & Farmer, A. (2001). Genetic risk factors as possible causes of the variation in European suicide rates. *The British Journal of Psychiatry, 179*(3), 194–196. doi:10.1192/bjp.179.3.194.

Milner, A., McClure, R., & De Leo, D. (2012). Socio-economic determinants of suicide: An ecological analysis of 35 countries. *Social Psychiatry and Psychiatric Epidemiology, 47*(1), 19–27. doi:10.1007/s00127-010-0316-x.

Mishara, B. L. (2006). Cultural specificity and universality of suicide. *Crisis: The Journal of Crisis Intervention and Suicide Prevention, 27*(1), 1–3. doi:10.1027/0227-5910.27.1.1.

Murray, C., & Lopez, A. (1996). *The global burden of disease: A comprehensive assessment of mortality and disability from diseases, injuries and risk factors in 1990 and projected to 2020.* Cambridge, MA: Harvard University Press. Available at: http://www.ennonline.net/resources/490.

Nock, M. K., Borges, G., Bromet, E. J., Cha, C. B., Ronald, C., & Lee, S. (2008). Suicide and suicidal behavior. *Epidemiologic Reviews, 30*(1), 133–154. doi:10.1093/epirev/mxn002.Suicide,

Noh, E. (2007). Asian American women and suicide. *Women & Therapy, 30*(3), 87–107. Retrieved from http://www.tandfonline.com/doi/abs/10.1300/J015v30n03_08.

Oliffe, J. L., Han, C. S. E., Ogrodniczuk, J. S., Phillips, J. C., & Roy, P. (2011). Suicide from the perspectives of older men who experience depression: A gender analysis. *American Journal of Men's Health, 5*(5), 444–54. doi:10.1177/1557988311408410.

Patel, V., Ramasundarahettige, C., Vijayakumar, L., Thakur, J. S., Gajalakshmi, V., Gururaj, G., et al. (2012). Suicide mortality in India: A nationally representative survey. *Lancet, 379*(9834), 2343–2351. doi:10.1016/S0140-6736(12)60606-0.

Pearson, V., & Liu, M. (2002). Ling's death: An ethnography of a Chinese woman's suicide. *Suicide and Life-threatening Behavior, 32*(4), 347–359. Retrieved from http://onlinelibrary.wiley.com/doi/10.1521/suli.32.4.347.22338/full.

Pearson, V., Phillips, M. R., He, F., & Ji, H. (2002). Attempted suicide among young rural women in the People's Republic of China: Possibilities for prevention. *Suicide & Life-threatening Behavior, 32*(4), 359–369. Available at: http://www.ncbi.nlm.nih.gov/pubmed/12501961.

Phillips, M. R., Li, X., & Zhang, Y. (2002). Suicide rates in China, 1995–99. *Lancet, 359*(9309), 835–840. doi:10.1016/S0140-6736(02)07954-0.

Platt, S., & Hawton, K. (2000). Suicidal behaviour and the labour market. In K. Hawton, & K. van Heeringen (Eds.), *The international handbook of suicide and attempted suicide*. Chichester: John Wiley & Sons, Ltd.

Pritchard, C. (1996). Suicide in the People's Republic of China categorized by age and gender: Evidence of the influence of culture on suicide. *Acta psychiatrica Scandinavica, 93*(5), 362–367. Available at: http://www.ncbi.nlm.nih.gov/pubmed/8792906.

Range, L. M., & Leach, M. M. (1998). Gender, culture, and suicidal behavior: A feminist critique of theories and research. *Suicide & Life-threatening Behavior, 28*(1), 24–36. Available at: http://www.ncbi.nlm.nih.gov/pubmed/9560164.

Robertson, J. M., & Fitzgerald, L. F. (1992). Overcoming the masculine mystique: Preferences for alternative forms of assistance among men who avoid counseling. *Journal of Counseling Psychology, 39*(2), 240–246. Available at: http://www.eric.ed.gov/ERICWebPortal/search/detailmini.jsp?_nfpb=true&_&ERICExt Search_SearchValue_0=EJ451099&ERICExtSearch_SearchType_0=no&accno=EJ451099.

Schmidtke, A., Bille-Brahe, U., De Leo, D., Kerkhof, A., Bjerke, T., Crepet, P., et al. (1996). Rates, trends and sociodemographic characteristics of suicide attempters during the period 1989–1992: Results of the WHO/EURO Multicentre Study on Parasuicide. *Acta Psychiatrica Scandinavica, 93*(5), 327–338. Available at: http://onlinelibrary.wiley.com/doi/10.1111/j.1600-0447.1996.tb10656.x/abstract.

Silverman, M. M., Berman, A. L., Sanddal, N. D., O'Carroll, P. W., & Joiner, T. E. (2007). Rebuilding the tower of Babel: A revised nomenclature for the study of suicide and suicidal behaviors. Part 2: Suicide-related ideations, communications, and behaviors. *Suicide & Life-threatening Behavior, 37*(3), 264–277. doi:10.1521/suli.2007.37.3.264.

Steen, D. M., & Meyer, P. (2004). Modernization and the male-female suicide ratio in India 1967–1997: Divergence or convergence? *Suicide & Life-threatening Behavior, 34*(2), 147–159. Available at: http://www.ncbi.nlm.nih.gov/pubmed/15191271.

Stillion, J. M., White, H., Edwards, P. J., & McDowell, E. (1989). Ageism and sexism in suicide attitudes. *Death Studies, 13*(3), 247–261. doi:10.1080/07481188908252302.

Strike, C., Rhodes, A. E., Bergmans, Y., & Links, P. (2006). Fragmented pathways to care. *Crisis: The Journal of Crisis Intervention and Suicide Prevention, 27*(1), 31–38. doi:10.1027/0227-5910.27.1.31.

van Bergen, D. D., van Balkom, A. J. L. M., Smit, J. H., & Saharso, S. (2012). "I felt so hurt and lonely": Suicidal behavior in South Asian-Surinamese, Turkish, and Moroccan women in the Netherlands. *Transcultural Psychiatry, 49*(1), 69–86. doi:10.1177/1363461511427353.

WHO (2012). World Health Organization: Suicide prevention (SUPRE). Available at: September 30, 2012, from http://www.who.int/mental_health/prevention/suicide/suicideprevent/en/.

Yip, P. S. (2001). An epidemiological profile of suicides in Beijing, China. *Suicide & Life-threatening Behavior, 31*(1), 62–70. Available at: http://www.ncbi.nlm.nih.gov/pubmed/11326769.

Yip, P. S. F., Liu, K. Y., Hu, J., & Song, X. M. (2005). Suicide rates in China during a decade of rapid social changes. *Social Psychiatry and Psychiatric Epidemiology, 40*(10), 792–798. doi:10.1007/s00127-005-0952-8.

Zaheer, J., Links, P. S., Law, S., Shera, W., Hodges, B., Tsang, A. K. T., et al. (2011). Developing a matrix model of rural suicide prevention. *International Journal of Mental Health, 40*(4), 28–49. doi:10.2753/IMH0020-7411400403.

Zhang, J., Conwell, Y., Zhou, L., & Jiang, C. (2004). Culture, risk factors and suicide in rural China: A psychological autopsy case control study. *Acta Psychiatrica Scandinavica, 110*(6), 430–437. doi:10.1111/j.1600-0447.2004.00388.x.

Zhang, J., & Xu, H. (2007). The effects of religion, superstition, and perceived gender inequality on the degree of suicide intent: A study of serious attempters in China. *Omega, 55*(3), 185–197. Available at: http://www.pubmedcentral.nih.gov/articlerender.fcgi?artid=3205909&tool=pmcentrez&rendertype=abstract.

11

MATRIX MODEL FOR SUICIDE PREVENTION

Focus on Canada and India

Paul S. Links, Juveria Zaheer, Rahel Eynan and Amresh Srivastava

Introduction

Studies have consistently shown differences in suicide rates and demographics between urban and rural areas in countries in several parts of the world, including English-speaking Western countries, Scandinavia, Eastern and Central Europe, and Asian countries including Japan, India, and Sri Lanka (Hirsch, 2006). Suicide research on epidemiology, service utilization and prevention strategies tend to focus on urban areas, resulting in a conceptualization of suicide which may not be applicable to rural populations (Hirsch, 2006). Rural areas have differing geographical, socioeconomic, political and cultural characteristics that must be considered in the development and implementation of evidence-based suicide prevention strategies. Many countries have identified rural suicide as a major public health concern and share common challenges in developing prevention strategies. Our earlier collaborations focused on the commonalities and differences found between suicide in Canada and China (Zaheer et al., 2011–12). This chapter describes the collaborative effort to understand suicide from an international perspective, focusing on Canada and India.

Collaborating across international boundaries can clarify the impact of culture as a causal factor in suicide. A comparison focusing on culture, social and political factors, beliefs and attitudes can improve understanding of other cultures while deconstructing one's own system to better understand needs, strengths and challenges related to suicide prevention. Feedback from others can serve as an alternative measure of the effectiveness of a country's policies, practices and ideas, while facilitating reflexive practice and the identification of assumptions underlying policies and practices (Bairstow, 2000). Lastly, Canada has a large population of Indian-born Canadians and Canadians of Indian descent, and cultural factors are important to suicide prevention for these groups.

The chapter begins by highlighting the demographic characteristics of suicide in the two countries. We then describe the essential elements of the matrix model for suicide prevention in rural areas and some specific research to demonstrate how the model may be applicable to studying these two different countries. Finally, the chapter ends with a description of plans for our initial steps in collaborating between Canada and India. Our collaboration includes completion of a needs assessment for suicide prevention and testing suicide prevention training for primary health care workers in the Mumbai region of India.

Suicide in Canada

In Canada for 2009, the national suicide rate was 11.5/100,000 with significantly more men dying by suicide than women at a rate of 3.2:1 (Statistics Canada, 2012; http://www.statcan.gc.ca/tables-tableaux/sum-som/l01/cst01/hlth66d-eng.htm; accessed August 28, 2012). Men have higher suicide rates than women in every age group, while women are at significantly greater risk than men for non-fatal suicide attempts (Langlois & Morrison, 2002). Rural and frontier areas of Canada have an overall suicide rate of 41 per 100,000, significantly higher than the overall rate (Hirsch, 2006). Rural farming communities have shown higher suicide rates than the national average (Pickett, King, Faelker, & Bienfeld, 1999), and Aboriginal populations in rural areas are at an even higher risk for suicide (Haggarty, Cernovsky, Bedard, & Merskey, 2008).

Major depressive disorder (MDD) is a major risk factor for suicidal behavior in Canada, with estimated rates of MDD in 65% of persons with suicidal behavior (Blackmore et al., 2008). Rural areas, however, have shown lower rates of 12-month prevalence of MDD than urban areas, after controlling for the effects of race, immigration status, working status and marital status; however, rural residents with MDD were significantly less likely to access mental health services (Wang, 2004). An investigation of suicidality in the Arctic Inuit community found high rates of suicidal ideation within the past week of the study (43.6%) and suicide attempts within the last month (30%), but did not find a significant relationship between depressed mood and suicidal behavior (Haggarty et al., 2008).

The most common method of suicide in Canada is suffocation, principally hanging or strangulation, followed by poisoning, which includes drug overdoses and inhalation of motor vehicle exhaust, followed by firearms (Langlois and Morrison, 2002). Females were much more likely to use poisonings and much less likely to use firearms than males (Langlois and Morrison, 2002). The evidence suggests that suicide in rural versus urban areas is more influenced by social and cultural factors and therefore, these factors must be considered along with mental illness when developing suicide prevention initiatives.

Suicide in India

In India, the number of suicides alone is equivalent to the total number of suicides in the four European countries with the highest number of suicides (Bertolote & Fleischmann, 2002). In the past three decades the rate of suicide in India increased by 43% and most recent official statistics indicate that 134,599 individuals died by suicide in 2010 (National Crimes Record Bureau (NCRB), 2010). One of the most recent estimates of the suicide rate in India came from a nationally representative mortality survey of deaths between 2001 and 2003; this survey provided an estimate of 187,000 deaths due to suicide in individuals aged 15 years or older (Patel et al., 2012). In contrast to the phenomenon observed in high-income countries where suicides rates increase with age, suicide in India is a problem among the young and middle-aged group. The majority of those who died by suicide (71%) were under the age of 44 years. Of the total deaths by suicide in individuals 15 years or older, about 40% of suicide deaths in men and about 56% of suicides in women occurred in young adults aged 15–29 (Patel et al., 2012). The overall aged-standardized suicide rate per 100,000 population at ages 15 years or older was 18.6 for men and 12.7 for women. At the national level the male–female ratio is 2:1, with 63% of suicides occurring among males. In women, the highest suicide rates are seen between the ages of 15 and 24 (109/100,000 population); however, in southern India, the suicide rates are as high as 148/100, 000, one of the highest rates in the world (Aaron et al., 2004). Across India, the suicide rate ranges from 0.5 to 45.9/100,000 population (Aaron et al., 2004). The majority of suicides (60%)

occur in rural areas (National Crimes Record Bureau (NCRB), 2010). The age-standardized death rates at age 15 and older were twice as high in rural compared with urban areas (Patel et al., 2012). Similar to suicides observed in other rural areas in other parts of the world, self-poisoning, involving the ingestion of agricultural pesticides accounted for nearly half of suicides in India. Self-poisoning was the leading method of suicide for both men (49%) and women (44%). Hanging was the second most used method in both men (35%) and women (26%).

Suicide reports from India highlight a complex array of risk factors that are associated with suicide among them: family problems and interpersonal relationship (29.2%) and illness (22.3%). Intertwined with these factors are characteristics of rural reality: low literacy level, poverty, failure of crops, growing costs of cultivation, heavy debt burden, unemployment, alcoholism, easy access to means of suicide, and poor access to emergency medical care (National Crimes Record Bureau (NCRB), 2010; Patel et al., 2012). Presently, there are approximately 3000 psychiatrists, 500 clinical psychologists, 400 psychiatric social workers, and 900 mental health nurses in India (Sinha & Kaur, 2011). Thus the ratio of mental health professional to population is extremely low. Government mental health programs are primarily directed towards the severely mentally ill. Issues such as suicide prevention are not specifically mentioned, suggesting they have a low priority and thus making these important services inaccessible to the community. Only 9% of 269 suicide decedents had been in contact with a mental health professional or family physician or were in treatment before their suicide (Gururaj, Isaac, Subbakrishna, & Ranjani, 2004). Considering the enormous socio-cultural plurality and economic disparities between developing and developed countries, interventions from Western countries are unlikely to be germane to the existing social realities of developing countries such as India (e.g. health care delivery practices).

Suicide prevention in India: complex socio-cultural challenges

The phenomenology of suicide behavior is quite different in India as opposed to Western countries. Many barriers exist related to understanding and studying suicide in India. The foremost challenge in moving forward on suicide prevention in India is the legal position of suicide, which is a punishable offense. This prevents people from reporting suicide to hospitals in order to avoid the legal problems, consequently leading to suicide being unreported and untreated. In addition, Jacob (2008) listed inefficient civil registration systems, non-reporting of deaths, variable methods of death certification and social stigma as obstacles to studying suicide.

In India, suicide is recognized as a social problem rather than a medical one; therefore, a response from the medical perspective is challenged as unhelpful. Milner and Sveticic (2012), in a review of published psychological autopsy studies, observed that about 66% of suicide cases remained without an axis I diagnosis in the studies examined, 37% did not have any sub-threshold/mild conditions to account for suicide. Similarly, Parkar, Nagarsekar and Weiss (2009) reported from a cohort of 94 women and 104 men that many patients (50% of women and 41.3% of men) did not fulfill the criteria for any diagnosis, or did so only for an adjustment disorder or a V-code. Manoranjitham et al. (2010) examined the relative contributions of psychosocial stress and psychiatric morbidity to suicides in a rural Indian population from the state of Tamil Nadu in southern India and found that ongoing stress and chronic pain significantly contributed to the model associated with suicides, and psychiatric morbidity did not enter the model. According to Jacob, suicide in India is generally associated with social and economic adversity, and cultural discord; thus, "psychiatric interventions aimed at recognizing and treating mental illness alone will not have a major impact on reducing suicide in the developing world" (2008, p. 104).

Instead, Jacob (2008) called for "population-based approaches" that included macroeconomic policies, programs to meet basic human needs, changing a culture that accepts suicide as a means to resolve personal misery, the restriction of pesticides, equity for women, and media guidelines for suicide reporting. Although Jacob (2008) also argued that the identification of high risk individuals in terms of their psychiatric diagnosis and need for treatment is unlikely to have any impact on the overall suicide rates in India, thus, it is unclear what the impact of improved recognition and treatment of common psychiatric diagnoses such as alcoholism and depression might be. Some recent attempts at suicide prevention with individuals identified as having psychiatric problems are discussed later in the chapter.

In spite of these complexities, training and education regarding individuals at risk are less than adequate for a range of people who might interface with these individuals at risk. While the Central and State Governments in India have been regularly conducting training programs for primary care physicians working in rural and urban areas (Behere & Behere, 2008), training opportunities for non-physician mental health professionals are lacking (WHO, 2001; Vijayakumar, 2010). The undergraduate medicine psychiatric curriculum has only recently been improved (Thirunavukarasu, 2007) but as the vast majority of suicides occur in rural areas, there is a dire need for training and services in these areas. Training of health and non-health professionals can change the negative attitudes (Srivastava & Tiwari, 2012) and facilitate intervention and referrals at the grass-root level. However, the training, particularly of other health professionals and staff beyond physicians, is far too inadequate to meet the requirements (Barua, 2009). Conducting learning needs assessment prior to implementation of training programs will help improve acceptance and adherence, and overcome challenges such as health care providers not having the requisite skills and expertise to implement a recommended action and to deliver or practice recommendations (Grant, 2002). We discuss our plans to carry out a needs assessment in Mumbai, India, at the end of the chapter.

The matrix model for suicide prevention

The matrix model of suicide prevention has been developed to address the risk factors for rural suicides through evidence-based interventions aimed at targeted populations (Zaheer et al., 2011–12). The matrix model of suicide prevention can be responsive to epidemiological, cultural and social variability within rural areas worldwide, while constructing a replicable protocol that can be evaluated in an evidence-based manner. The model will incorporate evidence for rural suicide prevention, examine the applicability of general suicide prevention measures to rural areas, and identify the impact of cultural, social, geographical, economic and gender factors which can mediate suicide risk in rural areas and may be common across several countries. The matrix model framework consists of four columns that address: rural risk factors for suicide, evidence-based interventions, targets of the intervention, and evaluation strategies.

The first column of the matrix model of rural suicide prevention will focus on targeting specific risk factors for rural suicide described in the literature, including limited access to care, social and geographic isolation, access to means, and stigma and cultural considerations (Hirsch, 2006). The second column of the matrix model focuses on identifying evidence-based interventions for suicide prevention, as described in the Mann et al. (2005) review. Communities can identify priorities based on their community profile and the model is flexible enough to address financial or infrastructure limitations. The third column of the matrix model will focus on the targets of the intervention. Each community will have a profile of high-risk populations, health care providers or community members, and mental health workers, and can select an appropriate target from the options identified in the matrix model. The fourth column will focus on the evaluation of the chosen targeted intervention, by providing a framework of appropriate, measurable outcomes geared to the intervention.

The ongoing cross-cultural collaboration has illustrated the importance of addressing shared risk factors for rural suicide. However, many differences exist in terms of system delivery, patterns of isolated populations, means of suicide, and cultural issues. The matrix model is designed to accommodate these differences within an evidence-based framework. We will apply the matrix model to both populations by identifying and describing the four identified risk factors for rural suicide, matching the risk factor with an evidence-based intervention, selecting the target of the intervention, and choosing the appropriate evaluation strategy.

First column: identifying risk factors for rural suicide

I Limited access to care

Rural areas may show differences in access to services compared to urban areas, often within the same country. A lack of access to services, including fewer mental health service providers, a lower quality of mental health care, less economic resiliency and undiagnosed and treated mental illness, contributes to the risk of suicide in rural areas (Pesonen et al., 2001; Judd, Cooper, Fraser, & Davis, 2006; Pearce, Barnett, & Jones, 2007; Razvodovsky & Stickley, 2009). Epidemiologic evidence suggests that discrepancies in rural versus urban mental health assessment and care may contribute to the pattern of suicide attempts and suicide in rural India and Canada. Interventions that improve rural health care providers' mental health assessments and management of individuals at risk for suicides and that surmount the risk factors for rural residents are urgently needed. While services can be difficult to access in rural areas of both countries, the role of health systems, attitudes to mental health and roles of mental health workers differ significantly, and need to be considered when choosing appropriate service-based suicide prevention interventions. Both Canada and India share a lack of trained clinicians in rural areas and face barriers in funding, training opportunities, and geographical access.

II Social and geographic isolation

Many countries have shown patterns of increasing suicide with increasing rurality and remoteness, suggesting that social and geographic isolation may be important risk factors for suicide in rural areas (Hirsch, 2006; Middleton et al., 2004). Geographic and social isolation may also limit the availability of social support in times of crisis; rural suicide victims are more likely to have lacked a close intimate relationship than urban suicide victims (Hirsch, 2006).

III Access to means

Rural areas often show differing patterns of methods used for suicide than urban areas, and these differences can be mediated by availability and cultural factors. For example, firearm use is often more common in rural areas in some countries, and as such is more accessible to individuals with suicidal ideation. This trend is seen in several countries, such as Finland, as hunting rifles are much more accessible in rural areas (Hintikka, Lehtonen, & Viinamaki, 1997). While firearm fatalities are less commonly seen in Asia, pesticide self-poisoning is a largely rural phenomenon and the most common method of rural suicide in countries including India and Sri Lanka. Approximately two-thirds of all acute pesticide poisonings in rural areas worldwide are suicidal acts, resulting in an estimated 2,000,000 cases of intentional pesticide poisoning and over 220,000 deaths annually (Hendin et al., 2008).

IV Stigma and cultural considerations

Rural and urban areas often have different conceptions of mental illness and suicide, and increased stigma and other cultural considerations may be risk factors for rural suicide. Although the eminent sociologist Emile Durkheim has been cited in arguments that rural social network and stability confer protection against suicide when compared to its urban counterparts, epidemiological evidence does not support this claim (Kushner & Sterk, 2005). Recent discussions and research on a rural ideology that often promotes a focus on family and community-oriented life, and mental disorders may be stigmatized, deterring rural patients from seeking treatment, and hence contribute to a higher rural suicide rate (Hirsch, 2006). Even when mental health services are available, rural individuals have lower rates of service utilization than their urban counterparts and may turn to physicians or religious leaders instead (Beautrais, 2003). Certain populations who are more likely to reside in rural areas are at increased risk for suicide, including indigenous people and farmers (Miller & Burns, 2008). Finally, culturally bound gender role stress has been linked to rural suicide. Studies have described male sex-role stereotyping and the ideology of self-reliance as a risk factor for suicide in Australian males (Robertson & Fitzgerald, 1992). Gender expectations have also been associated with suicide in rural women; in Sri Lanka, women in rural areas have lower rates of mental illness than in urban areas, but psychological autopsy studies suggest marital and in-law stress and social isolation as risk factors for a higher rate of suicide (Hendin et al., 2008).

Second column: evidence-based strategies for rural suicide prevention

The second column of the matrix model focuses on identifying evidence-based interventions for suicide prevention in order to provide an evidence-based framework for suicide prevention in rural communities addressing the specific risk identified in the first column (Mann et al., 2005). Communities can identify priorities based on their community profile and the model is flexible enough to address financial or infrastructure limitations. The review identified physician education, means restriction and gatekeeper education as interventions with the most evidence, and also reviewed the evidence for psychopharmacology, screening programs, psychotherapies and system collaboration. Although the studies reviewed tend to focus on urban populations, several strategies for suicide prevention have been tested in rural areas. In this section, we will present evidence-based strategies targeted on mediate risk factors for suicidal behavior in rural populations, including access to services, geographic and social isolation, access to means and stigma and cultural considerations.

I Evidence-based strategies for improving access to care

- *Physician education.* Mann et al.'s (2005) review of suicide prevention strategies indicated that physician education increases the number of diagnoses and treatment for depressed patients, and shows accompanying reductions in suicide. In rural areas, it can be difficult for people at risk for suicide to access mental health professionals, and education of general practitioners in high risk areas has been shown to reduce rates of suicide. A large-scale study in Hungary examined the results of a five-year depression-management educational program for GPs and their nurses, implemented through the establishment of a depression treatment clinic and psychiatrist telephone consultation service in the intervention region (Szanto et al., 2007). The annual suicide rate in the intervention region decreased from the five-year pre-intervention average of 59.7 per 100,000 to 49.9 per 100,000. Importantly, in rural areas, the female suicide rate in the intervention region decreased by 34% and increased by 90% in the control region.

- *Gatekeeper education.* Gatekeeper education can be defined as education and training to equip important persons in the community with the knowledge and skills to reduce stigma, facilitate discussion and identify and approach at-risk community members. It can be a key strategy to improving access to care in rural communities. Mann et al.'s (2005) review indicated that gatekeeper education can help reduce suicidal behavior, especially in situations where the roles of gatekeepers are formalized and pathways to treatment are readily available. In many rural communities, people are more likely to seek help from community leaders, including religious leaders and respected elders in the community (Beautrais, 2003). People in rural communities may have greater access to gatekeepers than mental health professionals and the gatekeepers can work to ensure that people at risk access services quickly.

- *Telecommunications.* Telecommunications can be defined as communication over a distance by cable, internet, telephone, or broadcasting. Technology-based interventions may provide assistance in overcoming the lack of mental health manpower in rural areas. Although Mann et al.'s (2005) review did not include telecommunications as an intervention with "most evidence," it may create new opportunities in suicide prevention, research and clinical practice (Krysinska & De Leo, 2007).

II Addressing geographic and social isolation

- *Integrated social programs.* Community-based interventions designed to reduce social isolation and to increase public awareness of suicide have been shown to reduce suicide rates in rural towns (Motohashi, Kanero, Sasaki, & Yamaji, 2007). A key example of reducing suicidal behavior through community-based interventions focused on reducing social isolation in a community-based intervention study for suicide prevention in six towns in the Akita Prefecture of Japan (Motohashi et al., 2007). In this study, public awareness-raising activities using a health promotion approach emphasizing the empowerment of residents and civic participation were conducted. Measures of promoting a sense of purpose among senior citizens and creating a community network were also taken. Suicide rates in intervention towns decreased from 70.8/100,000 in 1999 before the intervention to 34.1/100,000 in 2004, after the intervention. The suicide rate in control towns was 47.8/100,000 before the intervention and 49.1/100,000 after the intervention. Interventions included the creation of a community network to eliminate the sense of psychological isolation found in elderly people, including visits by nurses in snowy weather and to those who are home-bound. Other community-building activities included resident engagement in the research process, lecture meetings, and social awareness activities, such as theatrical performances.

- *Physician and health professional education.* In Motohashi, Kanero, Sasaki, and Yamaji's study, health professional education was also a component of an intervention designed to reduce social isolation. Interventions included a resident-based mental health survey and specialist training on suicide prevention for public health and welfare staff, which then engaged in mental health consultation activities and circulated through the town.

- *Telecommunications.* Interventions including telephone support and crisis hotlines may hold promise as interventions to reduce social isolation in rural populations at risk of suicide (Krysinska & De Leo, 2007). Luxton, June and Kinn (2011) identified three existing technologies that may have an impact on suicide prevention, though, empirical investigation of these strategies is still to be completed. Web-based suicide prevention programs provide around-the-clock access and also ensure the user privacy and anonymity. Outreach via e-mail is being utilized by the Samaritans in the UK and follow-up caring letters are being piloted in US military hospitals (Luxton et al., 2011). In the Netherlands 113Online is a combination of a website and a telephone help-line for suicidal persons, their relatives and bereaved next of kin. The services it provides include crisis intervention, self-tests and brief psychotherapy (Mokkenstorm, Huisman, & Kerkhof, 2012). Mobile devices and Smartphones are being used to assist recently discharged patients to access community services and resources; these new technologies can be effective in reducing homelessness and monitoring for suicide risk after discharge from inpatient care (Forchuk et al., 2008).

III Addressing access to means

• *Means restriction.* Mann et al.'s systematic review of suicide prevention suggests that restricting access to lethal methods decreases suicide by these methods. However, methods vary widely worldwide, and within geographic areas and demographic groups. Suicide prevention strategies should focus on restricting means for the most common methods of suicide within an area, and the possibility of substitution of methods requires ongoing monitoring, as does compliance with restrictions (Mann et al., 2005). Further, some means may lend themselves to restriction through legislation and education, whereas others may be very difficult to regulate.

• An example of a means restriction intervention in rural areas can be found in Sri Lanka. The country has seen a 700% increase in suicide since 1960, which researchers believe is strongly linked to the increased availability of pesticides secondary to the agricultural revolution (Eddleston & Phillips, 2004). Legislation has been enacted in Sri Lanka to regulate production, transportation, storage and sale of pesticides, and Sri Lanka has explored the introduction of locked boxes for pesticide (Hendin et al., 2008). These boxes are found on individual farms or at a central point in the village, and the keys are held by a trusted family member or respected community figure, incorporating aspects of gatekeeper education into means restriction interventions (Vijayakumar, Pirkis, & Whiteford, 2005). Hawton et al. (2009) evaluated the acceptability of these devices in rural Sri Lanka, providing 400 lockable storage devices to four villages, and conducted assessment interviews in rural households. Data on suicide and self-harm were also collected from local hospitals. Initially, only 1.8% of households had been locking up pesticides, and 72.5% of adults and 50.4% of households had easy access to pesticides for adults and children respectively. At 30 weeks, most informants in households reported using a box all the time, and most of the boxes were locked on inspection.

IV Reducing stigma

• *Gatekeeper education.* Although not specific to reducing stigma in rural areas, Knox et al.'s (2003) evaluation of the impact of the US Air Force suicide prevention program on risk for suicide and other outcomes that share underlying risk factors provides good evidence for efforts to target stigma as a modifiable risk factor for suicide. The intervention aimed to reduce stigma about help seeking for mental health and psychosocial problems, enhance understanding of mental health and change social norms and policies. Gatekeeper education was a key component of this strategy; the senior ranks of the Air Force strongly endorsed a radical change in social norms to decrease stigma and worked to sustain these newly stated values. Implementation of the program was associated with a sustained decline in the rate of suicide and other adverse events, including accidental death, homicide and family violence.

Third column: targets of the intervention

The third column of the matrix model will focus on the targets of the intervention. Each community will have a profile of high-risk populations, determined by epidemiological data, which should be targeted for interventions, specifically improving access to care or reducing stigma in these groups. Further, specific targets should be identified for interventions such as gatekeeper education – the community profile will determine the trusted members of the community who come into contact with at-risk subjects. Physician or health professional training interventions will have varying targets based on the primary points of access to care in the community.

Fourth column: evaluation of the strategies

The Kirkpatrick Model of Evaluation will provide a framework to assess the matrix model of rural suicide prevention. The Kirkpatrick Model is an effective and flexible way to measure the outcomes of the matrix model by focusing on four levels of evaluation (Kirkpatrick, 1975). The first level of the Kirkpatrick Model measures reactions, or the perceptions and opinions of the intervention, and is one useful way to evaluate physician and gatekeeper education programs. The second level of the model measures learning, or changes in knowledge, attitudes and skills, for example, interventions designed to reduce stigma in high-risk populations may apply this method of evaluation to measure changes in attitudes towards help seeking. The learning level may also measure knowledge in identifying people at risk for suicide and the symptoms of major depressive disorder in physicians and gatekeepers. Level three of the Kirkpatrick Model is used to measure transfer, or the transfer of behaviors in the real clinical environment. Transfer outcomes may be used to measure changes in pesticide availability, including lock-box utilization or restricted access to purchase pesticides. Finally, level four of the Kirkpatrick Model measures results, or the impact on patient outcomes, for example, reduction in suicide rates compared with a control community, or increased case-finding of at risk persons.

Recent suicide prevention initiatives in Canada and India

Gatekeeper education program to prevent subway suicides in Toronto, Canada

We participated in a developmental-sequential mixed method program evaluation of a gatekeeper education program with a large urban transit commission (Eynan, 2011). The objectives of the gatekeeper education program were (1) to improve positive attitudes toward suicide prevention and the suicidal patron; (2) to increase factual knowledge about suicide and suicide-risk warning signs; and (3) to enhance risk assessment and the intervention skills of staff directly intervening with distressed patrons. Although suicides in the subway were an uncommon event, the transit commission was committed to implementing and evaluating prevention programs that were supported by suicide prevention experts. From the program's inception, the transit commission understood that demonstrating significant reductions of suicides or suicide attempts per year, given the low base rate, was likely to never be demonstrated. However, the transit commission was very aware of the significant impact of suicides on the subway to patrons and staff.

The rationale for a sequential mixed-method approach to program evaluation that included individual interviews with staff following the intervention was enthusiastically supported. The purpose of the qualitative sub-study was to provide the commission information about how the program impacted staff and to obtain in-depth information about the perspectives of the staff regarding the training effects on their knowledge, skills, attitudes, and intervention abilities. The quantitative evaluation involved a repeated measures design testing the participant staff's knowledge, skills and attitudes pre to post training and at three months follow-up. Eligible employees were those staff who attended the workshops during the evaluation period. Some 307 of the 360 attendees (85.3%) of the education program completed the pre and post questionnaires; 150 of 347 (43.2%) attendees completed the follow-up questionnaires. Using a purposive convenience sampling strategy, 30 staff participated in the individual qualitative interviews. A semi-structured interview asked the participants following their participation about their ability to identify distressed patrons at risk for suicide, ability to engage patrons in a direct and open talk about suicide and their comfort and confidence to intervene.

The quantitative results demonstrated significant changes in participant staff's positive attitudes towards suicide prevention pre to post training and at three months follow-up (effect size post = 0.46; follow-up = 0.38; $p < 0.001$). The staff's knowledge of suicide procedures showed significant gains from prior to after the intervention and at three months follow-up (effect size post = 0.28; follow-up = 0.46; $p < 0.001$). The staff's general knowledge about suicide and suicide risk also significantly increased from prior to after the intervention and at three months follow-up (effect size post = 1.02; follow-up = 0.70; $p < 0.001$). Finally, the staff responsible for intervening with distressed patrons demonstrated enhanced intervention responses compared pre to post training and at three months follow-up (effect size post = 0.58; follow-up = 0.92; $p < 0.001$).

The subsequent follow-up interviews added crucial depth to the understanding of the program's value for staff participants. In terms of increased knowledge, one staff responsible for interventions commented on his ability to directly talk about suicide with patrons:

> Just in the way I approach someone, knowing that I am not going to instigate a suicide attempt just by bringing it up in the conversation. I was always trained that [when confronting a person] you just asked 'Is everything okay, you are not thinking of doing anything, are you?' The training taught me to ask directly: 'Are you here to commit suicide?'
>
> *(Constable)*

Another staff member spoke about the changes in his attitudes and his increased awareness:

> It made me understand the reasons, why they may be contemplating suicide. Prior to the course, inside of me, I was angry that they would be wanting this, to disrupt so many people's lives, to interrupt my job, and make my job more difficult. How could they! I would still do what I had to do, but now I tend to be more sympathetic, more concerned for their well-being.
>
> *(Supervisor)*

One staff member discussed the effects of the training to heighten his alertness when on duty:

> You are paying attention a bit more . . . now I walk the platform and if I see anything out of the ordinary . . . Well, just this morning I had a lady standing here for fifteen minutes. I approached her and asked her if she was okay, if there is anything that I can help her with . . . I may not have done that prior to the suicide training.

The use of a mixed-method approach to the program evaluation provided significant and meaningful evidence of the value of the gatekeeper education program (Kral, Links, & Bergmans,

2012). In particular, administrators for the transit commission appeared persuaded about the program's impact by the staff's description of their increased suicide prevention awareness. The transit commission was able to provide ongoing support for the program, in spite of knowing that the actual rate of suicides might or might not be affected. Although the rates of suicide will be analyzed and examined over the longer term, the mixed-method evaluation approach was successful in providing proximal feedback to judge the program's value. With increased awareness of the issue of suicide prevention throughout the organization, the transit commission has moved to actively look at installing barrier doorways on subway platforms to prevent patrons from accessing the subway tracks.

Blueprint for a National Suicide Prevention Strategy in Canada

Canada does not have a National Suicide Prevention Strategy. However, the Canadian Association for Suicide Prevention (CASP) released in October 2004 their Blueprint for a National Suicide Prevention Strategy. The second edition of the CASP strategy was released at their 2009 National Conference in Brandon, Manitoba (CASP, 2009). In spite of this effort, the Canadian government has not yet developed policies or procedures to implement a Canadian National Suicide Prevention Strategy. Ironically, the objectives of most strategies adopted around the world are based on expert consensus guidelines for national strategies for the prevention of suicide that were formulated at a meeting in Calgary and Banff, Alberta, and adopted by the UN in 1996 (CASP, 2009).The Blueprint includes the common themes found in suicide prevention strategies which include: public education, responsible media reporting, school-based programs, detection and treatment of depression and other mental disorders, attention to those abusing alcohol and drugs, attention to individuals suffering from somatic illness, enhanced access to mental health services, improvement in assessment of attempted suicide, postvention, crisis intervention, work and unemployment policy, training and education of health professionals and reduced access to lethal methods of suicide (Anderson & Jenkins, 2006).

Training for lay health workers in India

Patel and colleagues (2011) developed and tested a collaborative stepped-care intervention for depressive and anxiety disorders delivered by lay heath workers in primary care centers (the MANAS intervention). The study took place in Goa, a small state on the western coast of India. The primary outcome of the study was the decrease in prevalence of the common mental disorders over the 12-month period of the study. Secondary outcomes included changes in severity of symptoms, suicidal behavior and disability levels. The intervention involved a two-month training course for lay health workers with non–health care backgrounds and focused on psycho-education with more resource-intensive interventions reserved for those with severe disorders or those not responding to the simpler interventions. At six months follow-up, in terms of common mental disorders, the intervention had a significant effect on recovery versus the enhanced usual care in public but not in private facilities (Patel et al., 2010). At 12 months follow-up, Patel et al. (2011) found a significant impact of the intervention in public facilities with a 30% reduction in prevalence of the common disorders in these facilities versus those providing enhanced usual care. Also in the public facilities, there was a significant positive impact on the severity of symptoms with a decrease of about 50% versus a 30% decrease in the control condition. In terms of reported suicide plans or attempts over the 12-months follow-up, the public facilities versus the controls demonstrated a 36% reduction between the arms of the study. In terms of days suffering disability, the intervention arm in the public facilities reported four or five fewer disability days in the previous month than the control arm. However, no impact on any outcome was found in the participants cared for in private primary health care facilities. This study of interventions by lay health care workers has much promise, particularly as an impact was found on suicidal plans and behaviors and that the process indicators suggested that the psycho-educational aspects of the intervention were particularly responsible for the improvements found (Patel et al., 2011). The reasons for the differences between private and public facilities are still to be understood; however, Patel et al. favored the explanation that private care facilities provided more personalized client-centered care that cancelled out the impact of the intervention.

Brief intervention to reduce subsequent suicide behavior among attempters

Vijayakumar, Umamaheswari, Ali, Devaraj and Kesavan (2011) reported a randomized controlled trial on the effectiveness of a brief intervention for suicide attempters admitted to an intensive medical care unit of a general hospital in Chennai, India. The study was taken from data at the Chennai site that had been part of the WHO Multisite Intervention Study on Suicidal Behaviours (SUPRE-MISS). The intervention involved a one-hour psycho-educational session and follow-up at weeks 1, 2, 4, 7 and 11, plus follow-up at months 4, 6, 12, and 18 months after discharge and was compared to treatment as usual (TAU). The intervention led to a significant reduction in attempted suicides over the follow-up period; 8 in the intervention group versus 17 in TAU (OR =17.3; CI 10.8–29.7) and in suicides (1 versus 9 in the respective groups; OR 35.4; CI 18.4–78.02). The authors felt these results were consistent with the overall SUPRE-MISS study carried out in five sites around the world and spoke to the value of brief interventions plus extended follow-up. The study was limited because of problems with recruitment and follow-up, particularly in India where suicide continues to be a punishable offense. However, based on this work, future replications of this intervention are clearly warranted.

Next steps: the Mumbai Project

The overarching goal of the project is to foster international collaboration between Canada and India as previously successfully achieved between Canada and China (Law et al., 2011). The overall objective of this project is to conduct a comprehensive training needs assessment for suicide prevention among health care professionals in rural India. The goal is to identify gaps in training and services and facilitate the development of an effective professional training program aimed at enhancing competencies in risk assessment and management of individuals at-risk for suicide. Increasing the competencies of health care providers has the potential for intervention and prevention of suicide-related behavior among the rural Indian population.

A combination of qualitative and quantitative strategies will be applied to provide a more comprehensive understanding of the normative and prescribed learning needs. To identify the breadth of needs and regional practice patterns, formal and informal, planned and opportunistic approaches (Lewis & Lewis, 1991) will be utilized. (1) Environmental scans will examine existing sources of information to ensure the relevance of the training. The environmental scans will be external (i.e., region) and internal (i.e., hospital or institutions). External environmental scanning will use sources such as guidelines of care, literature searches, published reports from professional organizations or regulatory bodies, and medical core curricula. Internal environmental scanning will include conference calls, oral or written recommendations, chart audits, mission statements, and comments from in-house experts and department heads. (2) Gap analysis will compare performance with required competencies and will utilize self-assessments and objective knowledge and skill tests that will be developed to identify learning needs. (3) Critical incident reviews will explore prescribed (i.e. best practices) and unperceived needs by reviewing outcome of critical incidents, dimensions of patient–provider interactions, the efficacy of outcomes, and health care providers' reflection and perception. These reviews will identify roles, cohort vulnerabilities, and barriers in the service delivery system. Focus group interviews will be conducted to explore health care providers' perceived and expressed needs and help identify areas of discrepancies. (4) Consultations to evaluate the feasibility of integrating smart technologies in the training of health care providers in rural India will be conducted with key informants.

We will apply the Kirkpatrick Model (TKM) (1994) as a theoretical framework to guide the analyses and triangulate the qualitative and quantitative data. Using qualitative (e.g., content analysis) and quantitative (e.g., descriptive statistics) analyses techniques we would focus on identifying and measuring deficiencies and gaps in competencies (i.e., attitudes, knowledge, and skills) and educational activities. The theoretical framework will focus on the needs assessment outputs from health care professionals and measure four levels of interest: Level I: Satisfaction – the overall quality of their training, relevance to clinical utility, attitudes to suicide prevention (e.g. gap analysis, focus groups, surveys and environmental scans); Level II: Learning – acquired and existing competencies (e.g., critical incident reviews and gap analysis); Level III: Performance – the applications of skills in clinical settings (e.g. environmental scans, critical incident reviews); Level IV: Results – prioritizing learning needs and future directions.

Discussion

Our examination of suicide in Canada and India brings to light the many differences between the two countries. In spite of these differences, we have argued that our matrix model for suicide prevention will foster collaborations across cultures and nations that can have important synergistic benefits. In both countries, suicide prevention must be multi-determined and broadly based, focusing on the realities of local contexts. Yet the risk factors across both countries are driven by limited access to care for distressed individuals, social and geographic isolation, ready access to means, and stigma and cultural considerations. Although the role of psychiatric disorders and the risk of suicide clearly differ between the two countries, it cannot be concluded that interventions targeting common psychiatric disorders or patients identified at risk for suicide will not lead to reductions in the numbers of suicides. The overall rate reductions in both countries will require political and policy initiatives to address, for example, the inequities related to poverty and gender in India or experienced by Aboriginal communities in Canada. Selective prevention strategies remain to be tested, particularly the training of primary care providers, gatekeeper educational programs and targeted interventions for mental health patients at risk.

We have recognized from our previous collaborations between China and Canada that the processes of these collaborations are vital and rich learning experiences. The shared experience can lead to new, unanticipated opportunities to move suicide prevention forward across all cultures and nations.

Acknowledgements

Parts of this chapter have been adapted from:

Zaheer, J., Links, P. S., Law, S., Shera, W., Hodges, B., Tsang, A. K. T., et al. (2011). Developing a matrix model of rural suicide prevention. *International Journal of Mental Health, 40*(4), 28–49. doi:10.2753/IMH0020-7411400403.

References

Aaron, R., Joseph, A., Abraham, S., Muliyil, J., George, K., Prasad, J., Minz, S., Abraham, V. J., & Bose, A. (2004). Suicides in young people in rural southern India. *Lancet, 363*, 1117–1118.

Anderson, M., & Jenkins, R. (2006). The national suicide prevention strategy for England: The reality of a national strategy for the nursing profession. *Journal of Psychiatric Mental Health Nursing, 13*, 641–650.

Bairstow, K. (2000). Cross national research: What can we learn from inter-country comparisons? *Social Work in Europe, 7*(3), 8–13.

Barua, A. (2009). Need for a realistic mental health programme in India. *Indian Journal of Psychological Medicine, 31*(1), 48–49.

Beautrais, A. L. (2003). Subsequent mortality in medically serious suicide attempts: A 5-year follow-up. *Australian and New Zealand Journal of Psychiatry, 37*, 595–599.

Behere, P. B., & Behere, A. P. (2008). Farmers' suicide in Vidarbha region of Maharashtra state: A myth or reality? *Indian Journal of Psychiatry, 50*(2), 124–127.

Bertolote, J. M., & Fleischmann, A. (2002). A global perspective in the epidemiology of suicide. *Suicidolgi, 7*(2), 6–8.

Blackmore, E. R., Munce, S., Weller, I., Zagorski, B., Stansfeld, S. A., Steward, D. E., Caine, E. D., & Conwell, E. (2008). Psychosocial and clinical correlates of suicidal acts: Results from a national population survey. *British Journal of Psychiatry, 192*, 279–284.

CASP National Suicide Prevention Strategy (2009). Available at: www.suicideprevention.ca (accessed May 26, 2011).

Eddleston, M., & Phillips, M. R. (2004) Self poisoning with pesticides. *British Medical Journal, 328*, 42–44.

Eynan, R. (2011). Preventing suicides in the Toronto subway system: A program evaluation. Unpublished doctoral dissertation. University of Toronto, Toronto.

Forchuk, C., MacClure, S. K., Van Beers, M., Smith, C., Csiernik, R., Hoch, J., & Jensen, E. (2008). Developing and testing an intervention to prevent homelessness among individuals discharged from psychiatric wards to shelters and 'no fixed address'. *Journal of Psychiatric Mental Health Nursing, 15*, 7, 569–575.

Grant, J. (2002). Learning needs assessment: Assessing the need. *British Journal of Medicine, 324*, 156–159.

Gururaj, G., Isaac, M. K., Subbakrishna, D, K., & Ranjani, R. (2004). Case control study of completed suicides in Bangalore, India. *Injury Control and Safety Promotion, 11*, 3, 193–200.

Haggarty, J. M., Cernovsky, Z., Bedard, M., & Merskey, H. (2008). Suicidality in a sample of Arctic households. *Suicide and Life-threatening Behavior, 38*, 699–707.

Hawton, K., Ratnayeke, L., Simkin, S., Harriss, L., & Scott, L. (2009). Evaluation of acceptability and use of lockable storage devices for pesticides in Sri Lanka that might assist in prevention of self-poisoning. *BMC Public Health, 9*(69), 1–12.

Hendin, H., Phillips, M. R., Vijaykumar, L., Pirkis, J., Wang, H., Yip, P., Wasserman, D., Bertolote, J. M., & Fleischmann, A. (Eds.). (2008). *Suicide and suicide prevention in Asia*. Geneva: World Health Organization.

Hintikka, J., Lehtonen, J., & Viinamaki, H. (1997). Hunting guns in homes and suicides in 15–24 year-old males in eastern homes and suicides in 15–24 year old males in eastern Finland. *Australian and New Zealand Journal of Psychiatry, 31*, 858–61.

Hirsch, J. K. (2006). A review of the literature on rural suicide: Risk and protective factors, incidence, and prevention. *Crisis, 27*(4), 189–199.

Jacob, K. S. (2008). The prevention of suicide in India and the developing world: The need for population-based strategies. *Crisis, 29* (2), 102–106.

Judd, F., Cooper, A. M., Fraser, C., & Davis, J. (2006). Rural suicide: People or place effects? *Australian and New Zealand Journal of Psychiatry, 40*, 208–216.

Kirkpatrick, D. L. (1975). Techniques for evaluating training programs. In D. L. Kirkpatrick (Ed.), *Evaluating training programs*. Alexandria, VA: ASTD.

Knox, K. L., Litts, D. A., Talcott, W., Feig, J. C., & Caine, E. D. (2003). Risk of suicide and related adverse outcomes after exposure to a suicide prevention programme in the US Air Force: Cohort study. *BMJ, 327*, 1–5.

Kral, M. J., Links, P. S., & Bergmans, Y. (2012). Suicide studies and the need for mixed methods research. *Journal of Mixed Methods Research, 6*, 236–249.

Krysinska, K. E., & De Leo, D. (2007). Telecomunications and suicide prevention: Hopes and challenges for a new century. *Omega, 55*(3), 237–253.

Kushner, H., & Sterk, C. E. (2005). The limits of social capital: Durkheim, suicide, and social cohesion. *American Journal of Public Health, 9* (7), 1139–1143.

Langlois, S., & Morrison, P. (2002). Suicide deaths and suicide attempts. *Health Reports, 13*(2), 9–22.

Law, S. F., Liu, P., Hodges, B. D., Shera, W., Huang, X., Zaheer, J., & Links, P. S. (2011). Introducing psychiatry to rural physicians in China: An innovative education project. *American Journal of Psychiatry, 168*(12), 1249–1254.

Lewis, J. A., & Lewis, M. D. (1991). *Management of human service programs.* Monterey, CA: Brooks/Cole.

Luxton, D. D., June, J. D., & Kinn, J. T. (2011). Technology-based suicide prevention: Current applications and future directions. *Telemedicine and e-Health, Jan./Feb.,* 50–54.

Mann, J. J., Apter, A., Bertolote, J., Beautrais, A., Currier, D., Haas, A., Hegerl, U., Lonnqvist, J., Malone, K., Marusic, A., Mehlum, L., Patton, G., Phillips, M., Rutz, W., Rihmer, Z., Schmidtke, A., Shaffer, D., Silverman, M., Takahashi, Y., Varnik, A., Wasserman, D., Yip, P., & Hendin, H. (2005). Suicide prevention strategies: A systematic review. *JAMA, 294*(16), 2064–2074.

Manoranjitham, S. D., Rajkumar, A. P., Thngadurai, P., Prasad, J., Jayakaran, R., & Jacob, K. S. (2010). Risk factors for suicide in rural south India. *British Journal of Psychiatry, 196*, 26–30.

Middleton, N., Whitley, E., Frankel, S., Dorling, D., Sterne, J., & Gunnell, D. (2004). Suicide risk in small areas in England and Wales, 1991–1993. *Social Psychiatry and Psychiatric Epidemiology, 39*, 45–52.

Miller, K., & Burns, C. (2008). Suicides on farms in South Australia, 1997–2001. *Australian Journal of Rural Health, 16*, 327–331.

Milner, A., & Sveticic, J. (2012). Suicide in the absence of mental disorder? A review of psychological autopsy studies across countries. *International Journal of Social Psychiatry, 11*, May 11. [Epub ahead of print.]

Mokkenstorm, J. K., Huisman, A., & Kerkhof, A. J. (2012). Suicide prevention via the internet and the telephone. *Tijdschriftvoorpsychiatrie, 54*(4), 341–348.

Motohashi, Y., Kanero, Y., Sasaki, H., & Yamaji, M. (2007). A decrease in suicide rates in Japanese rural towns after community-based intervention by the health promotion approach. *Suicide and Life-threatening Behavior, 37*(5), 593–599.

National Crimes Record Bureau (NCRB) (2010). *Accidental deaths and suicides in India.* New Delhi: Ministry of Home Affairs, Government of India.

Parkar, S. R., Nagarsekar, B., & Weiss, M. G. (2009). Explaining suicide in an urban slum of Mumbai, India: A sociocultural autopsy. *Crisis, 30*(4), 192–201.

Patel, V., Ramasundarahettige, C., Vijayakumar L., Takur J. S., Gururaj, G., Suraweera, W., & Jha, P. (2012). Suicide mortality in India: A nationally representative survey. *Lancet, 379*, 2343–2351.

Patel, V., Weiss, H. A., Chowdhary, N., Naik, S., Pednekar, S., Chatterjee, S., Bhat, B., Araya, R., King, M., Simon, G., Verdeli, H., & Kirkwood, B. R. (2011). Lay health worker-led intervention for depressive and anxiety disorders in India: Impact on clinical and disability outcomes over 12 months. *British Journal of Psychiatry, 199*, 459–466.

Patel, V., Weiss, H. A., Chowdhary, N., Naik, S., Pednekar, S., Chatterjee, S., De Silva, M. J., Bhat, B., Araya, R., King, M., Simon, G., Verdeli, H., & Kirkwood, B. R. (2010). Effectiveness of an intervention led by lay health counselors for depressive and anxiety disorders in primary care in Goa, India (MANAS): A cluster randomized controlled trial. *Lancet,* Published online Dec. 14, 2010.

Pearce, J., Barnett, R., & Jones, I. (2007). Have urban/rural inequalities in suicide in New Zealand grown during the period of 1980–2001? *Social Science & Medicine, 65*, 1807–1819.

Pesonen, T. M., Hintikka, J., Karkola, K. O., Saarinen, P. I., Antikainen, M., & Lehtonen, J. (2001). Male suicide mortality in eastern Finland: urban-rural changes during a 10-year period between 1988 and 1997. *Scandinavian Journal of Public Health, 29*, 189–193.

Pickett, W., King, W. D., Faelker, T., & Bienfeld, N. (1999). Suicides among Canadian farm operators. *Chronic Diseases in Canada, 20*, 105–110.

Razvodovsky, Y., & Stickley, A. (2009). Suicide in urban and rural regions of Belarus, 1990–2005. *Public Health, 123*, 27–31.

Robertson, J. M., & Fitzgerald, L. F. (1992). Overcoming the masculine mystique: Preference for alternative forms of assistance among men who avoid counseling. *The Journal of Clinical Psychology, Counseling and Psychotherapy, 39*, 240–246.

Sinha, S. K., & Kaur, J. (2011). National mental health programme: Manpower development scheme of eleventh five-year plan. *Indian Journal of Psychiatry, 53*(3), 261–265.

Srivastava, M., & Tiwari, R. (2012). A comparative study of attitude of mental versus non-mental health professionals toward suicide. *Indian Journal of Psychological Medicine, 34*(1), 66–69.

Stats Canada (2012). Available at: http://www.statcan.gc.ca/tables-tableaux/sum-som/l01/cst01/hlth66d-eng.htm (accessed August 28, 2012).

Szanto, K., Kalmar, S., Hendin, H., Rihmer, Z., & Mann, J. J. (2007). A suicide prevention program in a region with a very high suicide rate. *Archives of General Psychiatry, 64*(8), 914–920.

Thirunavukarasu, M. (2007). Psychiatry in UG curriculum of medicine: Need of the hour. *Indian Journal of Psychiatry, 9*(3), 159–160.

Vijayakumar, L. (2010). Indian research on suicide, *Indian Journal of Psychiatry, 52*(1), S291–S296.

Vijayakumar, L., Pirkis, J., & Whiteford, H. (2005). Suicide in developing countries (3): Prevention initiatives, *Crisis, 26*, 120–124.

Vijayakumar, L., Umamaheswari, C., Ali, Z. S. S., Devaraj, P., & Kesavan, K. (2011). Intervention for suicide attempters: A randomized controlled study. *Indian Journal of Psychiatry, 53*(3), 244–248.

Wang, J. L. (2004). Rural-urban differences in the prevalence of major depression and associated impairment. *Social Psychiatry and Psychiatric Epidemiology, 39*, 19–25.

WHO (2001). *The world health report 2001: Mental health: new understanding, new hope.* Chapter 3: Solving mental health problems: p. 2. Available at: http://www.who.int/whr/2001/chapter3/en/index1.html (accessed Feb. 28, 2011).

Zaheer, J., Links, P., Law, S., Shera, W., Hodges, B., Ka Tat Tsang, A., Huang, X., & Lui, P. (2011–12). Developing a matrix model of rural suicide prevention: A Canada-China collaboration. *International Journal of Mental Health, 40*, 28–49.

EDITORIAL COMMENTARY

According to the World Health Organization (WHO), almost one million people die by suicide worldwide each year (WHO, 2012). While suicidal behavior is understood as a complex interaction of biological, psychological, social, cultural and geographical factors, psychiatric illness has been shown to be a major contributing cause. From a clinical perspective, a psychiatric evaluation, which includes the identification of factors that increase an individual's risk of suicide, and protective factors that reduce this risk, is considered a core component of a suicide risk assessment (Jacobs et al., 2003). However, due to low base rates of suicide and unique factors, it is not possible to predict suicide on an individual level (Pokorny, 1983, 1993). The goal of a suicide assessment is not to predict suicide, but rather to place a person along a continuum of putative risk, to appreciate the bases of suicidality and allow for a more informed intervention (Jacobs, Brewer, & Klein-Benheim, 1999).

Despite the difficulty in predicting suicide at the individual level, psychiatrists have an important role in caring for the suicidal patient, identifying and treating mental illness that contributes to suicide risk. Tackling suicide prevention, however, requires a broader focus than simply diagnosing and treating mental illness. In both clinical and research practice, the field of psychiatry has been limited by the focus on diagnosing mental illness at the expense of understanding the complex neurobiological and genetic causes of symptoms and dysfunction (Insel & Cuthbert, 2010). Importantly, however, a narrow focus on establishing and treating a psychiatric condition minimizes the important contribution of psychological, social and cultural factors which shape patient experience. The clinical and research interests of psychiatrists may fail to address the priorities of the patients and families they seek to treat (Thornicroft, Rose, Huxley, Dale, & Wykes, 2002). For example, while the National Institutes of Mental Health in the United States identify a discovery in the brain and behavioral sciences, charting mental illness trajectories, and the development of interventions focusing on the prevention, treatment and cure of mental illness as strategic objectives (NIMH, 2008), mental health service users may express differing priorities. In contrast to the NIMH objectives, Thornicroft et al.'s (2002) work with service users identified research priorities such as user involvement in all stages of mental health research, discrimination and abuse, social and welfare issues, arts as therapies and advocacy. It is to the benefit of psychiatrists, patients and the mental health system to consider all of these issues rather than privileging certain priorities over others.

Just as psychiatry must expand its focus from the diagnosis and treatment of mental illness to consider the role of biological factors and the ways in which emotional, behavioural and social elements play a role in patients' experiences, we must also take a broader view with respect to the prevention of suicide. As Marsha Linehan (2008) points out, the assumption that suicide is a symptom of a mental illness and the prevention of suicide requires the treatment of the underlying disease has guided the field of suicide prevention research. However, she reviews the evidence and argues persuasively that interventions designed to reduce the symptoms of mental illness have not been shown to reduce the incidents of non-fatal suicidal behaviour or death by suicide (Linehan, 2008). In order for psychiatrists to contribute to the field of suicide prevention, we must focus on the biological, psychological, social and cultural factors that contribute to this complex phenomenon. In this section, we see how psychiatrists can take a biopsychosocial approach in undertaking investigations to identify risk factors and warning signs for suicide and to develop and rigorously evaluate suicide prevention strategies informed by research findings.

From a biological standpoint, improved diagnosis and treatment of mental illnesses, specifically mood disorders, is a promising intervention in suicide prevention. Mann et al.'s (2005) review of suicide prevention strategies indicated that physician education increases the number of diagnoses and treatment for depressed patients, and shows accompanying reductions in suicide. From a psychological perspective, increased awareness of the emotional and behavioural antecedents of suicidal behaviour can be better understood through qualitative studies (Cleary, 2012; Hjelmeland & Knizek, 2010; Joe, Canetto, & Romer, 2008). From a social angle, gatekeeper education can help reduce suicidal behaviour, especially in situations where the roles of gatekeepers are formalized and pathways to treatment are readily available (Mann et al., 2005). Further, restricting access to lethal methods decreases suicide by these methods. However, methods vary widely worldwide, and within geographic areas and demographic groups. Suicide prevention strategies can take into account social factors by focusing on restricting means for the most common methods of suicide within an area (Mann et al., 2005).

In recent years, psychiatrists have begun to understand the importance of considering cultural factors in addition to a biopsychosocial approach. As Kirmayer (2006) outlines, cultural psychiatry advances the perspective that a multi-disciplinary approach is necessary to integrate culture as a feature of biology and to be aware of cultural constructions of biology, to attend to psychological processes while appreciating that our views are influenced by larger social discourses, and to critically examine the interaction of both local and global systems of knowledge and power. Kirmayer also highlights the dangers of privileging quantitative evidence-based medicine over cultural research. These issues are also important for psychiatrists to consider in suicide prevention research. Suicide is a complex outcome with many contributing risk factors, including mental illness, access to means, social stresses and isolation, lack of access to care, and stigma and cultural factors, and psychiatrists are striving to undertake research in these domains. Additionally, mental health care is moving from a fragmented, psychiatrist-dominated model to a collaborative, interdisciplinary approach incorporating the perspectives of health care providers, patients and their families (Rubin & Zorumski, 2012). Similarly, suicide research benefits both from the perspectives of multiple disciplines and international collaboration.

Not only do psychiatrists have a role in treating individual patients in their communities; they have an important responsibility to help elucidate the biological, psychological and social factors contributing to suicide. Psychiatrists can help address the risk of suicide of diverse populations, share research and experience across international boundaries and, collaborating with other professionals, evaluate suicide prevention strategies in a rigorous manner, advocate for the responsible use of resources, and contribute to policies and strategies in order to address this major public health concern.

References

Cleary, A. (2012). Suicidal action, emotional expression, and the performance of masculinities. *Social Science & Medicine, 74*(4), 498–505. doi:10.1016/j.socscimed.2011.08.002.

Hjelmeland, H., & Knizek, B. L. (2010). Why we need qualitative research in suicidology. *Suicide & Life-threatening Behavior, 40*(1), 74–80. doi:10.1521/suli.2010.40.1.74.

Insel, T., & Cuthbert, B. (2010). Research domain criteria (RDoC): Toward a new classification framework for research on mental disorders. *American Journal of Psychiatry, 167*(July), 748–751. Available at: http://works.bepress.com/charles_sanislow/2/.

Jacobs, D. G., Baldessarini, R. J., Fawcett, J. A., Horton, L., Meltzer, H., Pfeffer, C. R., & Simon, R. I. (2003). Practice guideline for the assessment and treatment of patients with suicidal behaviors. *American Journal of Psychiatry*. Available at: www.psych.org/psych_pract/treatg/pg/SuicidalBehavior_05-15-06.pdf.

Jacobs, D. G., Brewer, M., & Klein-Benheim, M. (1999). Suicide assessment: An overview and recommended protocol. In D. G. Jacobs (Ed.), *The Harvard Medical School Guide to Suicide Assessment and Intervention*. San Francisco: Jossey-Bass. Available at: http://www.amazon.com/gp/reader/0787943037/ref=sib_dp_pop_toc/104-0608046-7039127?%5Fencoding=UTF8&p=S009#reader-link.

Joe, S., Canetto, S. S., & Romer, D. (2008). Advancing prevention research on the role of culture in suicide prevention. *Suicide & Life-threatening Behavior, 38*(3), 354–62. doi:10.1521/suli.2008.38.3.354.

Kirmayer, L. J. (2006). Beyond the "new cross-cultural psychiatry": Cultural biology, discursive psychology and the ironies of globalization. *Transcultural Psychiatry, 43*(1), 126–144. doi:10.1177/1363461506061761.

Linehan, M. M. (2008). Suicide intervention research: A field in desperate need of development. *Suicide & Life-threatening Behavior, 38*(5), 483–5. doi:10.1521/suli.2008.38.5.483.

Mann, J. J., Apter, A., Bertolote, J., Beautrais, A., Currier, D., Haas, A., et al. (2005). Suicide prevention strategies: A systematic review. *JAMA: the journal of the American Medical Association, 294*(16), 2064–74. doi:10.1001/jama.294.16.2064.

NIMH (National Institute of Mental Health) (2008). *Strategic plan.*

Pokorny, A. D. (1983). Prediction of suicide in psychiatric patients: Report of a prospective study. *Archives of General Psychiatry, 40*(3), 249–57. Retrieved from http://www.ncbi.nlm.nih.gov/pubmed/6830404.

Pokorny, A. D. (1993). Suicide prediction revisited. *Suicide & Life-threatening Behavior, 23*(1), 1–10. Available at: http://www.ncbi.nlm.nih.gov/pubmed/8475527.

Rubin, E. H., & Zorumski, C. F. (2012). Perspective: Upcoming paradigm shifts for psychiatry in clinical care, research, and education. *Academic Medicine: Journal of the Association of American Medical Colleges, 87*(3), 261–265. doi:10.1097/ACM.0b013e3182441697.

Thornicroft, G., Rose, D., Huxley, P., Dale, G., & Wykes, T. (2002). What are the research priorities of mental health service users? *Journal of Mental Health, 11*(1), 1–3. doi:10.1080/096382301200041416.

WHO (2012). World Health Organization Suicide Prevention (SUPRE). Available at: http://www.who.int/mental_health/prevention/suicide/suicideprevent/en/ (accessed September 30, 2012).

PART III

Psychology

EDITORIAL INTRODUCTION

Psychology appears to be at a crossroads when it comes to suicide treatment and assessment. Edwin S. Shneidman founded the American Association of Suicidology in 1968 with a strong mission towards suicide prevention, however, psychology seems to have moved consistently towards assessment and away from treatment. When we were asking authors to come forward and provide us with submissions for this section, it was difficult to find researchers focusing on the prevention of suicide or the treatment of those who had made an attempt at suicide. The psychology section of this text demonstrates this reality. We feel that this trend needs to be questioned especially within psychology training programs with a recommended focus on both prevention and treatment .

Part III begins with Chapter 12 by John McIntosh that provides the most recent official figures for suicide in the United States. This chapter has identified that the modal suicide victim primarily remains white elderly males, though increases among the middle-aged have raised the risk in this group to high levels as well. While economic crises have often been proposed as the reason for recent increases, and specific anecdotal evidence supporting this factor are also presented, the author points out that the reasons for changes in suicide are not easily determined. The author posits that, based on the data presented, targeted prevention and intervention efforts might help address the high risk of men, the aged, the middle-aged, and military personnel. Possible method restriction measures, related particularly to firearms and poisons, might be effective to lessen suicides in the US population.

In Chapter 13, Ward-Ciesielski, McIntosh and Rompogren report on their study which measured attitudes towards therapists who lose patients to suicide. In their study it was found that therapists appear to inaccurately predict the reactions of the individuals who are left behind after a patient suicide. Both comparisons between therapist and student attitudes demonstrate that therapists believe that survivors have less positive attitudes and stronger negative attitudes toward them than were actually reported by the students. The results of the study could help with the development of appropriate postvention techniques that will foster professional growth rather than detrimental emotional responses among therapists who experience the loss of a patient to suicide.

Joseph S. Munson has contributed Chapter 14 that adds another important dimension to practitioner response to client suicide in examining the impact of client suicide on practitioner post-traumatic growth. Munson's research provides the field of psychology and suicidology with direction to shape further assumptions of how client suicides affect post-traumatic growth in clinicians. Specifically, this research added to current theory by showing that both PTSD and PTG can exist simultaneously in clinicians after a client suicide.

In Chapter 15, Perlman and Neufeld examine the necessity for and implications of high quality suicide risk assessment on psychological practice, policy, and research. The authors' examination of risk assessment points out that suicide risk assessment is not a singular event but, rather, an ongoing process that involves much more than the use of "tools" and "scores".

To conclude Part III, Séguin, Lesage, Renaud and Turecki present a novel Trajectory-Based model in the study of suicide in Chapter 16. The life calendar approach presented here, and for the first time in suicide research, adds to the identification of past (e.g., sexual or physical abuse and childhood separation) and recent (e.g., spousal separation) life events previously associated with suicide. It also attempts to quantify the burden these events may represent in each period of life.

12

USA SUICIDE

Epidemiology

John L. McIntosh

Introduction

Suicide is a significant mental and public health issue. The World Health Organization (2012) estimated in 2000 that nearly one million suicides took place worldwide. With a worldwide rate of 16 per 100,000 population, the rate in the United States of over 12 (2010 figures) is below the estimated international rate and can be described as moderate and not among the highest nations. However, as a large country, deaths by suicide in the USA represent an important matter. While suicidal behavior includes the broader spectrum of suicidal ideation, nonfatal suicidal acts (suicide attempts), and the effects of suicide deaths on the bereaved (see e.g., Jordan & McIntosh, 2011), the focus of this chapter will be on suicide mortality in the United States of America.

Currently in the USA (official data for the year 2010), there are over 38,000 suicide deaths annually (38,364; official Centers for Disease Control and Prevention [CDC] figures, 2012; McIntosh & Drapeau, 2012) and suicide ranks 10th as a cause of death (compared to 16th for homicide, $N = 16,259$ and a rate of 5.3). At that level this means that on average an American dies by suicide every 14 minutes (13.7 in 2010), with 105 (105.1) intentional deaths each day. Stated in the most comparable terms, however, the crude rate of suicide in 2010 was 12.4 per 100,000. That means that if a representative sample of 100,000 Americans were selected on January 1 and followed throughout the calendar year 2010, we would expect to observe that 12 or 13 would have died by suicide during the year. When placed in the context of all modes of death in the nation, suicide's 10th ranking represents a leading cause of US mortality. In fact, in 2009 (and continued in 2010) suicide became the leading cause of injury mortality, exceeding the previous leading cause, unintentional motor vehicle traffic crashes (Rockett et al., 2012). In addition, suicide deaths by those under 75 years of age led to over 1 million years of potential life lost (YPLL-75; 1,106,124, Centers for Disease Control and Prevention, CDC, 2012) and represent the 4th leading cause of death for YPLL in the USA.

Before describing the patterns and trends of suicide for important demographic factors, it is important to explain the figures that have appeared so far and will follow hereafter. The figures for deaths by suicide are based on official mortality statistics derived from death certificates. Therefore, those deaths for which the cause of death was classified as suicide by the coroner or medical examiner are the only deaths that are included. These data, compiled for deaths across the nation, are posted at CDC websites (e.g., www.cdc.gov/injury/wisqars/index.html).

The use of statistics in the field of suicidology has a long history (e.g., Durkheim, [1897] 1951). While they are a source of consistently compiled data and are the official figures, they are not without criticism and potential limitations (see, e.g., McIntosh, 1991, p. 57). It has been noted that these figures are likely a conservative estimate of the actual levels (Allen, 1984). The most current suicide data are for deaths occurring during the year 2010 and these figures (along with historical data for previous years) will be provided here.

Demographic variables

Over the history of suicidology, a large number of demographic variables have been studied. Problems and limitations with respect to research methodology and other issues exist for many of those variables and investigations. Thus, the focus of this chapter will be on those demographic variables that are available from official mortality data and have proven to be reliable and consistent in their relationship to suicide over time.

Gender/sex

Perhaps the most important individual variable associated with suicide risk is gender or sex. In particular, men die by suicide at levels nearly four times those of women, whether considering the number of deaths or the rate. In 2010, 30,277 men killed themselves and 8,087 women (male:female ratio of 3.7:1). Similarly the rates of suicide were 20.0 compared to 5.2 per 100,000 population for men and women, respectively (a ratio of 3.8:1). On average, there were 83 suicides by men and 22 by women each day in 2010. This gender difference in suicide has been observed consistently over time (see Figure 12.1; see also McIntosh & Jewell, 1986).

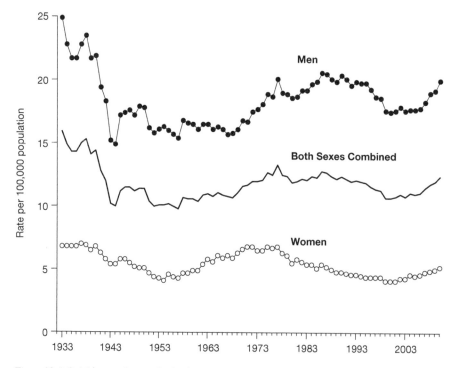

Figure 12.1 Suicide rates by gender in the USA, 1933–2010

Race/ethnicity

Race

In the USA, suicide is clearly highest among whites. When compared to all nonwhites combined into a single grouping, in 2010, whites represented 34,690 suicides while there were 3,674 among nonwhites. On an average day in 2010, there were 95 white deaths by suicide and 10 by nonwhites. Although the numbers lead to a ratio of 9.4:1, the risk of suicide as measured by the rate of suicide (per 100,000 population) was only 2.4:1 (14.1 vs. 5.8, white vs. nonwhite, respectively). This demonstrates the importance of the use of rates in determining suicide risk. The number of deaths must be placed in the context of the size of the population in which these deaths occur (direct comparability is possible because rates are calculated as a rate per unit of 100,000 population in each group). As observed for gender, racial differences in suicide over time have largely remained consistent (see Figure 12.2).

Suicide is a complex phenomenon and understanding of the risk associated with demographic variables is most often best described by the combination of variables rather than the individual variables alone. When gender and race are considered together, it is revealed that gender remains the most predictive variable, with men of both racial groupings demonstrating higher risk than women of either grouping. At the same time, whites show higher rates than their nonwhite

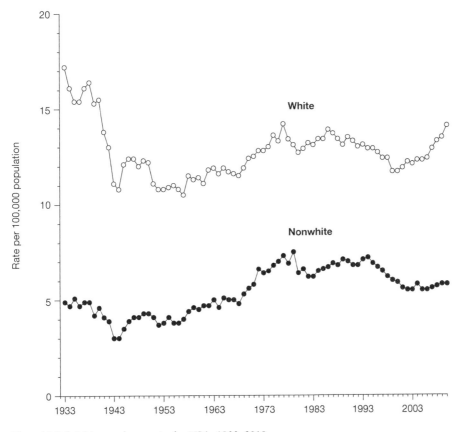

Figure 12.2 Suicide rates by race in the USA, 1933–2010

counterparts by gender. In 2010, white men (N = 27,422) had a suicide rate of 22.6 compared to nonwhite men (N = 2,855) at 9.4, and white women (N = 7,268) and nonwhite women (N = 819) with rates of 5.9 and 2.5, respectively. Therefore, those at highest risk for suicide are white men.

Ethnicity

There is considerable variation in US suicide rates by ethnicity. This diversity is most obvious within the nonwhite as a whole grouping discussed above. In particular, although suicide rates are consistently higher among the white population, rates for Native Americans/American Indians are only slightly lower than those for whites, though rates for Asian and Pacific Islanders and those for blacks are significantly lower and similar (see Figure 12.3). In 2010, the white rate (14.1) noted above can be compared to the slightly lower rate for Native Americans (N = 469) at 11.0 per 100,000 population, and those for Asian and Pacific Islanders (N = 1,061) and blacks (N = 2,144) of 6.2 and 5.1, respectively. The figure for Hispanics (who may be of any race) in 2010 (N = 2,661) was 5.3 per 100,000. Data for other racial/ethnic groups are not readily available (and/or the annual population figures with which to calculate rates are not available).

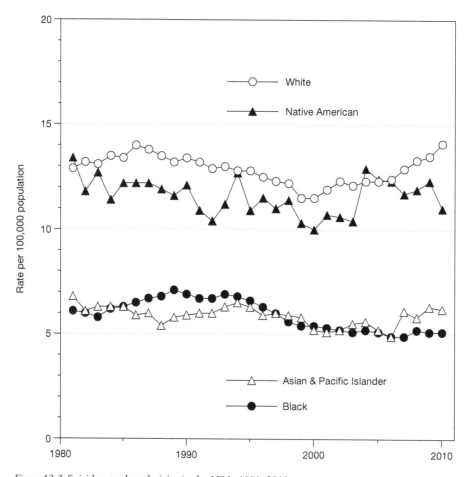

Figure 12.3 Suicide rates by ethnicity in the USA, 1981–2010

Age

While rates and risk have largely remained consistent over time for both gender and race, substantial changes in suicide rates have taken place across the years with respect to age and life periods. In fact, some of the greatest changes in suicide rates over long periods of time have occurred among various age groups. Changes in rates for two groups have taken place over several decades (i.e., the young 15–24 years and elders 65 years and above) and a more recent, now decade-long change has occurred in a third life period (i.e., midlife). Traditionally, which refers to the time periods of especially the 1960s and earlier, suicide rates could best be described as increasing with age, such that lowest rates were observed among the youngest age groups, and primarily in a linear fashion rates increased across the lifespan to their highest rates in late life. The major and substantial changes in suicide rates among the young, old, and middle-aged, however, have produced a pattern that can best be described as bimodal. That is, rates still are lowest in the youngest age groups but now peak in midlife, decline slightly in the early years of late life (i.e., among the young-old 65–74) and then increase again to a second peak among the old-old (75 and above; see Figure 12.4).

The large changes in rates noted for the three life periods deserve some individual attention. Perhaps the best known of the changes in suicide by age are those seen for young people

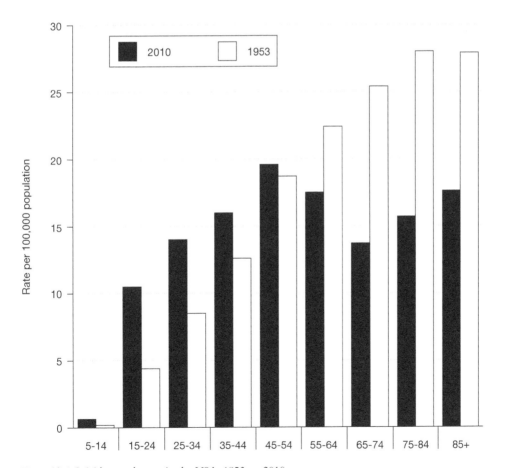

Figure 12.4 Suicide rates by age in the USA, 1953 vs. 2010

(McIntosh, 2000). Suicide is a leading cause of death among the young, ranking third for those aged 10–14 and 15–24 and second for those 25–34 years of age in 2010 (suicide ranked in the top four causes of death for all age groups 10–54 years in 2010). The young do not die from disease-related causes but rather from their own incautious behavior or that of others (accidents, homicides, and suicides being the top three causes of death, representing nearly 3 out of 4 [72.2% in 2010] of all deaths in those 15–24 years of age; McIntosh, 1993). The Years of Potential Life Lost statistic noted earlier predominantly reflects the deaths occurring in young age groups. Clearly, therefore, youth suicide is important with respect to suicide and its prevention. Regarding the changes in rates for youth, it is and has been often stated that suicide among young people (usually meaning the 15–24 years age group) has increased dramatically over time. While there is truth in this observation, the actual temporal pattern of changes is far more complicated and not often mentioned. It would be accurate to observe that suicide among those 15–24 years of age has increased substantially from the historical low levels in the 1950s. In fact, the 2010 suicide rate for this group (4,600 suicides) is 10.5 per 100,000 population compared to 4.0 in 1956: an increase of 163%. This is yet another demonstration of the importance of suicide among the young. It should be noted though, that youth suicide increased tremendously and rapidly from the low of the 1950s through the mid- to late-1970s followed mostly by three decades of stability and declining rates. Youth suicide most often exceeded the national rate from the mid-1970s through the early 1990s but has since been lower than the national rate for over a decade (see Figure 12.5) but still considerably higher than the 1950s through the early 1970s. The trend for elevated rates of suicide in young age groups has included those aged 25–34 as well, producing higher rates in comparison to those from the mid-1950s (see also Figure 12.4).

The second of the major age-related trends has been the most long-term, taking place since the 1930s and continuing through 2010. This change has been the large decline in suicide among US elders (see Figure 12.5). From a rate of over 45 per 100,000 in the 1930s (in 1933 during the Great Depression), the rate has consistently decreased (with only a brief increase for several years of the early-to-mid 1980s) to the current levels at 14.9 in 2010 (5,994 suicides). Despite these tremendous declines and increases for the young, older adults remain as they have been throughout the existence of official US mortality statistics, at levels of suicide higher than the nation and the young (the place of the elderly with respect to the middle-aged will be addressed below). That is, older adults are still among the highest risk for suicide in the nation and a demographic group under-represented among suicide prevention efforts (see McIntosh, Santos, Hubbard, & Overholser, 1994).

The last and most recent of the major demographic trends among age groups has been the increase in rates among those in midlife (those 45–64 years of age; see Figure 12.5; see e.g., Hu, Wilcox, Wissow, & Baker, 2008; Phillips, Robin, Nugent, & Idler, 2010). Since 2000, there has been a steady increase in suicide rates for the middle-aged (during a period of declining rates among virtually all other demographic groups until the past few years). This increase, along with the continuing declines for the old, have resulted in the rate at midlife being the highest across the lifespan currently (see Figure 12.4). While there is a bit more to this risk level, as will be noted below, these increases in middle-aged Americans deserve closer investigation and prevention attention as well.

While the aggregate age group rate trends noted above have greatly influenced the overall demographic picture of suicide rates over time, the use of disaggregated data is more revealing with respect to specific groups at high (and low) risk of suicide. In addition, these disaggregated figures show issues that may be hidden within the aggregate data. Thus, when suicide rates by age are considered simultaneously with gender (and race), better information about risk by age is observed. For instance, rates by age for men show a bimodal pattern of increases with age.

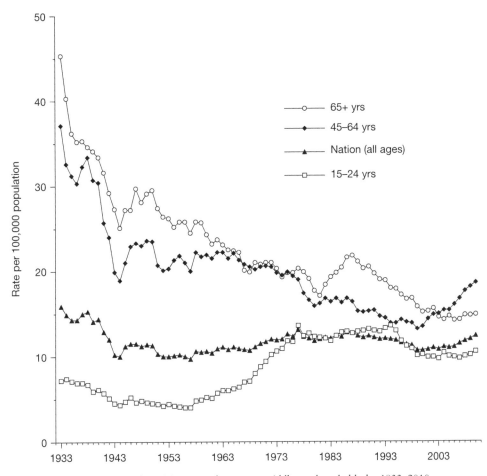

Figure 12.5 Suicide rates in the USA among the young, middle aged, and elderly, 1933–2010

While this is the same general description for the nation as a whole, men's rates are highest at all ages and while there is a peak in rates in middle age and a later peak in late life, the latter is clearly highest (instead of the midlife highest level for both genders combined). These patterns can be seen in Figure 12.6, along with the rates of suicide by age among women in the USA in 2010. As has always been the pattern for women, rates increase with age to midlife, peaking among women aged 45–54 years, followed by declines thereafter to low rates in late life. These disparate patterns by gender produce the highest differences between men and women in older adulthood and low differences in midlife.

As a final aspect of age differences, the additional consideration of age, gender, and racial differences in suicide reveal that whites of each gender follow the patterns just described for men and women by age respectively, but the rates for whites are higher than those for the corresponding aggregate gender–age groups (see Figure 12.7). By comparison, the pattern for nonwhites by age and gender shows lower rates than for whites of the same gender–age group across the lifespan, but also reveals: (1) the markedly higher risk for white males (particularly white males in late life); and (2) the peak in suicide rates for nonwhite males in young adulthood (25–34 years), with generally lower rates through the rest of adulthood. Therefore, these data by age indicate that the highest risk for suicide are elderly white males and the middle-aged.

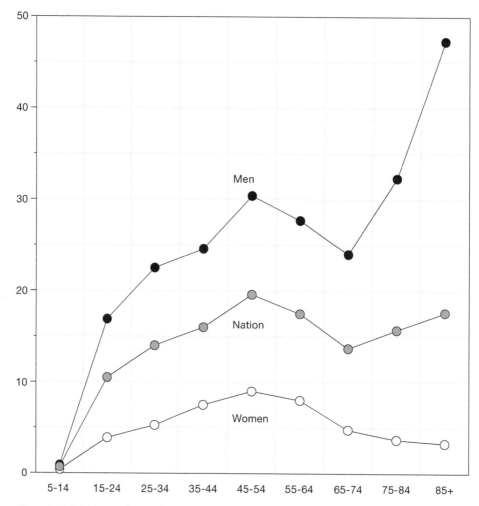

Figure 12.6 Suicide rates by gender and age in the USA, 2010

Marital status

Patterns of suicide by marital status underscore the importance of utilizing rates of suicide rather than raw numbers of deaths in making comparisons and determining risk among a population. As is apparent from Figure 12.8, the clearly highest number of suicides are by those who are married, followed by the single (never married) and then considerably lower numbers among the divorced and widowed. However, when taking into account the number of individuals of each of these marital statuses in the population (i.e., calculating a rate), it can be seen that the clearly *lowest rate* is among the population subgroup with the clearly *largest number* of suicides: the married. In fact, the rate for those who are single in the population is second lowest, with the widowed slightly higher, with the divorced representing the highest risk of suicide, at levels nearly twice those of the closest other group.

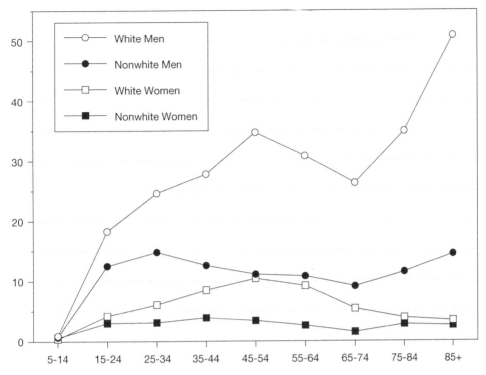

Figure 12.7 Suicide rates by gender, age, and race in the USA, 2010

Geographic patterns of suicide

The levels of suicide in the USA have been highly consistent over time, both in broader geographic terms as well as generally for individual states. Suicide rates are highest in the Western region of the nation and more specifically in the Mountain division, with the lowest rates in the Northeast region and its New England and particularly the Middle Atlantic divisions (see Figure 12.9). In fact, in 2010, every one of the eight individual states in the Mountain division ranked among the top ten in suicide rate (with Alaska, Oregon, and South Dakota, due to ties, completing the top 10). At the other extreme, 2010 is consistent with longstanding patterns where the Middle Atlantic states of New Jersey and New York rank 49th and 50th, respectively (the other Middle Atlantic state, Pennsylvania, ranks 33rd with a rate equal to the national figure), with the District of Columbia ranking 51st. Specific data by states, regions, and divisions (McIntosh & Drapeau, 2012) as well as by gender and for the young (15–24 years) and old (65 and above) may be found elsewhere (www.suicidology.org/stats-and-tools/suicide-statistics). Geographic patterns by gender and for the age groups young and old are highly similar to the national levels noted already.

Methods of suicide

Although declining consistently over time, firearms remain the most frequently employed method in US suicides. For the year 2010, firearms were utilized in 19,392 of the 38,364 deaths by suicide (50.5%). For the nation as a whole, hanging, strangulation, and suffocation represented more than 2 out of every 10 intentional deaths (9,493; 24.7%); while poisons, which includes solid,

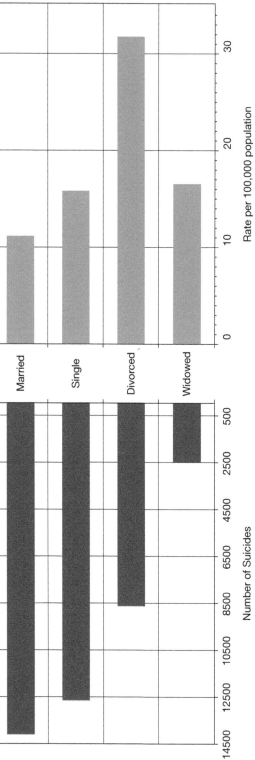

Figure 12.8 Suicides and suicide rates by marital status in the USA, 2010

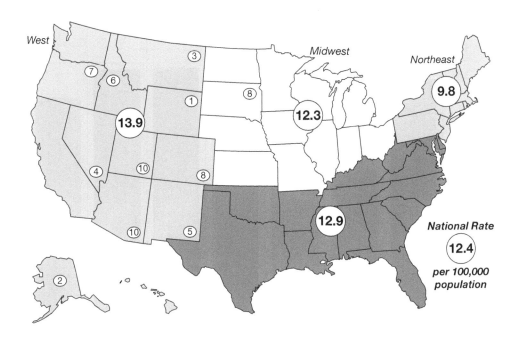

Figure 12.9 Regional suicide rates in the USA and Top-10 ranking states, 2010

liquid, and gas poisons, were almost 2 of every 10 suicides (6,599; 17.2%); and all other methods combined were less than 1 of 10 (2,880; 7.8%). Gender differences in suicide methods are apparent, with men using firearms as their most common method (16,962; 56.0%) while women most often used poisons (3,026; 37.4%). Suffocation ranked second for men (7,592; 25.1%) while firearms were second for women (2,430; 30.0%). Men infrequently used poisons in their suicides (3,573; 11.8%). Firearms as a suicide method increased consistently and dramatically in the USA from the end of the 1940s until approximately 1990 for the nation and for both men and women. In addition, since that time a consistent decline for each of these same groups can be seen for the subsequent two decades (through 2010; McIntosh, 2012).

Temporal cycles

Suicides follow consistent patterns related to their occurrence by months of the year/seasons as well as days of the week. These patterns have shown some small fluctuations over time but have been relatively consistent. It should be noted that the differences between particular days of the week or months of the year are often relatively small, but the patterns of highest and lowest are generally consistent. Although a study (Kposowa & D'Auria, 2009) provided data that implied that the day of the week of highest levels of suicides was Wednesday, McIntosh (2009) disputed these data and suggested that the result was most likely due to location errors of the variable in the data files employed. In fact, as McIntosh (2001 and 2004) has shown, the day of the week on which the highest number of suicides occurs has always been Monday (at least for the time period 1992–2010), followed essentially always by Tuesday, with the weekend lowest (Saturday and Sunday, with Friday lowest among the weekdays; see Figure 12.10).

Researchers even from the time of Durkheim ([1897] 1951) have compiled data on the seasonality of suicides (McIntosh, 2001 and 2004). Patterns in the USA for many years showed

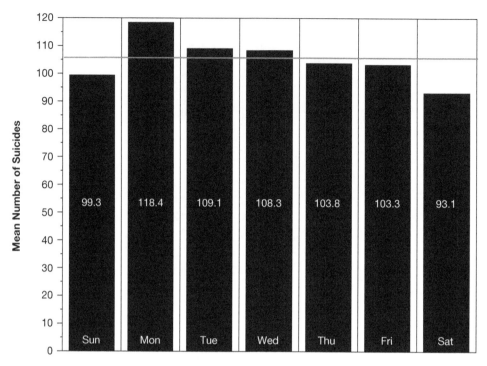

Figure 12.10 Suicides by days of the week in the USA, 2010

highest suicide levels in spring followed by fall months, with winter in particular (especially November and December) as well as fall being the lowest times for suicides. However, in recent years the numbers of suicides in the summer months have increased to levels similar to (and in some cases higher than) those in the spring months, so that presently the best description of highest levels of suicides are in the spring and summer months (see Figure 12.11).

Special consideration: suicide among military personnel

Although complete official suicide statistics for US military personnel are not readily available, recent developments in suicide in the military deserve attention at this time. Data providing information about suicide among military personnel are released by the various military branches, included among the variables compiled for 16 US states (available through CDC's WISQARS website, see CDC, 2012; e.g., Karch, Logan, McDaniel, Parks, & Patel, 2012), and provided in individual studies of military suicide. Traditionally, the suicide rate of military personnel has been lower than that for the corresponding groups in the population as a whole (e.g., Bagley, Munjas, & Shekelle, 2010). However, in the 1990s, to combat suicides among active military personnel, successful military suicide prevention programs were developed and instituted that were associated with the lowering of suicide rates in those military branches (e.g., Air Force: see Goldsmith, Pellmar, Kleinman, & Bunney, 2002, pp. 304–307, 436–438). Despite these promising early prevention efforts, in the past few years, suicide numbers and rates have increased in the military personnel of several branches, including veterans who have served in combat, active duty soldiers, and reservists. The explanations for these increases are not clear, though factors such as multiple deployments, PTSD and other mental health disorders, and traumatic brain injuries have all been

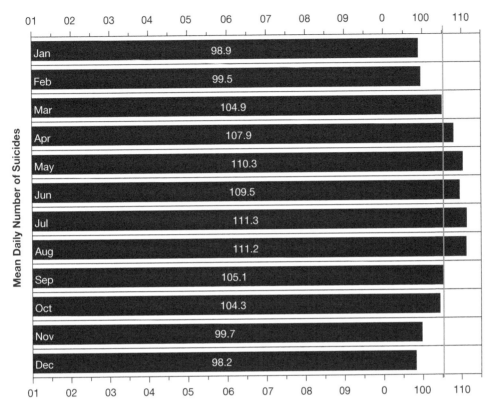

Figure 12.11 Suicides by months in the USA, 2010

noted as possible contributors. Concerted multiple efforts and numerous investigations have been instituted in the past few years in an effort to understand and prevent additional and future suicides and suicide attempts (e.g., Kuehn, 2009; Martin, Ghahramanlou-Holloway, Lou, & Tucciarone, 2009; Braswell & Kushner, 2012). The issue of suicide among members of the US Armed Forces is addressed in numerous sections and the prevention goals of the recently released *2012 National Strategy for Suicide Prevention* (Office of the Surgeon General and National Action Alliance for Suicide Prevention, 2012).

Conclusion

Providing the most recent official figures for suicide in the USA, this chapter has identified that the modal suicide victim primarily remains the same as in earlier times. That is, the highest risk group for suicide demographically is white elderly males, though increases among the middle-aged have raised the risk in this group to high levels as well. After approximately two decades of mostly declining suicide rates for nearly all demographic groups in the USA, recent increases among many groups have been noted.

While economic crises have often been raised as the reason for recent increases, and specific anecdotal evidence supporting this factor has been presented, explanations for changes in suicide are not easily determined. In fact, while correlational evidence might eventually demonstrate relationships, it should be noted that correlation does not necessarily indicate causation and more importantly, group findings (which are the nature of population-level demographic data) may not be relevant for individual risk or motivations. For example, noting that a suicide was a male or an older adult does not mean that their suicide was caused by either individually or even the combination of these two demographic characteristics. In other words, their suicide may well have been the result of forces totally unrelated to these demographic attributes. An additional caution about the use of population-level data relates to their usefulness in clinical decisions. For instance, although elderly African American women may be among the lowest risk population for death by suicide in the USA, a woman with those characteristics who presents to a clinician for assessment may well be determined by the clinician—based on clinical evidence, experience, judgment, and assessment—to be at higher risk for an imminent suicidal act than an elderly white male seen by the same clinician. Demographic figures can provide a component of assessment of individuals' risk of suicide but they are not strong enough alone to represent vital predictive power in the individual clinical setting. On the other hand, epidemiological data can provide important surveillance information regarding trends in deaths by suicide as well as identifying populations for whom preventive efforts are needed and among whom research and clinical evidence are encouraged to better understand the motivations to suicide and suggest possible prevention and intervention measures. In that regard, the data of this chapter suggest strongly, particularly when evaluated in terms of existing prevention approaches (which often do not involve many of the high-risk groups identified here, e.g., Lester, 2001; Maris, Berman, & Silverman, 2000, Chapter 21; Goldsmith et al., 2002, Chapter 8), that targeted prevention and intervention efforts might help address the high risk of men, the aged and middle-aged, and military personnel. Possible method restriction measures, related particularly to firearms and poisons, might also be effective to reduce the numbers of suicides in the population.

As demonstrated here, suicide is an important mental and public health issue. When these data are combined with those for suicide ideation and issues associated with the aftermath of suicide, the magnitude is seen to be considerably larger. For instance, in addition to the over 38,000 deaths by suicide, a nationwide Substance Abuse and Mental Health Services Administration (Centers for Disease Control and Prevention, 2011) survey found that in the past year (data for 2008–2009) alone 8.3 million Americans had serious thoughts of suicide (3.7% of the national population), 2.2 million had made a plan to kill themselves (1.0%), and 1 million had made an attempt on their lives (0.5%). Conservative estimates imply that over 230,000 individuals annually are affected by the suicide death of a significant other and at least 4.7 million individuals in the US population are bereaved by suicide (McIntosh & Drapeau, 2012).

Suicide is a multi-determined behavior, produced by multiple factors in combination and not by any single factor. These factors may include psychological (e.g., depression, hopelessness, burdensomeness, psychological pain), physical (e.g., illness, pain), social (isolation, loneliness), and cultural forces that may be addressed in prevention and intervention efforts to prevent suicide. Issues related to individual demographic characteristics (e.g., gender, race/ethnicity, life period, cohort experiences, etc.) may also be important in the suicides of individuals. Each of these factors represents potential issues that might be addressed to prevent individual suicides and in turn affect epidemiological patterns and trends.

Note on the text

Although not a duplication, this chapter updates the data for trends and levels presented in McIntosh (1991) with over two decades of figures as well as the addition of contemporary epidemiological issues.

References

Allen, N. H. (1984). Suicide statistics. In C. L. Hatton, & S. M. Valente (Eds.), *Suicide: Assessment and intervention* (2nd ed., pp. 17–31). Norwalk, CT: Appleton-Century-Crofts.

Bagley, S. C., Munjas, B., & Shekelle, P. (2010). A systematic review of suicide prevention programs for military or veterans. *Suicide and Life-threatening Behavior, 40,* 257–265.

Braswell, H., & Kushner, H. I. (2012). Suicide, social integration, and masculinity in the U.S. military. *Social Science & Medicine, 74,* 530–536.

Centers for Disease Control and Prevention (2011). Suicidal thoughts and behaviors among adults aged ≥18 years – United States, 2008–2009. *Morbidity and Mortality Weekly Report [MMWR], 60* (Whole No. SS-#13), October 21.

Centers for Disease Control and Prevention, National Center for Injury Prevention and Control (2012). *Web-based Injury Statistics Query and Reporting System (WISQARS),* September 18. Available at: www.cdc.gov/ncipc/wisqars [Fatal Injury Data].

Durkheim, E. ([1897] 1951). *Suicide.* New York: Free Press.

Goldsmith, S. K., Pellmar, T. C., Kleinman, A. M., & Bunney, W. E. (Eds.) (2002) Committee on Pathophysiology and Prevention of Adolescent and Adult Suicide, Board on Neuroscience and Behavioral Health, Institute of Medicine of the National Academies. *Reducing suicide: A national imperative.* Washington, DC: National Academies Press.

Hu, G., Wilcox, H. C., Wissow, L., & Baker, S. P. (2008). Mid-life suicide: An increasing problem in U.S. whites, 1999–2005. *American Journal of Preventive Medicine, 35,* 589–593.

Jordan, J. R., & McIntosh, J. L. (Eds.) (2011). *Grief after suicide: Understanding the consequences and caring for the survivors.* New York: Routledge.

Karch, D. L., Logan, J., McDaniel, D., Parks, S., & Patel, N. (2012). Surveillance for violent deaths: National Violent Death Reporting Systems, 16 states, 2009. *Morbidity and Mortality Weekly Report [MMWR], 60* (No. SS-#6), 1–43. September 14.

Kposowa, A. J., & D'Auria, S. (2009). Association of temporal factors and suicides in the United States, 2000–2004. *Social Psychiatry and Psychiatric Epidemiology, 45,* 433–445. doi: 10.1007/s00127-009-0082-9.

Kuehn, B. M. (2009). Soldier suicide rates continue to rise: Military, scientists work to stem the tide. *JAMA, 301,* 111–112.

Lester, D. (Ed.). (2001). *Suicide prevention: Resources for the millennium.* Philadelphia, PA: Brunner-Rutledge.

Maris, R. W., Berman, A. L., & Silverman, M. M. (Eds.) (2000). *Comprehensive textbook of suicidology.* New York: Guilford Press.

Martin, J., Ghahramanlou-Holloway, M., Lou, K., & Tucciarone. P. (2009). A comparative review of U.S. military and civilian suicide behavior: Implications for OEF/OIF suicide prevention efforts. *Journal of Mental Health Counseling, 31,* 101–118.

McIntosh, J. L. (1991). Epidemiology of suicide in the United States. In A. A. Leenaars (Ed.), *Life-span perspectives of suicide: Time-lines in the suicide process* (pp. 55–69). New York: Plenum Press.

McIntosh, J. L. (1993). Risk to life through the adult years. In R. Kastenbaum (Ed.), *Encyclopedia of adult development* (pp. 414–421). Phoenix, AZ: Oryx Press.

McIntosh, J. L. (2000). Epidemiology of adolescent suicide in the United States. In R. W. Maris, S. S. Canetto, J. L. McIntosh, & M. M. Silverman (Eds.), *Review of suicidology, 2000* (pp. 3–33). New York: Guilford Press.

McIntosh, J. L. (2001). Month, season and weekday variations in US suicide. Poster presentation at the annual meeting of the American Association of Suicidology, Atlanta, GA, April 19. Summary appears in J. L. McIntosh (Ed.). (2004). *Suicide 2001: Proceedings of American Association of Suicidology 34th annual conference* (CD-ROM; no pagination, Paper #P193, 2 pp.). Washington, DC: AAS.

McIntosh, J. L. (2009). "Suicide highest on Wednesday!" Really?! *NewsLink E-Community,* (quarterly newsletter of the American Association of Suicidology), *36*(2). Available at: http://app.e2ma.net/campaign/25465.ab393472b7d15dfceb661f2a2f1d04fe.

McIntosh, J.L. (2012). *U.S.A. suicide statistics for the year 2010: Overheads.* Washington, DC: American Association of Suicidology. Overheads of demographic variables and suicide include 78 slides. Available at: www.suicidology.com.

McIntosh, J. L., & Drapeau, C. W. (2012). *U.S.A. suicide 2010: Official final data.* Washington, DC: American Association of Suicidology, September 21. Available at: www.suicidology.org/stats-and-tools/suicide-statistics.

McIntosh, J. L., & Jewell, B. L. (1986). Sex difference trends in completed suicide. *Suicide and Life-threatening Behavior, 16,* 16–27.

McIntosh, J. L., Santos, J. F., Hubbard, R. W., & Overholser, J. C. (1994). *Elder suicide: Research, theory, and treatment*. Washington, DC: American Psychological Association.

Office of the Surgeon General (U.S. Department of Health and Human Services), & National Action Alliance for Suicide Prevention (2012). *2012 National Strategy for Suicide Prevention: Goals and objectives for action*. Washington, DC: HHS.

Phillips, J. A., Robin, A. V., Nugent, C. N., & Idler, E. L. (2010). Understanding recent changes in suicide rates among the middle-aged: Period or cohort effects? *Public Health Reports, 25,* 680–688.

Rockett, I. R. H., Regier, M. D., Kapusta, N. D., Coben, J. H., Miller, T. R., Hanzlick, R. L., Todd, K. H., Sattin, R. W., Kennedy, L. W., Kleinig, J., & Smith, G. S. (2012). Leading causes of unintentional and intentional injury mortality: United States, 2000–2009. *American Journal of Public Health,* published online ahead of print, 2012, *102,* e84–e92. doi:10.2105/AJPH.2012.300960.

World Health Organization. (2012). *Public health action for the prevention of suicide: A framework*. Geneva: WHO. Available at: www.who.int/mental_health/prevention/suicide/suicideprevent/en/ (accessed October 14, 2012).

13

ATTITUDES TOWARD THERAPISTS WHO LOSE PATIENTS TO SUICIDE

Erin F. Ward-Ciesielski, John L. McIntosh and Joscelyn Rompogren

Introduction

Providers across health care disciplines have the potential to encounter individuals who are suicidal and, as a result, to lose individuals under their care to suicide. This clinical inevitability is undeniably impactful and can have significant consequences for the treating professional, ranging from legal and professional repercussions to psychological and personal effects. In recent years, there has been a growing interest and increased research conducted on the topic of psycho-therapists who lose patients to suicide (e.g., Weiner, 2005; Dyregrov, 2011; Gutin, McGann, & Jordan, 2011). This body of evidence focuses almost exclusively on issues related to the experiences of the treating therapists at the time of the suicide (e.g., Gorkin, 1985). In particular, this research provides initial data concerning the personal and professional reactions to the suicide (e.g., Fox & Cooper, 1998; Farberow, 2005), possible ideas for postvention programs or courses (Kolodny, Binder, Bronstein, & Friend, 1979), as well as information and support for therapists in the event of a client suicide (Michel, 1997; Rycroft, 2005). However, though growing, current evidence remains sparse regarding the experiences of patient suicides for those impacted.

In an attempt to determine the prevalence of this clinical occurrence, Chemtob and colleagues investigated the frequency and impact of patient suicide among psychologists and psychiatrists (Chemtob, Hamada, Bauer, Torigoe, & Kinney, 1988b, and Chemtob, Hamada, Bauer, Kinney, & Torigoe, 1988a, respectively). They determined that 22% of psychologists and 51% of psychiatrists had experienced the loss of a patient to suicide and that "39 percent of [psychologists] who have lost one patient can expect subsequent [patient] suicide" (Chemtob et al., 1988b, p. 415), while 55% of psychiatrists could expect another suicide (Chemtob et al., 1988a).

Among the psychologists who had lost a patient to suicide, Chemtob, Hamada, Bauer, Torigoe, and Kinney (1988b) found that 49% reported post-traumatic symptoms. However, as would be expected, the reactions of therapists following a suicide encompass a wide variety of feelings, thoughts, and emotions. The most common of these reactions—including shock, disbelief, denial, sadness, anger, guilt, and anxiety—all seem to be a direct response to the death itself (Goldstein & Buongiorno, 1984; Chemtob et al., 1988b; Michel, 1997; Hendin, Haas, Maltsberger, Szanto, & Rabinowicz, 2004). As one of the first to explore this issue, Litman (1965) concluded that therapists react in a uniquely human fashion—as opposed to exhibiting a purely professional response—when confronting the suicide of a patient. From among the human reactions that all survivors of suicide have reported (e.g., Calhoun, Selby, & Selby, 1982; McIntosh, 1999; Jordan, 2001), guilt is prominent. Guilt experienced by therapists focuses on "self-questioning" (Litman, 1965, p. 573) and revolves around the therapist wondering if he or she did everything possible to prevent the suicide from taking place.

Not surprisingly, client suicides have more than emotional implications and can affect therapist-survivors' functioning in both their personal and professional lives. A meta-analysis of survivor literature showed that there is an overwhelming need for peer support, social networks, and professional help for those who experience the loss of someone to suicide, but these services may be overlooked when it comes to therapist-survivors (Dyregrov, 2011).

Alexander, Klein, Gray, Dewar, and Eagles (2000) surveyed 247 consulting psychiatrists in Scotland. Participants answered questions regarding the most distressing suicide they had encountered in their professional careers. Of these respondents, 33% admitted that the suicide had had an impact on their personal and daily lives, including experiences ranging from loss of sleep to preoccupation with the suicide itself. Alexander et al. also found that only 15% of the respondents had attended the patient's funeral, even though most of those who did attend described the occasion as helpful in reducing some of the more unpleasant reactions following the suicide. These researchers speculated that therapists may forgo this potentially grief-easing opportunity owing to fears and anxieties related to the reactions of the patients' families. Consistent with such an interpretation, Michel (1997) provided an account of his personal anxiety following the suicide death of a patient. After the client's death, he describes feeling afraid that the husband of that client would blame him for his wife's death and would ultimately come after and even kill him.

In an attempt to combine information from individual responses into a more general model of the therapist experience, Menninger (1991) found that "shock (feeling stunned or surprised), sadness (feeling loss or grief), anger, a sense of guilt ([feeling] regret), anxiety (feeling worried or fearful of criticism), and doubt about [their] competence (questioning their skills, feeling inadequate)" (p. 217) were the most frequently cited reactions experienced by a therapist over the loss of a client or patient to suicide. The set of responses that can be categorized as professional reactions (guilt, doubt about competence, etc.) seems to center on beliefs held by the therapist concerning his or her own inadequacy and failure.

These last aspects of therapist perceptions of inadequacy and doubt regarding competence or abilities are the most pertinent to the present study. The notion that those professionals who lose patients feel acute stress concerning their possible loss of professional standing in the eyes of their peers, the public, and the loved ones who survive the death appears as a common theme throughout the literature. These professionals worry that their colleagues, their supervisors, their institutions, and the family of the deceased will view them as incompetent failures or even as responsible for the death. These feelings of inadequacy or incompetence are likely to affect a therapist's responsibilities toward other clients, which may interfere with their ability to provide the best care. However, the experiences therapists go through in the aftermath of a client suicide may promote professional and personal growth if appropriate coping strategies are offered as a postvention (Valente & Saunders, 2002). There is currently a lack of resources for therapist-survivors that could be remedied by developing and enhancing support groups, supervision techniques, or workshops (one resource is a webpage at the American Association of Suicidology's site, www.suicidology.org/suicide-clinician-survivors).

While most attention in the literature has focused on psychologists and psychiatrists, other health care providers are similarly at risk of losing a patient to suicide and their reactions are documented in the literature. For instance, nurses and caregivers in a combat zone in Iraq have written about their experiences following the suicide of an individual with whom they were working (Valente & Saunders, 2002; Carr, 2011). While this chapter will focus on psychologists and other mental health care professionals, it is important to recognize that a wide range of health care professionals are working with individuals who may be at risk for suicide and for whom a patient's suicide death may be experienced. Thus, this study has implications and relevance to anyone who comes in contact with suicidal individuals in a helping capacity.

Despite the prevalence of experiencing the death of a patient by suicide, the majority of the small available literature remains focused on individual anecdotal experiences and reflections. There has only been one previous study conducted with an objective similar to the present one (Peterson, Luoma, & Dunne, 2002), and it served as a valuable resource for creating the survey used in this investigation. Peterson et al. surveyed survivors of suicide regarding their perceptions of the clinician treating their loved one at the time of their death by suicide. Of the 55 respondents, 42% believed the therapist had not told them all they wanted to know, and 48% believed the therapist had deceived them and withheld information. In addition, 72% thought the therapist had made mistakes while treating their loved one and 40% viewed the therapist as having held back information that might have been self-incriminating. Finally, 64% perceived the therapist as failing to do all he or she could have done in order to save the loved one's life. These results reflect an overwhelming sense of blame, anger, and distrust experienced by survivors of suicide toward the treating clinician. More extensive knowledge about survivor attitudes towards therapists could be used to develop comprehensive treatments for those who have lost a loved one to suicide.

Missing from previous research is how the colleagues, supervisors, institutions, families and general public view a therapist who loses a patient to suicide. Although basic to the situation of therapists as client suicide survivors, this specific issue has failed to receive much scholarly attention. The existing literature reveals that the professional may experience genuine anguish as a result of fears that he/she has failed in his/her therapeutic responsibilities to the patient. Nevertheless, attitudinal studies to determine the perceptions of therapists who have lost a patient to suicide are lacking. Therefore, this study hopes to begin a process that may help determine whether everyone (or anyone) else views the situation as a failure. That is, the present study aspires to investigate the instance of various attitudes (both negative and positive) toward therapist-survivors.

Specifically, this study seeks to identify attitudes the general population has toward therapists who lose patients to suicide. This preliminary investigation, in turn, will provide information about the frequency of serious negative reactions from the family and friends of the deceased. Based on the overall thrust of the literature, it is hypothesized that individuals who have had more experience with suicide (i.e., those who have lost a friend, relative, or loved one to suicide) will have more negative feelings toward therapists than those who have had less experience and exposure (i.e., those who have not lost anyone to suicide). Further, with respect to assessing the attitudes of therapists, it is hypothesized that those who have lost a patient to suicide will have less negative feelings toward fellow colleagues who have had the same experience.

Finally, in order to propel investigation on this topic, we were interested in the extent to which therapists' beliefs about how the loved ones of their deceased patients perceived them were representative of the actual attitudes held by the survivors. As there was no literature to guide our hypotheses, this was an exploratory aim of the study and the data from the general population and therapists in practice were compared.

Survey 1: Method

Participants

A total of 248 introductory psychology students (72 men and 173 women, 3 did not provide gender information; with a mean age of 23.2 years, $SD = 8.6$) at a Midwestern public university participated in the study (a total of 60 of these participants self-identified as losing someone to suicide; see Table 13.1). An announcement made about the study in each of the campus's introductory psychology classes acted as a means of soliciting participation. Links to the online survey (hosted by www.surveymonkey.com) were distributed and respondents received course credit for participating.

Materials and procedure

The study and its surveys were approved by the campus IRB. Questions within the survey primarily reflected Peterson et al.'s (2002) previous study of survivors' perceptions toward the therapists treating their loved ones at the time of the suicides. Using questions such as "Have you ever lost a friend, relative, or loved one to suicide?" and "Have you ever attempted suicide?," the survey's primary questions assessed the participants' level of experience with suicide. The responses to these primary questions determined which follow-up questions in the survey each respondent answered next. For example, if a participant answered that he *had* lost a friend, relative, or loved one to suicide, he would then answer a question about whether the individual who died by suicide had been in therapy at the time of the suicide.

Table 13.1 University participant demographic information

	(%)	N	M	SD
Have lost someone to suicide	24.19	60		
Parent	3.22	2		
Sibling	1.61	1		
Aunt/uncle	9.68	6		
Cousin	6.45	4		
Grandparent	4.84	3		
Significant other	0.00	0		
Best friend	0.00	0		
Other friend	51.61	32		
Other	22.58	14		
Time since suicide (in months)[a]			80.23	80.90
Age at time of suicide[a]			18.28	7.27
Feelings about therapy[b]			5.22	1.24
Feelings about therapists[b]			4.94	1.21
Attempted suicide (participant)[b]				
Yes	12.5	31		
No	87.5	217		

Notes: Ratings of feelings toward therapy and therapists are on a 7-point Likert-type scale with 1 indicating "extremely negative" and 7 indicating "extremely positive."

[a] N = 53. [b] N = 248.

Based on the responses to the two questions mentioned previously, the respondents answered between 9 and 28 questions (see Table 13.2). Therefore, the respondents' answers to the primary questions divided them into two categories: those who had lost someone to suicide and those who had not. Those who had lost someone (*N* = 60) answered questions about how they felt or would feel about a therapist treating their friend, relative, or loved one at the time of the suicide. For example, participants were asked to indicate the degree to which they blamed the therapist, how confident they felt in the therapist's abilities, how angry they felt, and how much they trusted the therapist. There were 13 attitudinal statements in all (see Table 13.3). The

Table 13.2 Demographic information for individuals who died by suicide (university participants)

	N	*(%)*
In therapy prior to death[a]	11	18.03
Yes, and in therapy at the time of suicide	6	11.48
Yes, but not in therapy at the time of suicide	4	6.56
No	34	55.74
Don't know	16	26.23
Suicide attempts prior to death by suicide[b]	12	21.43
Yes, multiple attempts	6	10.71
Yes, one attempt	6	10.71
No, never before	44	78.57
Risk of suicide was suspected by participant[b]		
Yes	9	16.07
No	47	89.93

Note. [a] N = 60. [b] N = 56.

Table 13.3 Mean attitudinal statement scores for university participant respondents

Attitudinal statement	Students who lost (in therapy)[a]	Students who lost (not in therapy)[b]	Students who have not lost[c]
Therapist failed	2.83	2.78	2.96
Reassured that therapist was treating	2.80	3.13	3.18
Betrayed by therapist	2.00	2.31	2.46
Trusted the therapist	2.83	3.15	3.21
Confident in the abilities of therapist	2.83	3.20	3.10
Outrage toward therapist	2.33	2.15	2.30
Secure knowing he/she was in therapy	2.33	2.95	3.16
Blamed the therapist	1.50	2.00	2.05
Grateful that therapist was treating	3.20	3.18	3.30
Anger toward therapist	2.00	2.58	2.62
Discouraged about effectiveness of therapy	3.33	3.28	3.38
Disappointed by therapist	2.67	2.98	3.07
Contempt toward therapist	2.00	2.80	2.60

Notes: Attitudes were measured on a 5-point scale (1 = *strongly disagree*, 5 = *strongly agree*).

[a] N = 6. [b] N = 55. [c] N = 185.

individuals who had not lost someone ($N = 188$) answered questions about how they *believed* they would have felt if they had lost someone to suicide and that person had been in therapy at the time of his or her death. These attitudinal questions were identical to those answered by participants who had lost someone to suicide, except that the wording was changed to indicate that they were *imagining* the loss of a loved one.

After these initial groupings of topics, the respondents answered a second question designed to divide them further: "Have you ever attempted suicide?" Participants who had not made a suicide attempt bypassed superfluous questions and finished the survey here, while those who had made a suicide attempt answered the question, "Were you in therapy at the time of your attempt?" Those individuals who were in therapy responded to questions similar to those asked earlier in relation to their respective feelings toward the therapist treating their loved one at the time of the loved one's death. Participants who were not in therapy at the time of their suicide attempt responded to questions regarding how they *believed* they would have felt if a therapist had been treating them at the time of the attempt. The final question of the survey asked all participants whether they were currently in therapy or had ever been in the past. The last page of the survey provided information containing the names and telephone numbers of various area mental health agencies, including bereavement services.

Survey 2: Method

Participants

Some 101 therapists (29 men and 72 women, mean age = 45.2, $SD = 14.2$, mean years in practice = 12.9, $SD = 9.2$) participated in the study. The names and addresses of therapists in Northern Indiana were collected from telephone directories and online searches. Agencies were contacted by telephone and every attempt was made to obtain information regarding the number of practicing therapists at the agency. A total of 417 surveys were mailed at the initial mailing; 21 surveys were returned owing to undeliverable addresses. The 101 surveys that were returned represented a 24.2% response rate.

Materials and procedure

A 43-item survey was presented in two forms: a link to a survey posted online (hosted by www.surveymonkey.com) and a paper copy. Therapists were given the option of either format. Nearly all ($N = 98$) completed the paper version.

Questions contained in the survey were selected based on information collected from previous studies that looked at the feelings and reactions of therapists following the death of a patient to suicide (Goldstein & Buongiorno, 1984; Chemtob et al., 1988a; Chemtob et al., 1988b; Michel, 1997; Hendin et al., 2004). Of the 43 total questions in the survey, each respondent answered between 15 and 30 questions. Similar to the university participant survey, depending on individual answers to primary questions, respondents were directed (automatically by the online survey or via written instructions on the paper one) through the survey (see Table 13.4). The survey began with questions to ascertain each therapist's level of experience with the suicide of a patient. Based on answers to this question ("Have you ever lost a client/patient to suicide?"), participants were divided into one of two groups: those who had lost a patient to suicide ($N = 33$) and those who had not ($N = 67$). Those who had lost a patient answered questions about how they felt following the suicide, how those closest to the deceased reacted to the therapist (i.e., the responding therapist), and how the respondent's colleagues reacted following the suicide. Those who had

Table 13.4 Therapist participant demographic information

	(%)	N	M	SD
Years in practice[a]			13.10	9.02
Predictability of suicide[b]			2.41	0.81
Preventability of suicide[c]			2.64	0.93
Lost a friend, relative, or loved one to suicide[a]	31.00	31		
Lost a patient to suicide[d]	32.67	33		
Time since last patient suicide (in years)[e]			8.73	7.78
Sought therapy following patient suicide[e]	12.12	4		
Had patient attempt suicide[b]	72.73	72		
Colleague patient suicide[f]	58.76	57		

Note. Ratings of predictability and preventability of suicide are on a 5-point Likert-type scale with 1 indicating "not at all" and 5 indicating "completely." [a] N = 100. [b] N = 99. [c] N = 98. [d] N = 101. [e] N = 33. [f] N = 97.

not lost a patient were presented with similar questions in which they were asked to *imagine* how they believe those closest to the person who died by suicide would react toward the therapist (i.e., the respondent) and how they *believed* their colleagues would react. The attitudinal questions presented to participants in both of these groups were almost identical to those described above in the university participant survey. However, instead of asking how they felt about a therapist, they were asked to rate how they believed the friends and family of the deceased felt about them. For example, therapists were asked to rate the level to which they believed the friends and family blamed (or would blame) them for the suicide, how angry the family was (or would have been) following the suicide, and how reassured the family was (or would feel) that their loved one was in therapy at the time of his or her death.

All participants were then presented with the question "Have you ever had a client/patient make a non-fatal suicide attempt?" Those respondents who had not had this experience (N = 27) were directed to the last questions of the survey, while those who had (N = 72) were presented with follow-up questions similar to those about patients who died by suicide. Finally, all participants were asked, "Have any of your colleagues in the field experienced the death of a client/patient by suicide?" Those who answered yes (N = 57) were presented with follow-up questions about how they responded to these colleagues. These attitudinal questions were similar in format to those described above, but included items that were more relevant to attitudes that might be expected within a work environment (e.g., the degree to which you supported the colleague, pointed out mistakes the colleague made, and referred fewer suicidal clients to the colleague; see Table 13.5). Those who answered no (N = 40) were asked how they *believed* they would respond to a colleague who lost a patient to suicide.

Results

The first study hypothesis was that university participants who had lost a friend, relative, or loved one to suicide would endorse more negative feelings toward therapists than individuals who had not experienced such a loss. Students were divided by whether or not they had actually lost a loved one to suicide. Owing to the small number of respondents who had lost someone who was in therapy at the time of death (N = 6), this subset of participants were omitted from analyses. Instead, the two groups used for subsequent comparisons each imagined the presence of a

Table 13.5 Mean attitudinal statement scores for therapist respondents

Attitudinal statement	Therapists who lost[a]	Therapists who have not lost[b]
Supported colleague	4.47	4.44
Felt the colleague was competent	4.25	4.13
Trusted decisions colleague made	4.16	4.04
Advised colleague	3.53	3.62
Pointed out mistakes colleague made	1.94	1.97
Rejected colleague professionally	1.83	1.89
Referred fewer suicidal clients to colleague	1.72	1.71
Blamed the colleague	1.50	1.52
Isolated colleague	1.41	1.46

Note. Attitudes were measured on a 5-point scale (1 = *strongly disagree*, 5 = *strongly agree*). [a] N = 31.
[b] N = 56.

therapist. The first group (those who had lost a loved one to suicide, but whose loved one was not in therapy at the time of death) imagined that a therapist treated their loved one who died by suicide, while the second group imagined both the death of a loved one by suicide and the presence of a therapist treating that loved one. The average of all negative attitude scores were not significantly different between students who experienced loss and those who did not, and the same was found for positive attitude scores. Thus, the data do not support this first hypothesis.

The second study hypothesis was that therapists who had lost a patient to suicide would endorse less negative feelings toward other therapists who have had the same loss than would therapists who had not lost a patient. In order to test this hypothesis, a factor analysis was first conducted on the data, but the three factors yielded by the factor analysis were not meaningfully related. Instead, independent samples *t*-tests compared each of the nine attitudinal statements to which therapists had responded regarding the way they believed they would react (or the way they had reacted) to a colleague who had lost a client or patient to suicide (Table 13.5). The first group consisted of therapists who had actually lost a client themselves (*N* = 31), while the second group of therapists had never experienced the loss of a client to suicide (*N* = 56). After utilizing a Bonferroni correction, none of the comparisons were statistically significant; thus, the data did not support this second hypothesis.

Finally, we were interested in the relation between the university participants' feelings toward therapists and what therapists expected others' feelings would be in the event of a patient suicide. Owing to the developmental stage of the surveys used and the lack of empirical literature addressing this question, there was no hypothesis regarding a specific relation between the responses given by university participants and those given by therapists. This analysis is considered a preliminary investigation of perceived and actual attitudes of survivors towards therapists.

An exploratory factor analysis was conducted using scores of all 13 attitudinal statements from the survey the students completed. Using the SPSS statistical software package (version 16), the factor analysis was rotated using a varimax rotation, and yielded two components (Table 13.6). The first component included attitudinal statements with negative target words (i.e., "anger" and "blame"), while the second consisted of positive statements (i.e., "trust" and "confident"). The word "contempt" was excluded from both factors due to its relatively low loading in either component.

After the attitudes were grouped, scores from all attitude statements in each factor were averaged to make one total mean score for negative attitudes and one total mean score for positive

Table 13.6 Exploratory factor analysis: rotated loadings

Variable	Therapist participants		University participants	
	Negative component	Positive component	Negative component	Positive component
Anger	.857		.810	
Outrage	.847		.750	
Blame	.829		.738	
Disappointed	.827		.696	
Discouraged	.790		.738	
Betrayed	.764		.768	
Failed	–		.766	
Secure		.874		.824
Grateful		.867		.733
Reassured		.756		.811
Trusted		.512		.667
Confident		–		.718

Note. Loadings of less than .40 are not included.

attitudes. An independent group's *t*-test was used to compare mean scores of each factor between students who have more experience with suicide and students who do not (i.e., those who have lost a loved one and those who have not).

To evaluate the relationship between student and therapist attitudes, an exploratory factor analysis was conducted to determine the factor structure of the attitudes therapists expected others to have toward them following a patient suicide. These variables were also rotated using a varimax rotation, and loaded into factors that were considered "negative" and "positive" (Table 13.6). Again, scores from all attitude statements in each component were averaged to make one total mean for negative attitudes and one total mean for positive attitudes (Table 13.7).

An independent group's *t*-test was performed to compare the negative attitude mean and the positive attitude mean between therapists and students. Only attitudinal statements that were grouped into the same components for both therapists' expectations and students' actual attitudes were used in this analysis. There was a significant difference in mean scores between therapists and students for both positive and negative factors: therapists rated positive attitudes significantly lower than students, $t(288) = -5.27$, $p < 0.001$, and they rated negative attitudes significantly higher than students, $t(292) = 6.492$, $p < 0.001$.

Discussion

To date, there has been a paucity of empirical investigation into the actual attitudes that suicide survivors have toward the therapist or other mental health professional involved in their loved one's treatment at the time of death (or, more generally, about therapists who have lost a patient to death by suicide). As such, this study of general population and therapist attitudes is an integral and necessary first step toward addressing the issue.

While neither hypothesis about the effect of losing a loved one or a patient to suicide was supported by the data obtained, the most interesting and significant finding of this study is that therapists appear to inaccurately predict the reactions of the individuals who are left behind after a patient suicide. Both comparisons between therapist and student attitudes demonstrate that

Table 13.7 Mean attitudinal statement scores for university and therapist respondents

Target word	Factor		Mean	
	Positive	Negative	Student[a]	Therapist[b]
Discouraged		Negative	3.35	3.38
Grateful	Positive		3.29	2.98
Trusted	Positive		3.20	3.00
Reassured	Positive		3.18	2.98
Confident	Positive		3.14	3.50
Secure	Positive		3.10	2.85
Disappointed		Negative	3.05	3.23
Failed		Negative	2.93	–
Contempt		Negative	2.62	2.82
Anger		Negative	2.60	3.20
Betrayed		Negative	2.42	2.84
Outrage		Negative	2.25	2.75
Blamed		Negative	2.05	2.92
Positive factor mean for all subjects			3.18	2.72
Negative factor mean for all subjects			2.65	3.40

Note. Attitudes were measured on a 5-point scale (1 = *strongly disagree*, 5 = *strongly agree*). [a] N = 235. [b] N = 55.

therapists believe that survivors have less positive attitudes and stronger negative attitudes toward them than were actually reported by the students. Thus, while the literature throughout the field would suggest that therapists should be concerned with the reactions of survivors and negative backlash following a patient suicide, the results from this study preliminarily indicate that this may not be the case.

Although this exploratory study has provided interesting questions upon which to base further investigation, it also has several limitations that are critical to consider when interpreting the results and planning future studies. First, because we had a very limited number of student participants who had lost someone to suicide and even fewer participants who had lost someone who was in therapy at the time of their death, we were unable to make anticipated comparisons. For instance, we had so few participants who had lost someone who was in therapy (N = 11) that we were unable to use these individuals in any analyses. Making comparisons between this group and those who had lost someone who was not in therapy would have been the ideal way to answer our first research question. Also, we were not able to compare the attitudes of students who had lost someone in therapy to the attitudes therapists expected these individuals to have as survivors. This would have been a preferable way in which to answer our third research question. Subsequent studies addressing this issue will benefit from recruiting participants in a way that increases the likelihood of including individuals who have lost someone to suicide, especially someone who was in therapy at the time of their death.

Second, there may be reason to question the comparison between the attitudes of therapists who have and have not lost a patient toward colleagues. Social desirability and discomfort admitting such a loss or poor memory about some past behavior may have been responsible for the limited variability in these responses. Unlike other areas of the survey where therapists were asked about their reactions following the death and the attitudes they believed survivors had toward them, there was very limited variability in the range of responses given on questions about attitudes and actions toward colleagues. Future projects would improve on the present study by addressing the potential for social desirability or recall biases in this section, in particular.

Despite these limitations, the information obtained through the use of these surveys is invaluable as a starting point from which to begin evaluating the types of realistic reactions that therapists can expect following the tragic and often traumatic death of a patient by suicide. Anecdotal reports on individual therapist experiences are important as a way to highlight the unfortunate fact that patient suicide is likely to be encountered by practicing therapists. However, the data are lacking on the extent to which these individual fears and expectations that are reported in anecdotal reports are, in fact, an accurate representation of the attitudes held by the general population. This study and the surveys developed for it provide one way to begin understanding the truth behind these fears and the extent to which they are more harmful than helpful for therapists following a patient suicide. This information can help with the development of appropriate postvention techniques that will foster professional growth rather than detrimental emotional responses among therapists who experience the loss of a patient to suicide.

Acknowledgements

An earlier report of some of the results of this study were presented at the April 2007 annual conference of the American Association of Suicidology, New Orleans, LA.

References

Alexander, D. A., Klein, S., Gray, N. M., Dewar, I. G., & Eagles, J. M. (2000). Suicide by patients: Questionnaire study of its effect on consultant psychiatrists. *British Medical Journal, 320*, 1571–1574. doi:10.1136/bmj.320.7249.1571.

Calhoun, L. G., Selby, J. W., & Selby, L. E. (1982). The psychological aftermath of suicide: An analysis of current evidence. *Clinical Psychology Review, 2*, 409–420. doi:10.1016/0272-7358(82)90021-6.

Carr, R. B. (2011). When a soldier commits suicide in Iraq: Impact on unit and caregivers. *Psychiatry, 74*, 95–106. doi:10.1521/psyc.2011.74.2.95.

Chemtob, C. M., Hamada, R. S., Bauer, G., Kinney, B., & Torigoe, R. Y. (1988a). Patients' suicides: Frequency and impact on psychiatrists. *American Journal of Psychiatry, 145*, 224–228.

Chemtob, C. M., Hamada, R. S., Bauer, G., Torigoe, R. Y., & Kinney, B. (1988b). Patient suicide: Frequency and impact on psychologists. *Professional Psychology: Research and Practice, 19*, 416–420. doi:10.1037/0735-7028.19.4.416.

Dyregrov, K. (2011). What do we know about needs for help after suicide in different parts of the world? A phenomenological perspective. *Crisis: The Journal of Crisis Intervention and Suicide Prevention, 32*, 310–318. doi:10.1027/0227-5910/a000098.

Farberow, N. L. (2005). The mental health professional as suicide survivor. *Clinical Neuropsychiatry, 2*, 13–20.

Fox, R., & Cooper, M. (1998). The effects of suicide on the private practitioner: A professional and personal perspective. *Clinical Social Work Journal, 26*, 143–157. doi:10.1023/A:1022866917611.

Goldstein, L. S., & Buongiorno, P. A. (1984). Psychotherapists as suicide survivors. *American Journal of Psychotherapy, 38*, 392–398.

Gorkin, M. (1985). On the suicide of one's patient. *Bulletin of the Menninger Clinic, 49*, 1–9.

Gutin, N., McGann, V. L., & Jordan, J. R. (2011). The impact of suicide on professional caregivers. In J. R. Jordan, & J. L. McIntosh (Eds.), *Grief after suicide: Understanding the consequences and caring for the survivors* (pp. 93–111). New York: Routledge.

Hendin, H., Haas, A. P., Maltsberger, J. T., Szanto, K., & Rabinowicz, H. (2004). Factors contributing to therapists' distress after the suicide of a patient. *American Journal of Psychiatry, 161*, 1442–1446. doi:10.1176-appi.ajp.161.8.1442.

Jordan, J. R. (2001). Is suicide bereavement different? A reassessment of the literature. *Suicide and Life-threatening Behavior, 31*, 91–102. doi:10.1521/suli.31.1.91.21310.

Kolodny, S., Binder, R. L., Bronstein, A. A., & Friend, R. L. (1979). The working through of patients' suicides by four therapists. *Suicide and Life-threatening Behavior, 9*, 33–46.

Litman, R. (1965). When patients commit suicide. *American Journal of Psychotherapy, 19*, 570–576.

McIntosh, J. L. (1999). Research on survivors of suicide. In M. Stimming, & M. Stimming (Eds.), *Before their time: Adult children's experiences of parental suicide* (pp. 157–180). Philadelphia, PA: Temple University Press.

Menninger, W. W. (1991). Patient suicide and its impact on the psychotherapist. *Bulletin of the Menninger Clinic, 55*, 216–227.

Michel, K. (1997). After suicide: Who counsels the therapist? *Crisis, 18*, 128–130. doi:10.1027/0227-5910.18.3.128.

Peterson, E. M., Luoma, J. B., & Dunne, E. (2002). Suicide survivors' perceptions of the treating clinician. *Suicide and Life-threatening Behavior, 32*, 158–166. doi:10.1521/suli.32.2.158.24406.

Rycroft, P. (2005). Touching the heart and soul of therapy: Surviving client suicide. *Women & Therapy, 28*, 83–94.

Valente, S. M., & Saunders, M. (2002). Nurses' grief reactions to a patient's suicide. *Perspectives in Psychiatric Care, 38*, 5–14. doi:10.1111/j.1744-6163.2002.tb00650.x.

Weiner, K. M. (Ed.). (2005). *Therapeutic and legal issues for therapists who have survived a client suicide: Breaking the silence.* New York: Haworth Press.

14

IMPACT OF CLIENT SUICIDE ON PRACTITIONER POST-TRAUMATIC GROWTH

Joseph S. Munson

Introduction

Since 1996 when Tedeschi and Calhoun first started researching this new construct called post-traumatic growth, researchers have observed positive outcomes to traumatic events including health traumas, chronic illnesses, HIV and AIDS, interpersonal abuse, bereavement, death of a loved one, natural or environmental disasters, war, and other adverse life events (Linley & Joseph, 2004). Post-traumatic growth has been observed in both men and women, across cultures, throughout the lifespan, and ranging in time from two weeks to eight years since experiencing the trauma (Tedeschi & Calhoun, 1996; Linley & Joseph, 2004; Sheikh, 2008).

The aim of Munson's (2009) study was to examine post-traumatic growth in clinicians after they have survived the suicide death of a client. Post-traumatic growth had not been researched in terms of how a suicide might affect positive change in the practitioner. The goal of this research was to give evidence that practitioners can also prosper after a client suicide. The findings of this study may help mental health clinicians to better understand the factors that contribute to practitioners' post-traumatic growth after a client's suicide.

Though the field of Suicidology has been slow to recognize positive outcomes that may arise from working with clients who are suicidal, there are documented positive aspects of this work. Richards (2000) focused on transference and counter-transference issues and found that 91% of the clinicians in her study believed that the connection that they had with the suicidal client was useful to that person. Other positive aspects included good record keeping, genuine listening, patience, loving support, de-emphasizing omnipotence, a good personal support system, and realizing an expected emotional response to their work (Richards, 2000). Resiliency, personal strength, relating well to others, and seeing new possibilities in life have been noted as positive outcomes related to working with suicidal clients.

Positive outcomes for therapists who work with clients who have experienced trauma have been described various ways in the literature. The valued subjective experiences that are most common include: well-being, contentment, satisfaction, hope, optimism, and happiness (Seligman & Csikszentmihalyi, 2000, p. 5). Specific individual traits such as courage, mindfulness, spirituality, wisdom, and interpersonal skill are related to positive outcomes. Group-level traits related to positive outcomes following trauma include responsibility, altruism, nurturance, work ethic, and civility (Linley, Joseph, Harrington, & Wood, 2006). There is also empirical evidence that practitioners develop religious and spiritual beliefs as a result of experiencing a trauma (Shaw, Joseph, & Linley, 2005). It is believed that the development of religious and spiritual beliefs provides a framework to aid in threatening situations, and thereby revealing positive outcomes to the trauma (Shaw et al., 2005). Specifically, religion and spiritual beliefs provide a philosophy of life as a framework for interpreting life's challenges and help in resolving concerns of suffering, death, and tragedy (Emmons, McCullough, & Tsang, 2003).

It is believed that most people are exposed to at least one traumatic experience during their lives (Ozer et al., 2003). Not everyone copes with traumatic events in the same way; some manage the trauma in a way they endure the acute distress and seem to move on to the next challenge with ease, and others seem to have greater difficulties in the process of recovery. Bonanno (2004), for example, differentiates between recovery and resilience where recovery implies a deficit in functioning or a threshold of psychopathology before a gradual return to pre-event coping, and resilience reflects the ability to maintain a stable equilibrium. Researchers have suggested that suicide presents more difficult bereavement than other types of losses because the death is unexpected, stigmatizing, and viewed as preventable (Bugen, 1977; Worden, 1991).

In developing a model of growth following trauma often referred to as growth through adversity, Linley and Joseph (2004) concluded that stressful and traumatic experiences that lead to perceptions of threat to one's life, uncontrollability, and helplessness are more likely to precipitate growth. Additionally, events that are dealt with by means of positive reinterpretation, acceptance coping, and effortful reflection among people, who are optimistic and experience high levels of positive affect, are likely to lead to reports of greater growth. This theory is substantiated by Bonanno and colleagues (2003) who described how some of the survivors of the World Trade Center disaster reported better adjustment, more active social networks, and were also rated as better adjusted by their close friends after the event.

Working with suicidal clients is complex and often difficult for practitioners. According to Hoff (2001), when clients are in crisis, there is no alternative for "simple, direct communication" by a caring person. However, responding to clients in crisis can leave the practitioner vulnerable to the vicarious stress related to working with clients in crisis. The experience of responding to a client who has just taken his/her own life, in particular, can place the practitioner in danger of being traumatized.

Crisis theory posits that stressors can present a danger for psychopathology or an opportunity for psychological growth (Caplan, 1964; Holahan & Moos, 1990). Previous literature claims that if one is exposed to a traumatic event (directly, secondarily, or vicariously), then one will be more susceptible to traumatic stress or PTSD (Figley, 1995; Stamm, 1999; Catherall, 2002; Salston & Figley, 2003). Constructivist self-development theory emphasizes the individual nature of trauma, including the idea that individuals construct the meaning that a particular trauma has for them based on specific factors. The theory outlines the various aspects of personality affected by trauma including: self-capacities, ego resources, psychological needs, related cognitive schemas, memory, and frame of reference (McCann & Pearlman, 1992).

More recently, however, there has been an increasing interest in those individuals who seem to do well after having experienced a traumatic experience. According to Scaer (2001), "Traumatic stressors are inherently subjective in valence; an event that generates traumatic stress for one individual may leave another psychologically unscathed." Individuals who do well after a trauma have been said to have "hardiness, resiliency, optimism, and self-efficacy" (Taylor & Brown, 1994). This alternative framework of examining positive effects following a negative event has addressed how individuals are changed and even how they prosper after a traumatic experience. Positive psychology has begun the change of focus from the preoccupation of negative effects of traumatic events to emphasizing and building positive qualities that contribute to the flourishing or optimal functioning of people (Seligman & Csikszentmihalyi, 2000).

Positive psychology is an encompassing term for the study of positive character traits, virtues, and strengths; with the aim of having a balanced empirical understanding of the complete human experience (Seligman et al., 2005). Positive psychology does not eliminate the value of understanding illness, dysfunction, and distress; instead, positive psychology intends to shift the basis of inquiry solely from a deficit-focus to including an asset-focus, which offers new ground for examination (Linley et al., 2006). In efforts to emphasize the synthesis of positive experiences after negative events, post-traumatic growth developed from a positive psychology conceptualization (Linley & Joseph, 2003; 2004; 2006). Post-traumatic growth is defined as positive change in self-perception, interpersonal relationships, and philosophy of life following a stressful or traumatic experience (Tedeschi & Calhoun, 1995).

Post-traumatic growth occurs "when in the context of loss, people may actively seek positives or gains to defend against mortality threats engendered by the experience, and if found, serve to promote the belief that life is meaningful" (Davis & McKearney, 2003). Growth is not necessarily the direct result of the traumatic event; it can be better understood as the individual's perspective in the aftermath of the event (Tedeschi & Calhoun, 2004). To some extent, the crisis can define the meaningfulness of the event based on how one's assumptions of the world, specifically one's safety, one's identity, and one's future, are challenged (Janoff-Bulman, 1992). Several models provide factors related to post-traumatic growth and distinguish it from other normative developmental processes. Tedeschi and Calhoun's (1996) research indicates that those who have experienced a traumatic event, such as a client suicide, compared to those who have not, report positive changes at a significantly higher level among survivors.

Using the post-traumatic growth model developed by Tedeschi and Calhoun (1996) as a framework, the Munson (2009) study aided in understanding practitioners' experiences as suicide survivors. The post-traumatic growth dimensions (i.e., new possibilities, relating to others, personal strength, appreciation of life, and spiritual change) will provide a basis for examining clinicians coping after a client suicide has been completed. Munson (2009) examined 117 practitioners who had lost a client to suicide (64 female, 53 male) during any point in their careers. This was accomplished through survey research utilizing the Professional Quality of Life Scale (ProQOL), the Post-Traumatic Growth Inventory (PTGI), and a Self-Report Questionnaire.

The outcomes of the study were mixed in that some of the expected relationships between variables were significant while others were not. Correlational analyses determined three significant relationships between post-traumatic growth and the hours spent working with suicidal clients at the time of a client suicide, compassion fatigue, and years of clinical experience. A simultaneous multiple regression analysis determined that time passed since last suicide completion was a significant predictor of post-traumatic growth. A MANOVA that was conducted to determine whether independent variables were significantly related to the subscales of the Post-traumatic Growth Inventory revealed no significant relationships.

The finding that practitioners with greater number of weekly hours working with suicidal clients at the time of the last client suicide was significantly positively correlated with higher post-traumatic growth, is consistent with the theory of Linley and Joseph (2004). These authors concluded that stressful and traumatic experiences that lead to perceptions of threat to one's life, uncontrollability, and helplessness are more likely to precipitate growth. Additionally, previous evidence has shown that growth can be achieved after an individual is impacted by an event that induces extreme stress (Bonanno et al., 2003). Results of the current study can also be compared to Kassam-Adams (1995) and Schauben and Frazier's work (1995), which identified personal growth, hope, and resiliency as positive outcomes by trauma counselors. Thus, this finding is in the direction that was expected based on current literature, which showed that increased impact events, such as working with higher amounts of suicidal clients and then losing a client to suicide, contribute to a greater opportunity for post-traumatic growth.

The finding that compassion fatigue is significantly positively related to post-traumatic growth was consistent with Figley's (1993) study in which he found that "the stress resulting from helping or wanting to help a traumatized or suffering person" leads to compassion fatigue. Therapists tend to place emphasis on drawing on their own personal qualities to help clients (Brown, 1987a). According to Tedeschi et al. (1998), the same personal qualities that place clinicians in danger of developing compassion fatigue can also help the clinician prosper and transform negative responses to post-traumatic growth. This study provides evidence that among clinicians who lose a client to suicide, those who have higher amounts of compassion fatigue also have higher post-traumatic growth.

Finally, Munson (2009) also showed that clinicians who have less clinical experience had a stronger relationship with post-traumatic growth. This finding is compared with Brown's (1987) research that concluded that trainees are more likely to experience a greater impact from a client's suicide than clinicians who have been in the field longer. Prior literature supports this finding by showing that a therapist in training will have a greater initial reaction to a client's suicide than his or her more experienced professional counterpart (Brown, 1987b; Chemtob, Hamada, Bauer, Torigoe, & Kinney, 1988; Kleespies, Penk, & Forsyth, 1993). For example, McAdams and Foster (2000) found that older and more experienced counselors reported less intense reactions to client suicide, or a lesser impact, thus minimizing the chance for post-traumatic growth. This finding could be further explained by the fact that clinicians who have been in the field longer usually are able to determine the clients they want to work with and work more in a supervisory capacity, therefore having less opportunities to be impacted by a client suicide.

Munson (2009) showed that the length of time since last client suicide was directly and positively related to predicting post-traumatic growth. The more time that had passed since the client suicide was completed was related to greater post-traumatic growth in the clinician. This finding that the more time that had passed since losing a client to suicide provided a positive PTG result could be seen as consistent with the old adage that "time heals all wounds." For example, Cadell, Regehr, and Hemsworth (2003) report that trauma is a precursor to change and growth, and as people attempt to re-establish equilibrium in their life, they are able to reflect on and re-evaluate themselves. Individuals who have experienced a traumatic event may be more aware of their own mortality and therefore appreciate life more than before the trauma event occurred. Research conducted by Linley and Joseph (2004) further showed that events dealt with by means of acceptance coping, positive reinterpretation, and effortful reflection among people who are optimistic and experience high levels of positive affect, are likely to lead to reports of greater growth. Tedeschi and Calhoun describe this aspect of post-traumatic growth as "meaning-making," through which trauma can in turn result in wisdom and growth from what was experienced.

Notable observations in the demographics of the sample population include participants who had a range of 0–40 years of experience, with a mean of 16.27 years; this variable was inversely correlated with post-traumatic growth and it could be interpreted that since the majority of the sample had about 15 years experience that the data was skewed towards a younger population, although it was not a bimodal sample distribution. The sample population ranged from obtaining 0–500 hours of specialized suicide training, with a mean of 46.74 hours; this variable shows that almost the entire sample had some specialized suicide training and the majority of the sample had an extreme amount. Participants also presented with a range of 0–50 hours a week of clinical contact with suicidal clients at the time of the suicide, with a mean of 11.87 hours, and a range of 0–50 hours of contact presently, with a mean of 5.86 hours; this variable shows a notable decrease in the average amount of hours that practitioners are working with suicidal clients on a weekly basis. This could provide evidence for the participants' significant correlation with compassion fatigue and with the impact that working with this population has on practitioners. Participants ranged from 0–9 completed suicides in the past five years, with a mean of 0.77

suicides. It is obvious that the majority of the sample had not lost a client to suicide in the last five years, which gives more reason to expand the sample population and to examine how post-traumatic growth is experienced with time. Participants also ranged from 0–29 years since the last completed client suicide, with a mean of 6.60 years. This variable was a significant predictor of post-traumatic growth and showed that the majority of the sample had lost a client to suicide after five years. This variable needs further examination from a longitudinal standpoint. Lastly, participants had a range of 0–98 score on the post-traumatic growth inventory, with a mean score of 34.31. This score appears low when compared to Tedeschi and Calhoun's (1996) study that had a mean score of 75 with a standard deviation of 21. That study limited their sample to within 12 months of experiencing a traumatic event, which again raises the question of the impact of time on post-traumatic growth. Other notable demographics show that the sample population was 89.7% Caucasian, 64% female, 48.7% professional counselors, and participants at the time of the suicide were working at a mental health outpatient center (29.1%) where after the suicide the majority of the sample was working in private practice (23.4%). These demographics give a broad scope of who the participants are and how diverse the sample is.

The findings of this study were consistent with prior research on post-traumatic growth. Greater amounts of clinical contact hours at the time of the last completed suicide were predictive of greater post-traumatic growth and are in the direction that was expected. Tedeschi and Calhoun (1995), Joseph and Linley (2004), as well as Cadell and colleagues (2003) reported that increased impact events, such as higher clinical contact with suicidal clients and then losing a client to suicide, contribute to a greater opportunity for post-traumatic growth. According to Davis and McKearney (2003), post-traumatic growth occurs "when in the context of loss, people may actively seek positives or gains to defend against mortality threats engendered by the experience, and if found, serve to promote the belief that life is meaningful." Growth is not necessarily the direct result of the traumatic event; it can be better understood as the individual's perspective in the aftermath of the event (Tedeschi & Calhoun, 2004). To some extent, the crisis can define the meaningfulness of the event based on how one's assumptions of the world, specifically one's safety, one's identity, and one's future, are challenged (Janoff-Bulman, 1992).

The finding that compassion fatigue is positively correlated with post-traumatic growth might be viewed as confounding when you examine the definitions of each construct separately. This relationship could be seen as counterintuitive. Compassion fatigue occurs when a therapist is exposed to clients' experiences and secondarily becomes victimized themselves through their own empathy for their client. Figley (2002a) describes compassion fatigue as "a function of bearing witness to the suffering of others." Post-traumatic growth occurs when an individual is able to move past a traumatic event and prosper from the experience. Findings of this study support the idea that clinicians can experience post-traumatic growth and compassion fatigue together. That is, a therapist can endure the traumatic experience of a client suicide, feel empathic fatigue, and then still be able to prosper in the aftermath. It is also important to understand that PTG and PTSD are not on the same continuum, they are thought to be independent of each other. Therefore, an individual would be able to experience distress and growth from the same event (Tedeschi & Calhoun, 2004). Calhoun and Tedeschi (1999) proposed that post-traumatic growth may be experienced at the same time as stress symptoms in the aftermath of a trauma and that some degree of distress and rumination is almost necessary to produce positive changes.

Practitioners' years of clinical experience were inversely related to post-traumatic growth. This finding could be theorized to mean that practitioners who are newer to the field could be impacted more by a client suicide than those clinicians who are more experienced in the field. Brown (1987b) and Chemtob et al. (1988) believed that psychiatrists experienced more suicides and higher risk clients early in their career from working in psychiatric and general hospitals because graduate programs required clinical training in these locations. Brown (1987) also reported that therapists seemed to change the way they practiced and changed their views about themselves in working with suicidal patients over time. This finding is supportive of post-traumatic growth theory, which suggests that individuals will change how they relate to others, find more personal strength, create new possibilities, experience spiritual changes, and find a new appreciation for life (Tedeschi & Calhoun, 1996).

Finally, the length of time passed since the last client suicide for a practitioner was a significant predictor of post-traumatic growth. It is believed that the confrontation of a trauma can shatter the world-view of a person and creates a need to cognitively and emotionally process the new trauma-related information (Janoff-Bulman, 1992). Hollon and Garber's research (1988) showed that new trauma-related information can only be processed in one of two ways: either assimilated within an existing model or the existing model must be accommodated to allow in the new information. According to Joseph and Linley's (2005) second factor of their model (accommodation versus assimilation), accommodation allows the individual to move beyond the pre-trauma baseline, since growth is defined as creating new world-views.

Munson's (2009) research provides the field of counseling and suicidology with direction to shape further assumptions of how client suicides affect post-traumatic growth in clinicians. Specifically, this research added to current theory by showing that both PTSD and PTG can exist simultaneously in clinicians after a client suicide. Also, this research added to theory by demonstrating that a client suicide may serve as a catalyst for clinicians to reach high levels of post-traumatic growth. Furthermore, the level of impact of the suicide, as measured by the early occurrence of the suicide in the clinician's career, may have a direct influence on the clinician's level of post-traumatic growth, at earlier and later periods of their professional career.

In counseling, active engagement with meaning-making can be very helpful as a coping strategy for clients, where clients learn to explore their sense of self, identity, roles and relationships, and perception of priorities since the traumatic experience (Sheikh, 2008). This can also be the case with practitioners. In most cases, after a trauma occurs, the individual's world-view has been shattered, giving them the opportunity to make new meaning out of life (Janoff-Bulman, 1992). Munson's (2009) findings show that practitioners are able to make new meaning of the traumatic event in the form of post-traumatic growth through their years of experience and through the amount of time that has passed since the client suicide. Practitioners who have less clinical experience have a strong relationship with post-traumatic growth, but practitioners who have more time that has passed also have a strong relationship with post-traumatic growth. For some clinicians who are early in their professional development, the traumatic experience of losing a client to suicide may have transformed their perspective, making them open enough to allow a new world-view that encompasses post-traumatic growth. In addition, for practitioners who have been in the field for a greater length of time since the suicide, it can be assumed that time has allowed them the opportunity to find meaning from their subsequent experiences. There is still more to learn about how the time continuum can affect mental health practitioners in the aftermath of a client suicide.

A suggestion for future research includes making specific distinctions between post-traumatic growth and the concept of resiliency. In future studies, there needs to be a comparison between those who are able to continue with life after a hardship or adversity versus those who are able to prosper and have a positive quality of transformation after a traumatic event (Tedeschi & Calhoun, 2004). Further examination of the personal, professional, and situational factors that lead one to resiliency versus advancing one to post-traumatic growth should be addressed in future research. A comparison between clinicians who have high and low levels of post-traumatic growth after a client suicide also is needed in future studies.

Lastly, it would be of interest to further examine the relationship between clinical support and clinicians' post-traumatic growth following client suicide. Even though it was not significant in this study, it makes sense to think that the amount of quality clinical supervisory support from others after a suicide would be highly valued to clinician survivors, especially considering the effectiveness of suicide survivor support groups as a way of mitigating the negative effects of losing a loved one to suicide. Coyne and Downey (1991) provided evidence that the role of social support is influential in the development of post-traumatic growth since it may provide acceptance and encouragement for the person to self-disclose their ruminations and feelings of the trauma. Also, social support satisfaction has been associated with post-traumatic growth (Park, Cohen, & Murch, 1996), but clinical support has not yet been validated. Another suggestion for future studies would be to examine pre-existing measures of clinical support and test those measures with clinician suicide survivors to see whether it is a good predictor of post-traumatic growth. The study of suicide survivors is still new and there is much more to learn about post-traumatic growth in clinicians who survive a client suicide. Because research with clinicians who have lost a client to suicide is new, there are many variables that have not been examined. Thus, there remains a need for a specific model that predicts post-traumatic growth in clinicians after a suicide.

References

Bonanno, G. (2004). Loss, trauma, and human resilience: Have we underestimated the human capacity to thrive after extremely aversive events? *American Psychologist, 59*, 20–28.

Bonanno, G., Noll, J., Putnam, F., O'Neill, M., & Trickett, P. (2003). Predicting the willingness to disclose childhood sexual abuse from measures of repressive coping and dissociative tendencies. *Child Maltreatment*, 8, 302–318.

Bonanno, G. A., Rennicke, C., & Dekel, S. (2005). Self-enhancement among high-exposure survivors of the September 11th terrorist attack: Resilience or social maladjustment? *Journal of Personality and Social Psychology*, 88(6), 984–998.

Brown, H. N. (1987a). Patient suicide during residency training: Incidence, implications, and program response. *Journal of Psychiatric Education, 11*, 201–206.

Brown, H. N. (1987b). The impact of suicide on psychiatrists in training. *Comprehensive Psychiatry, 28*, 101–112.

Bugen, L. (1977). Human grief: A model for prediction and intervention. *American Journal of Orthopsychiatry, 47*, 196–206.

Cadell, S., Regehr, C., & Hemsworth, D. (2003). Factors contributing to post-traumatic growth: A proposed structural equation model. *American Journal of Orthopsychiatry, 73*, 279–287.

Calhoun, L. G., & Tedeschi, R.G. (1999). *Facilitating post-traumatic growth: A clinician's guide*. Mahwah, NJ: Lawrence Erlbaum Associates.

Caplan, G. (1964). *Principles of preventive psychiatry*. Oxford: Basic Books.

Catherall, D. R. (2002). Secondary stress and the professional helper. Retrieved September 6, 2002 from http://www.ctsn-rcst.ca/Secondary.html.

Chemtob, C. M., Hamada, R. S., Bauer, G., Torigoe, R. Y., & Kinney, B. (1988). Patient suicide: Frequency and impact on psychologists. *Professional Psychology: Research and Practice, 19*, 416–420.

Coyne, J. C., & Downey, G. (1991). Social factors in psychopathology: Stress, social support, and coping processes. *Annual Review of Psychology, 43*, 401–425.

Davis, C. G., & McKearney, J. M. (2003). How do people grow from their experience with trauma or loss? *Journal of Social & Clinical Psychology, 22*, 477–492.

Emmons, R. A., McCullough, M. E., & Tsang, J. (2003). The assessment of gratitude. In S. J. Lopez, & C. R. Snyder (Eds.), *Positive psychological assessment: A handbook of models and measures* (pp. 327–341). Washington, DC: American Psychological Association.

Figley, C. R. (1993). Leaving the home from the war. *PsychCRITIQUES*, 38, 289.

Figley, C. R. (1995). *Compassion Fatigue: Coping with secondary stress disorder in those who treat the traumatized*. Levittown: Brunner/Mazel.

Figley, C. R. (2002a). Compassion fatigue: Psychotherapists' chronic lack of self-care. *Journal of Clinical Psychology, 58*, 1433–1441.

Figley, C. R. (2002b). *Treating compassion fatigue*. New York: Brunner-Routledge.

Hoff, L. A. (2001). *People in crisis: Understanding and helping* (5th ed.). San Francisco: Jossey-Bass.

Holahan, C., & Moos, R. (1990). Life stressors, resistance factors, and psychological health: An extension of the stress-resistance paradigm. *Journal of Personality and Social Psychology, 58*, 909–917.

Hollon, S. D., & Garber, J. (1988). Cognitive therapy. In L. Y. Abramson (Ed.), *Social cognition and clinical psychology: A synthesis* (pp. 204–253). New York: Guilford Press.

Janoff-Bulman, R. (1992). *Shattered assumptions: Towards a new psychology of trauma*. New York: Free Press.

Joseph, S., & Linley, P. A. (2004). Positive therapy: A positive psychological theory of therapeutic practice. In P. A. Linley, & S. Joseph (Eds.), *Positive psychology in practice* (pp. 354– 368). Hoboken, NJ: Wiley.

Joseph, S., & Linley, P. (2005). Positive adjustment to threatening events: An organismic valuing theory of growth through adversity. *Review of General Psychology, 9*, 262–280.

Kassam-Adams, N. (1995). The risks of treating sexual trauma: Stress and secondary trauma in psychotherapists. In B. H. Stamm (Ed.), *Secondary traumatic stress: Self-care issues for clinicians, researchers, and educators* (pp. 37– 48). Lutherville, MD: Sidran.

Kleespies, P. M., Penk, W. E., & Forsyth, J. P. (1993). The stress of patient suicidal behavior during clinical training: Incidence, impact, and recovery. *Professional Psychology: Research and Practice, 24*, 293– 303.

Linley, P. A., & Joseph, S. (2003). Trauma and personal growth. *The Psychologist*, 16, 135.

Linley, P. A., & Joseph, S. (2004). Positive change following trauma and adversity: A review. *Journal of Traumatic Stress, 17*, 11– 21.

Linley, P. A., & Joseph, S. (2006). The positive and negative effects of disaster work: A preliminary investigation. *Journal of Loss and Trauma*, 11, 229–243.

Linley, P. A., Joseph, S., Harrington, S., & Wood, A. M. (2006). Positive psychology: Past, present, and (possible) future. *The Journal of Positive Psychology*, 1, 3–16.

McAdams, C. R., III, & Foster, V. A. (2000). Client suicide: Its frequency and impact on counselors. *Journal of Mental Health Counseling, 22*, 107–121.

McCann, I. L., & Pearlman, L.A. (1992). Constructivist self development theory: A theoretical model of psychological adaptation to severe trauma. In D. K. Sakheim, & S. E. Devine (Eds.), *Out of darkness: Exploring Satanism and ritual abuse* (pp. 185–206). New York: Lexington Books.

Munson, J. S. (2009). Impact of client suicide on practitioner post-traumatic growth. (Doctoral dissertation). University of Florida, Gainesville, FL. Retrieved from ProQuest Dissertations, AAT 3367562.

Ozer, E. J., Best, S. R., Lipsey, T. L., et al. (2003). Predictors of posttraumatic stress disorder and symptoms in adults: a meta–analysis. Psychological Bulletin, 129, 52–73.

Park, C. L., Cohen, L. H., & Murch, R. L. (1996). Assessment and prediction of stress-related growth. *Journal of Personality, 64*, 71–105.

Richards, B. M. (2000). Impact upon therapy and the therapist when working with suicidal patients: Some transference and countertransference aspects. *British Journal of Guidance and Counselling, 28*, 325–337.

Salston, M. D., & Figley, C. R. (2003). Secondary traumatic stress effects of working with survivors of criminal victimization. *Journal of Traumatic Stress, 16*, 167–174.

Scaer, R. C. (2001). *The body bears the burden: Trauma, dissociation, and disease*. Binghamton, NY: The Haworth Press, Inc.

Schauben, L., & Frazier, P. (1995). Vicarious trauma: The effects on female counselors of working with sexual violence survivors. *Psychology of Women Quarterly*, 19, 49–64.

Seligman, M. E. P., & Csikszentmihalyi, M. (2000). Positive psychology: An introduction. *American Psychologist, 55*, 5–14.

Seligman, M. E. P., & Steen, T. A. (2005). Positive psychology progress: Empirical validation of interventions. *American Psychologist*, 60, 410–421.

Shaw, A., Joseph, S., & Linley, P. A. (2005). Religion, spirituality, and post-traumatic growth: A systematic review. *Mental Health, Religion & Culture, 8*, 1–11.

Sheikh, A. (2008). Post-traumatic growth in trauma survivors: Implications for practice. *Counseling Psychology Quarterly, 21*, 85–97.

Stamm, B. H. (1999). *Secondary Traumatic Stress: Self-care issues for clinicians, researchers, and educators*. Lutherville: Sidran Press.

Taylor, S. E., & Brown, J. D. (1994). Positive illusions and well-being revisited: Separating fact from fiction. *Psychological Bulletin*, 116, 21–27.

Tedeschi, R. G., & Calhoun, L. G. (1995). *Trauma and transformation: Growing in the aftermath of suffering*. Thousand Oaks, CA: Sage.

Tedeschi, R. G., & Calhoun, L. G. (1996). The Post-traumatic Growth Inventory: Measuring the positive legacy of trauma. *Journal of Traumatic Stress, 9*, 455–471.

Tedeschi, R. G., & Calhoun, L. G. (2004). Target article: 'Post-traumatic Growth: Conceptual foundations and empirical evidence'. *Psychological Inquiry, 15*, 1–18.

Tedeschi, R. G., Park, C. L., & Calhoun, L. G. (1998). *Post-traumatic growth: Positive changes in the aftermath of crisis*. Mahwah, NJ: Erlbaum.

Worden, J. (1991). *Grief counseling and grief therapy: A handbook for the mental health practitioner* (2nd ed.). New York: Springer.

15

SUICIDE RISK

Themes for high quality assessment

Christopher M. Perlman and Eva Neufeld

Introduction

High quality suicide risk assessment is paramount to promoting patient safety and recovery. This is emphasized when we consider the number of persons who attempt to die by suicide. Rates of death by suicide have risen since 1950 (WHO, 2003), but are far outnumbered by hospitalizations for suicide attempts and self-injury. In 2009, 17,000 Canadians were hospitalized following attempts to die by suicide (CIHI & Statistics Canada, 2011). The estimated lifetime prevalence of suicide ideation ranges from about 2% to 18% among nine countries (Weissman et al., 1999). Though acknowledging that not all suicides are avoidable or preventable, thorough suicide risk assessment is a key step in recognizing and addressing suicide risk as early as possible (Pridmore, 2012).

In patient safety literature, there is a lack of integration of best practice related to the suicide risk assessment process (Brickell & McLean, 2011). For instance, a lack of information and documentation about suicide risk were among the most common root causes of deaths by suicide in in-patient settings in the United States (Mills, Neily, Luan, Osborne, & Howard, 2006). Recognizing the need for suicide risk assessment as a standard health care practice, quality assurance organizations such as Accreditation Canada have established guidelines or Required Organizational Practices (ROP) promoting the use of high quality risk assessment in all health care settings (Accreditation Canada, 2011). While these frameworks often provide clear requirements that suicide risk assessment must be completed, specific information about the assessment process, itself, is often omitted. Thus, there is a need to integrate key aspects of suicide risk assessment into a framework for informing policy development, education, and best practice.

A number of resources exist describing aspects of suicide risk assessment, including clinical texts (Jacobs, 1999; Rudd et al., 2006), best practice guidelines (American Psychiatric Association (APA), 2003; Heisel et al., 2006; Registered Nurses' Association of Ontario, 2009) and summaries of risk assessment tools (Haney et al., 2012). However, few resources exist that integrate information on process and the use of assessment tools that may help inform practice. Therefore, the purpose of this research was to identify the key principles, processes, and tools to support high quality risk assessment in health care contexts.

Methods

This research was guided by a 15-member Pan-Canadian Advisory Panel on Patient Safety in Mental Health. The advisory panel consisted of clinicians, policy-makers, health care executives, quality and risk managers, patient representatives, and members of the Ontario Hospital Association and the Canadian Patient Safety Institute. The panel provided oversight to the development of the research approach, clarification of clinical or policy issues, consideration in the framing of research findings, and recommendations for reporting and dissemination. The research was carried out using a review of best practice, scientific, and clinical literature as well as stakeholder interviews.

Literature review

The literature review examined scientific articles, clinical literature, best practice reports, and other "grey" literature. Medical and social-sciences databases reviewed included the Cochrane Library, CINAHL, PubMed (Medline), PsycINFO, Google Scholar, and Scopus. Websites of professional practice organizations were also reviewed for relevant reports, guidelines, and/or research findings. References lists from germane articles were also reviewed. Articles were excluded if they were not specifically relevant to suicide risk assessment (e.g., pharmaceutical interventions). Articles that were included tended to fall into the following categories:

• suicide risk assessment tools/scales
• best practices in risk assessment
• general research on suicide risk
• quality indicators related to suicide risk assessment.

Stakeholder interviews

Interviews were conducted to gather information about suicide risk assessment in practice. Interviewees were recruited using a convenience sampling approach. The recruitment process gathered persons with experience from different regions in Canada, from different health care populations and sectors, and with different professional backgrounds. This sampling strategy yielded a list of 30 potential interview candidates. Nine persons declined an interview, resulting in 21 completed interviews.

The interviews used a semi-structured approach asking, broadly, about the stakeholder's recommendations for conducting high-quality risk assessment; familiarity, use, and recommendations for suicide risk assessment tools; and recommendations for policy, practice, and evaluation of suicide risk assessment.

The interviews were recorded and analyzed using a deductive framework based on pre-set research objectives (e.g., identification of processes for suicide risk assessment) (Pope, Ziebland, & Mays, 2000). The deductive framework incorporated familiarization and organization of key themes in the data.

The results from the literature review were integrated with the themes identified from the interviews as well as feedback from the advisory panel. This approach was favourable for organizing the information into an integrated resource to facilitate education, policy development, evaluation, and continuous quality improvement.

Findings

The findings are organized into two sections: (1) themes for the process of suicide risk assessment; (2) considerations for the use of risk assessment tools.

Process themes

Theme 1: Suicide risk assessment should focus on understanding the person, not predicting future behaviour

There has been debate in the literature about the predictive validity of suicide risk assessment based on a number of factors, including suicide ideation (Large et al., 2011; Mulder, 2011); Draper, 2012). Statistically, the prediction of suicide following risk assessment is almost impossible and may be of limited clinical value (Szmukler, 2012), yet assessing the likelihood that a person will attempt to die by suicide in the near future can address immediate safety needs. While a certain degree of liability exists (e.g., identify the safest care setting), risk assessment should be viewed as an integral part of a holistic therapeutic process (Lyons, Price, Embling, & Smith, 2000). A person-focused risk assessment offers greater opportunity to learn about the person's lived experience, needs, and distress to inform interventions that mitigate future risk.

Theme 2: Therapeutic rapport and relationship are integral

A threat to the quality of suicide risk assessment is that the process may become automated and focus solely on risk management instead of recognizing the person's unique distress to inform intervention (Mulder, 2011). Therapeutic relationships are based on active listening, trust, respect, genuineness, empathy, and clear communication with the person (American Psychiatric Association (APA), 2003; Registered Nurses' Association of Ontario, 2009). This relationship can help minimize feelings of shame, guilt, and stigma, thus creating a more open environment for discussion and assessment. A safe, comfortable, private, and non-authoritarian environment is also important (Bergmans, Brown, & Carruthers, 2007).

Theme 3: Integrating knowledge of potentiating risk factors, warning signs, and protective factors

There is an extensive epidemiological literature that has identified factors associated with, and predictive of, suicide and suicide-related behaviour. Lists of risk factors are limited in utility unless they are organized into a framework that can help inform risk identification and mitigation. Risk assessment requires differentiation between potentiating risk factors, warning signs, and protective factors.

Potentiating risk factors describe variables associated with suicid-related behavior but not directly predictive of suicide (Jacobs, 1999). Warning signs are more proximal indicators that may set in motion the process of suicide (Rudd et al., 2006; Rudd, 2008). Protective factors are those that may mitigate risk of suicide (Ali, Dwyer, & Rizzo, 2011). Together, these factors can inform the underlying origins of suicide, the conceptualization of risk, and aspects of the person's life that can be leveraged to help mitigate risk of suicide. A list of some prominent potentiating risk factors, warning signs, and protective factors can be found in Table 15.1.

Interplay exists between warning signs, potentiating risk factors, and protective factors in several ways. First, the absence of potentiating risk factors does not negate the presence of warning signs, and vice versa. The challenge is eliciting these factors in a way that informs both the safety

Table 15.1 Selected warning signs, potentiating risk factors, and protective factors of suicide

Warning signs
- Threatening to harm or end one's life
- Seeking or access to means such as pills, weapons, or other means
- Evidence or expression of a suicide plan
- Expressions of (writing or talking) ideation about suicide or a wish to die
- Hopelessness
- Rage, anger, seeking revenge
- Acting reckless, engaging impulsively in risky behaviour
- Expressing feelings of being trapped with no way out
- Increasing or excessive substance use
- Withdrawing from family, friends, society
- Anxiety, agitation, abnormal sleep patterns
- Dramatic changes in mood
- Expresses no reason for living, no sense of purpose in life

Potentiating risk factors
- Unemployed or recent financial difficulties
- Loss of personal relationships (e.g., divorced, separated, widowed)
- Social isolation
- Prior traumatic life events or abuse
- Previous suicide behaviour
- Chronic mental illness
- Chronic, debilitating physical illness

Protective factors
- Strong connections to family and community support
- Skills in problem solving, coping and conflict resolution
- Sense of belonging, sense of identity, and good self-esteem
- Cultural, spiritual, and religious connections and beliefs
- Identification of future goals
- Constructive use of leisure time (enjoyable activities)
- Support through ongoing medical and mental health care relationships
- Effective clinical care for mental, physical and substance use disorders
- Easy access to a variety of clinical interventions and support for help seeking
- Restricted access to highly lethal means of suicide

Note: Adapted from Rudd et al. (2006).

of the person and ongoing risk mitigation. Second, the identification of potentiating risk factors should engage further assessment. However, the presence of potentiating risk factors, alone, does not assume risk. Third, protective factors do not supersede evidence of warning signs. Instead, potentiating risk factors and protective factors may become focal points of interventions, once risk is abated. Overall, the presence and combination between risk factors, warning signs, and protective factors may present differently and should be treated using a person-centred approach.

Theme 4: Consideration for the person's life circumstance

It is important to consider the person's current and past life circumstance. The concept of *predicament suicide* was identified as a way to describe the circumstance where a person experiences a drastic or traumatic event (e.g., extreme financial loss) and is unable to identify a means to cope or escape other than suicide (Pridmore, 2009). Recognizing predicaments may be particularly important in primary and occupational health settings where recognition of a predicament triggers further suicide assessment.

Several considerations exist for persons of different ages. Among youth, for example, using normalization during risk assessment is more effective in eliciting open responses. Considerations for "contagion effects" are also important as youth are more likely to engage in suicide-related behaviour if their peers or family have died by suicide (Alie et al., 2011). Older adults may downplay or under-report risk factors or thoughts related to suicide, and often present with somatic symptoms (Heisel et al., 2006). For older adults, it is particularly important that risk assessment is performed in the context of a strong therapeutic relationship rather than simply going through check-list approaches for ensuring the safety and recovery.

Theme 5: Suicide risk assessment should be trauma-informed

It is important to consider how life events and circumstances have affected a person, rather than using stigmatizing approaches that blame the person for suicide behaviour. *Suicide is not about what is wrong with a person; it is about what has happened to a person.* For instance, among lesbian, bisexual, gay, transgendered, or queer communities, suicide risk is not the result of a person's sexual orientation. Instead, it may be related to traumatic life experiences such as taunting, discrimination, harassment, marginalization, and victimization. This example extends to cultural groups, including persons from Aboriginal communities where generations of cultural trauma and marginalization may contribute to feelings of hopelessness, depression, and grief (Chandler & Lalonde, 2004). Trauma-informed suicide risk assessment that utilizes empathy and culturally sensitive approaches avoids further stigmatization and marginalization within the assessment process.

Theme 6: Communication and documentation are essential

Communication and documentation are important for all health care issues and processes, yet in understanding and preventing suicide, experts agree that they are essential. Clear, non-stigmatizing communication with the patient, appropriate involvement of informal supports, and collaborative communication with other team members and supports are crucial to understanding suicide risk as well as ongoing monitoring and prevention (Granello, 2010).

Documentation is essential for ensuring the efficacy of suicide risk assessment. After initial and ongoing assessments, chart notes should clearly identify the patient's level of risk and plans for treatment and preventive care. This should be easily accessible for all clinical staff through transitions in staffing (e.g., shift changes). Chart notes need to include detailed risk assessment findings, previous psychiatric history, previous treatment received, and concerns expressed by family or friends. Documentation with recommendations for ongoing risk monitoring is also important for transfers between care settings, as persons who have been discharged from in-patient psychiatric care are at higher risk of suicide than the general population (Ho, 2003; Hunt et al., 2009).

Theme 7: Risk assessment relies on clinical judgement that can be informed by, but not based on, risk assessment tools

Suicide risk assessment involves consideration of multiple factors and contexts, making clinical experience an asset for navigating this process. Many clinicians rely on the clinical interview and observations to assess suicide risk. However, a number of tools have been designed to assist in the suicide risk assessment process.

Tools should be regarded as one aspect of the risk assessment process that informs, but does not replace, clinical judgement of risk (Barker & Buchanan-Barker, 2005). The use of tools in the risk assessment process should be person-focused, incorporated into the clinical interview, and be a part, rather than the focus of patient care. Reliance on check boxes of risk factors is insufficient in the risk assessment process. Rather, tools should be used in the context of an established therapeutic rapport, where the clinician conceptualizes risk with the patient and determines the best approach to manage it (Mulder, 2011).

Themes for selecting a tool for risk assessment

Theme 1: Intended use

The selection of a risk assessment tool can be difficult, given the complexity of suicide-related ideation and behaviour across patient populations and care settings (Brown, 2000). Risk assessment tools range from brief emergency screeners to global assessments of suicide risk embedded in larger mental health assessments. Selecting a risk assessment tool may depend on its intended utility. Tools with fewer items may serve better for screening and monitoring risk, while tools with more items may be preferable for research or in-depth risk assessment once a therapeutic relationship has been established.

Theme 2: Mode of administration

Risk assessment tools also vary by administration (e.g., self-report vs. clinician-administered). Determining which tool to utilize may depend on organizational policies, clinician's preferences, or the circumstances specific to the patient. Self-reported risk assessment tools may provide corroboration for clinical judgement, as well as offer opportunities for persons with difficulty communicating their distress to discuss their responses with their clinician. However, many suicidal patients will deny suicide-related ideation when asked, and are less likely to rate themselves as high on suicide rating scales (Joiner, Rudd, & Rajab, 1999). Clinician-administered risk assessment tools generally require more time and training to administer than self-report format, yet they offer opportunities for standardizing documentation of risk and facilitating continuity of care.

Theme 3: Technical considerations

The psychometrics of risk assessment tools assist in determining the quality of the instrument. Strong *reliability* of an assessment tool is an indication that it will produce consistent results (i.e., internal consistency) at different periods (i.e., test–retest reliability), and/or when completed by different assessors (i.e., inter-rater reliability). Strong *validity* is an indication that the tool measures what it intended to measure (i.e., content and construct validity), distinguishes between groups that share similar features (i.e., concurrent validity), performs similarly to other tools in the same risk assessment domain (i.e., convergent validity), yet it still discriminates between dissimilar constructs (i.e., discriminant validity).

Sensitivity and specificity of a risk assessment tool are a component of validity. Sensitivity is the ability of the tool to correctly identify persons who *are* at risk (i.e., reducing false-negatives). Specificity is the ability of the tool to correctly identify those who *are not* at risk (i.e., reducing false-positives). In general, it should be expected that some margin of error will exist when utilizing risk assessment tools and that a certain percentage of false-positives and false-negatives cannot be avoided (Mulder, 2011; Naud & Daigle, 2010).

It is firmly established that the ability to predict suicide is low (Simon, 2011). There is no evidence to support the use of risk assessment scores *as the sole basis* for decision-making on acute risk. Although risk assessment tool scores can never be 100% accurate, they can inform clinical judgement on the immediate care needs of the person. Many valid and reliable suicide risk assessment tools are available that measure outcomes relevant to subsequent risk of suicide, such as hopelessness, death ideation, and/or other precipitants of suicide-related behaviour (see Brown, 2000; Perlman, Neufeld, Martin, Goy, & Hirdes, 2011; Haney et al., 2012, for a complete review of tools). Gathering this corroborating information in the context of the therapeutic relationship can improve the overall quality of the suicide risk assessment process.

In addition to the considerations above, clinicians may wish to reflect on these additional issues when choosing a risk assessment tool:

1 How much time will the risk assessment tool take to complete?
2 Is the risk assessment tool designed for your patient population (e.g., children/youth vs. adult in-patient)?
3 Is the risk assessment tool easy to score?
4 Are the scores meaningful? Do they add to my understanding of my patients?
5 Does the risk assessment tool aid with risk screening, acute assessment, etc.?
6 Are items on protective factors and resiliency included in the risk assessment items?
7 Is training required prior to administering the risk assessment tool?
8 Is the risk assessment scale in the public domain, or is a user-fee required?

Theme 4: Setting-specific considerations for risk assessment tools

- *Primary care and non-psychiatric care settings.* In non-psychiatric care settings, clinicians need to determine the potential risk for suicide and whether a referral to specialized mental health or hospitalization is required. Risk assessment tools should provide a screening function to indicate the accumulation of risk factors, warning signs, and protective factors. Tools that may be useful include the SAD PERSONS (Juhnke & Hovestadt, 1995) and the Tool for Assessment of Suicide Risk (TASR; Kutcher & Chehil, 2007). Among persons caring for older adults (e.g., in home care services) the Geriatric Suicide Ideation Scale (GSIS; Heisel & Flett, 2006) may be useful. The same tool can be used to monitor persons who may not be at high risk, but have the potential to develop risk on an ongoing basis (e.g., presence of potentiating risk factor with no warning signs).
- *Community mental health settings.* In community mental health care, persons may be experiencing longstanding mental health symptoms that may include chronic suicidality. Here, the main task is to determine if suicide risk has changed. A recent negative predicament may initiate warning signs of suicidality, with or without potentiating risk factors. Simple questions for "checking in" with the person, asking about suicidal thoughts, whether a plan is in place, and whether the person feels unsafe, are part of ongoing screening and monitoring in outpatient settings.

    Risk assessment tools such as the interRAI Community Mental Health (Hirdes, 2011) include a global assessment of the person's mental health status and functioning while providing a summary risk score based on the Severity of Self-Harm Scale (SOS; Neufeld, Hirdes, & Rabinowitz, 2011). Other tools that provide screening and/or in-depth assessment may also be appropriate. These include, but are not limited to, the Nurses' Global Assessment of Suicide Risk (NGASR; Cutcliffe & Barker, 2004), the Scale for Impact of Suicidality-Management, Assessment and Planning of Care (SIS-MAP; Nelson, Johnston, & Srivastava, 2010), the

Suicide Probability Scale (SPS; Cull & Gill, 1988), and the Reasons for Living Inventory (RFL; Linehan, Goodstein, Nielsen, & Chiles, 1983).

Care teams in this setting should decide between self-report and clinician-administered risk assessment based on their therapeutic rapport with outpatients. This decision may be moderated by patients' willingness to discuss suicide, as well as cognitive functioning and ability to communicate.

- *Emergency departments in hospitals.* In emergency departments, risk assessment involves identifying risk and intent, prior to considering discharge. Brief emergency screening as well as clinical interview and consultation are important to this decision-making process. Tools such as the SOS scale embedded in the interRAI Mental Health (Hirdes et al., 2002) provide information on the recency of ideation or attempts, intent, and other information about risk of harm to others and self-care. This will provide a brief indicator of risk that should be accompanied by a full clinical interview and/or focused assessment of risk, particularly if any indication of risk is identified through initial screening on the SOS or other screening methods applied. Global risk assessment tools may help the emergency team determine suicidal intent and the person's next level of care (e.g., hospital admission, discharge to community).
- *In-patient mental health settings.* In in-patient mental health settings, risk of suicide may have been identified prior to, or upon admission. However, screening for suicide risk is still important among patients where risk of suicide may not have been immediately identified. A number of the screening tools, listed in points 1 and 2 above, could be considered for ongoing screening within inpatient mental health.

In several Canadian jurisdictions and internationally, the standardized use of the interRAI Mental Health assessment automatically includes initial screening for suicide risk among all persons admitted to care. Using the SOS score following the completion of the interRAI assessment, persons needing a global suicide risk assessment are identified and the care planning process to mitigate suicide risk is developed. The interRAI mental health assessments also include a care planning guide, the Suicidality and Purposeful Self-harm Clinical Assessment Protocol (Neufeld et al., 2011), that provides further information to guide the global risk assessment process and intervention planning.

Implications for practice, policy, and research

Suicide risk assessment tools are useful in providing additional information and corroboration to inform the clinical interview. Literature reviews of available suicide risk assessment tools generally indicate adequate to strong internal consistency and appropriate construct validity for domains related to suicide risk. However, no universal consensus is available to suggest the adoption of one single, most effective risk assessment tool. Further, not all clinicians agree that risk assessment tools are a required component of the risk assessment process; some favour the clinical interview and clinical judgement. Given the high stakes and the liability risks in certain jurisdictions, conducting risk assessments that are comprehensive in scope and that assess individual risk and protective factors is of critical importance (Heisel et al. 2006).

Consensus is available regarding the use of scores on risk assessment tools to inform the severity and complexity of patients' distress levels. In some instances, scores indicate an accumulation of risk factors or warning signs and may be useful in informing the intricacy of suicide risk. However, caution should be taken in how these scores are used in practice. The danger is that complete reliance on a single risk score may remove the holistic nature of clinical assessment in favour of efficiency and liability protection (Bergmand et al., 2007). Scores generated from risk assessment instruments may be less valuable than the actual content covered in the specific items themselves.

The underlying utility for suicide risk assessment tools is to gather additional information that can further inform on patients' degree of risk of suicide, corroborate findings from the clinical interviews, and tease out discrepancies in risk, if any. The inclusion of risk assessment tools may be a way to improve the overall quality of the suicide risk assessment process, as the use of tools adds further evidence to both detect and manage suicide risk.

This research has identified a number of themes related to the process of high quality risk assessment and considerations for working with risk assessment tools. These themes can be used in frameworks to support policy, education, evaluation, and further research at both organizational and health system levels.

Suicide risk assessment is not a singular event but, rather, an ongoing process. This process involves much more than the use of "tools" and "scores". Instead, risk assessment is a crucial aspect of the therapeutic process that is, in turn, part of a person's journey to recovery. Policies can support this in several ways. First, supports are needed for ongoing and appropriate training for care providers. Second, education and policy should describe the appropriate use of risk assessment tools that emphasize when and how they can be used to inform clinical judgement. Third, resources should be in place to support and facilitate clear communication and documentation of suicide risk.

Ultimately, identifying key principles and processes should rest on an evidence base that demonstrates how these activities actually mitigate and reduce future risk. To date, this research does not exist. Due to the critical nature of suicide, clinical trials may not be appropriate. Instead, analysis of quality improvement initiatives may be more appropriate (i.e., the effect of process adaptation on patient responsiveness, early identification of risk, and risk prevention). Research should also examine the development of quality indicators to monitor the quality of risk assessment. This is challenging given the need for an efficient way to gather data across organizations and jurisdictions. In jurisdictions without consistent data systems, a random sample chart review may provide the only evidence for process.

Conclusion

Suicide risk assessment is a complex process involving clinical decision-making that affects the safety, treatment, and recovery of persons in distress. While a degree of liability must be considered in terms of efficiently assessing all persons in health care settings, the nature of this assessment must always remain person-centred. Quality assurance organizations implement mandates to perform risk assessment, ultimately, to make health care a safer and more responsive setting to a person's needs. Thus, policies and practices for risk assessment that do not consider the person's unique life circumstance using a comprehensive assessment in the context of a therapeutic relationship need to be avoided. Ultimately, comprehensive approaches to suicide risk assessment need to be supported by an organizational culture and policies that recognize and encourage person-centred care.

Acknowledgements

This chapter is based on research that was funded by the Ontario Hospital Association (OHA) and Canadian Patient Safety Institute (CPSI) that was published as an online resource entitled *Suicide Risk Assessment: A Resource Guide for Canadian Healthcare Organizations* (Perlman et al., 2011). This guide is available online, free of charge, at www.oha.ca.

References

Accreditation Canada (2011). *Required organizational practice handbook.* Available at: http://www.accreditation. ca/uploadedFiles/Rop-handbook-April-2010-EN.pdf.

Ali, M. M., Dwyer, D. S., & Rizzo, J. A. (2011). The social contagion effect of suicidal behavior in adolescents: Does it really exist? *Journal of Mental Health Policy and Economics, 14,* 3–12.

American Psychiatric Association (APA) (2003). Practice guidelines for the assessment and treatment of patients with suicidal behaviours. *American Journal of Psychiatry, 160*(11), 1–60.

Barker, P., & Buchanan-Barker, P. (2005). *The tidal model: A guide for mental health professionals.* New York: Routledge.

Bergmans, Y., Brown, A. L., & Carruthers, A. S. H. (2007). Advances in crisis management of the suicidal patient: Perspectives from patients. *Current Psychiatry Reports, 9,* 74–80.

Brickell, T. A., & McLean, C. (2011). Emerging issues and challenges for improving patient safety in mental health: A qualitative analysis of expert perspectives. *Journal of Patient Safety, 7*(1), 39–44.

Brown, G. K. (2000). *A review of suicide assessment measures for intervention research with adults and older adults.* Bethesda, MD: National Institute of Mental Health.

Chandler, M. J., & Lalonde, C. E. (2004). Cultural continuity as a moderator of suicide risk among Canada's First Nations. In L. Kirmayer, & G. Valaskakis (Eds.), *The mental health of Canadian Aboriginal peoples: Transformations, identity, and community.* Vancouver, BC: University of British Columbia Press.

CIHI, & Statistics Canada (2011). *Health indicators 2011.* Ottawa: ON: CIHI, 2011. ISBN: 978-1-55465-900-5. Available at: https://secure.cihi.ca/estore/productFamily.htm?locale=en&pf=PFC1635.

Cull, J. G., & Gill, W. S. (1988*). The suicide probability scale.* Los Angeles: Western Psychological Services.

Cutcliffe, J. R., & Barker, P. (2004). The Nurses' Global Assessment of Suicide Risk (NGASR): Developing a tool for clinical practice. *Journal of Psychiatric and Mental Health Nursing, 11*(4), 393–400.

Draper, B. (2012). Isn't it a bit risky to dismiss suicide risk assessment? *Australia and New Zealand Journal of Psychiatry, 46:* 385.

Granello, D. H. (2010). The process of suicide risk assessment: Twelve core principles. *Journal of Counselling & Development, 88,* 363–370.

Haney, E. M., O'Neil, M. E., Carson, S., Low, A., Peterson, K., Denneson, L. M., Oleksiewicz, C., & Kansagara, D. (2012). *Suicide risk factors and risk assessment tools: A systematic review.* VA-ESP Project #05-225; 2012.

Heisel, M. J., & Flett, G. L. (2006). The development and initial validation of the Geriatric Suicide Ideation Scale. *The American Journal of Geriatric Psychiatry, 14*(9), 742–751.

Heisel, M. J., Grek, A., Moore, S. L., Jackson, F., Vincent, G., Malach, F. M., & Mokry, J. (2006). National guidelines for seniors' mental health: The assessment of suicide risk and prevention of suicide. *The Canadian Journal of Geriatrics, 9* (Suppl. 2), S65–S71.

Hirdes, J. P., Curtin-Telegdi, N., Rabinowitz, T., Fries, B., Morris, J., Ikegami, N., Yamauchi, K., Smith, T., Perez, E., & Martin, L. (2011). *interRAI Community Mental Health (CMH) assessment form and user's manual version 9.2.* Washington, DC: interRAI.

Hirdes, J. P., Smith, T. F., Rabinowitz, T., Yamauchi, K., Pérez, E., Telegdi, N. C., Prendergast, P., Morris, J. N., Ikegami, N., Phillips, C. D., Fries, B. E., & Resident Assessment Instrument-Mental Health Group (2002). The resident assessment instrument-mental health (RAI-MH): Inter-rater reliability and convergent validity. *The Journal of Behavioral Health Services & Research, 29*(4), 419–432.

Ho, T. P. (2003). The suicide risk of discharged psychiatric patients. *Journal of Clinical Psychiatry, 64,* 702–707.

Hunt, I. M., Kapur, N., Webb, R., Robinson, J., Burns, J., Shaw, J., et al. (2009). Suicide in recently discharged psychiatric patients: A case-control study. *Psychological Medicine, 39,* 443–449.

Jacobs, D. (1999). *Harvard Medical School guide to suicide assessment and intervention.* San Francisco: Jossey-Bass.

Joiner, T. E., Rudd, M. D., & Rajab, M. H. (1999). Agreement between self- and clinician-rated suicidal symptoms in a clinical sample of young adults: Explaining discrepancies. *Journal of Consulting and Clinical Psychology, 67,* 171–176.

Juhnke, G. A., & Hovestadt, A. J. (1995). Using the SAD PERSONS Scale to promote supervisee suicide assessment knowledge. *The Clinical Supervisor, 13*(2), 31–40.

Kutcher, S., & Chehil, S. (2007). *Suicide risk management: A manual for health professionals.* Malden, MA: Blackwell Publishing Ltd.

Large, M., Sharma, S., Cannon, E., et al. (2011). Risk factors for suicide within a year of discharge from psychiatric hospital: A systematic meta-analysis. *Australian and New Zealand Journal of Psychiatry, 45:* 619–628.

Linehan, M. M., Goodstein, J. L., Nielsen, S. L., & Chiles, J. A. (1983). Reasons for staying alive when you are thinking of killing yourself: The Reasons for Living Inventory. *Journal of Consulting and Clinical Psychology, 51*, 276–286.

Lyons, C., Price, P., Embling, S., & Smith, C. (2000). Suicide risk assessment: A review of procedures. *Accident & Emergency Nursing, 8*(3), 178–186.

Mills, P. D., Neily, J., Luan, D., Osborne, A., & Howard, K. (2006). Actions and implementation strategies to reduce suicidal events in the VHA. *The Joint Commission Journal on Quality and Patient Safety, 3*, 130–141.

Mulder, R. (2011). Problems with risk assessment. *Australian and New Zealand Journal of Psychiatry, 45*, 605–607.

Naud, H., & Daigle, M. S. (2010). Predictive validity of the Suicide Probability Scale in a male inmate population. *Journal of Psychopathology and Behavioral Assessment, 32*(3), 333–342.

Nelson, C., Johnston, M., & Srivastava, A. (2010). Improving risk assessment with suicidal patients: A preliminary evaluation of the clinical utility of the scale for impact of suicidality-management, assessment and planning of care (SIS-MAP). *Crisis, 31*, 231–237.

Neufeld, E., Hirdes, J. P., & Rabinowitz, T. (2011). Suicidality and purposeful self harm clinical assessment protocol. In J. P. Hirdes, N. Curtin-Telegdi, K. Mathias, C. M. Perlman, T. Saarela, & H. Kolbeinsson (Eds.). *interRAI Mental Health Clinical Assessment Protocols (CAPs) for use with community and hospital-based mental health assessment instruments: Derivation and application manual.* Version 9.1. Washington, DC: interRAI.

Perlman, C. M., Neufeld, E., Martin, L., Goy, M., & Hirdes, J. P. (2011). *Suicide risk assessment: A resource guide for Canadian healthcare organizations.* Toronto, ON: Ontario Hospital Association and Canadian Patient Safety Institute.

Pope, C., Ziebland, S., & Mays, N. (2000). Qualitative research in health care: Analysing qualitative data. *BMJ, 320*(7227): 114–116.

Pridmore, S. (2009). Predicament suicide: Concept and evidence. *Australasian Psychiatry, 17*, 112–116.

Pridmore, W. G. (2012). Suicide is preventable, sometimes. *Australasian Psychiatry.* 2012 July 6. [Epub ahead of print.]

Registered Nurses' Association of Ontario (2009). *Assessment and care of adults at risk for suicidal ideation and behaviour.* Toronto: Registered Nurses' Association of Ontario.

Rudd, M. D. (2008). Suicide warning signs in clinical practice. *Current Psychiatry Reports, 10*, 87–90.

Rudd, M. D., Berman, A. L., Joiner, T. E., Nock, M. K., Silverman, M. M., Mandrusiak, M., Orden, K., & Witte, T. (2006). Warning signs for suicide: Theory, research, and clinical applications. *Suicide and Life-threatening Behavior, 36*, 255–262.

Sanchez, H. (2001). Risk factor model for suicide assessment and intervention. *Professional Psychology and Practice, 32*, 352–358.

Simon, R. I. (2011). Improving suicide risk assessment. *Psychiatric Times, 28*(11). Available at: http://www.psychiatrictimes.com/risk-assessment/content/article/10168/2000387.

Szmukler, G. (2012). Risk assessment for suicide and violence is of extremely limited value in general psychiatric practice. *Australia and New Zealand Journal of Psychiatry, 46*(2): 173–174.

Weissman, M. M., Bland, R.C., Canino, G. J., Greenwald, S., Hwu, H. G., Joyce, P. R., Karam, E. G., Lee, C. K., Lellouch, J., Lepine, J. P., Newman, S. C., Rubio-Stipec, M., Wells, J. E., Wickramaratne, P.J., Wittchen, H. U., & Yeh, E. K. (1999). Prevalence of suicide ideation and suicide attempts in nine countries. *Psychological Medicine, 29*(1), 9–17.

World Health Organization (WHO) (2003). Suicide rates (per 100,000) by country, year, and gender. Available at: http://www.who.int/mental_health/prevention/suicide/suiciderates/en/.

16

TRAJECTORY-BASED MODELS IN THE STUDY OF SUICIDE

Monique Séguin, Alain Lesage, Johanne Renaud and Gustavo Turecki

Introduction

Suicide is a major public health concern and ranks among the top ten causes of death for individuals of all ages in most Western countries (WHO, 2005). Over the past 30 years, numerous studies have examined the relationship between suicide and mental disorders (Barraclough, Bunch, Nelson, & Sainsbury, 1974; Zhang et al., 2003). These studies have identified numerous clinical risk factors for suicide completion, including previous suicide attempts, male sex, family history of suicide, presence of psychiatric problems and inadequate treatment of mental disorders and addictive behaviours (Kim et al., 2003; Lesage et al., 2008; Renaud, Berlim, McGirr, Tousignant, & Turecki, 2008).

The standard method used to assess psychopathology in suicide completers is the psychological autopsy (Hawton et al., 1998). Under this proxy-based interview process, best informants provide data that serves to investigate a number of risk factors related to suicide death. Psychological autopsy studies have demonstrated that approximately 90% of suicide cases presented a psychiatric disorder (Hawton et al., 1998; Isometsa, 2001; Kim et al., 2003, Arsenault-Lapierre, Kim, & Turecki, 2004; Zouk, Tousignant, Séguin, Lesage, & Turecki, 2006; Lesage, Boyer, Grunberg, Loyer, & Chawky, 1994) or psychosocial difficulties (Hawton et al. 1998; Cheng, Chen, Chen, & Jenkins, 2000; Angst, Stassen, Clayton, & Angst, 2002).

That being said, for some clinical researchers, the identification of risk factors, especially psychosocial ones assessed at a single point in time, has hit a brick wall in terms of clinical utility (Mann, Watermaux, Haas, & Malone, 1999; Cassells, Paterson, Dowding, & Morrison, 2005). The investigation of suicide death could stand to benefit from the use of complementary methods especially in regard to the distribution of adversity over the life course.

Trajectory-based models

The importance of development, life events and biographical factors are widely recognized, as well as their impact on the development of pathology, which could eventually lead to the development of suicidal behaviours. For example, Compass et al. (1988) presented a framework for the development of depression involving a complex series of relationships between life events, negative and positive affectivity and stress-related variables, to the extent that the choice of coping strategies may be effective or not in lowering stress, depending on affectivity.

As for suicide research, a great deal of knowledge has been drawn from psychological autopsy methods. More recently, some variables have been capturing the attention of researchers and clinicians such as early adversity, violence and sexual abuse, which are considered to be among the most common risk factors associated with mental health problems and suicide attempts (Beautrais, 2010; Kessler, Davis, & Kendler, 1997; McGirr et al., 2009). That being said, most of the "well-established" risk factors such as mental health problems, presence of life events and the lack of mental health services occur at the end of the trajectory. We know little about the burden of adversity and how it accumulates over the years, its long-lasting and profound effect over the life course and how the complex series of developmental mechanisms involved in the suicidal outcome interact. In order to better conceptualize etiological models of suicide, two elements are required: (1) multi-determinism; and (2) interaction (Rutter, Kim-Cohen, & Maughan, 2006). Researchers are becoming increasingly interested in trajectory-based models, which integrate transitional processes like vulnerability, stress sensitivity and tolerance to adversity and examine dynamic aspects such as trajectory curves (Luthar & Brown, 2007; Zucker, 2006). A life trajectory implies a continual person–environment interaction (Karevold, Røysamb, Ystrom, & Mathiesen, 2009). Very few studies have specified trajectory as a continuous development of a life sequence, which necessarily involves transitions and turning points, not always accessible to quantitative measures. A life trajectory approach is a complex endeavour and should analyze multi-level risk factors (parenting, family dysfunction, negative life events, academic problems and professional and legal problems), their cumulative effects over time, and their varying consequences, for example, on the development of different types of mental health problems, during the life course perspective.

The life course method should be able to measure the burden of adversity to determine whether, on this basis, there exist differential profiles to, ultimately, arrive at a more targeted preventive intervention. That being said, it is important to know how to translate such biographical context into the meaningful account of life trajectories.

Our research group introduced the life-calendar method (Forest, Moen, & Dempster-McKain, 1996; Rutter, 2002b) in suicide research to shed more light on the longitudinal and cumulative impact of psychosocial factors.

The life-calendar method

The life-history calendar procedure, also referred to as narrative rating, is designed to elicit sufficiently detailed accounts of events to allow for coding that will help a panel of trained experts to evaluate their key characteristics. The interview method that uses the life trajectory calendar was borrowed from the life-history calendar research (Caspi, Moffitt, & Thornton, 1996; Ensel, Peek, & Lin, 1996). We developed a semi-standardized interview (available from the authors on request) and trained interviewers on its use. Prior experience (Tousignant, Séguin, Lesage, Chawky, & Turecki, 2003) in using the Life Events and Difficulties Scale (LEDS; Brown & Harris, 1978) and the Childhood Experience of Care and Abuse (CECA) instrument (Bifulco, Moran, Baines, & Brown, 1994) rendered us sensitive to the contextual aspects of life events and adversities to be covered using retrospective measures.

The life-calendar is used to map the events that mark an individual's trajectory in 12 spheres of life: place of residence, parent–child relationship, emotional-romantic relationships, adult family life, episodes of personal difficulty, academic life, professional life, social life, dimensions of losses/separations/departures, other social adversity, protective factors, help seeking/services, and drug use. For example, place of residence includes moving to another location and placement in foster homes. The parent–child relationship covers abuse, neglect and physical, sexual and household violence. With the help of a visual calendar, the approach serves contemporaneously to record the sequence and investigate event characteristics. Lists of questions addressing different themes and events are used to probe informants for narrative details. For each sphere, the interviewers identify whether the events were situational or permanent and determine their duration, intensity, frequency and context.

The life trajectory is reconstructed on the basis of events recalled by family and friends; we usually have access to medical and psychosocial reports obtained with the consent of participants. Written documents belonging to the deceased and the informants, including agendas and diaries, were also used if made available from the close relatives. That being said, despite the tremendous efforts deployed to gather data, the quality and quantity of information on the suicide victims were uneven, being at times too scant for the early childhood period or the last decade of life. Consequently, in some cases, part of the life trajectory remained incomplete. The events recalled were of public knowledge and were usually serious enough for the immediate family to notice and remember; however, informants might not have been privy to all of the deceased's personal and private events, setbacks, frustrations and letdowns. Nevertheless, numerous authors suggest that narrative-rating instruments help to increase the reliability and validity of the measurement of major stressful events (Brown & Harris, 1978; Dohrenwend, 2006). Studies have shown (Lin, Ensel, & Lai, 1997) that recall errors usually tend to under-report rather than over-report and that their impact tends to be greater for chronic and routine changes than for personal and family events.

After all the data was collected, each individual life trajectory was written up by the interviewers into a case vignette summarizing all the life events, their context, adversities, protective factors, psychopathology and service use. The research coordinator reviewed each interview, verified any inconsistencies in the narrative details and spot-checked the audiotape interviews. When details were found to be missing, we recontacted informants and corrected the interviews before the panel of raters coded the burden of adversity. Adverse events and types of event were tallied for each five-year segment. Each vignette was then submitted to the panel of raters, which was independent of the interviewers.

The raters were trained to evaluate the likely "contextual threat" of events by assessing their place within the respondent's developmental circumstances. The interviewers sought to accumulate sufficient narrative details about the life events to allow the trained raters to pass judgement on the key characteristics of the events (Dohrenwend, 2006). Our raters had prior experience with this type of narrative rating with the LEDS and CECA.

The panel rated each five-year period in terms of burden of adversity. This conceptualization was borrowed from the morbidity burden or low disease burden approach (Powers & Peckham, 1990; McGinnis & Foege, 1993; Forest et al., 1996) used to identify overall morbidity that seems to affect health. It is associated with the allostatic load concept that links psychosocial stress to the neurobiological and genetic dimensions of mental disorders and suicide (McEwen, 1998; Forrest & Riley, 2004). The rating scale used in this study was inspired by the scales developed by Brown and Harris for the LEDS (Brown, Andrews, Bifulco, & Harris, 1990). The LEDS rating includes four different coding intensity levels, and intra-pair coding agreement runs from 78% to 91% in samples with diagnoses of depression and schizophrenia (Brown & Harris, 1978).

Our panel evaluated the burden of adversity by taking into account the inventory of life events and the intra-category variability of events, using a scale of 1 to 6 to rate accumulation and concurrence of adversity throughout the individual's life at five-year intervals. The overall burden assessments ranged from severe (rating of 1 or 2), to moderate (3 or 4), to low (5 or 6). This evaluation took into consideration the number of risk factors, their importance, duration, and severity, the extent of the consequences, the concurrence of events and the counterbalancing protective factors. For example, a burden of 1 corresponded to multiple risk factors in each sphere of life prevailing over the entire five-year period, with absolutely no protective factors. Inversely, a burden of 6 corresponded to normal difficulties lasting a shorter period of time (less than one year) and affecting only one or two spheres of life, with presence of protective factors. Over the course of the research, we developed dictionaries to define variables and provide examples of cases for each codification in order to be consistent in the coding and minimize rating drifts by panel members. Intra-rater reliability was assessed as follows: in all cases the raters coded each trajectory independently before the consensus discussion. Intra-pair agreement for the 10 five-year segments ranged from 76% to 97%, and the lower agreement was found in the 0–5 age segment.

Data analysis

The life trajectory data analysis was conducted with a SAS group-based modeling of longitudinal data (Jones, Nagin, & Roeder, 2001; Nagin & Tremblay, 2001). The SAS-based Traj procedure (Nagin & Tremblay, 2005) provided the capacity: (1) to identify subgroups of persons who followed distinct trajectories; (2) to examine the pattern of variation and stability over time for the subgroups in question; and (3) to estimate the proportion of individuals in each group. In order to identify models with the optimum number of groups, we assessed models with two, three, and four groups. In so doing, we evaluated models with various specifications for stable, linear, quadratic and cubic shapes of the trajectory groups. For each group, the significance level for each parameter was given in the output. Also, the statistical procedure yielded the probability of each subject to be classified in other groups and assigned group membership based on the highest probability of classification. Together, these indices provided estimates of model fit.

Examples of life trajectory profiles

A first study conducted in New Brunswick examined the suicide death of 102 individuals of the 109 deaths after suicide that occurred over a 14-month period in 2002–2003. The procedure identified two categories of suicides by clustering subjects on the basis of longitudinal patterns of adversity (Figure 16.1). The first is characterized by early adversity and more Axis II disorders, and the second by late adversity associated with addiction disorders. Though a new method was used, the findings were rather consistent with previous findings. This should bolster the generalization of results.

Theories from developmental research may help to explain the two trajectories identified. First, some authors (Bifulco et al., 2002; Rutter, 2002a) have already suggested that childhood exposure to a harmful environment has profound effects on adult health and that childhood exposure to different types of abuse directly increases the risk of maladaptive attachment styles (Brière & Runtz, 1990; Bryant & Range, 1995; Rutter, 2002b) and mental disorders during adulthood (Kendler, Gardner, & Prescott, 2002). Individuals who followed trajectory 1 were all exposed to early adversity, especially physical and sexual abuse. In trajectory 1, we also noted a high number of prior suicide attempts (though this did not prove to be statistically significant), a higher number of addiction disorders and a higher number of Axis II psychopathologies. Over the last five years, we also observed an accumulation of personal problems, especially regarding difficulties between suicide victims and their children or the death of a close relative. Individuals who followed this life trajectory committed suicide at age 44 on average. Trajectory 1 was characterized by early burden of adversity coupled with multiple addiction disorders and later Axis II pathologies. This group was more likely to present comorbid disorders, which suggests

Burden of adversity

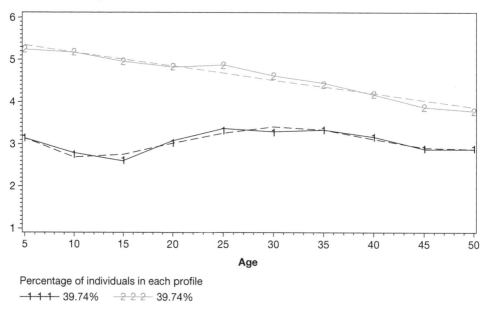

Percentage of individuals in each profile
—1–1–1— 39.74%   –2–2–2– 39.74%

Figure 16.1 Developmental trajectories and burden of adversity in two different suicide mortality groups

that some individuals never manage to overcome harsh early experiences and that the burden they bear grows over time.

Trajectory 2 was characterized by a reaction to major difficulties later in life. Individuals who fell under this second profile had fewer difficulties identified over the life span, except for the last five years, which suggests a later accumulation of difficulties. This second trajectory was marked by a slower decline over time and was accompanied and compounded by Axis I disorders such as mood disorders.

Youth and young adult suicide trajectories

In another study, we explored the unique developmental challenges and early adversity faced by youth and young adults who died of suicide. Sixty-seven suicide victims, the suicide group (SG), were compared with 56 living control participants with no suicidal ideations over the last year, the control group (CG), matched for age, gender and geographical region.

The results of this study with 67 suicide victims and 56 control participants indicate a difference in the SG trajectories compared to the CG trajectories. A good control group helps to measure the population distribution of risk factors and outcomes. Participants in the control group were not as exposed to hardship and did not develop as many mental health problems over time as the suicide group, but they were still not "very healthy". Indeed, 12% of the participants had experienced major mental health difficulties in the last 12 months prior to the study and 7% over the course of their lives (ranging from 14–29 years old), which is consistent with the data from epidemiological studies that indicate that 14% of children under 20 years of age have mental health problems (Canadian Community Health Survey, 2003). Some of the children in the control group had been exposed to hardship: 14% of the children aged between 0 and 4 years old, 18% of the children aged between 5 and 9 years old and 34% of the children aged between

10 and 14 years old had been exposed to abuse or physical/sexual violence. The change in the developmental trajectory of the children aged between 15 and 19 years old was consistent with the results found by other researchers. Caspi observed that during the period of "emerging adulthood" (i.e., ages 15–29), where most men and women become more socially dominant, warm, responsible, agreeable and emotionally stable, negative life events persist over time for some people. These normative developmental changes in personality functioning have been observed in multiple birth cohorts, in different Western nations, using both longitudinal and cross-sectional research designs (Roberts, Caspi, & Moffitt, 2003).

People in the suicide group had much more difficulty over the course of their lives, starting at an early age. The presence of difficulties within the parental relationship, characterized by the presence of neglect, discord and physical/sexual violence, is among the most important adverse events (Table 16.1). These early adversities, coupled with the lack of a protective adult relationship, identified by the number of separations from one or both parents before the age of 15, seem to place young children on a specific path, whereas possible familial biological predisposition pooled with the accumulation of adverse events will subsequently develop into mental health difficulties such as ADHD, the presence of mood disorders, substance abuse, dependence disorders and anxiety disorders, which will create even more difficulties in the professional domain, with financial and legal difficulties by the time they are teens and young adults.

Table 16.1 Life events comparison between the suicide group and control group

Life events	No.	(%)	No.	(%)	OR	CI95%	p
Age 0–4	67		56				
Discipline/neglect/ tensions in parent–child relationship	33	49.25	8	14.29	5.824	2.395–14.161	0.000
Sexual abuse/ physical-psychological violence of S	11	16.42	1	1.79	10.804	1.349–86.533	0.006
Age 5–9	67		56				
Discipline/neglect/ tensions in parent–child relationship	40	59.70	10	17.86	6.815	2.941–15.789	0.000
Sexual abuse/ physical-psychological violence of S	13	19.40	1	1.79	13.241	1.674–104.754	0.002
Academic difficulties	27	40.30	7	12.50	4.725	1.864–11.979	0.001
Relational difficulties	18	26.87	5	8.93	3.747	1.291–10.875	0.011
Negative experiences	11	16.42	2	3.57	5.304	1.123–25.046	0.021
Age 10–14[a]	67		56				
Discipline/neglect/ tensions in parent–child relationship	52	77.61	19	33.93	6.751	3.041–14.987	0.000

Table 16.1 Continued

Life events	No.	(%)	No.	(%)	OR	CI95%	p
Sexual abuse/ physical-psychological violence of S	12	17.91	1	1.79	12.000	1.508–95.474	0.004
Mental health problems	25	37.31	5	8.93	6.071	2.139–17.236	0.000
Academic difficulties	41	61.19	10	17.86	7.254	3.125–16.838	0.000
Relational difficulties	20	29.85	8	14.29	2.553	1.024–6.364	0.040
Legal difficulties	9	13.43	1	1.79	8.534	1.047–69.601	0.019
Age 15–19[b]	63		53				
Discipline/neglect/ tensions in parent– child relationship	48	76.19	19	35.85	4.920	2.285–10.593	0.000
Sexual abuse/ physical-psychological violence of S	10	15.87	1	1.89	9.649	1.195–77.914	0.011
Mental health problems	45	71.43	12	22.64	7.500	3.313–16.977	0.000
Academic difficulties	42	66.67	6	11.32	14.000	5.250–37.337	0.000
Professional difficulties	25	39.68	2	3.77	16.071	3.602–71.715	0.000
Relational difficulties	24	38.10	3	5.66	9.860	2.781–34.966	0.000
Financial losses	16	25.40	2	3.77	8.471	1.855–38.690	0.002
Legal difficulties	15	23.81	1	1.89	15.865	2.023–124.409	0.001
Age 20–24[c]	43		33				
Discipline/neglect/ tensions in parent– child relationship	26	60.47	9	27.27	3.312	1.393–7.873	0.005
Relationship difficulties with spouse	31	72.09	10	30.30	3.961	1.718–9.135	0.001
Mental health problems	38	88.37	7	21.21	9.172	3.627–23.195	0.000
Professional difficulties	28	65.12	3	9.09	12.684	3.596–44.734	0.000
Relational difficulties	24	55.81	3	9.09	9.860	2.781–34.966	0.000
Financial losses	22	51.16	4	12.12	6.356	2.037–19.825	0.001
Legal difficulties	14	32.56	3	9.09	4.667	1.267–17.188	0.013
Age 25–29[d]	7		5				

Notes: $N = 123$, Suicide Group ($N = 67$), Control Group ($N = 56$).
[a] In this age group, four people committed suicide at the ages of 13 and 14.
[b] In this age group, twenty people committed suicide between the ages of 15 and 19.
[c] In this age group, thirty-nine people committed suicide.
[d] Non-significant information for this age group.

Interestingly, not all suicide victims followed the same developmental trajectory (Figure 16.2). The result identifies two categories of suicides by clustering subjects on the basis of longitudinal patterns of adversity, in the manner suggested by the allostatic load theory (McEwen, 1998). Suicide victims characterized by Trajectory 1 seem to have been exposed to more severe adversity at an earlier age: 70–90% were exposed to a difficult parental relationship (defined by the presence of neglect, harsh discipline and much tension), and one fourth of the subgroup was placed in foster homes or in residential institutions. These children were 27 times more likely to have been exposed to the presence of physical and/or sexual abuse. The present study has included both physical and sexual abuse as a single item in the analysis because of limitations due to the small number of participants. That being said, ulterior research should investigate the effect of various abuse experiences separately given its importance in terms of mental health over the life span.

People identified by Trajectory 2 were characterized by the presence of family tension, discord and academic difficulties. They had early learning difficulties (48.6% in Trajectory II compared to 80% in Trajectory I), but less behavioural difficulties in school compared to the other subgroup. The absence of behavioural difficulties may have elicited less social stigmatization and therefore have created more social connections. An early pattern of behavioural adjustment (indicated by an absence of aggressive behaviour problems) may act as a protective factor to buffer a child from the future effects of social rejection by peers (Dodge & Pettit, 2003) at least in certain areas of life and for some time.

These two trajectories may have different etiological explanations. Trajectory 1 is clearly characterized by severe developmental difficulties and a lack of adult protection, starting at a very early age, creating a spiral of events and mental health problems throughout the life cycle. This profile is well understood and documented in the developmental literature. Trajectory 2, however, may be characterized by a slower decline over time possibly due to a less harmful

Burden of adversity scores

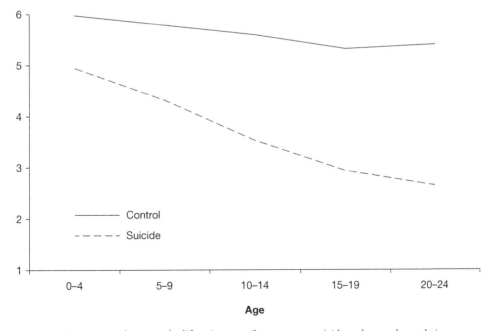

Figure 16.2 Comparison between the life trajectory of two groups: suicide and general population

environment coupled with adaptive efforts, which will wear out over time. These etiological differences should be better understood. For example, it is not clear if the difficulties observed in Trajectory 2 are explained by the different nature of childhood adversity or if the differences may be explained by other mechanisms such as a lack of ability in decision-making or the lack of ability to choose adapted coping strategies or the presence of some specific type of personality structure, such as greater emotional reactivity among certain participants. These difficulties may render people in this subgroup more sensitive to stressful environments, they may generate greater feelings of distress or may be attracted to a peer environment known to increase the risk of substance abuse, for example. These variables were not measured in our studies, which may be a limitation of our methodology, but should be considered in future similar studies.

Results from this study confirmed our hypothesis regarding a positive link between the presence of early violence as a predictor of cumulative difficulties over time in almost all areas of the life cycle and, consequently, of suicide death. The results suggest that too many children who are exposed to harmful environments may never manage to overcome harsh early experiences and that the burden they bear grows over time.

Conclusion

The life-calendar approach presented here and for the first time in suicide research adds to the identification of past (e.g., sexual or physical abuse and childhood separation) and recent (e.g., spousal separation) life events previously associated with suicide. It also quantifies the burden these events may represent over each period of life. Suicide rarely occurs "out of the blue" (Bebbington et al., 2009), but rather in a context of major difficulty and adversity, present from a very young age.

Regarding etiological suicide studies, a methodology assessing quantitatively the accumulation of the burden of psychosocial adversities over time would fit better with models of cumulative burden and allostatic load formulated for stress and diseases. It would also help to distinguish pathways to suicide that may represent the "wear and tear" of cumulative adversities from other pathways in which depression may play a greater role, not to mention the neurobiological abnormalities and genetic predispositions that may be associated with each of these (McEwen, 1998; Forrest & Riley, 2004). This would contribute to the refinement of suicide prevention strategies.

References

Angst, F., Stassen, H. H., Clayton, P. J., & Angst, J. (2002). Mortality of patients with mood disorders: Follow-up over 34–38 years. *Journal of Affective Disorders, 68,* 167–181.

Arsenault-Lapierre, G., Kim, C., & Turecki, G. (2004). Psychiatric diagnoses in 3275 suicides: A meta-analysis. *BMC Psychiatry, 4,* 37.

Barraclough, B., Bunch, J., Nelson, B., & Sainsbury, P. (1974). A hundred cases of suicide: Clinical aspects. *British Journal of Psychiatry, 125,* 355– 373.

Beautrais, A. L., Gibb, S. J., Faulkner, A., Fergusson, D. M., & Mulder, R. T. (2010). Postcard intervention for repeat self-harm: Randomised controlled trial. *British Journal of Psychiatry, 197*(1), 55–60.

Bebbington, P., Cooper, C., Minot, S., Brugha, T., Jenkins, R., Meltzer, H., & Dennis, M. (2009). Suicide attempts, gender and sexual abuse: Data from the 2000 British Psychiatric Morbidity Survey. *American Journal of Psychiatry, 166,* 1135–1140.

Bifulco, A., Brown, G. W., & Harris, T. O. (1994). Childhood experience of care and abuse (CECA): A retrospective interview measure. *Child Psychology and Psychiatry, 35,* 1419–1435.

Bifulco, A., Moran, P., Baines, R., & Brown, G. W. (2002). Exploring psychological abuse in childhood: Association with other abuse and adult clinical depression. *Bulletin of the Menninger Clinic, 66,* 3.

Brière, J., & Runtz, M. (1990). Differential adult symptomatologies associated with three types of childhood abuse. *Child Abuse and Neglect, 14*, 357–364.

Brown, G. W., Andrews, B., Bifulco, A., & Harris, T. O. (1990). Self-esteem and depression: I Measurement issues and prediction of onset. *Social Psychiatry and Psychiatric Epidemiology, 25*, 200–209.

Brown, G. W., & Harris, T. O. (1978). *Social origins of depression: A study of psychiatric disorder in women.* London: Tavistock.

Bryant, S., & Range, M. L. (1995). Suicidality in college women who report multiple versus single types of maltreatment by parents: A brief report. *Journal of Child Sexual Abuse, 4*, 87–94.

Caspi, A., Moffitt, T., & Thornton, A. (1996). The life history calendar: A research and clinical assessment method for collecting retrospective event-history data. *International Journal of Methods in Psychiatric Research, 6*, 101–114.

Cassells, C., Paterson, B., Dowding, D., & Morrison, R. (2005). Long- and short-term risk factors in the prediction of inpatient suicide: A review of the literature. *Crisis, 26*(2), 53–63.

Cheng, A. T., Chen, T. H., Chen, C. C., & Jenkins, R. (2000). Psychosocial and psychiatric risk factors for suicide: Case-control psychological autopsy study. *British Journal of Psychiatry, 177*, 360–365.

Compass, B. E., Malcarne, V. L., & Fondacaro, K. M. (1988). Coping with stressful events in older children and young adolescents. *Journal of Consulting and Clinical Psychology, 56*, 405–411.

Dodge, K., & Pettit, G. S. (2003) A biopsychosocial model of the development of chronic conduct problems in adolescence. *Developmental Psychology, 39*(2), 349–371.

Dohrenwend, B. P. (2006). Inventorying stressful life events as risk factors for psychopathology: Toward resolution of the problem of intracategory variability. *Psychological Bulletin, 132*(3), 477–495.

Ensel, W., Peek, M., & Lin, N. (1996). Stress in the life course: A life history approach. *Journal of Aging and Health, 8*, 389–416.

Forest, K., Moen, P., & Dempster-McKain, D. (1996). The effects of childhood family stress on women's depressive symptoms: A life course approach. *Psychology of Women Quarterly, 20*, 81–100.

Forrest, C., & Riley, A. (2004). Childhood origins of adult health: A basis for life-course health policy. *Health Affairs, 23*, 155–164.

Hawton, K., Appleby, L., Platt, S., Foster, T., Cooper, J., Malmberg, A., & Simkin, S. (1998). The psychological autopsy approach to studying suicide: A review of methodological issues. *Journal of Affective Disorders, 50*, 269–276.

Isometsa, E. T. (2001). Psychological autopsy studies: A review. *European Psychiatry, 16*, 379–385.

Jones, B., Nagin, D., & Roeder, K. (2001). A SAS procedure based on mixture models for estimating developmental trajectories. *Sociological Methods & Research, 29*(3), 374–393.

Karevold, E., Røysamb, J., Ystrom, E., & Mathiesen, K. S. (2009). Predictors and pathways from infancy to symptoms of anxiety and depression in early adolescence. *Developmental Psychology, 45*, 1051–1060.

Kendler, K., Gardner, C., & Prescott, C. (2002). Toward a comprehensive developmental model for major depression in women. *American Journal of Psychiatry, 159*, 1133–1145.

Kessler, R. C., Davis, C. G., & Kendler, K. S. (1997). Childhood adversity and adult psychiatric disorder in the US National Comorbidity Survey. *Psychological Medicine, 27*, 1101–1119.

Kim, C., Lesage, A., Séguin, M., Vanier, J., Lipp, O., Chawky, N., & Turecki, G. (2003). Patterns of comorbidity in male suicide completers. *Psychological Medicine, 33*, 1299–1309.

Lesage, A., Boyer, R., Grunberg, F., Loyer, M., & Chawky, N. (1994). Suicide and mental disorders: A case-control study of young men. *American Journal of Psychiatry, 151*, 1063–1068.

Lesage, A., Séguin, M., Guy, A., Daigle, F., Bayle, M. F., Turecki, G., & Chawky, N. (2008). Systematic services audit of all consecutive cases of suicide in New Brunswick, Canada. *Canadian Journal of Psychiatry, 53*(10): 671– 678.

Lin, N., Ensel, W., & Lai, W. (1997). Construction and use of the life history calendar: Reliability and validity recall data. In I. H. Gotlib, & B. Wheaton (Eds.), *Stress and adversity over the life course: Trajectories and turning points* (pp. 178–204). New York: Cambridge University Press.

Luthar, S. S., & Brown, P. J. (2007). Maximizing resilience through diverse levels of inquiry: Prevailing paradigms, possibilities and priorities for the future. *Development and Psychopathology, 19*, 931– 955.

Mann, J. J., Watermaux, C., Haas, G. L., & Malone, K. M. (1999). Toward a clinical model of suicidal behaviour in psychiatric patients. *American Journal of Psychiatry, 156*, 181–189.

McEwen, B. (1998). Protective and damaging effects of stress mediators. *Seminars in Medicine of the Beth Israel Deaconess Medical Center, 338*(3), 171–179.

McGinnis, J. M., & Foege, W. H. (1993). Actual causes of death in the United States. *Journal of the American Medical Association, 270*, 2207–2212.

McGirr, A., Alda, M., Séguin, M., Cabot, S., Lesage, A., & Turecki, G. (2009). Familial aggregation of suicide is explained by cluster B traits: A three-group family study of suicide controlling for major depressive disorder. *American Journal of Psychiatry, 166*, 1124–1134.

Nagin, D., & Tremblay, R. (2001). Analyzing developmental trajectories of distinct but related behaviors: A group-based method. *Psychological Methods, 6*, 18–34.

Nagin, D., & Tremblay, R. (2005). What has been learned from group-based trajectory modeling? Examples from physical aggression and other problem behaviors. *Annals of the American Academy of Political and Social Sciences, 602*, 82–117.

Powers, C., & Peckham, C. (1990). Childhood morbidity and adulthood ill health. *Journal of Epidemiology and Community Health, 44*, 69–74.

Renaud, J., Berlim, M. T., McGirr, A., Tousignant, M., & Turecki, G. (2008). Current psychiatric morbidity, aggression/impulsivity, and personality dimension in child and adolescent suicide: A case-control study. *Journal of Affective Disorders, 105* (1–3): 221–228.

Roberts, B. W., Caspi, A., & Moffit, T. E. (2003). Work experiences and personality development in young adulthood. *Journal of Personality and Social Psychology, 84*(3), 582–593.

Rutter, M. (2002a). Nature, nurture, and development: From evangelism through science toward policy and practice. *Child Development 73*, 1–21.

Rutter, M. (2002b). The interplay of nature, nurture and developmental influences: The challenge ahead for mental health. *Archives of General Psychiatry, 59*, 996–1000.

Rutter, M., Kim-Cohen, J., & Maughan, B. (2006). Continuities and discontinuities in psychopathology between childhood and adult life. *Journal of Child Psychology and Psychiatry, 47*, 276–295.

Tousignant, M., Séguin, M., Lesage, A., Chawky, N., & Turecki, G. (2003). Le suicide chez les hommes de 18 à 55 ans: trajectoires de vie [Suicide among men 18 to 55 years of age: Life trajectories]. *Revue Québécoise de Psychologie, 24*(1), 145–159.

World Health Organization (WHO) (2000). *World health report 2000. Health system: improving performance.* WHOSIS: World Health Organization Statistical Information System. Accessed 5 July 2005.

Zhang, J., Conwell, Y., Wieczorek, W. F., Jiang, C., Jia, S., & Zhou, L. (2003). Studying Chinese suicide with proxy-based data: Reliability and validity of the methodology and instruments in China. *Journal of Nervous and Mental Disorders, 191*(7), 450–457.

Zouk, H., Tousignant, M., Séguin, M., Lesage, A., & Turecki, G. (2006). Characterization of impulsivity in suicide completers: Clinical, behavioural and psychosocial dimensions. *Journal of Affective Disorders, 92*, 195–204.

Zucker, R. A. (2006). Alcohol use and the alcohol use disorders: A developmental–biopsychosocial systems formulation covering the life course. In D. Cicchetti, & D. J. Cohen (Eds.), *Developmental psychopathology* (2nd ed., pp. 620–656). Hoboken, NJ: Wiley.

EDITORIAL COMMENTARY

The psychology section, Part III, contains five chapters. We have an overview of the issue, a unique model of predicting suicidal ideation, suggestions for quality assessment, what others think of practitioners who lose patients to suicide, and the impact of suicide on practitioners.

In Chapter 12, John McIntosh provides an epidemiological study reviewing suicide in the USA. His data is current and extremely informative. Although he uses US data, the findings are similar to those in Canada and also Europe. His study supports the current understanding of suicide being a multi-faceted, complex issue. Interestingly he has identified that after many years of decreasing suicide statistics, the trend has begun to reverse, with suicide tending to increase across the USA, though the determinants for this remain elusive.

In Chapter 16, Monique Séguin et al. provide us with a new unique way of assessing those at risk for suicide. Within the trajectory based models they focus on the life-calendar model. This model uses specially trained professionals to reconstruct the individual's life into 12 spheres and uses these events within the spheres to determine the possible impact of the events on the person and the impact these events may have on suicidal ideation or threat. This model places suicide ideation and suicide attempt within the context of a person's life, as suicide rarely occurs outside of this context.

In Chapter 15, Chrisopher Perlman and Eva Neufeld address the issue of providing quality risk assessments. They argue that there is lack of integration across locations and disciplines and that there is a need for a coordinated suicide risk assessment tool. Their study includes a literature review and stakeholder interviews. Their findings are organized into themes and should be of special interest to the practitioner. Their focus on how the assessment process impacts on the patient is refreshing and an important reminder of the overall purpose of a suicide risk assessment.

In Chapter 13, Ward-Ciesielski et al. examine the perception that persons who had lost someone to suicide had about the therapist or caregiver who had provided care to the patient who died of suicide. They predicted that the feelings of those who had lost someone to suicide would be negative towards the therapist. There hypotheses were not supported as no differences were found between those who had lost someone to suicide and those who had not. The implications of these findings are important to practitioners who may be reluctant to accept patients who have a high potential for suicide.

We conclude the review of Part III with Chapter 14 by Joseph S. Munson that examines the impact of patient suicide on the practitioner. Findings indicate that the greater the time-distance from the suicide, the greater the potential for the clinician's growth. The implications of this are that clinicians can expect not only to experience some PTSD but also PTG in that they can experience personal growth through what are difficult and painful events.

It is clear from these chapters that further work is needed in all aspects of suicide research. We agree and support the notion that more rigorous scientific research needs to be conducted in areas such as suicide prevention (especially to gain some agreement on the factors that underlie suicide), person-centred assessment, and the impact on survivors. As a clinical psychologist, one of our editors feels strongly that psychology is moving too far into the development of impersonal assessment tools and is forgetting the needs of the person who is experiencing suicidal ideation. While such tools are indeed needed, it is important that we do not forget why the tools are being developed in that they are needed to guide treatment not merely to assess and pass the person along to someone else. The 'treatment' of suicide exhibits the characteristics of an assembly line, in one end of a psych ward and out the other, having been fully assessed but not treated. All too often treatment is passed to para-professionals or lay workers and is not conducted by professionals where it should be taking place. We encourage psychologists and psychological training programs to keep the person at the centre of any treatments or assessment model.

PART IV

Social work and allied health care disciplines

EDITORIAL INTRODUCTION

Allied health professionals play a unique and vital role in the clinical care of suicidal people and make contributions to the furtherance of clinically focused suicide research. Allied health professionals is a term that refers to a large group of health professionals that make up to 50–60% of the workforce in hospitals and clinics in the USA and Canada (University of California San Francisco, 2012; Association of Canadian Community Colleges, 2012). Despite comprising this large percentage of the workforce, a realistic appraisal of the scholarly, research contributions emanating from this group, indicates a very limited output. Part IV seeks in some small way to help to remedy that and contains five interesting chapters.

First, a contributing factor to the paucity of intervention research is the reluctance of researchers and Ethics Research Boards to include suicidal participants in their studies. This reluctance has been widely documented. Involving participants who are suicidal in research poses some ethical and pragmatic problems. Individuals who are perceived to be at risk for suicide are either excluded from the clinical trials or withdrawn during the trials. Few studies have examined the effects of research assessments on study participants' suicidality. In Chapter 17, Rahel Eynan et al. examine the impact of study assessments on the suicidality of study participants with a lifetime history of suicide attempts.

In Chapter 18, Yvonne Bergmans et al. reflect on the needs and factors necessary to create an intervention for people with recurrent suicide-related behaviours from the perspective of the lead co-creator and facilitator of the group intervention. It is noteworthy that this is one of a 'handful' of suicide intervention-focused studies; an area of literature that this is most lacking – and not only in allied disciplines but this is a critique that can be applied (accurately) to Suicidology *per se*.

Changing the focus somewhat though not entirely, we could not resist including Chapter 20, authored by Carlos Saravia. As one of the founders of the Portuguese Suicidology Association, a psychiatrist, clinician and researcher, he is well placed to take the reader on a 'historical, clinical tour' of suicidology. From Durkheim's sociological perspective, to pre-neurobiological psychodynamic views, to the importance of the cognitive model – it is fascinating to note that while his perspectives clearly draw on the Portuguese experience, there are clear and obvious similarities with experiences from other parts of the world; most notably the multi-dimensional nature of suicide. The differences are also noteworthy, reflecting that clinically focused suicidology research must also be cognisant of cultural nuance; the comments on the role of the family in Portugal, for example, may not necessarily translate to other countries with different cultural nuances.

In Chapter 19, Yvonne Bergmans and Rahel Eynan report on the results of a pilot study of a 20-week out-patient Psycho-social/Psycho-educational Intervention for people with Recurrent Suicide Attempts (PISA). The intervention targets potential risk factors and areas of deficit, including cognitive, affective and impulsivity known to characterize people with recurrent suicide-related behaviour. Once again, this is one of the few examples of suicide intervention studies that have been empirically tested and found to have utility.

And then in Chapter 21, Yvonne Bergmans et al. describe the pathways to transition that occurred for group participants under the age of 25 years who had experienced recurrent suicide attempts and participated in a PISA intervention, introduced in Chapter 18.

17

IS RESEARCH WITH SUICIDAL PARTICIPANTS RISKY BUSINESS?

Rahel Eynan, Yvonne Bergmans, Jesmin Antony,
John R. Cutcliffe, Henry G. Harder, Munazzah Ambreen,
Ken Balderson and Paul S. Links

Introduction

Suicide is a public health problem with extensive social, emotional and economic consequences. According to the World Health Organization, it is one of the leading causes of premature death worldwide (WHO, 2011) and claims the lives of approximately one million individuals annually. As a serious public health problem, suicide research is imperative, yet there are fewer empirical studies on suicide than on numerous less common causes of death (Mishara & Weisstub, 2005). There is a paucity of information about the efficacy of treatments for individuals with the highest-risk psychiatric disorders, and actively suicidal individuals (Vincent, 2003). Generally, intervention studies targeting mental disorders often have excluded individuals with a history of suicide attempts, or those perceived to be at current or future risk for suicide (Pearson, Stanley, King, & Fisher, 2001). While researchers agree that empirical investigations are needed to better understand suicide and to help develop effective prevention and treatment protocols (Pearson et al., 2001; Fisher, Pearson, Kim, & Reynolds, 2002; Lakeman & FitzGerald, 2009), there is a hesitancy among researchers to include individuals who are at high risk for suicide in research studies. Despite the fact that suicide research aims at examining the presence of the vulnerability manifested in suicide risk, the perceived burden of monitoring and managing suicidal crises, the ethical and legal implications, and potential consequences are often the rationales cited for the exclusion of high risk participants (Pearson et al., 2001; Jobes, Bryan, & Neal-Walden, 2009; Lakeman & FitzGerald, 2009). Concomitantly, there is a ubiquitous perception among researchers, health care professionals, and the public (Feldman et al., 2007; Meerwijk et al., 2010), that talking about suicide elevates the suicide risk and may result in the individual's attempt to end their life (Lakeman & FitzGerald, 2009).

Alternatively, there are a number of studies, which contend that while some participants may feel distressed when asked about suicidal ideation and suicidal behaviour, it does not contribute to an intensification in suicide risk nor does it result in long-term distress (Hahn & Marks, 1996; Parslow, Jorm, O'Toole, Marshall, & Grayson 2001; Henderson & Jorm, 1990; Jacomb et al., 1999). While even a small rate of increase in distress or depressive symptoms may be seen as a cause for concern, Reynolds, Lindenboim, Comtois, et al. (2006) reported that for 63 high-risk chronically suicidal women with Borderline Personality Disorder (BPD), distress and suicidality vary independently. In-depth questions about suicide caused no significant difference in the number of participants reporting an increase or decrease in suicidality, while 46% reported no change at all. Any reported elevation in suicide risk tended to be small with low-level interventions such as validating feelings or providing emergency number cards being sufficient for nearly all participants in their study.

A randomized control trial conducted by Gould et al. (2005) indicated no iatrogenic effect of screening questions that asked 2342 high school students about suicide. Being asked about suicidal ideation or behaviours appears to have been beneficial for students with depressive symptoms or histories of previous suicide attempts. A later study conducted by Cukrowicz, Smith and Poindexter (2010) involving participants with major depressive disorder, reported lowered suicide ideation at 1 month post-assessment and no suicide behaviour reported at both 1 month and 3 months post-assessment. A multi-centre, single-blind, randomized control trial, in primary care settings (Crawford et al., 2011) concluded that screening for suicidal ideation among individuals with signs of depression did not appear to induce feelings that life is not worth living. More recently, Rivlin, Marzano, Hawton, and Fazil's (2012) case-control study to assess the effects of participating in a research study compared 120 prisoners who made a recent medically serious suicide attempt (case group) and 120 prisoners who had not made a near-lethal attempt (control group). Interviews relating to the suicide attempt of the prisoners with a near-lethal attempt were conducted within four weeks of the attempt. Self-reported distress declined significantly in both groups after taking part in the interview. Males, in both groups, and females in the control-group reported that mood levels improved significantly after the interview. In the group of near-lethal attempters, 50% of the male prisoners reported an increase in mood at the end of the interview, 42% reported their mood remained the same, and 8% reported a decrease in mood. Similarly, 32% of the females with near-lethal attempts reported an improved mood, 40% reported their mood did not change, and 23% reported a decrease in mood after the interview. A small number of participants found the interview difficult and upsetting. Over 90% of the participants (both groups) indicated they were pleased that they had participated in the research.

Overall, there still remains a need for definitive research to indicate whether to include or not include suicidal individuals in research. Similar to the Reynolds et al. (2006) study, the purpose of this study was twofold: (1) to examine the the effects of research assessment interviews on self-harm and suicide urges of study participants who were recently discharged from an inpatient psychiatric service after being admitted with a current suicide attempt or a current suicide ideation with a lifetime history of suicidal behaviour; and (2) to describe the frequency with which clinical interventions were used to reduce suicide risk.

Procedure and methods

The examination of the post-assessment changes in participants' urges to self-harm and suicide is part of a larger prospective cohort study which examined the occurrence of post-discharge suicidal ideation and behaviour in a high-risk cohort of recently discharged patients. The participants were followed up prospectively for evidence of suicidal ideation and behaviour at 1, 3, and 6 months following discharge from an inpatient psychiatric service or short stay Crisis Stabilization Unit (CSU). The prospective cohort study was carried out between May 2007 and December 2009 and utilized a concurrent quantitative-qualitative methods design. The findings from the quantitative and qualitative studies were published separately elsewhere (Cutcliffe et al., 2012; Links et al., 2012). Herein we only report on the post-assessment changes in participants' self-harm and suicide urge ratings.

Participants were recruited from among patients with a lifetime history of suicidal behaviour admitted to the inpatient psychiatric service or to the short-stay (72 hours) CSU for a current suicide attempt or for current suicidal ideation with some level of intent to die. The history of suicide attempts was based on self-report or chart documentation. A suicide attempt was defined as "a potentially self-injurious behaviour with a nonfatal outcome, for which there is evidence (either explicit or implicit) that the person intended at some (nonzero) level to kill himself/herself" (O'Carroll et al., 1996). Self-harm is defined as a self-inflicted, potentially injurious behaviour for which there is evidence that the person does not intend to end their life (Silverman, Berman, Sanddal, O'Carroll, & Joiner, 2007).

Baseline assessments were conducted during participants' hospital admission after obtaining permission from their inpatient physician and a signature of informed consent. Assessment of psychopathological predictive factors, i.e., diagnosis, depression, hopelessness, impulsivity, alexithymia, problem solving deficits (described in detail elsewhere (Links et al., 2012)), and the participants' suicidal ideation were administered while in hospital or shortly after discharge. The study received research ethics approval from the hospital's Research Ethics Board.

Suicidal ideation at baseline

Baseline suicidal ideation was assessed during the participants' index hospital stay with the Scale for Suicide Ideation (SSI) (Beck, Kovacs, & Weissman, 1979). The SSI is a 21-item, interviewer-administered rating scale which measures the current intensity of patients' specific attitudes, behaviours, and plans to die by suicide on the day of the interview and during the preceding week. This scale has demonstrated internal consistency, inter-rater reliability, and concurrent validity (Beck et al., 1979) and adequate predictive validity significantly predicting eventual suicide (Brown, Beck, Steer, & Grisham, 2000).

Suicidal ideation at follow-up

To assess for evidence of suicidal ideation and behaviour after hospital discharge, the SSI (Beck et al., 1979) was administered at the 1, 3, and 6 months follow-up interviews. At the 6 months follow-up appointment, participants were asked to report on any self-injury events without intent to die or suicide attempts with intent to die during the 6 months post-index hospital discharge using the clinician-administered Lifetime Parasuicide Count (Linehan & Comtois, 1996).

Suicide risk assessment

Participants were assessed for suicide risk using a modified Washington Risk Assessment Protocol (UWRAP; Linehan, Comtois, & Murray, 2000). The six-item UWRAP Face Sheet and the Debriefing Form were reduced to a three-item risk-assessment which was administered at the start and at the end of each follow-up research assessment interview conducted at 1, 3 and 6 months. Participants were asked to self-rate their self-harm and suicide urges using the following questions:

1. Please rate your urges to self-harm on a scale of 0–7 (none to severe); 2. Please rate your urge to suicide on a scale of 0–7 (none to severe), and 3. Please rate your sense of control over any self-harm or suicide urges using a scale of 0–7 (out of control to in control).

A participant was considered to be at moderate or high risk requiring suicide risk intervention if he or she rated their "urges to self-harm" or "urges to suicide" as 4 or higher and indicated they were uncertain of their ability to control their urges. If the score was below 4 but the research associate had reasons to be concerned about the participant's ability to control their urges not to self-harm or suicide, clinical judgment prevailed.

Statistical analyses

Descriptive statistics (mean, standard deviation, quartiles) were calculated to characterize the patients at baseline with respect to demographics (i.e., age, sex, race/ethnicity, marital status), psychopathologic risk factors, and psychiatric co-morbidities, overall and by group. Comparisons between groups at baseline were conducted using a chi-square test, Fisher's exact test, *t*-test or Wilcoxon rank-sum test. A 95% (*p* <.05) significance level was adopted. All statistical analyses were conducted using the Statistical Package for the Social Sciences (SPSS, Version 15 for Windows, SPSS Inc., 2006).

Findings

Sample description

A total of 152 patients admitted to the inpatient psychiatric service met study criteria and were referred to the study coordinator. Of those, 120 (78.9%) consented to participate in the study. By the end of the study, 8 (5.3%) participants had withdrawn from the study and 9 (6%) were lost to follow-up. There were nearly equal numbers of male (63; 52.5%) and female (57; 47.5%) participants, and the mean age was 37.5 years (SD =11.1). The vast majority of participants (98; 81.9%) were admitted to hospital for a current suicide attempt, 22 (18.3%) were admitted for suicide ideation. Only 27 (22.5%) participants were admitted to inpatient services for their first-time suicide attempt, while the majority of participants (93; 78.5%) had a median number of two previous attempts (interquartile range = 2) over their lifetime.

The most common current psychiatric diagnoses among study participants were affective disorders (confirmed by SCID-I). Based on DSM-IV criteria 99 (90%) study participants met criteria for major depressive episode or bipolar disorder, while 12 (10.9%) met criteria for schizophrenic disorders. Two-thirds (74; 67%) of the study participants met criteria for Axis-II disorders (confirmed by SCID-II), and borderline personality disorder (BPD) was diagnosed in 36 (31.9%) of the participants.

Suicidal ideation

At baseline (*N* =119), SSI scores ranged from 10 to 31, with a mean score of 23.6 and standard deviation of 3.8. As indicated in Table 17.1, over the course of the study the SSI mean score significantly decreased from the observed baseline score (M_{Base} = 23.6 (SD = 3.8) vs. M_1 = 7.9 (SD = 9.0), *p* value < .0001; M_{Base} = 23.6 (SD = 3.8) vs. M_3 = 6.6 (SD = 7.8), *p* value <. 0001: M_{Base}= 23.6 (SD = 3.8) vs. M_6 = 5.7 (SD = 7.8), *p* value < .0001 at 1, 3 , and 6 months respectively). Of note, a high proportion of participants reported no suicide ideation (SSI score = 0) at the follow-up interviews at 1 month (40.0%), 3 months (44.8%), and 6 months (48.0%).

Changes in urges to self-harm following research interview

The magnitude and the direction of change were calculated by comparing pre- and post-assessment ratings. We examined a total of 290 research assessments which were conducted over a 6 months period of study. As indicated in Table 17.1, throughout the study period, only nine

Table 17.1 Changes in self-reported ratings of suicidality and control over period of assessment

Measure/Time	Pre-assessment Ratings Mean (SD)	Post-assessment Ratings Mean (SD)	Δ	Patterns of Changes Increase N (%)	Decrease N (%)	No change N (%)
Month 1 (N = 99)						
Urges to self-harm	1.31(1.7)	1.13 (1.7)★	−0.18	3 3.0	16 16.2	80 80.8
Urges to suicide	1.36 (1.8)	1.14 (1.6)★	−0.22	2 2.0	14 14.1	83 83.8
Sense of control	6.06(1.2)	6.19(1.2)	+0.13	12 12.1	4 4.0	83 83.8
Month 1 (N = 95)						
Urges to self-harm	1.06(1.5)	1.01 (1.5)	−0.05	6 6.1	6 6.1	83 87.4
Urges to suicide	1.08 (1.6)	1.06(1.6)	−0.02	7 7.4	7 7.4	81 85.3
Sense of control	6.03(1.3)	6.17(1.3)	+0.14	11 9.2	3 3.2	81 85.3
Month 6 (N = 96)						
Urges to self-harm	.74 (1.3)	70 (1.2)★	−0.04	0 0	4 3.3	92 95.8
Urges to suicide	.91(1.5)	85(1.5)★	−0.06	0 0	5 5.2	91 94.8
Sense of control	6.36(1.1)	6.42(1.1)	+0.06	7 7.3	2 2.1	87 90.6

Note: ★Based on paired sample *t-* test *p* value <.05.

research interviews (9/290, 3.1%) resulted in an increase in the urges to self-harm following the study interview. In the vast majority of research interviews there was no change in the pre-post self-harm ratings (255/290, 87.9%). A decrease in self-harm urges rating was reported following 26 interviews (26/290, 9%).

Overall, as indicated in Table 17.1, the pre- and post-assessment interview self-harm ratings were at the low end of the scale indicative of low urges to self-harm. Throughout the study period the mean rating was below 2.0 (on an 8-point scale ranging from "0" = none to "7"= severe). Comparison of post-assessment ratings from the first follow-up study interview (1 month) to the last (6 months) shows a slight decrease did occur in the self-harm urges ratings over the course of the study (M_1 = 1.13 (SD = 1.7) vs. M_6 = .7 (SD = 1.2).

Nine participants indicated an increase in their self-harm urges following the assessment interview. The overall increase in self-harm urges ranged from 1 to 4 with a mean increase of 1.8 (SD = 1.1) and a median of 1. As indicated in Table 17.2, a significant increase in the mean self-harm urges score is reported after the 1 month and 3 months assessment interviews (Δ_1 = +2.0; M_{pre} = 1.0 (SD = 1.0) vs. M_{post} = 3.0(SD = 2.7), *p* value = .005; Δ_3 = +1.7; (M_{pre} = 2.0 (SD = 2.0) vs. M_{post} = 3.7 (SD = 2.0), *p* value = .004, respectively). None of the participants reported an increase in self-harm urges following the 6 months interview. Only three (3/9, 33.3%) of the participants who reported an increase in their self-harm urges following a study interview had rated their post-assessment self-harm urges as greater than 4. Interventions were offered to those participants identified as high-risk (discussed in detail in the Interventions section).

During the study period, 26 participants indicated their self-harm urges decreased following the study interview. The overall decrease in ratings ranged from -1 to -7 and the mean decrease was -1.7 (SD = 1.6) with a median of 1. As indicated in Table 17.2, the comparison of pre- and post-assessment ratings of those participants who have indicated a decrease in their self-harm

Table 17.2 Changes in self-reported urges to self-harm or suicide after the follow-up assessment interview

Measure/ Time	Increase		Δ	p value	Decrease		Δ	p value	No change	
	Pre	Post			Pre	Post			Pre	Post
Urges to self-harm										
Month 1	1.0	3.0	+2	0.1	2.4	.94	−1.46	0.0001	1.1	1.1
(N=99)	(1.0)	(2.7)			(1.9)	(1.9)			(1.6)	(1.6)
Month 3	2.0	3.7	+1.7	0.004	3.2	.67	−2.53	0.0026	.84	.84
(N = 95)	(2.0)	(2.0)			(2.1)	(.8)			(1.3)	(1.3)
Month 6					2.5	1.5	−1	0.046	.66	.66
(N = 96)					(1.3)	(1.3)			(1.2)	(1.2)
Urges to suicide										
Month 1	1.5	3.0	+2	0.32	2.9	1.0	−1.9	0.001	1.1	1.1
(N = 99)	(.7)	(2.7)			(2.0)	(1.2)			(1.7)	(1.7)
Month 3	1.0	4.0	+3	0.01	3.3	1.0	−2.3	0.034	.83	.83
(N = 95)	(2.3)	(2.3)			(2.2)	(1.5)			(1.4)	(1.4)
Month 6					1.8	.8	−1	0.025	.86	.86
(N = 96)					(.45)	(.45)			(1.5)	(1.5)

urges shows a statistically significant decrease in self-harm urges following the 1, 3 and 6 months assessment interviews (Δ_1 = − 1.5, p = <.0001;Δ_3 = -2.5, p = .026; Δ_6 = -1.0, p = .046, respectively). Among those who reported a decrease in their self-harm rating, two (2/26, 7.7%) participants had rated their post-assessment self-harm urges to be greater than 4.

As noted earlier, the vast majority of study participants (87.9%) did not report any changes in their self-harm urges following the study interviews. Their post-assessment ratings ranged from 0 to 7, and had a low mean score which decreased during the course of the study from 1.1 (SD = 1.6) to .66 (SD = 1.2). Thirteen (13/255, 5.5%) of the "no change" follow-up interviews had self-harm ratings greater than 4.

Changes in urges to suicide following the research interview

The same descriptive data was also examined for ratings of suicide urges. As shown in Table 17.1, throughout the study period, only nine research interviews (9/290, 3.1%) resulted in an increase in the urge to suicide following the study interview. Similar to the pattern seen with self-harm urges, the vast majority of research interviews resulted in no change in the pre-post suicide urges ratings (255/290, 87.9%), while a decrease in suicide urges ratings was reported following 26 study interviews (26/290, 9%).

Overall, as indicated in Table 17.1, the pre- and post-assessment interview suicide urges ratings were at the low end of the scale, indicative of low urges to suicide. Throughout the study period, the mean rating was below 2.0 (on an 8-point scale ranging from "0" = none to "7" = severe). Comparison of the suicide urges post-assessment ratings from the first follow-up study interview (1 month) to the last (6 months) shows a slight decrease occurred in the suicide urges ratings over the course of the study (M_1= 1.14 (SD = 1.6) vs. M_6 = .85 (SD = 1.5)). Nine participants indicated an increase in their suicide urges following the assessment interview. The overall increase in suicide urges ranged from 1 to 4 with a mean increase of 2.0 (SD = 1.2) and a median of 2. As indicated in Table 17.2, a significant increase in the mean suicide urges score is reported after the 1- and 3-months assessment interview (at 1 month: Δ_1 = +2.0; M_{pre}= 1.5 (SD = .7) vs. M_{post} = 3.5 (SD = .7), p value = .32; at 3 months: Δ_3 = +3.0; M_{pre} = 1.0 (SD = 2.3) vs. M_{post}= 4.0 (SD= 2.3), p value .01, respectively). None of the participants reported an increase in suicide urges following the 6 months interview. Of the nine participants who had reported an increase in their suicide urges following the assessment interviews five (5/9, 55.6%) had an elevated post-assessment score (> 4). Interventions were offered to those participants identified as high-risk (discussed in detail in the Interventions section).

During the study period, 26 participants indicated their suicide urges decreased following the study interview. The overall decrease in ratings ranged from -1 to -7 and the mean decrease was -1.8 (SD = 1.7) with a median of 1. As indicated in Table 17.2, the comparison of pre- and post-assessment ratings of those participants who have indicated a decrease in their suicide urges shows a statistically significant decrease in suicide urges following 1, 3 and 6 months assessment interviews (Δ_1 = − 1.9, p = <.001; Δ_3 = -2.3, p = .034; Δ_6 = -1.0, p = .025, respectively). Only one participant from among those who reported a decrease in their suicide urges (1/26, 3.9%) had rated their urges to suicide after a follow-up interview as greater than 4. The vast majority of study participants (87.9%) did not report any changes in their suicide urges following the study interviews. Their post-assessment ratings ranged from 0 to 7, and had a low mean score which decreased during the course of the study from 1.1 (SD = 1.6) to .66 (SD = 1.2). Sixteen (16/255, 7.8%) of the "no change" follow-up interviews had suicide ratings greater than 4.

Changes in self-reported control over self-harm and suicide urges following assessment interview

Following the post-assessment interviews, 92.7% of the participants rated their level of control over their self-harm and suicide urges as ≥ than 5 (on an 8-point scale ranging from "0" = out of control to "7" = in control). As indicated in Table 17.1, risk assessment protocols over the 6 month period of the study indicated the vast majority of post-assessment interviews reflected no change in the participants' ability to control their self-harm and suicide urges (255/290, 87.3%). An examination of the data indicates both pre- and post-assessment scores are at the high end of the scale and are indicative of a high level of control over self-harm and suicide urges. Over the course of the study, only 9 participants (9/290, 3.1%) indicated their sense of control over their urges had weakened after the study interview. None of the decreases in control, however, were statistically significant (p = .2; p = .06; p = .2, respectively). Conversely, 10.3% of study assessments (30/290) reported a greater sense of control over participant urges following the study interview. The increases in self-control over self-harm and suicide urges were statistically significant at the 1, 3 and 6 months study interviews (at 1 month: M_{pre} = 4.9 (SD = 1.4) vs. M_{post} = 6.4 (SD = 0.7), p value = .01; at 3 months: M_{pre} = 6.2 (SD = 1.0) vs. M_{post} = 6.4 (SD = 0.7), p value = .01, at 6 months: M_{pre} = 6.6 (SD = .8) vs. M_{post} = 6.7 (SD = 0.7), p value = .008, respectively).

Interventions

A participant was judged as a high risk for suicidal behaviour if they rated the "urge to self-harm" or the "urge to suicide" as 4 or greater, or based on the research associate's clinical judgment after administering the SSI. Eighteen (18%) study participants required some clinical intervention to lower the risk of suicidality. Nine (9%) participants required "soft" intensity interventions (e.g., validation of feelings, de-escalation) at one of their follow-up interviews (3.1%; 9/290). These interventions were provided by the research associate who used mood improvement strategies and de-escalation techniques and did not require clinical investigator involvement.

Of the 90 assessment interviews carried out throughout the study period, 13 high-intensity interventions were initiated (4.5%; 13/290) for nine study participants. Of the nine requiring clinical intervention, two (22%) required intervention at two assessment interviews (1 and 3 months; 1 and 6 months) while one study participant required intervention at all three assessment interviews (1, 3 and 6 months).

Of the 13 who were referred to the emergency psychiatric service, five (38.5%, 5/13) were assessed by emergency psychiatry personnel and discharged home, six (46.2%, 6/13) were kept in the short stay unit for ≤ 72 hours, and two (15.4%, 2/13) were admitted to the psychiatric in-patient unit.

Participants who required clinical intervention reported much higher suicidal ideation throughout the study period as measured by the SSI compared to the rest of the sample (at 1 month: M = 7.2 (SD = 8.5) vs. M 21.2 (SD = 9.8), p value=.003; at 3 months: M = 5.9 (SD = 7.1) vs. M = 25.7 (SD = 1.5), p value <.001; at 6 months M = 4.5 (SD = 6.3) vs. M = 25.0 (SD = 3.3), p value <.001) (see Table 17.3).

Factors associated with high-intensity intervention

There were no statistically significant differences between participants who required high-intensity intervention following their study interview and those who did not in Axis I or II

Table 17.3 Differences in post-assessment changes between participants who required intervention and the rest of the sample

Time/Measure	Sample		High intensity intervention		P value	
	Pre	Post	Pre	Post	Pre	Post
1 month						
Self-harm urges	1.2 (1.7)	1.0 (1.5)	3.6 (1.5)	4.2 (1.3)	.002	.001
Suicide urges	1.2 (1.6)	1.0 (1.4)	4.4 (2.1)	4.4 (2.1)	.001	.001
Sense of control	6.2 (1.0)	6.3 (1.0)	3.6 (1.9)	4.2 (1.6)	.001	.001
Suicidal ideation	7.2 (8.5)		21.2 (9.8)		.003	
3 months						
Self-harm urges	1.0 (1.5)	1.0 (1.5)	3.0 (1.0)	2.3 (0.6)	.016	.035
Suicide urges	1.0 (1.6)	1.0 (1.6)	3.0 (2.7)	3.3 (2.5)	.155	.232
Sense of control	6.1 (1.2)	6.3 (1.2)	3.3 (2.3)	3.3 (2.1)	.018	.004
Suicidal ideation	5.9 (7.1)		25.7 (1.5)		<.001	
6 months						
Self-harm urges	0.6 (1.1)	0.5 (1.0)	3.6 (1.7)	3.6 (1.7)	.001	.001
Suicide urges	0.7 (1.4)	0.7 (1.3)	4.0 (1.2)	4.0 (1.2)	.001	.001
Sense of control	6.5 (1.0)	6.5 (1.0)	4.4 (1.8)	4.6 (1.8)	.003	.002
Suicidal ideation	4.5 (6.3)		25.0 (3.2)		<.001	

Note: At 1 month: Sample N = 94, Intervention N = 5, At 3 months: Sample N = 92, Intervention N = 3, At 6 months: Sample N = 91, Intervention N = 5.

diagnoses with the exception of Post-Traumatic Stress Disorder (PTSD). A greater proportion of study participants who required high-intensity intervention following their study interview met criteria for a current PTSD episode (N = 6/9, 66.7% vs. N = 36/110, 32.70%, p = .025). However, there were no statistically significant differences between participants in the sub-group who required high intensity intervention following their study interview and those who did not in psychopathological predictive factors, i.e., depression severity, hopelessness, impulsivity, alexithymia, problem solving deficits (described in detail elsewhere (Links et al., 2012)) and the reason for the index hospital admission. The majority of study participants in both groups (those who required high intensity intervention and those who did not) had previously been admitted for recurrent suicide attempts (58.9% vs. 77.8%).

At baseline, there were no statistically significant differences in suicidal ideation, based on Scale for Suicidal Ideation mean scores, between the sample and the nine participants who required high-intensity intervention (M = 23.4 (3.8) vs. M = 24.1 (4.0), p value = 0.8); however, participants who required high-intensity intervention had a much higher score at the 1, 3 and 6 months assessment interview (see Table 17.3). A statistically significant larger proportion of study participants who required intervention reported at least one self-harm incident during the 6 months study period compared to the rest of the sample (7/8, 87.5% vs. 31/89 34.8%, p value < .001) and those who required intervention engaged in a significantly greater number of self-harm behaviours (M = 0 .88 (SD = 0.35) vs. M = 0 .35 (SD = 0.48), p value = .008).

Conclusion

Suicidal individuals are often excluded from research based on the idea that suicide risk will increase if one talks about suicide (Lakeman & FitzGerald, 2009; Pearson et al., 2001; Reynolds et al., 2006). To explore the validity of this belief, our study examined the effects of suicide assessment interviews on study participants' reported self-harm and suicide urges over a 6 month period. A total of 103 participants with suicide ideation and/or behaviour who were recently discharged from an inpatient psychiatric service were assessed at 1, 3 and 6 months post-discharge.

The primary finding of our study is that the vast majority of suicidal participants reported no changes in self-harm or suicide urges following assessment interviews (255/290, 87.9%) and in some cases, even reported a decrease in post-assessment suicide risk (26/290, 9%). In other words, the inclusion of suicidal participants in research interviews rarely increased suicide risk in this population. Only a small proportion of study participants (9/290, 3%) reported an increase in their self-harm or suicide urges following their assessment interview. Moreover, there was a decline in the number of participants who reported an increase in suicidality over time. By the end of the 6 month follow-up period, none of the participants reported an increase in suicide risk post-assessment, comparable to the findings of Cukrowicz, Smith and Poindexter (2010).

Based on our research experience and those reported by others (Rivlin et al., 2012; Reynolds et al., 2006), the decline in reported suicidality over time may be due to the therapeutic and cathartic effect of the assessment interviews, including both the content of the research interview and the relationship formed between the interviewer and interviewee. A second factor that may have contributed to this decline is that, with time, participants may have become more familiar with and therefore less reactive to the assessment interview process. In the end, it is difficult to determine whether or to what extent the therapeutic effect of the interview or the interviewer, habituation, or post-assessment diminished anxiety contributed to the findings. Further research is required to better understand the impact of these factors.

As mentioned earlier, instances of elevated risk following study assessments were rare in our study. When determining whether a participant was in need of risk management intervention, four factors were considered, including the modified UWRAP self-harm and suicide ratings, the suicide ideation assessment, the participants' perceived sense of self-control and the research associate's clinical judgment. The use of multiple factors helped ensure that the presence of elevated suicide risk was identified and appropriate steps were taken. In most cases, minimal intervention strategies (validation, de-escalation) were sufficient to reduce potentially negative consequences. In the few more acute cases, however, "high-intensity" intervention was required. Similar to Reynolds et al.'s (2006) study, we found that compared to the rest of the sample, the sub-group of participants who required intervention following their study assessment interviews reported elevated self-harm and suicide urges and a lesser ability to control those urges throughout the course of the study. This group also reported twice the number of previous suicide attempts than reported by the rest of the sample. While the suicide ideation scores of the non-intervention sub-sample decreased significantly over the course of the 6 months study, the scores of those participants who required intervention remained unchanged from their baseline scores. This suggests that elevated suicidal ideation and perceived low self-control are a combination of factors that may contribute to the need for intervention.

Individuals in the high-risk group did not differ from the rest of the sample in psychopathology or Axis I or II diagnoses, with the exception of PTSD. The majority of participants who required intervention endorsed symptoms which are consistent with a PTSD diagnosis. Further exploration is needed to assess the extent in which PTSD acts as an indicator of elevated suicide risk.

In alignment with Reynolds et al. (2006) and Cukrowicz et al. (2010), our findings demonstrate that suicide research with participants with a history of suicidality can be conducted safely without the fear of elevating their suicide risk with the following provisos:

- The research associate must be well trained in being able to identify elevated risk (i.e., through suicide assessments, participant ratings, personal judgment).
- An appropriate "safety net" (Cutcliffe, 2002) protocol must be in place and ready to be implemented prior to recruitment of participants. This protocol has two elements:
  - It must outline the safety measures to be instituted in the case of elevated risk, including names and locations of individuals trained and competent in risk assessment.
  - It must provide a list of available treatment resources should the need arise for the participant subsequent to the visit.

Cutcliffe (2002) further suggests that forewarning participants in an information letter gives the option not to reply to the offer of participation. As well, reiterating the possibility of arousal of emotions in the consent form allows a second and "in person" opportunity for the person to decline or defer participation.

Overall, our work has expanded on previous research (Gould et al., 2005; Reynolds et al., 2006; Cukrowicz et al., 2010; Crawford et al, 2011; Rivlin, et al., 2012) sharing limited generalizability. Sampling and measurements in this study make it unique. Our sample included, in almost equal numbers, both genders (males: 52.5%, females: 47.5%) recruited from among patients who were admitted to the inpatient psychiatric service or the CSU for a suicide attempt or current suicidal ideation with a lifetime history of suicidal behaviour, i.e., individuals at high risk of suicide. Nearly two-thirds of our sample (59.2%) was admitted for a current suicide attempt. In addition, unlike Reynolds et al. (2006), our sample was not limited to participants who met criteria for BPD. The most common diagnosis in our study was affective disorders

(90%) and only 31.9% of participants met criteria for BPD. Limiting the study to participants of BPD would have limited the findings.

Despite our best efforts, however, our study did have limitations. Based on our clinical experience, we differentiated between the urge to self-harm and the urge to suicide, recognizing that these two urges represent discrete behaviours with distinct intents. Thus, we modified the UWRAP (Linehan et al., 2000) and focused only on two questions: the first enquiring about self-harm urges, and the second about suicide urges. A limitation of the study was that the psychometric properties of this modified UWRAP scale were not established and therefore we cannot comment on its validity and reliability.

While we relied on this brief UWRAP scale to assess the magnitude of change in the pre- and post-assessments, participants were also rigorously assessed for their suicidal ideation on the assessment day and the preceding week regardless of their self-reported suicidal urges. Nonetheless, we only examined the proximal effects of the assessments and did not evaluate the distal effects in the weeks following the interview. Given that 39.4% of our sample engaged in self-harm and suicide attempts, there may be a need for longer monitoring period.

Another consideration is that data was not systematically collected on the time it required to provide "soft" intensity intervention or higher-level intensity interventions throughout the study, thus, we cannot comment on the extent of the burden placed on clinical and administrative management of the research. Future studies are needed to investigate the extent to which unscheduled interventions with highly suicidal participants burden researchers.

Overall, our findings provide robust evidence that in a sample of highly suicidal individuals, inquiring about suicidal ideation rarely increased self-harm and suicide urges. The few participants who required some intervention had elevated levels of suicide ideation and behaviour at baseline and almost all reported symptoms of PTSD. This study reinforces the notion that research involving high risk suicidal individuals is possible when study protocols are well planned and executed by trained assessors and clinicians who are able to identify participants at risk and provide intervention if necessary.

Acknowledgments

The research team wishes to offer their thanks to the Canadian Institutes for Health Research who generously supported this research (funding reference number MOP82835).

References

Beck, A. T., Kovacs, M., & Weissman, A. (1979). Assessment of suicidal ideation: The scale for suicide ideation. *Journal of Consulting and Clinical Psychology, 47,* 343–352.

Brown, G. K., Beck, A. T., Steer, R. A., & Grisham, J. R. (2000). Risk factors for suicide in psychiatric outpatients: A 20-year prospective study. *Journal of Consulting and Clinical Psychology, 68,* 371–377.

Crawford, M. J., Thana, L., Methuen, C., Ghosh, P., Stanley, S. V., Ross, J., Gordon, F., Blair, G., & Bajaj, P. (2011). Impact of screening for risk of suicide: Randomised control trial. *The British Journal of Psychiatry, 198,* 379–384.

Cukrowicz, K., Smith, P., & Poindexter, E. (2010). The effect of participating in suicide research: Does participating in a research protocol on suicide and psychiatric symptoms increase suicide ideation and attempts? *Suicide and Life-Threatening Behavior, 40*(4), 535–543.

Cutcliffe, J. R. (2002). Ethics committees, vulnerable groups and paternalism: The case for considering the benefits of participating in qualitative research interviews. In J. Dooher, & R. Byrt (Eds.), *Empowerment and participation: Power, influence and control in health care.* London: Quay Books.

Cutcliffe, J., Links, P., Harder, H., Balderson, K., Bergmans, Y., Eynan ,R., Ambreen, M., & Nisenbaum, R. (2012). Understanding the risks of recent discharge: The phenomenological lived experiences – existential angst at the prospect of discharge. *Crisis, 33*(1), 21–29.

Feldman, M. D., Frank, P., Duberstein, P. R., Vannoy, S., Epstein, R., & Kravitz, R. L. (2007). Let's not talk about it: Suicide inquiry in primary care. *Annals of Family Medicine, 5*(5), 412–418.

FIsher, C. B., Pearson, J. L., Kim, S., & Reynolds, C. F. (2002). Ethical issues in including suicidal individuals in clinical research. *IRB: Ethics and Human Research, 24*(5), 9–14.

Gould, M. S., Marrocco, F. A., Kleinman, M., Thomas, J. G., Mostkoff, K., Cote, J., & Davies, M. (2005). Evaluating iatrogenic risk of youth suicide screening programs. *Journal of the American Medical Association, 293*(13), 1635–1643.

Hahn, W. K., & Marks, L. I. (1996). Client receptiveness to the routine assessment of past suicide attempts. *Professional Psychology: Research and Practice, 27*, 592–594.

Henderson, A. S., & Jorm, A. F. (1990). Do mental health surveys disturb? *Psychological Medicine, 20*, 721–724.

Jacomb, P., Jorm, A. F., Rodgers, B., Korten, A. E., Henderson, A. S., & Christensen, H. (1999). Emotional response of participants to a mental health survey. *Social Psychiatry and Psychiatric Epidemiology, 34*, 80–84.

Jobes, D. A., Bryan, C. J., & Neal-Walden, T. A. (2009). Conducting suicide research in naturalistic clinical settings. *Journal of Clinical Psychology, 65*, 382–395.

Lakeman, R., & FitzGerald, M. (2009). The ethics of suicide research: The views of ethics committee members. *Crisis, 30*(1), 13–19.

Linehan, M. M., & Comtois, K. A. (1996). *Lifetime Parasuicide History (LPH)*. Department of Psychology, University of Washington: Seattle, WA.

Linehan, M. M., Comtois, K. A., & Murray, A. (2000). The University of Washington Risk Assessment Protocol (UWRAP). Unpublished manuscript, University of Washington: Seattle, WA.

Links, P. S., Nisenbaum, R., Ambreen, M., Balderson, K., Bergmans, Y., Eynan, R., Harder, H., & Cutcliffe J. (2012). Prospective study of risk factors for increased suicide ideation and behavior following recent discharge. *General Hospital Psychiatry, 34*(1), 88–97.

Meerwijk, E. L., van Meijel, B., van den Bout, J., Kerkhof, A., de Vogel, W., & Grypdonck, M. (2010). Development and evaluation of a guideline for nursing care of suicidal patients with schizophrenia. *Perspectives in Psychiatric Care, 46*(10), 65–73.

Mishara, B. L., & Weisstub, D. N. (2005). Ethical and legal issues in suicide research. *International Journal of Law and Psychiatry, 28*, 23–41.

O'Carroll, P. W., Berman, A. L., Maris, R. W., Moscicki, E. K., Tanney, B. L., & Silverman, M. M. (1996). Beyond the Tower of Babel: A nomenclature for suicidology. *Suicide and Life-threatening Behavior, 26*(3), 237–252.

Parslow, R. A., Jorm, A. F., O'Toole, B. I., Marshall, R. P., & Grayson, D. A. (2001). Distress experienced by participants during an epidemiological survey of post-traumatic stress disorder. *Journal of Traumatic Stress, 13*, 465–471.

Pearson, J. L., Stanley, B., King, C. A., & Fisher, C. B. (2001). Intervention research with persons at high risk for suicidality: Safety and ethical considerations. *Journal of Clinical Psychiatry, 62*(Suppl. 25), 17–26.

Reynolds, S. K., Lindenboim, N., Comtois, K. A., Murray, A., & Linehan, M. M. (2006). Risky assessments: Participant suicidality and distress associated with research assessments in a treatment study of suicidal behavior. *Suicide and Life-threatening Behavior, 36*(1), 19–34.

Rivlin, A., Marzano, L., Hawton, K., & Fazil, S. (2012). Impact on prisoners of participating in research interviews related to near-lethal suicide attempts. *Journal of Affective Disorders, 136*, 54–62.

Silverman, M. M., Berman, A. L., Sanddal, N. D., O'Carroll, P. W., & Joiner, T. E. (2007) Rebuilding the Tower of Babel: a revised nomenclature for the study of suicide and suicidal behaviors. Part 2: suicide-related ideations, communications, and behaviors. *Suicide and Life-threatening Behaviors, 37*(3), 264–277.

Vincent, C. (2003). Understanding and responding to adverse events. *New England Journal of Medicine, 348*, 1051–1056.

World Health Organization (2011). *Mental health: Suicide rates per 100,000 by country, year and sex (table as of 2009)*. August 1. Available at: http://www.who.int/mental_health/prevention/ suicide_rates/en/.

18

CREATING AN INTERVENTION FOR PEOPLE WITH RECURRENT SUICIDE ATTEMPTS

Yvonne Bergmans, Keehan Koorn, Rahel Eynan and Colleen Pacey

Introduction

This is the first of a two-chapter submission that focuses on our Psychosocial/Psychoeducational Intervention for People with Recurrent Suicide Attempts (PISA). Part one (this chapter) provides the background story to the development of the PISA project (also known in some locations as Skills for Safer Living (SFSL)), and part two (Chapter 19) focuses on the results of the intervention to date. Accordingly, this chapter will provide the reader with an introduction to the development of the PISA/SFSL. It begins with the identified need, followed by attitudes and assumptions of the person working with this group. Finally, the last section articulates the basics of structure, inclusion and assessment. To date, the intervention has been delivered at four sites in Ireland, three community sites in Southern Ontario, and at two outpatient hospital sites in Toronto, Canada.

The need for the intervention

Suicide and self-injury create significant health care costs in Canada and the USA. It is estimated that for every suicide in the United States, there are 22 emergency department (ED) visits and five hospitalizations for suicide-related behaviours (http://mentalhealth.samhsa.gov/publications/allpubs/SMA01-3517/ch7.asp. Aug. 20, 2009). In Canada, in 2004, suicide and self-harm were the leading cause of injury death overall (28%) and the leading cause (88%) of intentional injury deaths (3,616), hospitalizations (69%), and permanent partial disability (83%). Suicide and self-harm accounted for 9% of all injuries resulting in hospitalization. There were 18,210 hospitalizations and 41,930 non-hospitalization treatments. Intentional self-injuries accounted for 4% of all ED visits due to injuries. For nearly 4,000 (3,879) individuals, their self-harm resulted in permanent partial disability and 199 suffered total permanent disability. An analysis of injury costs by intent shows that suicide and self-harm accounted for 12% of total injury costs, 7% of direct injury costs, and 19% of indirect injury costs in Canada in 2004. The direct and indirect costs of suicide and self-harm came to $2,442 billion. In 2004, suicide and self-harm were among the leading causes of death by injury in Ontario per capita (8.2 per 100,000 population), accounting for 22% of all injury deaths. Some 10% of all hospitalizations were due to injuries as a result of suicide and self-harm: 7052 individuals required hospital treatment and 16,045 received non-hospital treatment. For over 1,000 individuals (1,409) the self-harm behaviour resulted in permanent partial disability and 76 suffered total permanent disability (http://www.smartrisk.ca/downloads/research/publications/burden/EBI-Em-Final.pdf. p. 84, accessed September, 2012). Approximately 16% of those who attempt to end their lives will re-attempt suicide within the first year following their first event (Owens, Horrocks, House, 2002; Colman, Yiannakoulias, Schopflocher et al., 2004).

Attempted suicide and death by suicide are also expensive in terms of emotional, physical and psychological costs for everyone involved. A conservative estimate of six individuals being personally affected by each suicide, would translate to close to 2.5 million Canadians being affected annually by suicide and suicide-related behaviours (http://www.casp-acps.ca/Publications/blueprint%20final%20september.pdf). In Japan, the direct production loss of bereaved family members who lost a loved one to suicide was estimated at approximately US$197 million in 2006 alone (Chen, Lee, Chang, & Liaoh, 2009). It remains unknown how many classmates, coworkers, colleagues, immediate and extended family members have been affected by suicide and self-injury, including lost work time, reaching out to social supports, and financial support to their loved one whether before or after a death by suicide.

Suicide intervention research

Hjelemand and Knizek (2010) point out that suicidology research tends to fall into three categories: (1) epidemiological; (2) (neuro)biological; and (3) intervention studies, with a primary emphasis on explanations and cause–effect relationships. According to White (2005), we continue to work with "imperfect knowledge", using current measurement tools that are potentially inadequate for observing and understanding meaningful changes for suicidal people. We require an understanding that goes beyond our current knowledge of cause-effect explanations so often found in the suicidology literature with its focus on risk factors and warning signs (Hjelemand & Knizek, 2010). Linehan (2008) suggests that treatments targeting suicidal behaviour are more efficacious than those targeting a "presumed underlying disorder" (p. 484). Similarly, Leenaars (2004) suggests that psychotherapy for those who have attempted suicide needs to be person-centred therapy not mental disorder-centred therapy (p. 221), further suggesting that the need for multi-modal, long-term interventions is "critical" (p. 223). The research, by and large, shows a large gap in the experience of those who have attempted to end their lives, and/or have repeatedly tried to end their lives. This could then seriously impact how intervention is created, delivered, and/or facilitated.

Why focus on people with recurrent suicide attempts?

Several studies have found that people who made repeated attempts have been identified as:

- having a greater number of DSM-IV Axis I diagnoses with an earlier onset of psychiatric disorders;
- elevated levels of suicidal ideation, depression, hopelessness, and perceived stress;
- poorer social problem-solving skills;
- a history of childhood maltreatment;
- family histories of suicide attempts and psychiatric illness;
- alcohol and substance abuse issues (Rudd, Joiner, and Rajab, 1996; Forman, Berk, Henriques et al., 2004; Rosenberg, Jankowski, Sengupta et al., 2005).

It is suggested that not only are those who engage in repeated suicide attempts at higher risk for dying, they are also identified as a potentially "unique population" (Gibb, Andover, & Miller, 2009) across the illness spectrums as suggested by some of the factors listed above.

The background story

The PISA/SFSL intervention arose from the concerns of mental health department management and staff. The need was to develop a group intervention to try to stem the tides of people with recurrent attempts repeatedly coming to the emergency department (ED). This was evident from the sheer numbers of people who had repeatedly attempted suicide presenting to the ED and the general frustration and helplessness the ED staff felt in trying to deal with repetitive suicide-related behaviours and self-injury (McElroy and Sheppard, 1999; Spence, Bergmans et al., 2008; Bergmans, Spence et al., 2009). The aim of the intervention was to address domains the literature identified as challenging: affect (Linehan, Armstrong, Suarez et al., 1991; Levine, Marziali, & Hood, 1997; Dieter et al., 2000), behaviour (Bender, Gordon, Bresin et al., 2011), and cognition (Marzuk, Hartwell, Leon et al., 2005; Pitman, 2007). Affective challenges included managing emotional dysregulation, and addressing observed deficits in emotional literacy including naming and describing emotions. Behavioural challenges included impulsivity preventing individuals from keeping themselves safer while experiencing crises. Finally, cognitive challenges were in the area of problem solving, particularly while experiencing emotional crises. The aim of the intervention was to enhance awareness and skills levels in the areas of affect, behaviour and cognition so individuals could keep themselves safer.

The goal

The goal of this intervention is not to cure people, or to have them expect to never have a suicidal thought or attempt again. We cannot make suicidal thinking go away, however, we can identify skills and strategies to help steer the behaviour away from acting unsafely and towards acting more safely. The goal is ultimately to reduce the duration, intensity and frequency of suicide attempts and for the person to recognize their own moments of control and choice to live life as safely as they are able. This goal is grounded in the beliefs that:

- by voluntarily coming to group, the person is either curious or un/consciously wants to change;
- people want to and do have the ability to make changes;
- people don't 'like' being suicidal. Rather, they may not have the skills and/or awareness to know how to live differently.

People want their pain to end, even if just for a moment (Dieter, Nicholls, & Pearlman, 2000) and in moments of no or less distress, they are capable of learning new skills that will help them to tolerate and/or ease their pain in moments of increased vulnerability and fragility.

Stepping stones to creating an intervention: attitudes and assumptions on the part of the professional

Multiple attitudes and lessons have been taken into consideration when moving toward creating an intervention and these have been characterised as:

- Keeping it real
- the three Cs.

The cloak of professionalism: keeping it real

Paying attention to one's own strengths and challenges as a therapist is an ongoing process that requires vigilance and continuous reflection in order to be effective in the work. Ultimately, we want to work from our surplus and not our core (see the reply to article, Aksunai, n.d.: http://bitchmagazine.org/post/love-and-afrofeminism-is-the-self-care-movement-individualist-or-revolutionary-feminist-magazine-women-caregiving). At the end of the day, or week, our work needs to be invigorating and energizing to our souls. This is not to deny that there will be times when we feel exhausted and spent, yet, can we still say, "even in my tired state, I like what I'm doing and want to get up in the morning and go to work"? It is our responsibility to identify when we are no longer able to inherently identify that we like the work we do. The assumption here is that without passion, interest, flexibility, curiosity, and openness, we may be merely delivering rather than participating and engaging in the intervention. If as professionals we are not participating and enjoying what we're doing, there is a high potential for not being genuinely engaged with the "self", the participants or the intervention. It is not a crime, and more likely a credit, to identify that a particular intervention or population is not within the realm of one's interest or skill set. While skills can be learned, an inherent interest and genuine engagement or, as Minkoff (2012) suggests, attachment to the intervention one is doing, requires more than learning the cookbook of intervention skills.

We are socialized into our professions and the question arises, "Who am I as a professional and as a person? What does it mean to act or be a professional?" When I find myself donning the "professional cloak", it usually represents a feeling of the need to protect myself from a perceived feeling of vulnerability or fragility. If I observe and reflect on myself in this position, I realize that I am removed from the people I am working with and for. There is an invisible barrier whereby I am not engaged as myself, rather, I have chosen to engage with people from a completely rational, cognitive place. I am protecting my emotional vulnerability. I am only partially present. By remaining curious, empathic, respectful, ethical, and working with integrity, I can be myself and work in a professional setting. It is not an either/or, rather, it is an "and". I can say "I don't know." I can feel unsure or overwhelmed and ask colleagues for support. In remaining in and practising this stance, you don't have to be the "hero" struggling alone in the dark alone with a person whom you are really worried about or feel helpless around. It is therapeutically helpful to say "I'm sorry" if you have said or done something wrong in the therapeutic setting. Furthermore, in the words of Barbara Coloroso (1994): "Mean what you say, say what you mean and do what you say you're going to do" have been instrumental in providing clear, consistent and caring language both with colleagues and participants.

Ultimately, for some people, it is the relationship with the clinician and/or group that keeps them alive (Linehan, 1993, p. 6). Yalom and Leszcz (2005) remind us that, "The basic posture of the therapist to a participant must be one of concern, acceptance, genuineness, empathy. *Nothing, no technical consideration, takes precedence over this attitude*" (p. 117, original emphasis).

The three Cs

In working with people who have had recurrent suicide attempts, it needs to be recognized that as clinicians, we are working with imperfect knowledge (White, 2005), and as such, there needs to be an acknowledgement that some people may die by suicide. We do not have the power to "make" them want to live nor to stop their attempt(s) to end their lives. Our assumption that participants have the capacity to engage in the three Cs: competency, control and choice, can be challenged by a loss to suicide. Alternatively, clinicians may feel like the only hope that exists is what they themselves are holding on behalf of the person. Oftentimes the capacity within the person is hidden. As such, the skills need to be taught with the recognition that, in times of crises, as one person stated, "Ya gotta know that when the emotions go up there, the brain got left behind a long time ago!" (participant in Group 5, see Chapter 20). The greatest professional challenge I have experienced has been to titrate my hope. To be too hopeful for a person who is in the pit of despair runs the risk of the person feeling invalidated or not understood. It is dissonant to their internal experience. Sometimes when a person identifies that they have lost or are losing hope, our response will be "We (I) will carry the hope until such time as you are able to carry it for yourself."

Learning from the experts

Our greatest teachers are our participants, colleagues, and mentors. We are the professionals and participants are the experts in their experience; when we come together, we are both learners and teachers of and to one another. I cannot assume to know what is right for a particular person or what will or won't work. It is my role to walk with them on their journey, not to "make" them live or "make" them better. As a learner, I take what the person has to teach me seriously. I am an accompanier who sometimes has to take the lead and at other times has to follow or walk alongside. It is my responsibility to ask questions in order to find the balance of what is called for, when, with a particular person with respect to the level of involvement and direction the person would like to take, to remain as safe as possible. It has become a rare occurrence when I think and actively take any control away from the person in order to fulfill my professional and ethical duties regarding the risk of imminent harm that someone could inflict upon themselves. The interaction and intervention are interdependent where we come together as 'we'.

How we view the person: stigma or strength?

Too often the people whom we work with are put in the position of "other". Some are more stigmatized than others by virtue of their diagnoses, behaviours, or in some cases our transference/counter-transference to the situation, person or issues. Often working under the medical model lens, the deficit is the focus while paying minimal or no attention to the competency inherent in survival to this point in people's lives. Working with people who have attempted to end their lives can arouse our greatest fears and, for others, personal stories and experiences may engender questions about choices to live or die, seeing the act of suicide as a right or wrong. As facilitators, paying attention to the language we use when speaking about the person with colleagues may provide us with clues: is the person referred to as "just a (name diagnosis/cutter, etc.)"?; is hearing their name met with "Ughhh! Not her/him again!" These attitudes and responses place the person or population in the position of "less than" or "less able than". Consider a night of no sleep, multiple personal issues piling up in a single month, improper eating or lack of exercise and an under-resourced workplace. As professionals, our human needs and pressures can slowly tap at the shield of 'professional', perhaps leaving us feeling less tolerant, de-skilled, exhausted, vulnerable and not as fully engaged as we would like to be. Hence, it is safer, easier or even a survival strategy to widen the gap between us and them. It does not mean we are less capable, it means we are run-down, exhausted, frustrated, etc. Some professionals may become depressed and need "professional help". This is a reminder that we are square in the middle of being human and "not less than". Our participants are human and experience times of despair in a way that some of us might never experience. They have endured, survived and are able to tell their stories, and agree to work as hard as they can to try and help themselves.

The motivation to try to live life more safely is a testament to their inner courage, strength and capacity. In remaining accountable to each other, facilitators and participants are challenged and invited to hold no judgments of right or wrong regarding the choices that have been made to survive. The bottom lines of the intervention are to connect the participant to having the choices to make the decision to live, and create a space and place where they will be accepted as human with full regard and respect for who they are as a human being.

The intervention: deliver vs. participate and facilitate

As facilitators, we do not 'deliver' an intervention. We participate in and facilitate a group intervention. It is a process in which we are working out, together, what will be most relevant and related to the experiences of participants. At the initial start of providing this group intervention, I was encouraged to use an already existing protocol. I found it was not my language, not me being authentic. It was the delivery of "a program". Our first participants took their roles as learners and teachers seriously. They let us know "This isn't working for us!" Together we began to co-create an intervention that they could relate to with skills they found they needed, that the literature supported, and that we could manage. After 14 years of providing the program to 60+ groups, we continue to co-create each group with the people in the room. Their experiences, skills, insights, and previous learning are all added to the foundational content to make it "their group". Over the years, materials have been re-written to have more meaning for the population as a whole, handouts have been tweaked, new material has been brought in by participants and added to the guide, and some materials have been discarded.

It is a blend of process and content with the latter being quite fluid in the placement of its delivery based on the needs and issues raised by participants at their check-in where we discuss "skills used, challenges, and 'aha' moments" since we last met. Content from our guide's first module is generally covered as a base in the first month and from then on, content is delivered as it arises. Homework is offered as an invitation to consider, reflect upon, try, discuss. This reflects our conscious choice not to participate in the potential power struggle, the residual shame, guilt of 'feeling like a bad student' or adding to the unwritten rules or expectations of shoulds of authority figures. We are dealing with adults and hence expect that people will do what has meaning for them and is reflective of their own process. To decline the invitation is a choice which must be accepted without judgment.

The team

The interprofessional team is the 'juice' that keeps facilitators fuelled and accountable. Working with people from different professional backgrounds, training, skills, gender, cultural backgrounds is an enormous benefit to doing this work. I can't expect myself to know everything, nor to have the most up-to-date training in the most recent efficacious treatment protocols. However, usually someone else on the team does, and it's often the students from varying professions who are an integral part of the team.

To undertake this group, two facilitators are the minimum. To do it by yourself is extremely challenging and nerve-wracking, and if one member is particularly fragile on a given day, it is sometimes frightening. It can be done; however, don't expect to be able to do a lot of intensive work for the rest of the day.

We meet prior to group for 15 minutes to go over anything that has come up for participants during the week, and to check in with one another in terms of energy. This time is also used to strategize who might be best able to respond to a particular person due to an alliance or skill that others on the team might feel they don't have. Finally, the pre-group meeting is used to discuss topics to address from the previous week or content we would like to introduce.

Integral to the team at this stage in our development is the volunteer peer facilitator. The peer facilitator is an individual who has participated in two groups, taken a year away from the group to integrate what was learned in their daily lives, and is still participating in their own therapy. We have found that on some occasions, it is the peer facilitator who carries more credibility than the professionals, as it is they who can oftentimes say things to a participant that are more easily received than if said by a 'professional'. We have recently added four groups per year in a community outside of the large metropolitan city and renamed the intervention to "Skills for Safer Living" to provide a more accurate description for community members what the intervention is about. The facilitation team consists of a mental health professional working for a community mental health organization, a hired person with lived experience regarding suicide attempts, and a hired peer who is 'learning' the intervention; the latter two work for a peer support-run organization for people with lived experience of mental illness. It has been noted that peer facilitators who did not disclose previous suicide attempts to the group have, to date, tended to focus more on the content pieces/modules rather than the process.

After each group session the team meets to debrief, discuss potential content for the following week and air any concerns they may have about particular group member(s). It is decided at this time who will contact group members who were absent from the session without notice or follow up if there were any concerns regarding a particular individual. All of the facilitators meet with a co-supervisor on a weekly basis for one hour of supervision. To date, this has been a psychiatric consultant who is not a facilitator in order to: (1) provide an 'outsider' perspective; (2) assist in the discussions of transference/counter-transference; (3) provide a psychiatric perspective regarding clinical issues that may be interfering or contributing to a person's progress or challenges; and (4) pay attention to content 'drift'. The out-of-town groups meet weekly with YB, sometimes accompanied by a psychiatrist via video conference initially made possible by a community granting agency. Groups overseas meet via teleconference with YB every 4–6 weeks.

Overall the team members can expect to devote a minimum of 3 hours per week to the intervention. At the very basic, 15 minutes pre and post group, 1.5 hours in group and 1 hour team supervision on a weekly basis. In some jurisdictions, prior to meeting with the larger supervision group, small teams will meet independently for an hour per week. Being the person responsible for the intervention includes additional time for minutes to be taken, photocopying to be done, checking in with participants who were absent or who were perceived by the team as being at higher risk than usual. Peer facilitators can be enormously helpful in many of these areas, as well as task sharing among team members, providing they have been given the time in their work day.

Inclusion criteria

People who report two or more lifetime attempts are eligible for the intervention. The key is that the person identifies having had attempts. It is not unusual for a professional to comment, "Well, it really wasn't serious." The frame of reference is not the externalized, observable 'seriousness' of the attempt such as medical/physical results as accorded by a hospitalization or serious medical event, rather, it is the person's unique and experienced emotional/psychological intent that resulted in a behavioural expression of their wish to die.

People who are experiencing active psychoses; have recently assaulted another person for which charges have been laid; do not have stable housing; are unhoused, are unable to attend group sober; and/or have a high degree of narcissism with paranoia are participants for whom the intervention has not been found to be helpful. Once housing is procured, some level of sobriety is attained, and/or the person with the psychotic episodes are stabilized, people are welcome to re-apply if suicide-related behaviours remain an issue for them.

Assessment

A full assessment is done prior to participating in the groups. Basic socio-demographic questions are asked; persons on their networks of support; strengths, hobbies and goals are also included in the assessment. There is a focus on suicide-related behaviour with attention paid to self-injury to determine how the individual understands the similarities and/or differences between the two, if they engage in both. Participants are asked what dying or ending their lives would do for them; how it might be helpful. This provides an inroad to understanding what meaning suicide has for the person, with example answers being: "to end the pain"; "to end this miserable life"; "to get out of my horrible situation"; "so I won't have to worry any more"; "it's the only control I have"; "to give other people some peace because I'm just too much to handle". With respect to self-injury, the range of responses has included: "to let the bad out"; "to release the pain"; "to get other people to see how bad I feel inside because I have no words"; "to prevent myself from killing myself"; "to punish myself for what's happened". It is key to understand the suicide-related behaviours and self-injury from the perspective of the individual. Although participants are asked their diagnoses, the focus of the intervention is on the behaviour. The belief is that the behaviour is a form of communication for which the person has no words available.

Intent to die, beliefs about dying by suicide in the future, worst attempt, hospitalizations, reasons for living, and how a person has managed to remain alive up to this point are all discussed in the assessment. A previous peer facilitator suggested that for those engaging in suicide-related behaviours, intent could be better measured through the awareness or belief that the person thinks (1) they could die; (2) wants to die or (3) will die. This allows for a better understanding of where death lies on the spectrum between life and death. While the majority of individuals identify with "could or want to die", a minority of individuals identify that they do not wish to die. The person's present level of commitment to die or live at this time does not impact whether or not they participate in the group.

Socialization in the mental health field may have engendered a medical model lens, or a focus on deficits that need to be fixed. A participant remarked, "Why is it when you guys get us in to treatment, you never ask what are the parts about myself that I like? Why does it feel like I'm such a '(bad word)' that everything about me needs to change?" This was a reminder that the assessment needs to include strengths, likes and dislikes, hobbies and friends. If they cannot remember strengths, friends, etc. or answer "none", the person will be asked to look backwards, "What were they when you were well?" "What did you used to like to do that you find you don't do any more?" Strengths are the foundation to re-acquainting the person with their competencies and are articulated and reinforced from the initial meeting through to graduation from the intervention.

Intervention content and process

The weekly struggle in many groups has been to find the balance between process and content. The content/skills that are discussed arise out of the check-in of skills, challenges and "aha moments" experienced by group members in the past week. The first four sessions rely fairly heavily on introducing the language and basics to keeping oneself as safe as possible and the remaining 16 weeks build from there. There have been some groups which are more concrete and want a "lesson" to be formally introduced each week and others prefer the new skill/concept to arise out of the discussions. To prepare an agenda is helpful for some people. However, sticking to what the facilitators want irrespective of what arises during check-in negates the underlying assumption that this is the participants' group, so changes in focus need to be negotiated with participants. The key we found is that facilitators need to be flexible and know the content so it can be presented when the issue arises. This usually will take two cycles of co-facilitation for it to feel more natural. Nonetheless, after 60+ groups, even the person who wrote the guide gets "stuck" in not knowing which direction to go next. Interprofessional and peer co-facilitators are key in those moments.

Manualization and guides

There has been a strong push for manualization of interventions over the past decade. This is the result of research foci and is an attempt to maintain fidelity and transferability of a particular intervention across locations and sites. Contrary to trends, the PISA/SFSL guide is a guide, not a manual. Each group has its own personality. Each group will bring its own needs, strengths and skills. In this vein, the guide provides the content and skills with the understanding that it remains a living document. The foundational concepts remain consistent, yet the delivery, metaphors, and strategies utilized to explain and 'teach' them are permeable and to be used as they pertain to the needs of the group. As noted earlier, metaphors, articles, and stories might change based on the training, experiences, and creative ideas of participants and co-facilitators. A recent example is the use of the words "emotional hangover", the experience of feeling fragile, exhausted and raw after a group session or after an intense emotional experience. A colleague who is an addictions specialist proposed to the supervision team that this might not be the best term to use for those who have experienced substance abuse issues. A week later another member of the supervision team proposed "emotionally sore", like one would feel in their muscles after a work-out. It's not a bad thing, it means you've had a good workout and now you have to be gentle with the sore areas. It is open discussions like these that keep the intervention living/changing and relevant to the people who are using it and working with it.

References

Aksunai (n.n.). Give from your surplus, not your core. Available at: http://bitchmagazine.org/post/love-and-afrofeminism-is-the-self-care-movement-individualist-or-revolutionary-feminist-magazine-women-caregiving (accessed September 4, 2012).

Bender, T. W., Gordon, K. H., Bresin, K., & Joiner, T. E. (2011). Impulsivity and suicidality: The mediating role of painful and provocative experiences. *Journal of Affective Disorders, 129*, 301–307.

Bergmans, Y., Spence, J. M., Strike, C., Links, P., Ball, J. S., Rhodes, A. E., Rufo, C., Watson, W. J., & Eynan, R. (2009). Repeat substance using – suicidal clients – how can we be helpful? *Social Work in Health Care, 48*(4), 420–431.

Chen, Y. Y., Lee, M. B., Chang, C. M., & Liaoh, S. C. (2009). Methods of suicide in different psychiatric diagnostic groups. *Journal of Affective Disorders, 118*(1–3), 196–200.

Colman, I., Yiannakoulias, N., Schopflocher, D., Svenson, L. W., Rosychuk, R. J., Rowe, B. H. for the ED Atlas Group (2004). A population-based study of medically treated self-inflicted injuries. *Canadian Journal of Emergency Medicine, 6*, 313–20.

Coloroso, B. (1994) *Kids are worth it!* New York: Penguin.

Dieter, P. J., Nicholls, S. S., & Pearlman, L. A. (2000). Self injury and self capacities: Assisting an individual in crisis. *Journal of Clinical Psychology, 56*, 1173–1191.

Forman, E. M., Berk, M. S., Henriques, G. R., Brown, G. K., & Beck, A. T. (2004). History of multiple suicide attempts as a behavioral marker of severe psychopathology. *American Journal of Psychiatry, 161*, 437–443.

Gibb, B. E., Andover, M. S., & Miller, I. W. (2009) Depressive characteristics of adult psychiatric inpatients with a history of multiple versus one or no suicide attempts. *Depression and Anxiety, 26,* 568– 574.

Hjelemand, H., & Knizek, B. L. (2010). Why we need qualitative research in suicidology. *Suicide and Life-threatening Behavior, 40*(1), 74–80.

Leenaars, A. (2004). *Psychotherapy with suicidal people: A person-centered approach.* Chichester: John Wiley & Sons Ltd.

Levine, D., Marziali, E., & Hood, J. (1997). Emotion processing in borderline personality disorders. *The Journal of Nervous and Mental Disease, 185,* 240–246.

Linehan, M. (1993). *Cognitive-behavioral treatment of borderline personality disorder.* New York: Guilford Press.

Linehan, M. (2008). Suicide intervention research: A field in desperate need of development. *Suicide and Life-threatening Behavior, 38*(5), 483–485.

Linehan, M., Armstrong, H. E., Suarez, A., Allmon, D., & Heard, H. (1991). Cognitive-behavioural treatment of chronically parasuicidal borderline patients. *Archives of General Psychiatry, 48,* 1060–1064.

Marzuk, P. M, Hartwell, N., Leon, A. C., & Portera, A. C. (2005). Executive functioning in depressed patients with suicidal ideation. *Acta Psychiatrica Scandinavica, 112,* 294–301.

McElroy, A., & Sheppard, G. (1999). The assessment and management of self-harming patients in an accident and emergency department: An action research project. *Journal of Clinical Nursing,* 8(1), 66–72.

Minkoff, K. (2012). Changing the world, health, hope and recovery. Thursday, December 6, 2012, presentation at St. Michael's Hospital, Toronto, Ontario.

Owens, D., Horrocks, J., & House, A. (2002) Fatal and non-fatal repetition of self-harm: Systematic review. *British Journal of Psychiatry, 181,* 193–199.

Pitman, A. (2007). Policy on the prevention of suicidal behaviour: One treatment for all may be an unrealistic expectation. *Journal of the Royal Society of Medicine, 100,* 461–464.

Rosenberg, H. J., Jankowski, M. K., Sengupta, A., Wolfe, R. S, Wolford, G. L., & Rosenberg, S. D. (2005). Single and multiple suicide attempts and health risk factors in New Hampshire adolescents. *Suicide and Life-threatening Behavior, 35,* 547–557.

Rudd, M. D., Joiner, T. E., & Rajab, M. H. (1996). Relationships among suicide ideators, attempters and multiple attempters in a young adult sample. *Journal of Abnormal Psychology, 105,* 541–550.

Spence, J. M., Bergmans, Y., Strike, C., Links, P. S., Rhodes, A. E., Spence, J. M., Watson, W. J., Eynan, R., & Rufo, C. (2008). Managing the substance using-suicidal male who presents repeatedly to the ED. *Canadian Journal of Emergency Medicine, 10*(4), 339–346.

White, J. (2005). *Preventing suicide in youth: Taking action with imperfect knowledge.* Vancouver: University of British Columbia Press.

Yalom, I. D., & Leszcz, M. (2005). *The theory and practice of group psychotherapy.* New York: Basic Books.

19

WHAT CHANGES?
WHAT DOES IT MEAN?

A clinical intervention for people with recurrent suicide attempts

Yvonne Bergmans and Rahel Eynan

Introduction

There has been a call for practical and comprehensive interventions that would target persons with recurrent suicide-related behaviour (Hawton & Kirk, 1998; Links, 1998; Livesley, 2000; Pitman, 2007): however, as suicidal behaviour and suicide are still rare clinical outcome events, establishing treatment efficacy is challenging (Leitner, Barr, & Hobby, 2008). Research utilizing outcome measures that go beyond the outcome of suicide or suicide-related behaviour might have more utility, according to Pitman (2007). She recommended that intermediate measures that reduce potential risk factors for suicide-related behaviour, such as depression and hopelessness, could be used as feasible yet important proxy outcome measures.

This chapter reports on the results of a 20-week outpatient intervention, the Psychosocial/Psychoeducational Intervention for Persons with Recurrent Suicide Attempts (PISA), and known in one community as Skills for Safer Living, on risk factors and areas of deficit known to characterize persons with recurrent suicide-related behaviour (Bergmans & Links, 2002; 2009). The nomenclature by Silverman, Berman, Sanddal et al. (2007a; 2007b) will be used throughout this chapter, with particular focus on suicide-related behaviour, defined as

> a self-inflicted, potentially injurious behavior for which there is evidence (either explicit or implicit) either that (a) the person wished to use the appearance of intending to kill himself/herself in order to attain some other end; or (b) the person intended at some undetermined or some known degree to kill himself/herself. Suicide-related behaviors can result in no injuries, injuries or death.
>
> *(Silverman et al., 2007a, p. 272)*

The authors further explain that suicide attempts are defined as a "self-inflicted, potentially injurious behavior with a nonfatal outcome for which there is evidence (either explicit or implicit) of intent to die. A suicide attempt may result in no injuries, injuries or death" (Silverman et al., 2007a, p. 273).

Recurrent suicide-related behaviour

People with recurrent suicide-related behaviour have been reported as having a variety of diagnostic comorbidities that include combinations of depressive illness, substance abuse, bulimia nervosa, anxiety disorders, depression, and higher rates of alcohol dependence, BPD, and/or bipolar disorder (Anderson, Barter, McIntosh et al., 2002; Horesh, Orbach, Gothelf et al., 2003; Michaelis, Goldberg, Singer et al., 2003; Ystgaard, Hestetun, Loeb et al., 2004). Rudd, Joiner and Rumzek (2004) reported that a childhood history of anxiety disorder or major depressive disorder predisposed a person both to later multiple suicide attempts and personality psychopathology; further, they noted that for women, exhibiting recurrent suicide attempts was a function of having childhood anxiety disorders, not mood disorders. Forman, Berk, Henriques et al. (2004) found that multiple suicide attempters vs. single attempters had more severe psychopathology, suicidality and interpersonal difficulties when assessed following presentation to the emergency department after an attempt. Taken together, these findings indicate that persons with recurrent suicide-related behaviour are not characterized by one diagnosis, but more so by the magnitude and breadth of their psychopathology.

A variety of psychological deficits and potential risk factors alongside the complex combinations of comorbidities have been identified in this population. These include problem-solving deficits, cognitive rigidity, hopelessness, alexithymia, negative self-evaluation, and negative affectivity (Marzuk, Hartwell, Leon et al., 2005; Pruessner, Baldwin, Dedovic et al., 2005; Williams, Barnhofer, Crane et al., 2005). For those identified with BPD and recurrent suicide-related behaviours, instability and/or the following: deficits in emotion regulation, decreased levels of emotional awareness, difficulty in problem solving, or difficulties in managing interpersonal relationships have been evidenced (Linehan, Armstrong, Suarez et al., 1991; Levine, Marziali, & Hood, 1997; Kern, Kuehnel, Teuber et al., 1997; Dieter, Nicholls, & Pearlman, 2000; Pitman, 2007). Neurobiological factors may also contribute to some of the identified deficits and/or psychological factors (van Heeringen, 2003; Bostwick, 2005; LeGris & van Reekum, 2006). Given these factors, we specifically chose to study variables that reflect potential personal risk factors or psychological deficits associated with recurrent suicide-related behaviour that purportedly could be changeable as targets for our intervention. The potential risk factor domains chosen were: *affective* (alexithymia) because of its relationship to emotional awareness, depression (Taiminen, Saarijarvi, Helenius et al., 1996), self-injurious behaviour and suicide attempts (Polk & Liss, 2007; Horesh, Levi, & Apter, 2012); *cognitive* (hopelessness, life satisfaction, problem solving); and *impulsivity*.

A Psychosocial/Psychoeducational Intervention for People with Recurrent Suicide Attempts (PISA)/Skills For Safer Living (SFSL)

PISA/SFSL is a 20-week psychosocial /psychoeducational group intervention program developed for clients with a history of recurrent suicide attempts. (This chapter will provide an outline of the intervention however, for a more in-depth discussion, the reader is invited to refer to "A description of a psychosocial/psychoeducational intervention for persons with recurrent suicide attempts" (Bergmans & Links, 2002) or Chapter 18 in this volume.

The group intervention targets skills or coping strategies to lessen the potential risk factors or psychological deficits associated with recurrent suicide-related behaviour. People with a lifetime history of two or more suicide attempts self-referred or were referred after a suicide crisis from a variety of in-hospital or community resources. Participation in the group is based on the presence of recurrent suicide attempts as identified by the person and is not based on the presence of a particular psychiatric diagnosis. People with an active psychotic disorder or a recent history of interpersonal violence are excluded from the program. Participants are expected to have an individual therapist in the community while participating in the group. There are no restrictions regarding whether or not people participate in other treatments, for example, entering specific programs for eating disorders, substance abuse.

Methods

To date, 62 groups have been completed across five Canadian sites. Two of the sites were outpatient hospital locations and three were community-based joint projects with the Canadian Mental Health Association and the Self Help Alliance. Six groups (66 registered participants) were held at the community locations with one underway at the time of this writing; 55 group interventions were held in an inner city hospital located in downtown Toronto. Of the 349 participants (238 women and 111 men), who began the 62 group intervention, 249 (71.1%) completed all 20 weeks and 12 (3.4%) are currently participating.

As indicated in Table 19.1, participants' age ranged from 16–71 years of age with the mean age being 36 years (SD = 11.4). The age of onset of suicide-related ideation was 16.8 years (SD = 9.8; range, 2 to 61 years). The mean age of first recalled suicide-related behaviour was 21.02 years (SD = 10.7; range, 4 to 62 years). The majority of participants (66.9%) were single, nearly a quarter (23.7%; 83/349) had less than a high school education, and 28.9 % (101/349) had completed university. Nearly a quarter (24.2%; 85/349) were employed either full- or part-time and 28.9% (101/349) lived on their own with no support, while 22.9% (79/349) reported living with family or friends. Nearly half of the group participants (48.4%; 169/349) lived in shelters, boarding homes, the street, group homes, supportive housing units or the information was not obtained.

Participants reported various psychiatric diagnoses (see Table 19.2). The most frequent reported diagnoses were unipolar depression (63.5%) and Borderline Personality Disorder (BPD) (43.2%) followed by Bipolar Disorder (25.8%) and Post Traumatic Stress Disorder (PTSD) (20%). The study received ethics approval from St. Michael's Hospital Research Ethics Board, and all participants provided signed informed consent. Participants were not financially compensated for participation in the program.

Design and procedures

From the start, the group intervention has continued to be an ever-changing and evolving pilot project. Thus, beginning in 2000, over a three-year period, various measures have been added. Consequently, the number of respondents differs for each measure. To measure the change resulting from the group intervention in areas identified as deficits or risk factors for clients with recurrent suicide-related behaviour: cognition, affect, and impulsivity, a pre-post study analysis was conducted.

Participants were given the pre-group measures at the first session, and the post-group measures were given at the second-to-last session. All measures were completed by participants at home and returned the following week. Within the affective, cognitive, and impulsivity domains, the following measures were given.

Table 19.1 Sample characteristics

	Number of respondents		Number of respondents
Gender	249 (100%)	Children	236 (95.9%)
M	81 (32.5%)	No	165 (66.3%)
F	168 (67.5%)		
Marital status	222 (89.2%)	Thinking will die	175 (70.3%)
Single	176 (70.7%)	by suicide with plan	
Partnered	41 (16.5%)	Yes	102 (40.9%)
		No	59 (23.7%)
		Not sure	14 (5.6%)
Employed	238 (95.6%)	Current medical follow-up	243 (97.6%)
Yes	68 (27.3%)	No	44 (17.7%)
No	143 (57.4%)		
Long-term disability	26 (10.4%)		
Currently in school	220 (88.3%)	Current allied health follow-up	233 (93.5%)
Yes	26 (10.4%)	No	94 (37.8%)
No	194 (77.9%)	Yes	107 (42.9%)
Grade completed	226 (90.8%)	Forensic history	217 (87.1%)
< high school completed	54(21.9%)	No	168 (67.5%)
High school	74 (37.8%)		
Post-secondary	69 (27.7%)		
Graduate program	9 (3.6%)		
Reported substance use	235 (94.4%)	Housing	206 (83.7%)
Current use	100 (40.1%)	On own	75 (30.1%)
Previous history of use	60 (24.1%)	With family member(s)	56 (22.5%)
Current use reported		Subsidized	22 (8.8%)
No	72 (28.9%)	Supportive/boarding/ Group homes, etc.	50 (20.0%)
Previous treatment for substance use	222 (89.1)	Child Welfare involvement as a child	218 (87.5%)
Yes	58 (23.3%)	Adopted	14 (5.6%)
No	147 (59%)	Yes	31 (12.4%)
		No	173 (69.5%)

		Mean, median	Range	Standard deviation
Age	249 (100%)	37.1; 36	16–71	11.64
Age of recalled onset of feelings	218 (87.5%)	16.9yrs; 14.0yrs	2–61yrs	10.11
Age of recalled first attempt	228 (91.5%)	21.0yrs; 18.0yrs	4–61 yrs	10.6

Table 19.2 Participants' self-reported diagnoses at intake

Axis I	No.	(%)*
Depression	159	(66.5)
Bipolar disorder	70	(29.3)
Anxiety/panic	62	(25.9)
Post-traumatic stress disorder	47	(19.6)
Eating disorder	33	(13.8)
Obsessive compulsive disorder	18	(7.5)
Alcohol and/or drug dependence and or abuse	14	(5.8)
Schizophrenia	13	(5.4)
Axis II		
Borderline personality disorder	121	(50.6)
Antisocial personality disorder	4	(1.6)
PD-NOS/other PD	23	(10.1)
Other	96	(38.4)

Notes: PD-NOS: Personality Disorder Not Otherwise Specified. Participants (N = 239).
*Numbers do not total 239 because of multiple responses.

Affective

The 20-item Toronto Alexithymia Scale (TAS-20) is a self-report questionnaire containing items that are rated on a 5-point Likert-type rating scale from 1 (strongly disagree) to 5 (strongly agree) with five items inversely scored. It is hand scored with a maximum score of 100. It uses cutoff scoring: ≤51 = non-alexithymic, scores of 52 to 60 = moderately alexithymic, and scores ≥ 61 = highly alexithymic. The TAS-20 was chosen because it has three subscales, a three-factors structure that is theoretically consistent with the alexithymia construct and captures concepts relevant to identified deficits in emotional awareness: (1) difficulties identifying feelings; (2) difficulties describing feelings; and (3) externalization of emotion. The TAS-20 has been used in a variety of populations, including psychiatric outpatients, and previous evidence supports the convergent, discriminant, and concurrent validity of the TAS-20 (Taylor, Bagby, Ryan et al., 1990; Bagby, Parker, & Taylor, 1994). The Beck Depression Inventory (BDI) is a self-report questionnaire consisting of 21 items each with four possible responses that assesses different aspects of depressive symptomatology (Beck, Ward, Mendelsohn et al., 1961). Each response is assigned a score ranging from zero to three, indicating the severity of the symptom. The maximum possible score is 63. A score of <15 = Mild Depression, a score 15–30 = Moderate Depression, and a score >30 = Severe Depression. The BDI has demonstrated excellent psychometric characteristics, with a split-half reliability of 0.93, and excellent convergent and predictive validity, e.g., significantly predicting suicide ideation and eventual suicide (Beck, Ward, Mendelsohn et al., 1961; Beck, Steer, Kovacs et al., 1985).

Cognitive

The Beck Hopelessness Scale (BHS) is a 20-item true–false self-report questionnaire designed to assess negative attitudes about the future. Scores range from 0 to 20. The scale has been shown to have high internal consistency (Kuder-Richardson-20 coefficient alpha = 0.93) and a relatively high correlation with clinical ratings of hopelessness (r = 0.74) in a population of 294 hospitalized patients with recent suicide attempts (Beck, Weissman, Lester et al., 1974).

The Satisfaction With Life Scale (SWLS) is a self-administered 5-item scale which is designed to assess the self-identified cognitive-judgmental aspects of global life satisfaction. The items are rated on a 7-point Likert-type scale from 1 (= strongly disagree) to 7 (= strongly agree). Scores range from 5 to 35. It has demonstrated acceptable reliability, with high internal consistency, and test–retest reliability over periods of 2 months (r = 0.82) and 4 years (r = 0.54), respectively. The SWLS has demonstrated convergent and discriminant validity, relating positively with other measures of well-being, relating negatively with measures of distress, and yielding no significant relationship with emotional intensity (Pavot & Diener, 1993).

The Problem Solving Inventory (PSI) is a 32-item self-report scale designed to capture the person's perception of his or her own problem-solving behaviours and attitudes (Heppner & Petersen, 1982). The PSI inventory uses a 6-point Likert-type format (1= strongly agree to 6 = strongly disagree) and consists of three factors related to self-perception of problem-solving: confidence (self-assurance while engaging in problem-solving activities), personal control (determines the extent of control one has over their emotions and behaviours while solving problems), and approach-avoidance style (a general tendency to either approach or avoid problem-solving activities). High scores indicate general negative self-appraisal while lower scores reflect greater perceived problem-solving abilities. Joiner, Pettit, Perez et al. (2001) reported test–retest reliabilities from their previous research; coefficient alphas for the total scale were 0.93, and for three factor subscales they ranged from 0.76 to 0.87.

Impulsivity

The Barratt Impulsiveness Scale (BIS), often used in the investigation of impulsive behaviour, is useful in identifying impulsivity and evaluating the influence of this dimension on client performance without the influence of confounding factors such as anxiety traits (Barratt, Stanford, Kent et al., 1997). The 30-item BIS-11 describes common impulsive or non-impulsive (for reverse scored items) behaviours and preferences. Items are scored on a 4-point scale (1= rarely/never to 4 = almost always/always) without relation to any specific time period (a trait measure of impulsivity). Twelve items are reverse-scored, a design feature to avoid response sets. Higher summed scores for all items indicate higher levels of impulsivity. The BIS-11 consists of three sub-scales related to attentional impulsiveness (task-focus, intrusive thoughts, and racing thoughts), motor impulsivity (tendency to act on the spur of the moment and consistency of lifestyle), and non-planning impulsivity (careful thinking and planning and enjoyment of challenging mental tasks).

Data analysis

All pre- and post-responses were analyzed using descriptive statistics (frequencies, mean, median, and standard deviation). To assess the impact of the group intervention on the post-intervention we used mean scores paired sample *t* tests. Data were analyzed using SPSS 15.0 for Windows.

The percentage of change in mean scores of post-intervention scores, and pre-intervention scores were also calculated. A percentage change is a way to express the magnitude of change in a variable and it represents the relative change between the old value and the new one. The percentage of change was calculated by subtracting the pre-intervention mean score from the post-intervention score and dividing by the pre-training score and multiplying the result by 100.

Since participants were not refused the group intervention if they chose not to participate in the research, completion rates for pre and post measures do not correspond to the number of participants who completed the group intervention. Additionally, it also needs to be acknowledged that measures were introduced over time as the intervention evolved and questions became more focused. The number of completed pre-group and post-group measures are as follows:

TAS-20, N = 111; SWLS, N = 100; BIS, N = 93; BDI, N = 58; BHS, N = 83; and PSI, N = 75.

Results

Nearly two-thirds (249; 71.1%) of the participants "graduated" from the 20-week group intervention with 12 (3.4%) still participating in the intervention. Those who graduated had a mean attendance of 75.24% of the scheduled sessions (median, 80; mode, 90; range, 10 to 100). Of those who withdrew and did not complete the group intervention 18 (7.2%) returned at a later date to complete the intervention. As such, their data were incorporated into the present analysis. Some 89 individuals (26.4%) withdrew prior to completion of the 20 weeks group intervention. Reasons for withdrawal included: potential problems with readiness for the group (13.4%), extraneous health, treatment, and life issues (40.4%); and no reason given or lost to follow-up (29.2%).

Pre-group and post-group measures and paired *t*-test scores are presented in Table 19.3.

Table 19.3 Comparisons of pre- and post-group affective, cognitive, and impulsivity scores

	n	*Pre-intervention*	*Post-intervention*	*p value*
Affective				
TAS-20				
Difficulties identifing feelings	110	24.9 (6.5)	22.7 (7.0)	<.001
Difficulties describing feelings	110	17.8 (4.8)	16.8 (5.2)	0.015
Externally oriented thinking	111	20.8 (5.3)	18.9 (5.5)	<.001
TAS-20 Total score	111	63.7 (13.2)	57.9 (15.0)	<.001
BDI		36.5 (11.7)	31.5 (14.6)	0.002
Cognitive				
PSI				
Personal confidence	74	39.9 (12.2)	37.7 (10.2)	N.S.
Avoidance approach style	75	53.9 (13.1)	55.8 (10.6)	N.S.
Personal control	75	13.6 (8.3)	15.9 (7.5)	0.008
PSI Total score	75	115.0 (29.4)	119.0 (22.0)	N.S
BHS	83	14.8 (5.1)	20.9 (2.3)	<.001
SWLS	100	10.3 (5.5)	12.4 (7.3)	<.001
Impulsivity				
BIS Total score	93	76.1 (12.7)	73.7 (12.0)	0.026

Affective

Prior to participating in the group intervention 79.1% of the participants had TAS-20 scores indicative of moderate (total scores = 52–60) or high alexithymia (total scores ≥ 61). Nearly two-thirds of the participants (60%) had TAS-20 scores ≥ 61 and scores ranged between 61–90. Post-group intervention the proportion of participants who were moderately or highly alexithymic declined to 70.1% and the proportion of those highly alexithymic dropped to 50%.

As indicated in Table 19.3, there were statistically significant differences between the pre- and post-intervention scores. The pre-intervention TAS-20 total mean of 63.7 (SD = 13.2) dropped to 57.9 (SD = 15.0) post-intervention ($p < .001$). Overall, this indicated a shift from high alexithymia (> 60) to moderate alexithymia (range, 52–60). The percentage of change in the mean scores from pre-intervention to post-intervention was 9.1%. Overall, a statistically significant decrease in the three TAS-20 subscales is observed.

BDI scores 20–28 are considered to indicate a moderate depression while scores 29–63 reflect severe depression. The proportion of participants who endorsed symptoms consistent with severe depression declined post-intervention 77.1% to 62.3%. Conversely, the proportion of participants who endorsed symptoms of minimal depression post-intervention increased from 4.8% to 14.5%. As indicated in Table 19.3, there was a statistically significant decrease in the post-intervention BDI mean scores (36.5 (SD = 11.7) vs. 31.5 (SD = 14.6), $p. = .002$). While the percentage of change between pre- and post-intervention was 13.7%, the overall BDI mean score post-intervention remained in the severe depression range (29–63).

Cognitive

There was no statistically significant difference in the post-intervention total mean score of the PSI (115.0 (SD = 29.4) vs. 119.0 (SD = 22.0), p = N.S.). However, the extent of control one has over their emotions and behaviours while solving problems increased significantly post-intervention (13.6 (SD = 8.3) vs. 15.9 (SD = 7.5), $p = .008$). The percentage of change in the Personal control over emotions and behaviours post-intervention increased by 16.9%.

Results of the BHS indicated significant reductions in hopelessness from pre-intervention to post-intervention (14.8 (SD = 5.1) vs. 12.8 (SD = 5.9), $p = .002$). The decrease in hopelessness represents a decrease of 13.5%: however, hopelessness scores remained moderate, reflecting a chance of suicide (range 9–14).

Pre-intervention, the majority of the participants (53.3%) indicated they were extremely dissatisfied with their life (SWLS score < 9). Post-intervention the proportion of those extremely dissatisfied with their life decreased to 46.4%. While the global life satisfaction increased significantly post-intervention (10.3 (SD = 5.5) vs. 12.4 (SD = 7.3), $p <.001$) and the pre- to post-intervention percentage of change was 20.4%, the score remains within the range of moderately dissatisfied with one's life.

Impulsiveness

There was a significant decrease in BIS total mean score post-intervention (76.1 (SD = 12.7) vs. 73.7 (SD = 12.0), $p = .026$. The percentage of change was 3.2%. Aside from the non-planning subscale, BIS-11 subscales showed significance in the reduction from the beginning to the end of the intervention.

Discussion

Considering the complexities of suicide, understanding what defines a lessening of suicide risk for an individual might reside upon that particular individual. The results from this ongoing pilot study reflect that overall, for those who completed the 20-week intervention, there were significant statistical changes found in the potential risk factors and/or deficit areas that are identified as characteristic for those with recurrent suicide attempts. General life satisfaction, more emotional literacy, less depression and hopelessness and a perception of better problem-solving abilities were reported as per the self-administered evaluations. Despite these changes, overall scores remain within severe or moderate ranges, likely reflecting the magnitude of challenges that persons with recurrent suicide-related behaviour are observed to manifest (Rudd, Joiner, & Rajab, 1996). It also needs to be noted that despite the statistically significant changes observed, not all participants' scores changed, or changed in the positive direction. These are findings which are not often analyzed or reported and which, due to resource limitations, are not reported in this chapter. A 20-week intervention is a relatively short period of time in the larger timeline of clients' lives and although significant changes were observed, it is difficult to know at this time if, with time, further gains will be made. We need to be cognizant that when utilizing only quantitative data, results do not necessarily reflect, or might have little to do with the experience of the changes the participants perceive or understand. Developing Moroz-Franklin's (2002) suggestion, perhaps it is the participation in the intervention group that allows participants to perceive themselves more able to manage their struggles rather than the actual struggles changing. As noted elsewhere (Bergmans, Langley, Links et al., 2009) and suggested by Joiner (2005), knowing that one is not alone in having issues with suicidality may be one of the key factors in reducing the experience of isolation and marginalization; a concept familiar to group therapy, universality, as noted by Yalom (1995; Yalom & Leszcz, 2005).

Perhaps we are asking different questions of the information being given through quantitative questionnaires. Qualitative and anecdotal evidence suggests that with support, some clients who have participated in this intervention do go on to live safer and productive lives (Bergmans, Carruthers, Ewanchuk, James et al., 2009; Scrivener, 2011; Ana Cara, 2012; Selfhelpalliance, 2012; Weidner, 2012). The PISA/SFSL intervention might be only one of several possible steps toward further reduced risk of suicide in persons with recurrent suicide-related behaviour. To assume a one-size-fits-all would deny the complexity of (1) each individual; and (2) of suicide. It is thus suggested that interventions need to meet the needs of the client at the time and if a particular modality is not appropriate at one given period in their lives, it does not suggest it will never be appropriate. With time, maturity, skill development, awareness and integration, a person may be more ready and able for a particular modality at different times on their journey as witnessed by the 18 people who left and came back.

The TAS-20 has been a useful measure of the difficulties with emotional processing that are characteristic of individuals with recurrent suicide-related behaviour and has been able to capture change following a time-limited intervention. This intervention targets emotion-processing difficulties and focuses on teaching emotional literacy, identifying and describing how one is feeling, and learning alternatives to suicide-related behaviour in response to emotional distress. In this focus, it provides a language that goes beyond the word "suicide" with the intent being that those who are being asked to help will be able to hear "not safe" or "afraid" more calmly than "suicide" or "die". Our results showed that with a focus on teaching the language of emotion, alexithymia scores changed significantly. It could be suggested that a person who is neither able to identify or describe his or her emotions might be more prone to acting out distress. Without a language, feelings overwhelm or flood cognitive functions. Izard (2002) suggested that in times of emotional flooding, emotion will be the driver taking a "low road", or noncognitive move to action – a process that occurs within milliseconds. These results suggest that the TAS-20 is a useful measure to capture the emotional-processing deficits found in persons with recurrent suicide-related behaviour and, more importantly, the measure may be sensitive to change that results from psychosocial interventions.

This ongoing pilot study has several limitations which are also areas for future research. Challenges in resources impacted the following. (1) Sample sizes for each measure are both limited and vary between measures. Sample loss was affected by non-completion of both pre-group and post-group measures in part, hindered by our ability to aggressively pursue data collection of those who did not return measures at the end of group. It was also hampered by the staggered introduction of the questionnaires. (2) Failure of participants to respond to items within the measures was also a challenge, consistent with the use of self-report scales (Shrive, Stuart, Quan et al., 2006). (3) Being unable to systematically diagnose group participants, it remains unclear if this intervention is more appropriate for individuals with particular struggles than others. Time constraints, restrictions of who can apply in some granting agencies, institutional demands, clinical caseloads can all seem insurmountable in the life of an allied clinical researcher trying to do intervention with people who are at high risk for dying by suicide. The fact remains, a future randomized controlled trial would assist in addressing the issues of limited measures, lack of a control group, and lack of outcome data on suicide-related behaviour. It is our hope that future research will be able to focus on demonstrating the efficacy of the PISA/SFSL in reducing future suicide-related behaviour.

Conclusion

The PISA/SFSL pilot study continues to demonstrate that a 20-week group intervention has led to significant reductions in the cognitive, affective, and impulsivity deficits and potential risk factors associated with suicide-related behaviour. This suggests that this short-term intervention might be the first of many steps toward engaging clients with recurrent suicide-related behaviours to seek longer-term help for problems associated with a high risk for suicide.

References

Anna, Cara, (2012). More from Canada: Talking with Judy James. October 19. Available at: http://whichtools.wordpress.com/2012/10/19/more-from-canada-talking-with-judy-james/ (accessed October 20, 2012).

Anderson, C., Barter, F. A., McIntosh, V. V., et al. (2002). Self-harm and suicide attempts in individuals with bulimia nervosa. *Eating Disorders, 10*, 227–243.

Bagby, R. M., Parker, J. D., & Taylor, G. J. (1994). The Twenty-Item Toronto Alexithymia Scale-I: Item selection and cross-validation of the factor structure. *Journal of Psychosomatic Research, 38*, 23–32.

Barratt, E. S., Stanford, M. S., Kent, M. A., et al. (1997). Neuropsychological and cognitive psychophysiological substrates of impulsive aggression. *Biological Psychiatry, 41*, 1045–1061.

Beck, A. T., Steer, R. A., Kovacs, M., et al. (1985). Hopelessness and eventual suicide: A 10 year prospective study of patients hospitalized with suicidal ideation. *American Journal of Psychiatry, 142*, 559–563.

Beck, A. T., Ward, C. H., Mendelsohn, M., et al. (1961). An inventory for measuring depression. *Archives of General Psychiatry, 4*, 561–571.

Beck, A. T., Weissman, A., Lester, D., et al. (1974). The measurement of pessimism: The hopelessness scale. *Journal of Consulting Clinical Psychology, 42*, 861–865.

Bergmans, Y., Carruthers, A., Ewanchuk, E., James, J., Wren, K., & Yager, C. (2009). Moving from full-time healing work to paid employment: Challenges and celebrations. *Work, 33*, 389–394.

Bergmans, Y., Langley, J., Links, P., & Lavery, J. V. (2009). The perspectives of young adults on recovery from repeated suicide-related behavior. *Crisis, 30*(3), 120–127.

Bergmans, Y., & Links, P. S. (2002). A description of a psychosocial/psychoeducational intervention for persons with recurrent suicide attempts. *Crisis: Journal of Crisis Intervention and Suicide Prevention, 23,* 156–160.

Bergmans, Y., & Links, P. S. (2009). Reducing potential risk factors for suicide-related behavior with a group intervention for clients with recurrent suicide-related behavior. *Annals of Clinical Psychiatry, 21,* 17–25.

Bostwick, J. M. (2005). The stress axis gone awry: A possible neuroendocrine explanation for increased risk of completed suicide. *Primary Psychiatry, 12,* 49–52.

Dieter, P. J., Nicholls, S. S., & Pearlman, L. A. (2000). Self-injury and self capacities: Assisting an individual in crisis. *Journal of Clinical Psychology, 56,* 1173–1191.

Forman, E. M., Berk, M. S., Henriques, G. R., et al. (2004). History of multiple suicide attempts as a behavioral marker of severe psychopathology. *American Journal of Psychiatry, 161,* 437–443.

Hawton, K., & Kirk, J. (1998). Problem-solving. In K. Hawton, P. M. Salkovskis, J. Kirk, et al. (Eds.), *Cognitive behaviour therapy for psychiatric problems: A practical guide* (pp. 406–426). New York: Oxford Medical Publications.

Heppner, P. P., & Petersen, C. H. (1982). The development and implications of a personal problem solving inventory. *Journal of Counseling Psychology, 29,* 66–75.

Horesh, N., Levi, Y., & Apter, A. (2012). Medically serious versus non-serious suicide attempts: Relationships of lethality and intent to clinical and interpersonal characteristics. *Journal of Affective Disorders, 136,* 286–293.

Horesh, N., Orbach, I., Gothelf, D., et al. (2003). A comparison of the suicidal behavior of adolescent inpatients with borderline personality disorder and major depression. *Journal of Nervous and Mental Disorders, 191,* 582–588.

Izard, C. E. (2002). Translating emotion theory and research into preventive interventions. *Psychological Bulletin, 128,* 796–824.

Joiner, T., Jr, Pettit, J. W., Perez, M., et al. (2001). Can positive emotion influence problem-solving attitudes among suicidal adults? *Professional Psychology-Research and* Practice, 32, 507–512.

Joiner, T. (2005). *Why people die by suicide.* Cambridge, MA: Harvard University Press.

Kern, R. S., Kuehnel, T. G., Teuber, J., et al. (1997). Multimodal cognitive-behavior therapy for borderline personality disorder with self-injurious behavior. *Psychiatric Services, 48,* 1131–1133.

LeGris, J., & van Reekum, R. (2006). The neuropsychological correlates of borderline personality disorder and suicidal behaviour. *Canadian Journal of Psychiatry, 51,* 131–142.

Leitner, M., Barr, W., & Hobby, L. (2008). *Effectiveness of interventions to prevent suicide and suicidal behaviour: A systematic review.* Health & Community Care Research Unit, Liverpool University. InfoTech UK Research. Scottish Government Social Research. January 11, 2008. Available a: http://www.scotland.gov.uk/Publications/2008/01/15102257/0. Accessed February 21, 2008.

Levine, D., Marziali, E., & Hood, J. (1997). Emotion processing in borderline personality disorders. *Journal of Nervous and Mental Disorders, 185,* 240–246.

Linehan, M. M., Armstrong, H. E., Suarez, A., et al. (1991). Cognitive-behavioral treatment of chronically parasuicidal borderline patients. *Archives of General Psychiatry, 48,* 1060–1064.

Links, P. S. (1998). Developing effective services for patients with personality disorders. *Canadian Journal of Psychiatry, 43,* 251–259.

Livesley, W. J. (2000). A practical approach to the treatment of patients with borderline personality disorder. *Psychiatric Clinics of North America, 23,* 211–232.

Marzuk, P. M., Hartwell, N., Leon, A. C., et al. (2005). Executive functioning in depressed patients with suicidal ideation. *Acta Psychiatrica Scandinavia, 112,* 294–301.

Michaelis, B. H., Goldberg, J. F., Singer, T. M., et al. (2003). Characteristics of first suicide attempts in single versus multiple suicide attempters with bipolar disorder. *Comparative Psychiatry, 44,* 15–20.

Moroz Franklin, T. (2002). The impact of the P.I.S.A intervention: Clients' perspectives of P.I.S.A. Unpublished Master's thesis, York University, Canada. Presented at Symposium: Bergmans, Y., Links P.S., Goulard G., Miki, N., Quastel, A., Cook M., Franklin, T.M. The Impact of a Psychosocial/ Psychoeducational Intervention for Persons with Recurrent Suicide Attempts. The VIII International ISSPD Congress, Florence, Italy. October 12, 2004.

Pavot, W., & Diener, E. (1993). Review of the Satisfaction with Life Scale. *Psychological Assessment, 5,* 164–172.

Pitman, A. (2007). Policy on the prevention of suicidal behaviour: One treatment for all may be an unrealistic expectation. *Journal of the Royal Society of Medicine, 100,* 461–464.

Polk, E., & Liss, M. (2007). Psychological characteristics of self-injurious behavior. *Personality and Individual Differences, 43*, 567–577.

Pruessner, J. C., Baldwin, M. W., Dedovic, K., et al. (2005). Self-esteem, locus of control, hippocampal volume, and cortisol regulation in young and old adulthood. *Neuroimage, 28*, 815–826.

Rudd, M. D., Joiner, T. E. Jr, & Rajab, M. H. (1996). Relationships among suicide ideators, attempters and multiple attempters in a young-adult sample. *Journal of Abnormal Psychology, 105*, 541–550.

Rudd, M. D., Joiner, T. E. Jr, & Rumzek, H. (2004). Childhood diagnoses and later risk for multiple suicide attempts. *Suicide and Life-threatening Behavior, 34*, 113–125.

Scrivener, L. (2011). People who attempted suicide as youths trace their recovery. *The Toronto Star* on the web, 3 December. Available at: http://www.thestar.com/news/gta/article/1096524—people-who-attempted-suicide-as-youths-trace-their-recovery (accessed June 14, 2012).

Selfhelpalliance (2012). Skills For Safer Living Support Group Testimonials, 28 March. Available at:http://www.youtube.com/watch?v=0H98e2fA1Dk (accessed 12 April 2012).

Shrive, F. M., Stuart, H., Quan, H., et al. (2006). Dealing with missing data in a multi-question depression scale: A comparison of imputation methods. *BMC Medical Research Methodology, 6*, 57.

Silverman, M. M., Berman, A. L., Sanddal, N. D., et al. (2007a). Rebuilding the Tower of Babel: A revised nomenclature for the study of suicide and suicidal behaviors. Part I: Background, rationale, and methodology. *Suicide and Life-threatening Behavior, 37*, 248–263.

Silverman, M. M., Berman, A. L, Sanddal, N. D., et al. (2007b). Rebuilding the Tower of Babel: A revised nomenclature for the study of suicide and suicidal behaviors. Part II: Suicide-related ideations, communications, and behaviors. *Suicide and Life-threatening Behavior, 37*, 264–277.

Taiminen, T. J., Saarijarvi, S., Helenius, H., Keskinen, A., & Korpilahti T. (1996). Alexithymia in suicide attempters. *Acta Psychiatrica Scandinavica, 93*, 195–198.

Taylor, G. J., Bagby, R. M., Ryan, D. P., et al. (1990). Validation of the alexithymia construct: A measurement-based approach. *Canadian Journal of Psychiatry, 35*, 260–267.

van Heeringen, K. (2003). The neurobiology of suicide and suicidality. *Canadian Journal of Psychiatry, 48*, 292–300.

Weidner, J. (2012). Program teaches survivors coping skills for a better life, 20 January. Available at: *The Record* on the web: http://www.therecord.com/article/658197 (accessed 4 May 2012).

Williams, J. M., Barnhofer, T., Crane, C., et al. (2005). Problem solving deteriorates following mood challenge in formerly depressed patients with a history of suicidal ideation. *Journal of Abnormal Psychology, 114*, 421–431.

Yalom, I. D. (1995). *The theory and practice of group psychotherapy* (4th ed.). New York: Basic Books.

Yalom, I. D., & Leszcz, M. (2005). *The theory and practice of group psychotherapy* . New York: Basic Books.

Ystgaard, M., Hestetun, I., Loeb, M., et al. (2004). Is there a specific relationship between childhood sexual and physical abuse and repeated suicidal behavior? *Child Abuse & Neglect, 28*, 863–875.

20

SUICIDE

Towards a clinical portrait

Carlos B. Saraiva

Sociological and epidemiological introduction

For Émile Durkheim (1897), the term suicide is applied to all cases of death resulting directly or indirectly from a positive or negative act practiced by an individual, an act which the victim previously knew would have such an outcome. Suicide would result from the changes in the rural world, that is, it would present itself as a consequence of industrialization, qualifications, civilization. The French sociologist valued two dimensions in the attempt to understand the phenomenon of suicide: integration and regulation. Integration meant the social relation which connects the individual to the group and regulation the degree of external constraint on people, the common norms people live under. A theorist of social facts, which should be regarded as things, and of a collective consciousness, for the author, any human behavior, from feeling to thinking or acting was determined by society. Hence, the macro social facts were essential to the understanding of the phenomenon of suicide, disregarding everything that goes on in the psyche of the individual as an isolated member of society.

The empirical theories of Durkheim basically relied on the variation of suicide rates already registered in France in the 19th century. Among other comparisons, he observed differences between married and single individuals, rural and urban dwellers, as well as Catholics, Protestants and Jews. He mentioned the cohesive forces of religion, of the collective normative, of tradition and honor. He introduced the seminal concept of anomie, that is, the loss of norms, safety, stability and support, as a consequence of the pathological state of society. For example, an excluded and outcast individual would feel left out of the organic solidarity owed to those who belong to a whole, as happens with unemployed and divorced people. From this viewpoint would result the concept of anomic suicide (low social regulation), to which three other types would be joined: egoistic suicide, as in those who were depressed (low social integration), altruistic suicide, as in the case of the Hindu widowers who practiced sati in India, that was declared illegal in 1892 and nowadays is still a rare occurrence in remote villages (high social integration), and fatalistic as happens with prisoners or individuals who are surrounded (high social regulation). More than a hundred years later, it is still, nowadays, a classic division, which the social and economic crisis of the beginning of the 21st century has revived, mainly when one mentions anomie and its relation to depression, hopelessness and despair. In fact, there is now a new anomie: hopelessness, dissatisfaction and bitterness facing the failed expectations of well-being. In many countries one is even confronted with the question of children having the possibility of a harsher life than their parents, which seemed unthinkable some time ago. However, one must recognize that even in the 1980s, some works had warned of the signs of a new anomie that would appear in the West later on, particularly in Europe, in a very clear way: unemployment, the rise in divorce, more women working out of their homes, the increase in the old-age population, higher addiction to alcohol, more homicides, and a decrease in religious practices (Sainsbury, Jenkins, & Levey, 1982).

With the development of sociological studies on suicide later in the 20th century, still before World War II, a compromise appeared, between the social variables and the dimensions of the psyche, to understand the phenomenon of suicide. This confluence came both from sociology and psychoanalysis. Therefore, it is possible to find references to suicide even of sociological origin, such as escapist, aggressive, religious or ludic, among others.

In terms of epidemiology, when one focuses on the last 25 years, one finds the huge impact of the fall of the Berlin Wall (1989) and the collapse of the Soviet Union (1991). These historical facts reveal a harsh reality: the high rates of suicide (deaths by suicide/100,000 inhabitants/year) above 30 in Lithuania, Russia and Belarus, and above 20 in Slovenia, Hungary, Estonia, Ukraine and Latvia. On the WHO world map of suicides, the countries with the highest rates >13 can be seen in red. And others appear there too: France, China, Japan, Sri Lanka, New Zealand, Uruguay. Ten years ago we described four types of suicide patterns: (1) an upward-sloping pattern (e.g., males, Hungary, Spain, Slovenia); (2) a downward-sloping pattern (e.g., Ireland, the UK, Albania); (3) a convex pattern (e.g., males, Lithuania, Finland, Romania); and (4) a uniform pattern (e.g., males, Norway). Albania was the only European country where a downward-sloping pattern was found for both males and females (Veiga & Saraiva, 2003).

In the specific case of Portugal, there is evidence of an upward-sloping pattern. Taking into account that it is a relatively small country, with 11 million inhabitants, it presents one of the most intriguing asymmetries in suicide rates. In the North, the rate is 3, in the South, the rate is 30. The global rate is around 10. The answer to such a discrepancy is both sociological and psychiatric. The profile of a suicidal individual is of a man over 45 years old, divorced or widowed, unemployed or retired, living in greater Lisbon or in the South, with a reduced income, low qualifications, depressed and alcoholic, with a previous history of suicide attempts, socially isolated, with multiple affection-related problems, frequently with other persistent organic diseases associated, with no religious practice, a melancholic personality, and scarce medical and social support. The most common suicide methods are hanging, shotgun, pesticide poisoning and jumping. The most critical period seems to obey a seasonable pattern, from May to July (Saraiva, 2006).

Brief aspects of the psychodynamic models before the era of neurobiology

An understanding and explanation of psychiatry through the neurobiological models emerged after World War II, with an emphasis on the Nordic countries and the USA. Previously, one had the force of dynamic models which always tried to find answers to the psyche of suicidal agents. *Mourning and Melancholy* by Sigmund Freud, published in 1917, in the middle of World War I, and *Beyond the Pleasure Principle*, published in 1920, are frequently referred to as starting points for the conceptualization of the death instinct (thanatos) as opposed to the sexual instinct (libido). This means that after Freud had acknowledged the existence of episodes of cruelty during the war, he started to give less importance to his theories of sexuality and to value other aspects as well. On the other hand, the idea of a sadistic superego and a masochist ego would later on appear in his work, *The Ego and the Id* (1923) where one can perceive the importance of guilt in suicidology.

Ten years after, during the so-called second psychoanalytic generation, there was a surge of interest by several authors who deepened the issue of suicide. Among them principally Karl Menninger, Melanie Klein, Gregory Zilboorg, Alfred Adler, Karen Horney, Erich Fromm, and Harry Stack Sullivan. Menninger would be linked to the theory of the three wishes, which would be applicable to all suicidal people: to kill, to be killed and to die. From the instinct of aggression to the wish to return to the maternal womb, going through masochist submission. Melanie Klein considers suicide as a selective attack on the bad part of the object in order to preserve the good part which would be valuable to the Self. Zilboorg values an ethno-cultural model of identification with the dead one in the process of mourning, which gives an impulse to the wish of a suicide for reunion. Adler refers to suicide as a failure, a sign of social pathology, of lack of social cooperation. Horney emphasizes suicide as the consequence of a neurotic personality due to childhood conflicts and lack of love. Fromm interpreted suicide as a result of the objectification of the human being within his/her pessimistic view of life. Sullivan refers to suicide as an act of hostility and aggression towards the inner and the outer side of the individual, like a message to the oncomers.

From the third psychoanalytic generation, more than thirty years later, authors like Donald Winnicott, Heinz Kohnut and Coimbra de Matos also refer to suicide. Winnicott (1971) values the relationship with one's mother as essential to the organization of one's ego and its consequent mechanisms of defense. Kohut (1977) stresses the absence of continuous empathy of the parents as a non-protective factor. Matos (1982) emphasizes the narcissistic vulnerability, intolerance to pain and loss, collapse of omnipotence, and the wish for fusion.

Importance of the cognitive model to the understanding of the suicidal ideation

For the cognitive model, the most important feature is the meaning that the individual attributes to life's events and to the environment. Thus, there is primarily a value given to subjectivity, of how emotions and feelings are lived and to which one responds this way or the other. Aaron T. Beck has been an unsurpassable investigator of this theme since the 1960s. From a variety of theories the author values, besides hopelessness, a cognitive triad, schemas and distortions. In the cognitive triad, there is a negative vision of the self, of the world and of the future (e.g., "I am worthless, I am a failure; the world outside is hostile and dangerous; I have no hope for the future"). In the schemas, there is the emergence of ideas, experiences and patterns of behavior and also of relatively stable beliefs which, in the face of certain adversities may not duly support the individual. In the distortions, errors of evaluation and interpretation occur, in the face of facts which may generate suffering and disturbed responses (e.g., arbitrary inference, catastrophization, maximizing the negative, dichotomous thinking). This last issue of dichotomous thinking is, indeed, very relevant, mainly in impulsive young people with a suicidal tendency. Sometimes, the absolute radicalization of black or white may trigger a serious suicidal behaviour. Such psychological insufficiencies reveal that it is necessary to teach people how to use the adequate psychological tools.

Hopelessness, as well as the pain of an intrinsic pessimism, represents an interesting construct, which is the origin of the Hopelessness Scale of Beck and colleagues, a useful working tool in the investigation of suicide and even in clinical practice (20 questions, maximum score = 20). Since the 1980s, diverse theories either from the research area of psychiatry or psychology have associated hopelessness with other variations such as diathesis (vulnerabilities), stress or even cognitive rigidity. This has allowed the establishment of a bridge to the strategies of coping in order to, for example, solve problems. Many of these patients will say that they are crushed by a threatening pile of problems. Under this cognitive-behaviorist approach, it makes sense that in the interview with a potential suicidal person, one can help build a hierarchy of problems as well as list the reasons for living and the reasons for dying.

Later, in the 1990s, Beck defined the Theory of Modes, establishing a more global vision of the suicidal ideation. Modes are formed by schemas related to memories, life experiences, ways of living, and problem solving. The construct encloses sub-organizations of the personality where one can find not only the cognitives, but also the affectives, the motivational, and the behavioral components (e.g., "My life has reached a dead end; nobody cares for me; I cannot cope with this pain any longer; they will be better off without me"). Therefore, training to understand the suicidal ideation, besides the cognitive approach and the value attributed to internal triggers (e.g., thoughts) and to external ones (e.g., circumstances) is important. The Theory of Modes was developed by Beck's colleagues, like David Rudd, in his Fluid Vulnerability Theory in 2006. From this theory, one can infer that the suicidal crises are limited in time and that their triggering factors are fluid and not static.

Williams et al. (1996; 2006) consider suicide to be a reaction against stress experienced by an individual in a situation that he/she considers a trap without escape, and that, at the same time, expresses hopelessness and the inability to solve problems. These authors also developed the overgeneralization theory, that is, a deficit of cheerful autobiographical memories of reasons to live in the face of empirical evidence of the occurrence of traumatic events both in childhood and adolescence.

The observation of the emotional dysregulation of the suicidal patients was inspirational to the works of Marsha Linehan in the 1990s in her view of her Dialectical Behavior Therapy. This is a model more oriented to borderline personality disorder. The self-injuries are interpreted as life-saving behaviors, however, denouncing a maladaptive coping. The main goals are working on the dialectical aspects of the mind and getting to know the aptitude deficit in the solution of problems. Two sub-systems were defined: environmental and behavioral. The former consists of supports and suicidal models; in the latter there are affective and cognitive elements. Therapy includes individual and group sessions.

More recently new theories and therapies have been presented to fight depression and suicidal ideation, some of them originating in cognitive-behaviorist therapy, such as the Mindfulness-based Cognitive Therapy (Segal, Williams, & Teasdale, 2002), and others of dynamic inspiration, exemplified in the Mentalization-based Treatment of Borderline Personality Disorders (Bateman & Fonagy, 2004) and in the Goal-directed Action Therapy (Valach, Michel, Young, & Dey, 2006). Another curious theory is the Interpersonal-Psychological Theory of Thomas Joiner (2005), which is particularly interesting because it revives some of Roy Baumeister's concepts (1990), such as guilt and identity. According to this theory there is a disconnection and isolation of the suicidal, a form of social alienation, which essentially results from three constructs: (1) the feeling of not belonging; (2) a feeling of being a burden to the family; and (3) the loss of the fear of death.

Therefore, these attempts to understand the suicidal mind as a whole help the psychotherapeutic strategies in order to reduce the frequency and intensity of negative emotions, reduce feelings of self-denigration and self-criticism, and better manage interpersonal situations.

Suicidal behaviors are multifaceted and multi-determined

Suicidal behaviors include not only concepts which are difficult to define but also borders which are complicated to establish. Really, we observe a big umbrella, from the suicidal ideation to the completed suicide going through the suicide attempt, from non-suicidal self-injury to automutilation. From a more neurobiological perspective it is known that at the epicenter of this set of behaviors one can find the brain or the body, or, under a more organic perspective, the mind. In fact, the conceptual complexity of mental schemas is dynamic, not static. Precisely because of that, a person feeling hopeless for a long time may, in a moment of despair, wish for two worlds simultaneously: to live and to die. He/she may transitorily overcome the fear of the unknown, but their supreme goal is to really stop suffering. It is very common that the cognitive ambivalence may provoke a lack of balance in the individual right to the end, just as Erwin Stengel highlighted 50 years ago through the example of the cry: "I want to die, do something for me!" This aspect becomes very important when contrasted with the Pre-Suicide Syndrome by Walter Poldinger from the 1960s, in which a third phase of serenity is conceptualized, one which preceded the suicide act, which would be something exceptional, from our point of view. From our own experience we have met frustrated suicidal patients who employed potentially lethal methods who, during the act or immediately thereafter, intensely grab at life.

Edwin Shneidman's cubic model is an ingenious conceptualization and a way of perceiving that there are multiple factors with an impact on the individual. A small cube of 125 (5x5x5) represents the confluence of a maximum of pain, disturbance and pressure (Shneidman, 1988). The inspiration for this model came from previous work in which the author pointed out essentially three levels of suicide intentionality, four levels of lethality and ten commonalities of suicide. In the intentionality he distinguished a conscious from an unconscious role and also accident. In lethality he admitted levels, from high (e.g., jumping from high places) to non-existent (e.g., aggression). The ten commonalities of suicide, the common psychological features in human self-destruction are:

i   The common purpose of suicide is to seek a solution.
ii   The common goal of suicide is cessation of consciousness.
iii   The common stimulus in suicide is intolerable pain.
iv   The common stressor in suicide is frustrated psychological needs.
v   The common emotion in suicide is hopelessness-helplessness.
vi   The common cognitive state in suicide is ambivalence.
vii   The common perceptual state in suicide is constriction.
viii   The common action in suicide is aggression.
ix   The common interpersonal act in suicide is communication of intention.
x   The common consistency in suicide is with lifelong coping patterns.

To sum up, this is a general and deep perspective of what suicide is about.

Another highly important feature, impulsivity, works like a trigger for the acting out. If one considers, together with this, a previous inoculation of the internality of the locus of control, to the detriment of externality, the occurrence of suicide is more likely to happen. This is due to the lower probability of chance, of fortune or bad luck being able to determine survival. In fact, from a classical point of view, and to make it simple, it is possible to admit that an action can lead to suicide if basically there are three conditions: lethality, feasibility, and intentionality. The first two are related to the choice of method and the probability of timely help and the last has to do with will, consciousness, memories. These previous considerations are substantially linked to the great works of the psychologist and thanatologist Shneidman, when he very briefly refers to the suicide scenario: psychological pain, loss of self-esteem, constriction of the mind, isolation, despair and egression. This last feature contains the only imagined gateway to stop the suffering of unbearable mental pain, the so-called "psychache."

Major depression and more

Nothing comes out of the void, therefore one refers to the suicidal process. There is always a narrative, a story to be told, sometimes the death of loved one, a divorce, a cancer, any other meaningful loss. In other episodes there is no explanation coming from the vital surge, as has happened with endogenous depressions. Credit must be given to the dynamic authors, namely those from the second psychoanalytic generation already mentioned, who talk or refer to the symbolism of suicide, for example, as a message for those who stay. When one goes deep into the study of the suicidal process, it is common to find several childhood and adolescence traumas or other painful life events, mainly physical, emotional, and sexual abuse, abandonment experiences, and continuous rejection by key persons in the young people who attempted suicide (Saraiva, 1999).

Some more vulnerable temperamental traits have been pointed out, besides the already mentioned impulsivity and low self-esteem: ambition, perfectionism and identity confusion (Orbach & Iohan-Barak, 2009). The impulsivity is genetically inscribed and is common in patients with borderline and anti-social disorders. Low self-esteem, difficult to measure, seems to portray a kind of vulnerability. The ambition towards a high aspiration, if it is not satisfied, may lead to suicide as an escape. Perfectionism is related to obsessive individuals in whom strictness is a feature, the difficulties of adapting to change are clearly visible and the threshold of frustration is low. There is still an approach to narcissists, individuals who do not tolerate day-to-day failure or criticism. They mix the tree with the forest and can interpret a below par day, any ordinary frustration as a personal defeat. That can be potentially very dangerous. Identity confusion is a highly complex aspect mainly connected with the Self of the borderline. A strained relationship not only with one's own image "in the mirror," but also with the other, with the world, with the future, impregnated with chronic feelings of emptiness, and others of rage, or unpredictable affections. It is all about a real inner disturbance which generates great suffering. To be borderline is to be embodied with a high depression risk of suicidal behavior.

Since the pioneer studies of psychological autopsies in the USA by Robins et al. (1959), there has been a disturbing belief that major depression, present in more than a half of suicides described in the majority of the studies, is just a mood disorder. As if it was not also a problem of rhythms, time, affections, pleasure. Besides depression, Shaffer et al. (1996) highlighted three other major dangers, mainly for young people: drug addiction, aggressiveness and loneliness. However, the rush to try and understand the nosographic picture of the patient, even when one is dealing with experienced professionals, together with the transversality of symptoms, dangerously ignores the validation of the narrative and that neither contributes to a better knowledge of the suicidal process nor to the building of the therapeutic alliance (Michel & Jobes, 2011). Therefore, it is essential to validate the suffering and a therapist who does not understand the importance of this aspect is not working within the basic therapeutic relation in suicidology.

Hopelessness, in good time brought by cognitivists to suicidology, seems to be a more relevant feature than depression itself, facing the nature and persistence of the construct. Principally in times of economic crisis, similar to what has been happening in the West at present, since 2008, hopelessness has acquired a huge social visibility. If there is a feeling of exclusion associated, without horizons or projects, it is not necessary to go deep into Durkheim's sociology to understand that the risk of suicide rises. Man is an animal who needs proximity, being touched, being looked at and if there is absence of caring or love, then he suffers. Everybody knows the higher susceptibility of men to the loss of income and social status, unemployment and work conflicts, and of women to affective loss, or conflicts within the family. But while the former group do not immediately look for help, dragging the situation on, sometimes drinking excessively or using self-medication, women activate mechanisms of help more quickly, be it within the family, with friends, religion or medical support.

The controversy of some decades ago about which was the highest risk of suicide, whether unipolarity or bipolarity, nowadays seems clear. It is more serious to be bipolar. These patients feel episodically mischaracterized, without the energy and hyperactivity given by the feelings of pleasure and power. Also from the clinical point of view, one knows the events that in the beginning may provoke the acting out. In hypomania what one finds is a hyposomnia which is not felt like discomfort, but like one more opportunity for action. Therefore, it is particularly important to supervise the bipolar depressive patients in the three to six months after hospital discharge. When one focuses on symptoms, there is one which belongs to the sphere of certain objectivity and which can easily be mentioned: insomnia. In the depressed patients it is one of the problems which generate more anguish. That is why one of the primary preoccupations of the therapists is to prescribe sleeping medicines. Sedation is important. Dawn activation can be a further risk. It has been known, since the 1950s, that about 10% of the severely depressed patients who were hospitalized commit suicides later. As previously mentioned, in the depressed patients, the preoccupation with nightly sedation has priority, according to our own experience of more than thirty years (Saraiva, 2006). Some means, whether antipsychotics, antidepressants or even anxiolytics, are efficient in these cases: clozapine, quetiapine, mirtazapine, trazodone, clonazepam, among others. This does not exactly exclude an antidepressant medication in a stronger association, in efficient therapeutic doses, among which the SSRIs (e.g., escitalopram, citalopram, fluoxetine, fluvoxamine, paroxetine, sertraline) and even antidepressants with a double action like the SNRIs, exemplified in duloxetine and venlafaxine. Noradrenergic and dopaminergic antidepressants (e.g., bupropion, reboxetine), even though capable of improving anedhonia, are frequently not indicated in suicidal cases because of the risk of pre-activation of the bettering of mood. At present, it is unusual to use tricyclic antidepressants (e.g., amitriptiline, clomipramine) owing to the risk of toxicity and lethal effect in overdoses, principally with impulsive patients. The classic neuroleptics (e.g., chlorpromazine, flupenthixol, haloperidol, pimozide) are still indicated in special circumstances. Meanwhile the atypical antipsychotics (e.g., asenapine, aripiprazol, clozapine, olanzapine, paliperidone, quetiapine, risperidone, sertindol, ziprasidone, zotiapine), in spite of the risk of metabolic syndrome, obesity and hypersomnolence, came to be preferred owing to their better tolerability and lower risk of tardive dyskinesia, independent of comparisons of its efficiency. The neuroleptics and antipsychotics depot IM administered (e.g., haloperidol, flupenthixol, fluphenazine, risperidone, zuclopenthixol) have been found to be very useful in cases of difficult compliance, like some psychoses, bipolar depression type I, or even cases of borderline personality disorder. Mood stabilizers began to be used, not only the classic ones (e.g., carbamazepine, lamotrigine, lithium, valproate) but also the second generation antipsychotics with this new indication (e.g., asenapine, aripiprazol, olanzapine, quetiapine). In fact, it was known from clinical empirics that in bipolar rapid cycling patients, the undue and excessive use of antidepressants enhanced the cyclic episodes.

A curious speculation is due to the alleged ketamine immediate antidepressive effect after a single low dose administration, like a magic drug. This issue is highly controversial and needs more studies in order to know neurobiological pathways and to clarify the "synaptogenesis" hypothesis. In a brief historical note, from the 1950s onwards, and through the studies of post-mortem brains in the USA and the methodology of psychological autopsies more consistently implemented by Shneidman in the USA, it was possible to perceive the relevance of the depressive syndrome in the genesis of suicide. The suicide neurobiological model received new impact after the works carried out in Sweden by authors such as Marie Asberg and her colleagues in the 1970s in individuals who had survived suicidal attempts using violent methods. These investigations studied the cerebrospinal fluid of those patients and that allowed the postulation of the serotonergic model of suicide.

Later on it became clear that the brain regions reached by suicidality were not only restricted to the initial hypothesis from over 50 years ago which had to do with brainstem alterations, but also with the hippocampus, the hypothalamus, the amygdala, and the pre-frontal cortex.

With the development of neurosciences and genetics, more than three dozen candidate genes that may be involved in suicidality have been found until now. Among them, the most well-known and numerous are those of the serotonergic system (e.g., 5-HTT Gene, TPH1 Gene, TPH2 Gene, 5-HTR1A Gene, 5-HTRB Gene, 5-HTR2A Gene, 5-HTRC Gene, 5-HTR5A Gene). Other systems have been studied: noradrenergic, dopaminergic, gabaergic, glutamatergic, nitric oxid, neurotrophines. Among these, of particular interest is the deficit of BDNF (brain-derived neurotrophic factor) and the p75NTR Gene (p75 neurotrophine receptor). One is dealing with a fashionable research with surprising results every year which need to be replicated for a better consistency of the knowledge of the suicide genetics.

Other psychiatric disorders, besides major depression, have been reported as relevant to the phenomenon of suicide: schizophrenia, post traumatic stress disorder, addictions, including alcoholism, panic, anorexia, bulimia, among others. Once again, the methodology of psychological autopsies appears a means to determine the enlightenment of the suicidal process, its nosological and nosographic frames. Thus it will be easier to understand what happened in cases of equivocal deaths. In fact, there are a few questions to be answered: "What type of death? Why suicide? Why at that moment?" The aim is to decrease the number of undetermined deaths and bring suicide rates closer to reality. In terms of the European Union, Estonia and Portugal are among the countries with a higher register of undetermined deaths, higher than 10% of the total number of deaths. It is easy to verify that some of those deaths should have been registered as suicides. So, the closeness of forensic medicine to psychiatry and to public health is inevitable for a deeper knowledge of the suicidal process. From this collaboration one should also value psychopathologies and comorbidities. A depressed and alcoholic individual is a common association. A schizophrenic and addicted individual is also a common association. And so on.

In the particular case of schizophrenia, suicide is more frequent in the first years of the disorder, when facing the prominence of positive symptoms (e.g., delusions, hallucinations). When the syndrome evolves to the negative symptoms (e.g., affective flattening, apathy), the risk of suicide seems to diminish but one poses the question of the differential diagnosis with depression, a rather controversial theme. The suicidal methods of the schizophrenic individuals are usually violent, with a small margin for survival. The other anxiety disorders like post traumatic stress disorder and panic frequently cross paths with addictions, including alcohol and psychotropics abuse. One cannot also exclude a comorbidity with depression in the development of the suicidal process.

On the other hand, we know that many youth suicides occur at the interface with accident and it is precisely the psychological autopsy that will clarify the contours of that death. Did they leave any written message? Did they warn that they would enter a cloudy state of consciousness and that everything could happen? Were there similar episodes in the past? Obviously we are referring to suicidal behaviors with alteration of the state of consciousness, even completed suicides, some using violent methods (e.g., jumping, slashing of the throat), provoked not only by the abuse of illegal substances but also by legal substances sold in smartshops, amphetamines-type, psilocibine-type, mescaline-type, of which some examples are salvia, magic mushrooms, bath salts and a dangerous fertilizer, mephedrone, with potential for causing delusions, hallucinations and delirium. This issue with the smartshops is now triggering a heated debate over the conflict between the legality of certain commercial interests and harmful effects to the public health.

Final considerations

The key to the treatment of the suicidal ideation cannot be based only on psychotropics. It is not possible to understand utopia taken to the absurd that if one put lithium in the drinking water or administered SSRIs or clozapine to the population indiscriminately, one would solve the problem of suicide. Or still the possibility of applying electroconvulsive therapy to people with suicidal ideation and planning suicide.

A systemic perspective about people must be valued, by developing supporting mechanisms, diminishing tensions, lowering the emotional over-involvement and the hypercriticism of the expressed emotion (Santos, Saraiva, & Sousa, 2009). The question of family is very important. It is healthy to have an exchange of affection and not excessive cohesion to allow individualization and respect. Escapes from stress are needed, such as hobbies, sports, socialization, traveling. Therefore, it is necessary to create an affective proximity and to create alternatives. This aspect goes beyond the framework of medical sciences and is related to social sciences, also to political power, with the fight against social exclusion, isolation, unemployment, poverty, because despair is always lurking.

From another perspective, training in suicidology is essential, especially for general practitioners, in order that they may recognize early warning signs. Attention to visible behavior, to posture, to isolation, to attitudes. For example, giving away valuable objects and written messages to relatives or friends, like suicide notes. One of the principal myths is to think that someone who declares he/she will commit suicide will not do it. Three in every four suicidal individuals warned of their intention beforehand, in an explicit or metaphoric way. One should also pay special attention to the screening of suicidal ideas in specific high risk groups (addictive substances abusers, including alcoholics, police officers or even the military during or after a war). The suicidal individual is always a sufferer. Rare cases of suicide in public places, episodically reported by the media, frequently relate to revolt with a political meaning, as in Tibet, Tunisia, and recently Greece.

It is also necessary to intervene efficiently and early in the issue of prevention. The SOS centres, beyond all doubt efficient in the lowering of suicide rates, have an important role in the fight against loneliness, anguish and despair. This model exists almost all over the world, with a meritorious work. Churches, because of their vocation to promote religion and spirituality, are of great relevance. On the Internet, some regulation of pro-suicide sites should be attempted, as well as the creation of more pro-life sites. In schools a more consistent and specialized presence of psychologists with knowledge of suicidology should exist. In the media self-regulation should be established, according to the WHO methods of "how to release suicide news." This way, sensationalism could be controlled, as well as the revealing of disturbing details, sometimes as front-page news, in order to avoid the Werther effect (Phillips, 1974). If necessary, more legislation should be issued, in a more prohibitionist attitude.

To decrease the probability of death through the use of certain suicide methods, there should be efficient regulation of the commercialization and storage of pesticides, restriction on the acquisition of guns, installation of barriers or fences in high places, among others. Also particular attention must be paid to survivors in a mourning process after the suicide of a relative or friend. Frequently those people are vulnerable and suffering, mainly on certain key dates (Werlang & Botega, 2004). One has to be alert. The aim is to develop the idea of a project and continue to any possible horizon.

References

Bateman, A. W., & Fonagy, P. (2004). Mentalization-based treatment of BPD. *Journal of Personality Disorders, 18,* 36–51.

Baumeister, R. (1990). Suicide as escape from self. *Psychological Review, 97,* 90–91.

Beck, A. T. (1996). Beyond belief: A theory of modes, personality and psychopathology. In P. M. Salkovskis (Ed.), *Frontiers of Cognitive Therapy* (pp. 1–25). New York: Guilford Press.

Beck, A. T., Weissman, A., Lester, D., & Trexler, L. (1974). The measurement of pessimism: The Hopelessness Scale. *Journal of Consulting and Clinical Psychology, 42,* 861–865.

Durkheim, E. (1897). *Le Suicide.* Paris: Alcan.

Joiner, T. (2005). *Why people die by suicide.* Cambridge, MA: Harvard University Press.

Kohut, H. (1977). *The restoration of the self.* New York: International University Press.

Linehan, M. (1993). *Cognitive behavioral treatment of borderline personality disorder.* New York: Guilford Press.

Matos, C. (1982). Razões da Morte. Morte da Razão – Abordagem psicanalítica do suicídio. *Jornal do Médico, 110,* 1994.

Michel, K., & Jobes, D. A. (2011). *Building a therapeutic alliance with the suicidal patient.* Washington, DC: American Psychological Association.

Orbach, I., & Iohan-Barak, M. (2009). Psychopathology and risk factors for suicide in the young: Theoretical and empirical. In D. Wasserman & C. Wasserman (Eds.), *Oxford textbook of suicidology and suicide prevention: A global perspective* (pp. 633–641). Oxford: Oxford University Press.

Phillips, D. (1974). The influence of suggestion on suicide: Substantive and theoretical implications of the Werther effect. *American Sociological Review, 39,* 340–354.

Poldinger, W. (1969). *Die Abschatzung der Suizidalität.* Bern: Huber.

Robins, E., Murphy, G., Wilkinson, J., Gassner, S., & Kayes, J. (1959). Some clinical considerations in the prevention of suicide based on a study of a 134 successful suicides. *American Journal of Public Health, 49,* 888–899.

Rudd, M. D. (2006). Fluid vulnerability theory: A cognitive approach to understanding the process of acute and chronic suicide risk. In P. T. Ellis (Ed.), *Cognition and suicide.* Washington, DC: American Psychological Association.

Sainsbury, P., Jenkins, J., & Levey, A. (1982). The social correlates of suicide in Europe. In R. Farmer & S. Hirsch (Eds.), *The suicide syndrome.* London: Croom Helm.

Santos, J. C., Saraiva, C. B., & Sousa, L. (2009). The role of expressed emotion, self-concept, coping, and depression in parasuicidal behavior: A follow-up study. *Archives of Suicide Research, 13,* 358–367.

Saraiva, C. B. (1999). *Para-Suicídio.* Coimbra: Quarteto.

Saraiva, C. B. (2006). *Estudos sobre o para-suicídio: O que leva os jovens a espreitar a morte.* Coimbra: EA.

Segal, Z. V., Williams, J. M. G., & Teasdale, (2002). *MBCT for depression: A new approach preventing relapse.* New York: Guilford Press.

Shaffer, D., Gould, M. S., Fischer, P., Trautman, P., Moreau, D., Kleinman, M., & Flory, M. (1996). Psychiatric diagnosis in child and adolescent suicide. *Archives of General Psychiatry, 53,* 339–348.

Shneidman, E. (1985). *Definition of suicide.* New York: Wiley.

Shneidman, E. (1987). A psychological approach to suicide. In G. R. Vandenbos & B. K. Bryant (Eds.), *Cataclysms, crises, and catastrophes: Psychology in action* (pp. 147–182). Washington, DC: American Psychological Association.

Shneidman, E. (1988). Some reflections of a founder. *Suicide and Life-threatening Behavior, 18*(1), 1–12.

Shneidman, E. (1992). A conspectus of the suicidal scenario. In R. W. Maris, A. L. Berman, J. T. Maltsberger & R. I. Yufit (Eds.), *Assessment and prediction of suicide* (pp. 50–64). New York: Guilford Press.

Stengel, E. (1964). *Suicide and attempted suicide.* Harmondsworth: Penguin Books.

Valach, L., Michel, K., Young, R. A., & Dey, P. (2006). Suicide attempts as social goal-directed systems of joint careers, projects and actions. *Suicide and Life-threatening Behavior, 36*(6): 651–660.

Veiga, F. A., & Saraiva, C. B. (2003). Age patterns of suicide: Identification and characterization of European clusters and trends. *Crisis, 24*(2), 56–67.

Werlang, B. G., & Botega, N. J. (2004). *Comportamento suicida.* Porto Alegre: Artmed.

Williams, J. M., Barnhoffer, T., & Crane, C. (2006). The role of overgeneral memory in suicidality. In T. E. Ellis (Ed.), *Cognition and suicide.* Washington, DC: American Psychological Association.

Williams, J. M., Ellis, N. C., Tyers, C., Healy, H., Rose, G., & MacLeod, A. K. (1996). The specificity of autobiographical memory and imagebility of the future. *Memory & Cognition, 24,* 116–125.

Winnicott, D. (1971). *Playing and reality.* New York: Penguin Books.

21

MOTIVATION, RESISTING, CONSIDERING AND ACCEPTING

A qualitative study investigating young adults' participation in an intervention group for people with recurrent suicide-related behaviours

Yvonne Bergmans, John Langley and Paul S. Links

Introduction

Recurrent suicide-related behaviour is associated with greater levels of psychopathology (Forman, Berk, Henriques, Brown, & Beck, 2004), increased risk of death by suicide (Beautrais, 2003) and can occur across a spectrum of mental illnesses (Oquendo, Baca-Garcia, Mann, & Giner, 2008; Nock, Hwang, Sampson et al., 2009). Perry, Fowler, Bailey et al. (2009) note that the transition away from suicide-related behaviours can take many years. There is a paucity of work exploring the challenges and benefits of group interventions for people with recurrent suicide attempts. It remains that there is "little precedent" for specialized group therapy targeting people with recurrent suicide attempts (Yalom & Leszcz, 2005, p. 478) and, yet, the power of group therapy has been shown time and again (Marziali, Munroe-Blum, McCleary, 1997; Yalom & Leszcz, 2005; Befort, Donnelly, Sullivan, Ellerbeck, & Perri, 2010). Group interventions for people who experience recurrent suicide-related behaviours are often targeted for a specific diagnostic group such as Dialectical Behaviour Therapy for people identified with Borderline Personality Disorder (Linehan, 1993) or depression in older adults (Heisel, Duberstein, Talbot, King, & Tu, 2009), each identifying efficacy yet, specifically targeting high risk suicide-related behaviours is not well delineated.

Missing elements throughout the suicidology literature are the voices of those who might still be experiencing suicide-related behaviours and the voices of people who have experienced recurrent suicide attempts (Lakeman & FitzGerald, 2008; Spirito, Boergers, & Donaldson, 2000). Studies of the process of transition away from suicide attempts do not discern people with recurrent attempts from those with ideation or single attempts (Paproski, 1997; Hoover & Paulson, 1999; Fergusson, Beautrais, & Horwood, 2003; Everall, Bostik, & Paulson, 2006; Bostik & Everall, 2007), nor have people who might be currently engaging in suicide-related behaviours been included in these studies.

Studies investigating young people's transitions away from suicide-related behaviours note that seeking help has been identified as a challenge. Everall, Bostik, et al. (2006) suggest that the experience of shame contributes to both keeping negative emotions a secret and keeping participants away from seeking help. Others have suggested that help-seeking behaviours have been viewed as a sign of weakness by young people who will attempt to minimize symptoms to appear "normal" (Wisdom, Clarke, & Green, 2006; Burke, Kerr, & McKeon, 2008; Gilchrist & Sullivan, 2006). More significantly, it has been reported that help-seeking is inhibited among those who think of ending their lives (Rudd, Joiner, & Rajab, 1995; Deane, Wilson, & Ciarrochi, 2001; Rickwood, Deane, Wilson, & Ciarrochi, 2005). Furthermore, Everall, Altrows, and Paulson's (2006) work identifies that social support is central to a young person's healing, and it is emotional processing that often contributes to an increased sense of agency and sense of control.

The PISA/SFSL intervention is a multimodal group intervention based on a model of suicide-related behaviour being related to the person's deficits in processing emotion, problem-solving and interpersonal relationships. The intervention focuses on support and education in the areas of personal safety, emotional literacy, interpersonal relationships, and problem solving. All participants identify having had recurrent (two or more) suicide attempts (Bergmans & Links, 2002; 2009). The intervention is for people who are 16 years or older who self-identify as having had two or more suicide attempts. Principles of the intervention include: validation of the struggle, hope, the client as "expert", solution talk, and realistic expectations (Bergmans & Links, 2002). The goal of the intervention is to reduce intensity, duration and frequency of crisis episodes through the development of identifying choice and control in situations where death is the primary perceived option. Choices are offered through particular skill development in emotional literacy, becoming aware of personal rights, and emotional de-escalation strategies in an attempt to keep oneself as safe as possible. The group is co-facilitated by a peer facilitator (someone who is a minimum of a year away from having participated in the groups; is still in active therapy; is identified as being 'stable' in terms of suicide-related behaviours); and licensed professionals from a health care discipline, along with graduate level students.

The intervention has previously reported a change in affective, cognitive and impulsivity factors known to be part of the challenges/deficits that people with recurrent suicide attempts encounter (Bergmans and Links, 2002; 2009). This chapter expands on previous findings on transitioning away from recurrent suicide attempts for young adults (Bergmans, Langley, Links, & Lavery, 2009). It re-examines more closely the experienced pathways within the intervention process that participants identified as being meaningful. The 2009 paper discussed the process of transition where participants related experiences from their experience of multiple interventions over time. This analysis focuses on the process as it related to this specific intervention. In this chapter, a suicide attempt is a "self-inflicted, potentially injurious behaviour with a nonfatal outcome for which there is evidence (either explicit or implicit) of intent to die. A suicide attempt may result in no injuries, injuries or death" (Silverman, Berman, Sanddal, O'Carroll, & Joiner, 2007, p. 273). Suicide-related behaviour is defined as "a self-inflicted, potentially injurious behaviour for which there is evidence (explicit or implicit) that the person intended at some undetermined or some known degree to kill himself/herself and can result in no injuries, injuries or death" (Silverman et al., 2007, p. 272).

Method

Sample

Participants were young adults who had been between 18 and 25 years of age at their initial assessment for admission into the intervention. Each participant had completed one 20-week cycle of the group intervention. Of 32 young adults who were eligible to participate, five had moved out of the province, two had died by suicide, six did not respond to attempted contact or could not be located. One individual with a serious drug addiction was excluded from the study because the person was judged too impaired to be interviewed. Nineteen participants were contacted through their previously identified preferred means of contact: 10 by letter through regular post, seven through e-mail, and two by telephone. Participants received a follow-up telephone call with a thorough description of the study and an invitation to participate and be interviewed based on their availability. Sixteen people who had completed the intervention between 6 months and 6 years prior to the interview agreed to participate. Two refused and one cancelled the interview and was subsequently unable to be contacted. Prior to the first qualitative interview, agreement to participate was confirmed and signed consent was obtained. Ethics approval was granted by the St. Michael's Hospital Research Ethics Review Board.

Data collection

Sixteen interviews were conducted by one of the principal investigators (YB) and lasted 45 minutes to 2 hours. Interviews followed a guide based on the recovery literature and the interviewer's experience with this population, and included themes of family, care-providers, experience of suicidality, interventions, etc. Interviews became more focused as themes became more evident. New areas of inquiry were introduced to participants only after discussion with the research team. The interview used a conversational style, and allowed participants to lead the discussion into the areas they identified as important (Patton, 2002).

Data analysis

This study is a secondary analysis of a Grounded Theory study investigating transitions from recurrent suicide attempts for people between the ages of 16 and 65 years. A fuller account of the initial study can be found in Bergmans, Langley, Links and Lavery (2009). In this analysis the experience of the process specific to the PISA/SFSL intervention is examined. The revisiting of the data in this analysis undertook a thematic analysis method chosen for its flexibility. The underpinning theoretical framework is that of essentialist/realism which allows for the reporting of experiences, meanings and the reality of participants (Braun & Clarke, 2006).

Interviews were audio-recorded, transcribed verbatim and checked for accuracy. Members of the research team, including clinical students and fellows, read each of the interviews and came together to discuss themes and patterns noted in each interview. This allowed for discussion and interpretation from varying viewpoints, given that the team consisted of representation from the disciplines of sociology, psychology, psychiatry and social work.

Results

Study participants included 14 women and 2 men. Table 21.1 describes basic sample characteristics, and Table 21.2 reflects the suicide history.

Time since completion of the intervention ranged from 6 months to 6 years (mean = 26.9 months; median-mode = 24 months). Eleven (68.7%) participants reported no suicide-related behaviour since completion of the intervention. The remaining participants identified a reduction in their suicide-related behaviours over time. There was no evidence to support a relationship between time since intervention completion and suicide-related behaviours.

Table 21.1 Sample characteristics at time of study interview

Age at time of study	M = 25.8 (SD = 3.4)
Marital Status: single	N = 15 (94%)
Employment: full or part time	N = 4 (25%)
High school completion and/or some post secondary	N = 9 (56%)
Living arrangements: Living at home	N = 4 (25%)
History of childhood maltreatment	N = 16 (100%)

Table 21.2 Suicide history of the participants

Age of first recalled thoughts of ending one's life	M = 12.9 (SD = 3.02)
Age of first attempt	M = 15.1 (SD = 2.67)
Number of attempts	M = 7.8 (SD = 7.46)

Entry to group: motivation

The experience of the process of the group intervention began with Entry in to the Group, followed by the experience of being in the intervention group and life after the intervention. Study participants attributed the motivation for participating in the group intervention to external or internal factors or a combination of both. The external factors included making a family member, friend, employer or care-provider happy or, feeling a sense of indebtedness that they make the effort. These were in an attempt to be seen as acceptable by the other person whether it be a family member, employer or therapist:"I owed it to her (therapist) to have tried" (part. 12).[1]

> Honestly, when they gave me that list, I'm, like, fine, I'll go through the motions, I'll do what they want me to do so I can get back to work.
>
> *(part. 10)*

> When I was doing it for other people, it was because I wanted them to be happy . . . cause I thought that's what they wanted.
>
> *(part. 9)*

For some, the combination of what another person said and their perception of such commentary served to motivate them to participate: "she [mom] said if I didn't get help, then she was going to get me locked up" (part. 15).

The internal factors identified by study participants were related to an unfavourable perception of themselves or their lives: all contained high degrees of negative self-evaluation "incompetent" (part. 9), "worthless, of no value" (part. 13), "hurting, scared" (part. 4), "chaotic" (part. 14; 7; 11), "living in a zone" with no connection to self or other (part. 3).

Study participants were also motivated by their perception of how others might view them. Each term carried pejorative and stigmatizing projections of themselves. They identified not wanting to be seen by others as: "crazy" (part. 3), a "freak" (part. 10), "just nuts" (part. 4), or "I didn't want to look like a basket-case" (part. 16).

The coping strategy that participants discussed using to move through their daily lives and into the initial phase of joining the group was wearing a "mask" to avoid rejection or deal with their fears: "I couldn't wear my mask down because I was afraid that I was going to be rejected and unloved again" (part. 3); "a million different masks . . . to hide myself . . . that something was wrong with me and I didn't know what" (part. 16). The "masks" of protection and suspicion entered into the group room and remained throughout the initial weeks of group participation.

Attending the group: resisting, considering and accepting

Resisting

Many participants identified feeling anger throughout the initial stage of group. This anger was identified by many as stemming out of an internalized belief that the group intervention was not going to, could not, or should not work for them, and for some, it was compounded by the attitude that group facilitators were less than optimal: "I had to probably hear it [personal rights and ability to tolerate emotions] like at least sixty thousand times before I even considered you guys weren't just being jerks" (part. 4), ". . . first time I used them [skills] like 'they're crazy, they don't know what they're talking about'" (part. 10). Some participants identified taking a "one step removed" position, or going through the motions for an outside "gain" or seeing that what was being discussed might be useful for others and not for them:

> I didn't really believe that I could change . . . I went because of my conscience . . . I was, like, "yeah, I can see how that would be useful" before I would be around to use them, [skills] which at that point I really didn't think I was going to be, so it was kind of, like, "nice idea".
>
> *(part. 12)*

> Oh, yeah, I'm just going to go and do this so that they'll let me work.
>
> *(part. 10)*

Considering

"Considering" that the intervention might hold some value evolved through the interplay of the attitudes of facilitators, the wisdom and experiences of peer facilitators, and being with others with similar struggles. A key component clearly articulated by a participant was that facilitators: "be open to them, accept them for who they are and what they're saying, believe them. Let them know that they're believed" (part. 3).

The peer facilitators, graduates of the program at least two years further along in their journey, were recognized as having "had the same kind of experiences . . . I think that actually gave me some hope to start on" (part. 10). Peer facilitators were instrumental in their ability to "translate" and articulate concepts and skills into living practice, "nice to hear somebody say . . . 'well, this is how it worked for me'" (part. 10).

Considering also involved seeing oneself, perhaps for the first time, through the pain of another, "it was too real, too much all at once, I was overwhelmed and at the same time kind of relieved because it meant that I wasn't crazy, it meant that I wasn't different" (part. 16).

Considering one's own experience and witnessing the perspective of another also held some impact:

> We weren't diagnostically bounded, you know, which diagnosis it was . . . I thought that was good too, actually. . . having a mixed group kind of helps, at least, like, it helped me come out of my own brain a little bit . . . made me, like, wonder about other people and different experiences and other problems, and it kind of, like, gave

me a teeny, teeny bit of distance from my own, and also the whole thing, like, I wasn't all on my own.

(part. 4)

People who had it a lot worse than I did were smiling.

(part. 2)

Accepting and engaging

Accepting and engaging refers to the stage when participants begin to see themselves, their abilities, and potentially their lives from a different perspective. It is in this stage that participants become engaged in the group intervention and consider the possibilities of what the group intervention might do for them. While latching on to concepts or a particular strategy, the sense of inclusion and actively engaging with a concept or strategy/skill was articulated by all of the study participants. The particulars differ for each participant:

The first thing that I latched onto was the whole idea that I had personal rights, and I remember the first time I went through the session, the whole deal with me was the fact that I had them.

(part. 4)

The main thing is the array of choices that you guys presented, . . . but for me it was the volume of choices that finally convinced me that I did have one . . . once you have like an entire buffet table . . . you can't still say you have no choices, you can say you don't like any of them, but (laughing) you can't say they're not there.

(part. 4)

When I was back at your group, I didn't feel that I could ask for help because I didn't feel I was worth of any help.

(part. 3)

Instead of like an outcast, I felt . . . like I belonged somewhere at the time I didn't know where and I still don't completely know where but I do belong somewhere.

(part. 2)

This is a safe environment for all and everybody has a right to feel safe here and just the fact that I felt that inclusion.

(part. 8)

Actively engaging in the intervention went beyond being part of the intervention group, it also led to engaging with the possibility that life might be possible: "making the choice to live is going against everything, you know, I've told myself for eight or nine ten years" (part. 13). "I wasn't self-injuring every day and I was, like, 'oh, well, maybe this stuff is going to work'" (part. 10).

There were participants who had little memory of the specific PISA/SFSL group and others who had to return a few time before they were able to complete the group. For these participants, motivation may have been curtailed by internal factors or by poor facilitator/member dynamics:

I wasn't ready to come face to face with it . . . if you put me face to face with the facilitators of that I wouldn't remember them, I can't, like that's a blur to me, but I do remember that there was a lot of chaos in that group between the people and the clients and the facilitators. I didn't, it could have just been chaos in me but it felt in the group that there wasn't really direction.

(part. 1)

After the group: continuing the journey: skills, awareness and hope

Study participants identified the development of skills, awareness and hope. While hope may have been instilled, and skills may have been learned, they may not have been utilized or fully believed until well after finishing the group intervention.

Obviously that I got something out of here and I wouldn't have made it, I wouldn't have come back if there didn't, if there wasn't something that clicked, that I kept coming back, so there was something that came that attracted me to come back so . . . obviously if there was something that was important said in the group that held my interest or held my or held me there to believe that something is going to change.

(part. 3)

Okay, there's all these, like, techniques and these tools and things like that, um, that even though I had a very hard time applying at the time, I guess, it is kind of made me feel better (laughing) to know that there was, there was a whole bunch of things that I could do when I'm ready (laughing).

(part. 11)

Many participants indicated the concepts and skills had continued to be a presence in their lives, and for some, full application or understanding might be "scattered" (part. 8) some years later. One participant noted, that although introduced and discussed in the PISA/SFSL group, it was only six years and many therapeutic interventions later that: "like, one of the last things that I knew, like, one of those major things I was beginning to understand is that I don't deserve to be treated like crap on a regular basis" (part. 11).

Discussion

The group intervention for individuals who have experienced recurrent suicide attempts was identified by young group participants as having a role in their journey of transitioning away from recurrent suicide attempts. Study participants were able to engage in and tolerate the group process. Most were able to eloquently describe and articulate the journey through the PISA/SFSL intervention group.

Participation in the intervention was seen by these 16 individuals to be motivated by internal and external factors. Fear of consequences if they did not participate played a significant role for many; fear of being "locked up", fear of being perceived as "crazy" or fear that they would not be seen as acceptable. The coping strategy identified by the majority of the participants was to wear "masks" in order to move through their worlds, hoping to prevent someone finding out "there's something wrong with me." This points to the internalized and social stigma surrounding perceptions of being "different", perceptions of mental illness, perceptions of suicide-related behaviours. This fear and/or previous experience of potentially stigmatizing actions against or toward them resulted in the majority arriving to the group intervention wearing those masks, and for some it was the mask of anger, for others, the mask of resistance.

Resistance was identified as the consideration that the facilitation team were "jerks" and/or an internal belief that "this" wasn't going to work. As the group is in its initial formation, facilitators need to be cognizant of this resistance born out of a fear, and for many, the experience of rejection or being perceived as "less than". This would suggest that when working with this client population, the group facilitator plays a pivotal role in creating, at the start of the group intervention, a place of safety and inclusion.

Through the progression of group, seeing the possibility that there may be some value to participation began to occur through presentation of some of the concepts and/or skill utilization. The key was that it had to resonate for the individual, thus returning to the belief that the content has to hold meaning for participants in order for them to consider that it might have some value. Albeit cautiously, accepting themselves as participants in the group and being active group members occurred after participants had passed through their resistance and considered how things might be different for them. This in turn instilled some level of hope that things might have the potential of being different; believing oneself to be capable and competent; being worthy of respect and caring. The installation of hope and each participant's comment on the sense of belonging and inclusion, ascribe to the curative factors of group: universality and instillation of hope as noted by Yalom and Leszcz (2005). When considering Everall et al.'s (2006) finding that social support is central to a young person's healing, perhaps a significant feature of the PISA/SFSL intervention is that it creates a place of belonging and commonality. Furthermore, it could be interpreted that the focus on emotional literacy is concordant with Everall et al.'s (2006) suggestion that it is emotional processing that often contributes to an increased sense of agency and sense of control.

Once completing the PISA/SFSL intervention, the journey toward life continued for all. Named challenges included remembering and utilizing concepts and skills. Remembering one's right to live and be respected with self-awareness, insight, and further skill development occurred through further therapeutic interventions whether they were individual or group therapy.

Clinical implications

Group intervention can be an effective model for this population with the recognition that, as Yalom and Leszcz (2005) point out, the therapeutic factors of universality, hope, and acceptance may be the most important therapeutic factors at the initial stages of group. Over time, cohesion allows for more interpersonal learning and self-understanding. In the same way that clients are being coached to "tolerate the distress" (Linehan, 1993), facilitators need to "tolerate the distress" as participants move through their journey. When young adults enter into the group, they are fearful, participate for reasons which may be unclear to them at the time, believe they are incapable of making changes, and perceive themselves as failures. Supporting the literature noted earlier, the first hurdle for the participants in this study was to come to the group. They supported previously noted evidence that "looking normal" holds great meaning and this in turn promotes the wearing of masks in order to cope. The clinician could then anticipate resistance through either behaviour or 'masks' in the initial stages of group. It is the clinician's role to invite and encourage the mutual creation of an environment that balances these expressions of fear and unworthiness with acceptance, belief, and readily utilizable skills and concepts that hold meaning for participants. It is also important to recognize that the fear of seeing oneself in another participant could be comforting and/or frightening. This warrants the potential discomfort of being identified during the initial assessment interview with the client so there is some forewarning.

A key skill for clinicians is to "translate" the behaviours in the room to the emotional content driving those behaviours. This includes developing a common language; being aware of non-verbal language occurring for participants; teaching the words that more accurately describe the feelings and differentiating 'suicide' as a behaviour that may be driven by emotions and thoughts. It is also key for clinicians to acknowledge their own fears through regular supervision and to recognize that the use of the word 'suicide' does not always mean suicide is the foregone conclusive outcome.

Motivation, resisting, considering and accepting were the psychological processes that appeared to be at play for these participants. By virtue of some participants identifying they either did not remember or were not able to use the skills used at the time they were group participants suggests that considering, accepting and using what was learned does take time as the journey of life continues for these young people.

Limitations

The sampling frame in this study was limited, thus, the findings may be limited to this group only. Steps were taken to ensure the findings of this study were reflective of participant experiences. Experienced clinicians played a significant role through all of the stages of data collection and analysis. Participants and the Community Advisory Panel members had the opportunity to examine and provide input on our evolving model as it progressed. Future studies could compare responses from a group for others considered to be a high risk population to respondents from the PISA/SFSL groups. It would be important to invite participants from other PISA/SFSL groups to participate in a similar study to discern if the above findings hold, particularly with groups outside of the greater Toronto area and with facilitators who were not part of the initial creation of the intervention. The same could be said, if resources are available, to have an interviewer who is not familiar with the intervention. Similarly it would interesting to include participants over the age of 25years to identify if they experience the same progression through a group for people with recurrent suicide-related behaviours. It is unknown how the results might differ had there been more participants, given that only 50% of those under the age of 25 years who had graduated the program participated in the study. More male participants would also have been preferable. Had participants who chose not to participate given feedback for their reasons for not participating, it would have further enriched these findings. It could be said that participant bias would be a key issue in this study. If we are to work with people from their experience and with what they bring to intervention, working with their bias contributes to further evolution of intervention. This bias helps to create a balance to ensure intervention is client-centred and content that holds meaning for participants.

This study resulted out of a pilot study of the PISA/SFSL groups and provides a small first step. Ultimately, the value of the model will be determined by the reader/clinician who finds a new appreciation for the issues discussed in this chapter (Polkinghorne, 2006) and the extent to which our findings provide useful direction in clinical practice.

Conclusion

The young people in this study identified that a group specifically created for people with recurrent suicide attempts can play a significant role in the transition away from recurrent suicide attempts. Entering into a group intervention, as reported by participants in this study, is a mammoth task. It means publicly acknowledging to someone else and strangers, that a person has engaged in trying to end their lives. It is an "outing" to strangers that is the first risk many will take to trying to learn to live life more safely, hence self-guardedness and protection may be the presenting mask. Motivation, resisting, considering and accepting were the psychological

Stage of Group	Psychologial Feature	Contributing Factors

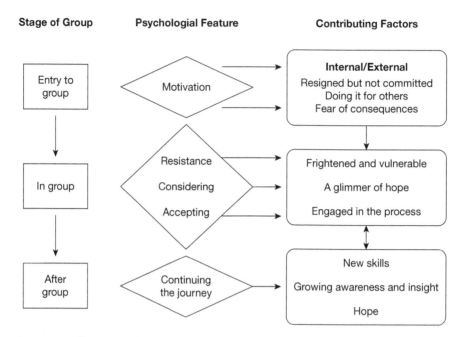

Figure 21.1 The journey through group and beyond

processes that appeared to be in play for these participants while they were participants. This is not to say they accepted everything that was offered or discussed. The 16 participants each had unique skills or awareness they took away with them. This serves to remind clinicians that just because we say something repeatedly, it does not mean it is being taken in, understood and/or remembered. The PISA/SFSL group is one step along the journey to healing (Figure 21.1). It is important that we continue to offer and investigate interventions for this high risk population. Their lives may depend on it.

Acknowledgements

We would like to thank Dr. Jim Lavery for his contributions to earlier drafts of this chapter.

Note

1 Part. = participant.

References

Beautrais, A. L. (2003). Subsequent mortality in medically serious suicide attempts: A 5 year follow-up. *Australian and New Zealand Journal of Psychiatry, 37*, 595–599.

Befort, C. A., Donnelly, J. E., Sullivan, D. K., Ellerbeck, E. F., & Perri, M. G. (2010). Group versus individual phone-based obesity treatment for rural women. *Eating Behaviors 11*, 17.

Bergmans, Y., Langley, J., Links, P. S., & Lavery, J. V. (2009). The perspectives of young adults on recovery from repeated suicide-related behavior. *Crisis: The Journal of Crisis Intervention and Suicide Prevention, 30*, 120–127.

Bergmans, Y., & Links, P. S. (2002). A description of a psychosocial/psychoeducational intervention for persons with recurrent suicide attempts. *Crisis: The Journal of Crisis Intervention and Suicide Prevention, 23*, 156–160.

Bergmans, Y., & Links, P. S. (2009). Reducing potential risk factors for suicide-related behavior with a group intervention for clients with recurrent suicide-related behavior. *Annals of Clinical Psychiatry, 21,* 17–25.

Bostik, K. E., & Everall, R. D. (2007). Healing from suicide: Adolescent perceptions of attachment relationships. *British Journal of Guidance & Counselling, 35,* 79–96.

Braun, V., & Clarke, V. (2006). Using thematic analysis in psychology. *Qualitative Research in Psychology, 3*(2), 77–101.

Burke, S., Kerr, R., & McKeon, P. (2008). Male secondary school students' attitudes towards using mental health services. *Irish Journal of Psychological Medicine, 25,* 52–56.

Deane, F. P., Wilson, C. J., & Ciarrochi, J. (2001). Suicidal ideation and help negation: Not just hopelessness or prior help. *Journal of Clinical Psychology, 57,* 901–914.

Everall, R. D., Altrows, K. J., & Paulson, B. L. (2006). Creating a future: A study of resilience in suicidal female adolescents. *Journal of Counseling and Development, 84,* 461–471.

Everall, R. D., Bostik, K. E., & Paulson, B. L. (2006). Being in the safety zone: Emotional experiences of suicidal adolescents and emerging adults. *Journal of Adolescent Research, 21,* 370–392.

Fergusson, D. M., Beautrais, A. L., & Horwood, L. J. (2003). Vulnerability and resiliency to suicidal behaviours in young people. *Psychological Medicine, 33,* 61–73.

Forman, E. M., Berk, M. S., Henriques, G. R., Brown, G. K., & Beck, A. T. (2004). History of multiple suicide attempts as a behavioral marker of severe psychopathology. *American Journal of Psychiatry, 161,* 437–443.

Gilchrist, H., & Sullivan, G. (2006). Barriers to help-seeking in young people: Community beliefs about youth suicide. *Australian Social Work, 59,* 73–85.

Heisel, M. J., Duberstein, P. R., Talbot, N. L., King, D. A., & Tu, X. M. (2009). Adapting interpersonal psychotherapy for older adults at risk for suicide: Preliminary findings. *Professional Psychology: Research and Practice, 40,* 156–164.

Hoover, M. A., & Paulson, B. L. (1999). Suicidal no longer. *Canadian Journal of Counselling, 33,* 227–245.

Lakeman, R., & FitzGerald, M. (2008). How people live with or get over being suicidal: A review of qualitative studies. *Journal of Advanced Nursing, 64,* 114–126.

Linehan, M. (1993). *Cognitive-behavioral treatment of borderline personality disorder.* New York: The Guilford Press.

Marziali, E., Munroe-Blum, H., & McCleary, L. (1997). The contribution of group cohesion and group alliance to the outcome of group psychotherapy. *International Journal of Group Psychotherapy, 47,* 475–497.

Nock, M. K., Hwang I., Sampson, N., Kessler, R.C., Angermeyer, M., Beautrais, A., et al. (2009). Cross-national analysis of the associations among mental disorders and suicidal behavior: Findings from the WHO world mental health surveys. *PLoS Medicine* 6(8) e1000123. Available at: http://www.plosmedicine.org/article/info%3Adoi%2F10.1371%2Fjournal.pmed.1000123 (accessed 18 November 2009).

Oquendo, M. A., Baca-Garcia, E., Mann, J. J., & Giner, J. (2008). Issues for DSM-V: Suicidal behavior as a separate diagnosis on a separate axis. *American Journal of Psychiatry, 165,* 1383–1384.

Paproski, D. L. (1997). Healing experiences of British Columbia First Nations women: Moving beyond suicidal ideation and intention. *Canadian Journal of Community Mental Health, 16,* 69–89.

Patton, M. Q. (2002). *Qualitative research and evaluation methods* (3rd ed.). Thousand Oaks, CA: Sage Publications, Inc.

Perry, C. J., Fowler, J. C., Bailey, A., Clemence, A. J., Plakun, E. M., Zheutlin, B., et al. (2009). Improvement and recovery from suicidal and self-destructive phenomena in treatment-refractory disorders. *The Journal of Nervous and Mental Disease, 197,* 28–34.

Polkinghorne, D. E. (2006). An agenda for the second generation of qualitative studies. *International Journal of Qualitative Studies on Health and Well-Being, 1,* 68–77.

Rickwood, D., Deane, F. P., Wilson, C. J., & Ciarrochi, J. (2005). Young people's help-seeking for mental health problems. *Australian e-Journal for the Advancement of Mental Health, 4*(3). Available http://www.auseinet.com/journal/vol4iss3suppl/rickwood.pdf (accessed 2 February 2009).

Rudd, M. D., Joiner, T. E., & Rajab, M. H. (1995). Help negation after acute suicidal crisis. *Journal of Consulting and Clinical Psychology, 63,* 499–503.

Silverman, M. M., Berman, A. L., Sanddal, N. D., O'Carroll, P. W., Joiner, T. E., Jr. (2007). Rebuilding the Tower of Babel: A revised nomenclature for the study of suicide and suicidal behaviors: Part II: Suicide-related ideations, communications and behaviors. *Suicide and Life-threatening Behavior, 37,* 264–277.

Spirito, A., Boergers, J., & Donaldson, D. (2000). Adolescent suicide attempters: Post-attempt course and implications for treatment. *Clinical Psychology & Psychotherapy, 7,* 161–173.

Wisdom, J. P., Clarke, G. N., & Green, C. A. (2006). What teens want: Barriers to seeking care for depression. *Administration and Policy in Mental Health and Mental Health Services Research, 33,* 133–145.

Yalom, I. D., & Leszcz, M. (2005). *The theory and practice of group psychotherapy.* New York: Basic Books.

EDITORIAL COMMENTARY

Allied health professionals play a unique and vital role in clinical care and furtherance of clinical research. Allied health professionals (AHP) is a term that refers to a large group of health professionals that make up to 50–60% of the workforce in hospitals and clinics in the USA and Canada (University of California San Francisco, 2012; Association of Canadian Community Colleges, 2012). Due to their sheer numbers, AHPs are considered to be central to the delivery of health care around the world and are found working jointly with physicians, nurses and pharmacists in delivery of patient care. Definitions of allied health professions vary across countries and contexts, but generally indicate that they are health professions distinct from medicine, dentistry, optometry, and nursing (Arena, Goldberg, Ingersoll, Larsen, & Shelledy, 2011). Some definitions only include health care providers that require registration by law to practice, but usually all allied health professions require a post-secondary degree or higher qualifications. In the United States Code of Federal Regulations (CFR, Title 42: Public Health), allied health is defined by exclusion. The Allied Health Professional Development Fund (AHPDF) of Ontario, which provide grants for professional development opportunities lists the following AHP as eligible professions: Physiotherapists, Occupational therapists, Respiratory therapists, Audiologists, Speech-Language Pathologists, Dieticians, Medical Laboratory Technologists, Pharmacists, and Medical Radiation Technologists. They are involved in the delivery of health or related services pertaining to identification, evaluation and prevention of diseases and disorders, dietary and nutrition services, and health system managements. Ambulatory health care settings are by far the largest employer of allied health workers: almost half (49.4%) of all allied health workers are employed in ambulatory care, with 28.7% and 21.9% employed in hospital and nursing care, respectively (Help Wanted: Will California Miss Out on the Next Billion-Dollar Growth Industry?).

Each of the allied health professions is ethically accountable for bringing a theoretically sound and evidence-based approach to problem solving in health care (Arena et al., 2011). Although the allied health professions are diverse, there is a pervasive effort to establish and promote clinical research to develop and evaluate effective treatment methods which are evidence-based to support the quality, effectiveness, and efficiency of clinical practice across the professions (Kronenfeld, Stephenson, & Nail-Chiwetalu, 2007). All of the AHPs are making unique contributions to clinical research. Inasmuch as these disciplines are rooted in practice, their contributions to research are inherently clinical. This means that, at a macro level, clinical research in allied health is very much "applied" research.

While there is a developing research presence from the allied health professions, there is a disparity in the amount of research published across these professions. As Arena et al. (2011) indicated, a PubMed query conducted using allied health profession search terms for the years, 2006–2011 found more than 80,000 publications for nursing: however, only 45,623 publications by physical therapists and 6,250 publications authored by occupational therapists.

To ascertain the state of clinical knowledge related to suicide risk factors and effective treatments, Joe and Niedermeier (2008) conducted the first comprehensive study of social work's contribution to the suicide literature. Their findings reveal that despite recent increases to the study of suicide by social work researchers, they have contributed limited evidenced-based knowledge on the treatment or prevention of suicide or suicide-related behaviours in the two and half decades reviewed. Less than 8% of the total number of social work-related research studies published on suicide reported on effective interventions. Hence, one in every 13 of the studies that included suicide or suicide-related behaviour addressed development of effective interventions. The findings also reveal that most of the studies had significant methodological flaws (Joe & Niedermeier, 2008). Most of the reviewed intervention studies failed to accurately describe the elements that comprise the intervention and, thus, cannot be replicated. The low specificity used to measure change renders the findings questionable. Furthermore, some studies lacked control groups, did not have randomized participants or had small sample sizes, thus, the findings cannot be generalized (Joe & Niedermeier, 2008).

So while acknowledging the limited contributions thus far, the aim of Part IV is to help to remedy some of these gaps in the literature and illuminate the clinically focused research contributions of allied health professionals with suicidal clients. In their search for contributors the editors of this section conducted several extensive electronic and manual searches for suicide research published in peer-reviewed journals of social work and allied health professions in our pursuit of contributors related to clinical practice and effective interventions. Our literature search in Medline, PsychoINFO, Social Work Abstracts, CINAHL included the following terms: social work, psychiatric social work, allied health occupations, physiotherapy, occupational therapy, speech-language pathology, clergy, pastoral care, chaplaincy services, respiratory therapists in combination with the following key words suicide, suicide ideation, suicide attempts. We restricted our time frame search to work published between January 1995 and May 2012. We found 179 articles, 146 were published prior to 2000 and 33 articles were published between the years 2000–2005. Of these 33 articles found, authors declined contributing their work on clinical applications/research or were inappropriate for inclusion in this section of the book. It can be argued perhaps that the reluctance we experienced is suggestive of a wider level of interest; this might in part explain why the scholarly output of allied health professionals could withstand further development.

One of the greatest challenges to suicide prevention can be attributed to the paucity of empirical research – particularly clinically focused research. The paucity of empirical evidence applies to all allied professions working in the field of mental health. Research among all allied professions is often small-scale and self-funded. Many of the studies are done for post-graduate programmes rather than projects undertaken as part of coherent properly funded programmes of research that add new empirical theoretical and methodological knowledge.

Social workers are the largest occupational group of mental health professionals (Manderscheid et al., 2004); hence, they are well positioned to intervene with suicidal clients. However, overall, they lack the knowledge derived from well-controlled methodological rigorous studies to effectively implement evidence-based interventions with suicidal clients.

Clinical research in allied health has played a key cross-cutting role through collaboration. While the contributions are considerable, more can be achieved if identified barriers could be addressed. Principal barriers to the development of clinical research by allied health professionals lie in the area of training, mentoring, and funding. Moreover, many allied professionals have heavy caseloads or are restricted by the amount of work they have to accomplish in a day, leaving little time for research.

Little is known about factors necessary for effective intervention. More research is needed to determine the optimal components of successful interventions. Intervention studies that rectify the methodological limitations in earlier studies and provide evidence-based interventions are essential. Allied health research needs to develop empirical clinical knowledge which incorporates the distinctive concepts, viewpoints, and practices of their discipline to successfully intervene with suicidal clients. Allied health professionals need to be critically involved in clinical research to improve clinical practice, particularly when there are several accepted approaches to prevent, diagnose, treat, or monitor a given condition, and to develop practice guidelines (Sox, 2010). Clinical research can be used to demonstrate the augmented benefit of an allied health intervention to standard medical care.

So as a last note, we strongly encourage our colleagues and peers to make substantive contributions to this critical area of research and practice – there is certainly room for and a desire for such scholarly work.

References

Arena, R. A., Goldberg, L. R., Ingersoll, C. D., Larsen, D. S., & Shelledy, D. (2011). Research in the allied health professions: Why fund it? *Journal of Allied Health, 40*(3), 161–166.

Help Wanted: Will California Miss Out on the Next Billion-Dollar Growth Industry? Report, http://www.calhealthjobs.org. Retrieved 2012-12-19.

Joe, S., & Niedermeier, D. M. (2008). Social work research on African Americans and suicidal behavior. *Health and Social Work, 33*(4), 249–257.

Kronenfeld, M., Stephenson, P. L., & Nail-Chiwetalu, B. (2007). Review for librarians of evidence-based practice in nursing and the allied health professions in the United States. *Journal of Medical Library Association, 95*(4), 394–407.

Manderscheid, R. W., Atay, J. E., Male, A., et al. (2002). Highlights of organized mental health services in 2000 and major national and state trends. In R. W. Manderscheid & M. J. Henderson (Eds.), DHHS Pub. No. (SMA) 3938. Center for Mental Health Services: Mental Health, United States, Rockville, MD: Substance Abuse and Mental Health Services Administration; 2004.

Sox, H. C. (2010). Defining comparative effectiveness research: The importance of getting it right. *Medical Care, 48,* S7–S8.

University of California San Francisco, Advancing the Allied Health Professions. Futurehealth.ucsf.edu. http://www.futurehealth.ucsf.edu/Public/Center-Research/Home.aspx?pid=88 (accessed 19 Dec. 2012).

PART V

Suicide survivors

EDITORIAL INTRODUCTION

In his final and fourth poem from *The Four Quartets*, T. S. Eliot wrote, "We shall not cease from exploration / And the end of all our exploring / Will be to arrive where we started / And know the place for the first time", and these four lines describe well how the use of applied research (through the fulfilment of Eliot's suggestion that we will "know the place for the first time") can create a positive change for the human condition. All too often research studies are revisits to and updates on topics resulting in confirmation of original research by previous explorers of that subject. Part V represents an effort to promote a new generation of explorers to advance into the subject of bereavement following suicide. These new explorers do "know the place for the first time" because they are not burdened with an agenda or a need to protect a conclusion they have already made. They are new eyes studying the effects that a cause of death as historic as death itself (suicide) can create for humankind.

Melinda M. Moore and Joseph S. Munson have each contributed chapters on their research into Post Traumatic Growth following suicide. Munson studied the impact of client suicide on clinicians (Chapter 14 in this volume) and in Chapter 24 Melinda M. Moore studies the impact on those who have lost someone to suicide. The potential for growth to be an outcome from such a loss is an understudied area in the literature. These chapters provide the reader with new information with which to approach the bereaved and clinicians who serve the deceased. The title of Chapter 24, by Moore, "Can Good Come From Bad?" captures the essence of traumatic loss by suicide that has eluded so many. Moore had enlisted the field of Positive Psychology to explore for the first time new outcomes following suicidal losses that will be encouraging to the readers.

In Chapter 25, David Miers and his colleagues present research into parental bereavement (the population most often seeking services) following a child's suicide. The researchers identified the critical resources needed by parents to survive (and perhaps grow) from their loss. The findings of this research show benefits that can be predicted for parents that seek a clinical setting for help. The research provides clearer directions for clinicians who are working with parents of children who suicide, equipping them with the tools needed to survive the journey.

In Chapter 23, Tanetta Anderson delves into the impact suicide has on peer relations. Peers are often disenfranchised from the bereavement spectrum while paradoxically viewed as high risk for suicidal behavior following loss. Anderson describes both clinical and social implications for the peer survivors through her qualitative research. In this approach, the reader hears the voices of those who have had long-term challenges dealing with others who just do not understand their grief. This chapter lets us appreciate how the pain and sadness that go untreated can grow and deepen within anyone exposed to a peer who takes his or her life.

In Chapter 26, Chris P. Shields and his research group examine the qualitative characteristics of bereavement for mothers in Northern Ireland. The team systematically reviewed the qualitative aspects of suicide bereavement and then shifted their focus to mothers who are making meaning of their loss to suicide. As a complement to his chapter, I return to this theme and draw upon the report produced by a noted suicide prevention activist in Northern Ireland, Mr. Patrick McGreevy. I have used this for the basis of my commentary as the information provided by McGreevy is an overview of how applied research can be imported from innovative practices internationally to then create local programs and national reforms to reduce the impact of suicide in Northern Ireland. Accordingly, Shields et al.'s chapter and McGreevy's report (see Editorial Commentary on p. 326), enable the reader to see how the micro and macro can complement each other to change social interactions around bereavement following suicide.

Regina Aguirre and Laura Frank Terry report in Chapter 22 on the very successful launch of their Active Postvention Model (APM) known internationally as the LOSS Team (Local Outreach to Suicide Survivors). Included in the chapter are the impact on the community of survivors and the impact on LOSS Team members providing the needed service. The service area includes a large and complex set of jurisdictions in the state of Texas. The program is providing responses both rural and urban, to a sprawling and busy section of America between Dallas and Fort Worth.

22

THE LOSS TEAM:
AN IMPORTANT POSTVENTION
COMPONENT OF SUICIDE
PREVENTION

Results of a program evaluation

Regina T. P. Aguirre and Laura Frank Terry

Introduction

At least six (Andriessen, 2009) to ten people (Jordan & McMenamy, 2004) are left behind to grieve each suicide—though the bereaved by suicide, also termed suicide survivors, would note this is a gross underestimate. The excruciating effects of suicide on survivors is perhaps best illustrated by studies indicating that suicide survivors are often at increased risk for suicide themselves—between 2 and 10 times that of the general population (Qin, Agerbo, & Mortensen, 2002; Prigerson, 2003; Runeson & Åsberg, 2003; Kim et al., 2005). Given this statistic, it is easy to understand Shneidman's (1972) suggestion that postvention—activities that come after the suicide to alleviate its impact on those bereaved—both assists the bereaved in their grief process and serves as suicide prevention for the next generation. The most common form of postvention for suicide survivors is the suicide survivor support group (e.g. Cerel, Padgett, Conwell, & Reed, 2009) but there is often a long period—up to four-and-a-half years (Campbell, Cataldie, McIntosh, & Millet, 2004)—between the death and the survivor accessing these or other grief support services. Additionally, it is estimated that only 25% of survivors seek help (Dyregrov, 2002; Provini, Everett, & Pfeffer, 2000).

An approach to connecting survivors to services is the active postvention model (APM), often referred to as Local Outreach to Suicide Survivors (LOSS) Team, where volunteer team members—usually survivors of suicide themselves—meet with new survivors shortly after the death to provide support and referrals (Cerel & Campbell, 2008). However, there is a lack of research on the effectiveness of the APM (Aguirre & Slater, 2010). In an effort to assist survivors of suicide in the local community and expand the research on the APM, a LOSS Team program was developed in Tarrant County, Texas. The LOSS Team began serving the community in April 2011 and this chapter summarizes the results of the evaluation of its first year of programming.

Literature review: does the research support that suicide survivors are at an increased risk?

There is a growing body of evidence that some suicide survivors do develop suicidal ideation and many psychological autopsy studies reveal that people who have suicided have themselves been survivors of one or more loved one's suicides. For example, in a study of adolescent suicide survivors, Prigerson (2003) found that, compared to peers grieving a non-suicide loss, they were five times more likely to have suicidal ideations. Qin et al. (2002) found similar results in a study of suicide survivors of family members, finding that they had increased risk even after controlling for the respective families' history of mental illness. Finally, Runeson and Åsberg (2003) found that the suicide rate was significantly higher among relatives where the death was by suicide as opposed to some other cause of death.

Why might suicide survivors become suicidal?

The majority of the research on suicide survivors indicates that they face a more complicated bereavement than peers bereaved by other causes of death. These "complications" include increased risk of developing mental illness (e.g., post-traumatic stress disorder, anxiety, depression); self-blame, guilt and shame often magnified by social stigmatization of suicide and the unanswerable "Why?"; and relationship struggles (Campbell, 2001; Jordan, 2001; Mitchell, Gale, Garand, & Wesner, 2003; Runeson & Åsberg, 2003; Jordan & McMenamy, 2004; Kaslow & Aronson, 2004; Mitchell, Kim, Prigerson, & Mortimer, 2005; Parrish & Tunkle, 2005). But, the question remains: Why would those so deeply affected by a loved one's suicide consider the same fate for themselves and their loved ones?

There are many theories of why people die by suicide: two are of particular importance for understanding the suicide survivor's experience: (1) Baumeister's (1990) Escape Theory (Aguirre & Slater, 2010); and (2) the Interpersonal Theory of Suicide (ITS) (Van Orden et al., 2010). Baumeister's (1990) Escape Theory posits that suicide is the culmination of the struggle to escape an unbearable situation. After experiencing one or multiple stressful life events, a person develops hopelessness—often indicated in suicide (e.g., Goldsmith, Pellmar, Kleinman, & Bunney, 2002), resulting in a numbing of emotions. While attempting to cope with the unbearable pain from the situation, the person may try different ways of escaping, including alcohol and other substance use. If positive events do not occur and social supports do not intervene, the person may choose suicide as the ultimate escape (Baumeister, 1990). Applying the theory to suicide survivors, there are several negative life events for the survivor: (a) stress before the suicide occurred (e.g., relationship difficulties); (b) the suicide itself; (c) the funeral and settling the estate; and (d) the suicide survivor's grief process including feelings of stigma, shame, isolation, self-blame, and psychache—intolerable psychological pain (Shneidman, 1996; Aguirre & Slater, 2010, p. 530), like those indicated in Baumeister's (1990) theory.

The ITS (Van Orden et al., 2010) is another effective explanation of how being a suicide survivor may increase one's risk for suicide. According to ITS, there are three constructs that interact, resulting in risk. These are thwarted belongingness—loneliness and absence of reciprocal care; perceived burdensomeness—liability and self-hatred; and the acquired capability for suicide. Becoming a survivor of suicide creates the perfect storm. Though prior, the survivor may have had a healthy level of belongingness in social and familial networks, these supports may either withdraw or change in quality (Cerel, Jordan, & Duberstein, 2008). Begley and Quayle (2007) found that many survivors close themselves off from others due to an increased unease in social situations. Suicide is still a stigmatized death (Sudak, Maxim, & Carpenter, 2008) to which survivors often react with self-blame and perceive that others blame them (Jordan, 2008)—resulting in the liability and self-hatred dimensions of perceived burdensomeness. Finally, exposure to a loved one's suicidal behavior and eventual suicide may result in an acquired capability for suicide: "Exposure to others who have engaged in suicidal behavior may activate habituation to the fear of suicidal behavior, thus accounting for clustering of suicidal behavior as a byproduct of elevated acquired capability" (Van Orden et al., 2010, p. 587).

How might postvention be preventive?

Shneidman's understanding of the psychache that accompanies every suicide was likely what fueled his suggestion that postvention is prevention for the next generation (Shneidman, 1972). This suggestion acknowledges that suicide survivors inherit their suicided loved ones' psychache (Aguirre & Slater, 2010) as evidenced by the growing body of literature on suicide survivors' complicated bereavement. Suicide postvention activities may include grief support activities such as individual therapy and support groups for survivors; and outreach to survivors aimed at connecting them to the aforementioned grief support services through linkages with other survivors in the community who provide encouragement and support (APM). The primary benefit of postvention services is alleviating psychache and is an example of how grief support services may intervene in the suicide survivor's quest for escape from the intolerable situation fitting with Baumeister's theory (1990). A secondary benefit of the survivor support group and the outreach to new survivors by other survivors (APM) is engendering a feeling of belongingness among a cohort of survivors—addressing one of the three components in the ITS (Van Orden et al., 2010) and thus reducing risk for suicide.

Method

To evaluate the impact of the first year of the LOSS Team's existence in Tarrant County (TC), a program evaluation was conducted with approval from the Institutional Review Board. Phenomenology was used as the philosophical approach since the goal was to capture the lived experience (Moustakas, 1994) of the survivors, team members, and police staff in the LOSS Team process. A purposive sample was drawn for phenomenological interviews and included participants in the following categories: (1) survivors receiving a LOSS Team outreach; (2) survivors who linked to services in TC prior to the LOSS Team's establishment; (3) LOSS Team members; and (4) a counselor from one of the two police departments that refer to the LOSS Team.

The impact of the LOSS Team services delivered in TC was measured in two ways: (1) time elapsed between death and access of services—measured quantitatively through case notes of those receiving a LOSS Team contact; and (2) an examination of the role of the LOSS Team in the grief process—investigated through phenomenological interviews. Interviews with survivors focused on the grief process, others' reactions to the suicide, which services they were using, how and when they linked to those, and their perceptions of the LOSS Team. During interviews with survivors who linked to services in Tarrant County prior to the LOSS Team's establishment, an excerpt from a documentary explaining the LOSS Team and how it functions was shown to provide context for the question regarding perceptions of the LOSS Team. Interviews with team members and the police department representative focused on their perceptions of the LOSS Team's impact in the community. The second author conducted the interviews; she is not a member of the LOSS Team nor has she attended a LOSS Team training. These characteristics provided for an etic (outsider's) voice in collecting and analyzing data to reduce bias. Data were analyzed using a constant comparative approach and triangulation between the two authors over multiple sessions. The first author provided an emic (insider's) voice in data analysis since she has been extensively trained in LOSS Team procedures, was a volunteer at the Baton Rouge Crisis Intervention Center where the LOSS Team began, and is a co-founder of TC's LOSS Team.

Program description

The TC LOSS Team was born out of concern in the mental health community related to linking survivors to resources. In the summer of 2010, the Suicide Prevention Coalition of Tarrant County (SPC-TC) discussed concern after a suicide in an apartment complex. The person who found the deceased did not know the deceased but was still profoundly affected. The apartment complex staff was trying to locate services for this survivor and had difficulties, despite there being two survivors of suicide support groups in TC, until they stumbled upon someone who was also a member of the SPC-TC. The first author of this chapter was in attendance and knew well of the LOSS Team concept. She explained it and the SPC-TC unanimously decided to develop the program.

The TC LOSS Team was begun as a pilot program through collaboration between the SPC-TC and the Innovative Community Academic Partnership (iCAP) initiative of the University of Texas at Arlington's School of Social Work. The LOSS Team is a team of volunteers who are survivors of suicide and/or mental health professionals. Through referrals from local police departments and others in the community, the team provides supportive services on-scene when the deceased is found or in the week after (delayed contact) to people who have lost a loved one to suicide. The team is devoted solely to the new survivors: answering questions, offering comfort, and explaining available community services. The program began serving Arlington, Texas, in April of 2011 after training with LOSS Team's creator, Dr. Frank Campbell. Since, the program has expanded to serve all of TC.

Results

Impact of the LOSS Team activities on survivors: quantitative results

Over the first 14 months of the LOSS Team's existence, the LOSS Team has had direct contact with 68 survivor familial and social networks.[1] These outreach activities have been in the forms of phone, email and face-to-face contact; 58 (85%) of these networks have received information about community resources and resource books[2]; the status of access to services is known to 45[3] (78%) of the survivor networks receiving resources. Twenty-nine (64%) of these survivors have accessed some form of grief support services, e.g., support group or individual counseling on average within 34 days of the LOSS Team initial contact with survivor (range 1–120 days with 79% of those accessing services within 30 days).

Impact of the LOSS Team activities on survivors: qualitative results

Eight survivors, two team members and one counselor from a referring police department participated in phenomenological interviews to assess the impact of the LOSS Team on the grief process. Themes related to the impact of the LOSS Team were commonly voiced among survivors who did and did not receive a LOSS Team outreach; these were echoed by LOSS Team members and the police department's referring counselor. These themes are presented with supporting quotations from the participants and include: (1) the decreased time in connecting with resources; (2) the impact of the LOSS Team members being survivors themselves; (3) the importance of multiple visits with the LOSS Team; (4) the impact of on-scene activities of the LOSS Team to the survivors; and (5) the role of the LOSS Team to the police department.

Decreased time in connecting with resources

Both survivors who experienced the LOSS Team outreach and survivors who did not receive the LOSS Team outreach (their loss occurred before the LOSS Team's formation in Tarrant County) all agreed that the LOSS Team's ability to connect survivors to resources quickly is an important and impactful service. One survivor without a LOSS Team contact noted: "Basically as far as the resources itself. You know, knowing the facts and the experiences would have helped me seek counseling a lot faster than I did. And as far as you know, you had a loss, you don't know what you're going to be doing next or anything of that nature too."

Impact of the LOSS Team members being survivors themselves

One of the strengths of the LOSS Team in both its conception (Cerel & Campbell, 2008) and TC is that many members are themselves survivors; in TC, the LOSS Team tries always to have one of the responding team members be a survivor. The importance of this characteristic emerged during interviews with survivors, team members and the referring police department counselor; this speaks to a "connection" that is formed between the team member and the new survivor when the survivor learns of the shared tragedy. A survivor who received a LOSS Team contact and also had a non-LOSS Team survivor in his life noted:

> One of my coworkers, um, he doesn't work here anymore, but his wife also died of suicide and so, he knew about SOS [Survivors of Suicide Support Group] and was able to, you know . . . my boss, soon after my wife passed away, he arranged a meeting with him and me. So I met him at a coffee shop and we talked for an hour or two. Yeah, we talked about our experiences and things.

A LOSS Team member, who is herself a survivor, shares her perception of the newly bereaved's reaction to learning that she is a survivor:

> And, um, Frank [Campbell] does say, and he was right, that when you tell the survivor about your loss and a brief . . . I just say: "I'm here and I want to help you. And I do want you to know that I lost my mom and my sister to suicide." That's all you say. But he's [Frank Campbell] right . . . that lady just looked at me and then she caught my eye and it was just, like, "Oh, my gosh!" Yes, I think it definitely helps to be a survivor.

A staff member from one of the referring police departments also echoed this importance:

> And so what I think is good about the LOSS Team is that they really, truly, could validate his [survivor referred to LOSS Team] emotions and feelings. And say: "Yeah, you're right; you should be mad. Yeah, you're right; you should be sad and this is why."

Importance of multiple visits with the LOSS Team

This theme has two sub-themes: the importance of follow-up visits and the importance of meeting both on-scene and later with the survivor. As part of the TC LOSS Team procedures, there are several follow-up visits with survivors—in-person or via phone depending on the survivor's preference. The various reasons for the importance of this element became clear through the interviews with survivors. One survivor, who received a LOSS Team contact and who considered taking his own life shortly after his loss, noted: "Yeah, nothing is going to help. The only thing that is really important is to make sure that they're not alone for the first three weeks. Make sure no one is alone." A survivor who did not receive a LOSS Team contact suggested:

> Maybe even a phone call. Because the first week, you're getting all the phone calls and after that you're just blind-sided; there's nobody. All those . . . it all stops. And it might be a good time when you start realizing, the walls are talking; that this is real. They just disappear.

Related to on-scene and later follow-ups, to date, whether the LOSS Team goes on-scene is at the discretion of the referring police departments and thus, the majority of contacts have been delayed rather than on-scene for the Team's safety. The Team has wondered if delayed is "just as good" since there has been success in reducing the time between the death and accessing services. The interviews with survivors indicate that both on-scene and delayed follow-up visits are necessary. Many of the survivors without an on-scene LOSS Team visit indicated that if the LOSS Team had been on-scene, they would not have remembered and would certainly not have been able to think about accessing the services discussed. Most of them indicated not remembering much from the time when they found the body and dealt with the police investigation. However, most of them also indicated the benefits of having a LOSS team member there with new survivors for a different reason: support. They indicated necessary follow-up later related to accessing services when the survivor could think more clearly. A survivor who found his wife and received a delayed LOSS Team contact describes his experience on-scene that illustrates the role a LOSS Team member could have played in his situation:

> And I saw that he [the police officer] had a gun on his side and I was begging him to go ahead and kill me right then, you know. So, yeah, I live in an apartment so they dragged me out of the apartment and set me on the stairs and I was just in a really big mess, um, they told me that I'm going to sign some papers.

In such a situation, LOSS Team members could have been sitting with this devastated survivor, and could have empathized and shared his or her own survivor experience, which, as noted above, is a very important aspect of the LOSS Team's impact on survivors.

Impact of the LOSS Team's on-scene activities for the survivors

Related to the importance of both an on-scene and follow-up presence is the significance of certain on-scene activities of the LOSS Team. These activities were specifically the LOSS Team's role in making connections for survivors and in helping them consider whether or not to see the body of their loved one. Making connections for survivors with their loved ones was not something the TC Loss Team originally had in the responding protocol. However, during an on-scene call, the LOSS Team members found themselves calling next of kin, children's schools, survivors' places of employment, etc. to assist family members in managing the chaos of their new reality. One survivor noted:

It would be helpful to make sure that, if a LOSS Team member was there, to make sure there were connections made between you and your family or friends to make sure you are not alone for the first few weeks.

Similar to connecting survivors to family members or friends, discussing the desire to see a loved one's body was not a specific element of outreach the team had in its response procedures but is clearly an important one to add. A survivor who regrets not seeing her loved one's body notes: "I don't know if I would have listened in that moment; I don't know. But if there might have been someone who seemed sincere, who might have said, 'Now you might want to think about seeing him . . .'" Contrastingly, a survivor who did see her son's body and is grateful said: "If I hadn't found my son myself, I know my mind, and I would have always pictured in my mind a more gruesome sight than what it was."

The role of the LOSS Team to the referring police department

A phenomenological interview with a referring counselor from one of the police departments we serve indicated that the LOSS Team fills an important role. Specifically, the Team has been able: (1) to provide services to survivors when the police department has not been able to due to protocols in the death investigation process—especially the case for murder-suicides; and (2) to provide long-term follow-up for survivors beyond the scope of the police department's crisis intervention role. The following are accounts from the qualitative interview describing two such incidents. Related to a murder-suicide:

> We had a horrific murder-suicide; I involved the LOSS Team in that particular situation because . . . there were some political reasons why I did that as well. We're dealing with an actual homicide and we're dealing with a suicide. We're dealing with the homicide piece, which is a crime element and we're dealing with a very angry [homicide] survivor there. The wife . . . is not going to take too kindly for us working both sides of the fence . . . As a matter of fact she actually said in my office: "I don't want to talk about the suspect's family; I don't care about the suspect's family; I don't want them to talk to me; if y'all are talking to them, then we're going to end our stuff here." . . . And that's immediately when we contacted the LOSS Team and said: "Look, you know, this family is devastated" . . . so I think the LOSS Team was able to get them hooked up with a lot of different resources that we just really couldn't provide at that time.

Another instance where a survivor who found his best friend's body needed care beyond the police department's scope:

> I think in his situation there were a couple of different things that happened. You know, he has a drinking issue . . . he was trying to outreach to his friend's family; sister kind of cut him off; didn't really want to have any kind of contact with him . . . So now he feels like, "I've lost my family; I've lost my great friend; I have this drinking problem . . ." What started to happen is right around 9.30, 10 o'clock every single night here [police department] for probably a good month, we would get a call from him. And they wouldn't be 10-minute calls; they would be hour-, hour-and-a-half-long calls . . . it started getting to the point, unfortunately, and I hate to say it, that we couldn't spend an hour-and-a-half or two with him. We would recognize his phone number

on caller ID and we would just let it go to voicemail. But again that's kind of a crummy thing . . . I contacted the LOSS Team . . . What has happened since, I think is a pretty phenomenal thing . . . you know he's going through counseling now; he's cleaned up a little bit of his drinking . . . he is really thriving in that setting. You know he got to the point where he wanted to end his own life . . . He had no family and I think he's almost kind of adopted the LOSS Team as his new extended family . . . he was talking about very specific reactions to a suicide, very specific feelings and emotions related to that suicide . . . they [the LOSS Team] know about grief counseling; they know all of the steps of the grief thing; but I think that with him, he really needed somebody to say, "Yeah, you're right," and validate his feelings . . . And so I think that was what was good about the LOSS Team is that they really, truly, could validate his emotions and feelings.

Discussion

This chapter presents the program evaluation results of Tarrant County LOSS Team's first year of programming. LOSS Team was developed to both assist survivors in the community and to contribute to the research on the Active Postvention Model (APM) of connecting survivors of suicide with services. In this evaluation, findings include that time elapsed between the suicide and accessing services did decrease from an estimate of 4.5 years without an APM like the LOSS Team (Campbell et al., 2004) to an average of 34 days; similar to the results of Cerel and Campbell's (2008) evaluation of the first LOSS Team with an average of 39 days. Perhaps more importantly, though, were the findings related to the significant impact of the LOSS Team's activities on survivors' grief processes.

The qualitative portion of the program evaluation was conducted using phenomenology to capture the lived experiences of survivors, the LOSS Team members, and a referring counselor from one of the police departments we serve. Through these interviews, it was learned that the LOSS team serves an important role in helping survivors connect to life-saving resources that engender belongingness. Specifically, three of the survivors interviewed noted being suicidal after becoming survivors. The LOSS Team helped them connect with therapy, grief support services and with other survivors. Additionally, all of the survivors interviewed noted that the LOSS Team's assistance with connecting with other survivors, grief resources, and their own support networks was paramount in their grief process. In support of Shneidman's (1972) suggestion that postvention activities such as the LOSS Team are suicide prevention, these connections are positive events in survivors' experiences that may alleviate the hopelessness contributing to the desire for escape through suicide (Baumeister, 1990). Also, connections with family members, LOSS Team members who are survivors, and especially other survivors in a support group setting engender belongingness, alleviating one of the three constructs of suicide risk in the Interpersonal Theory of Suicide (Van Orden et al., 2010). Thus, it is recommended that other LOSS Teams join Tarrant County's LOSS Team in evaluating the impact of their important work with survivors using a mixed methods approach to provide support for and understanding of the importance of this postvention work in the prevention of suicide.

Notes

1 Survivors do not exist in a vacuum but rather in the familial and social networks of the deceased. In the majority of the cases in our LOSS Team work, we are in contact with one survivor who indicates to us that the information and resources will be shared with a network of surviving family, friends, and sometimes larger entities such as schools.

2 In addition to a pamphlet listing local support groups and counselors, survivors are provided with copies of *Touched by Suicide* by Michael F. Myers and Carla Fine and the *SOS Handbook* by Jeffrey Jackson. When children are involved, survivors also receive *But I Didn't Say Goodbye* by Barbara Rubel.

3 Some of our survivors have not been available for follow-up contact due to address changes, requests not to be contacted after initial resource provision, or confidentiality (e.g., military and veteran responses).

References

Aguirre, R. T. P., & Slater, H. (2010). Suicide postvention as suicide prevention: A discussion of the need for postvention and the current efforts in the United States to expand postvention. *Death Studies, 34*(6), 529–540. doi:10.1080/07481181003761336.

Andriessen, K. (2009). Can postvention be prevention? *Crisis, 3*, 43–47.

Baumeister, R. (1990). Suicide as escape from self. *Psychological Review, 97*, 90–113.

Begley, M., & Quayle, E. (2007). The lived experience of adults bereaved by suicide. *Crisis, 28*, 26–34.

Campbell, F. R. (2001). Living and working in the canyon of why. *Proceedings of the Irish Association of Suicidology, Ireland, 6*, 96–97.

Campbell, F. R., Cataldie, L., McIntosh, J., & Millet, K. (2004). An active postvention program. *Crisis, 25*, 30–32.

Cerel, J., & Campbell, F. R. (2008). Suicide survivors seeking mental health services: A preliminary examination of the role of an active postvention model. *Suicide and Life-threatening Behavior, 38*(1), 30–34.

Cerel, J., Jordan, J., & Duberstein, P. (2008). The impact of suicide on the family. *Crisis, 29*, 38–44.

Cerel, J., Padgett, J., Conwell, Y., & Reed, G. (2009). A call for research: The need to better understand the impact of support groups for suicide survivors. *Suicide and Life-threatening Behavior, 39*, 269–281.

Dyregrov, K. (2002). Assistance from local authorities versus survivors' needs for support after suicide. *Death Studies, 26*, 647–668.

Goldsmith, S., Pellmar, T., Kleinman, A., & Bunney, W. (Eds.) (2002). *Reducing suicide: A national imperative.* Washington, DC: National Academies Press.

Jordan, J. (2001). Is suicide bereavement different? A reassessment of the literature. *Suicide and Life-threatening Behavior, 31*, 91–102.

Jordan, J. (2008). Bereavement after suicide. *Psychiatric Annals, 38*, 676–685.

Jordan, J., & McMenamy, J. (2004). Interventions for suicide survivors: A review of the literature. *Suicide and Life-threatening Behavior, 34*, 337–349.

Kaslow, N. J., & Aronson, S. G. (2004). Recommendations for family interventions following a suicide. *Professional Psychology: Research and Practice, 35*, 240–247.

Kim, C. D., Seguin, M., Therrien, N., Riopel, G., Chawky, N., Lesage, A. D., et al. (2005). Familial aggregation of suicidal behavior: A family study of male suicide completers from the general population. *American Journal of Psychiatry, 162*, 1017–1019.

Mitchell, A. M., Gale, D. D., Garand, L., & Wesner, S. (2003). The use of narrative data to inform the psychotherapeutic group process with suicide survivors. *Issues in Mental Health Nursing, 24*, 91–106.

Mitchell, A. M., Kim, Y., Prigerson, H. G., & Mortimer, M. K. (2005). Complicated grief and suicidal ideation in adult survivors of suicide. *Suicide and Life-threatening Behavior, 35*, 498–506.

Moustakas, C. (1994). *Phenomenological research methods.* Thousand Oaks, CA: Sage Publications.

Parrish, M., & Tunkle, J. (2005). Clinical challenges following an adolescent's death by suicide: Bereavement issues faced by family, friends, schools, and clinicians. *Clinical Social Work Journal, 33*, 81–102.

Prigerson, H. G. (2003, May). Suicidal ideation among survivors of suicide. Paper presented at the Survivors of Suicide Research Workshop Program, NIMH/NIH Office of Rare Diseases and the American Foundation for Suicide Prevention, Bethesda, MD.

Provini, C., Everett, J., & Pfeffer, C. (2000). Adults mourning suicide: Self-reported concerns about bereavement, needs for assistance, and help-seeking behavior. *Death Studies, 24*, 1–20.

Qin, P., Agerbo, E., & Mortensen, P. (2002). Suicide risk in relation to family history of completed suicide and psychiatric disorders: A nested case–control study based on longitudinal registers. *The Lancet, 360*, 1126–1130.

Runeson, B., & Åsberg, M. (2003). Family history of suicide among suicide victims. *American Journal of Psychiatry, 160*, 1525–1526.

Shneidman, E. (1972). Foreword. In A. Cain (Ed.), *Survivors of suicide* (pp. ix–xi). Springfield, IL: Charles C. Thomas.

Shneidman, E. (1996). *The suicidal mind.* New York: Oxford University Press.

Sudak, H., Maxim, K., & Carpenter, M. (2008). Suicide and stigma: A review of the literature and personal reflections. *Academic Psychiatry, 32*(2), 136–142.

Van Orden, K. A., Witte, T. K., Cukrowicz, K. C., Braithwaite, S. R., Selby, E. A., & Joiner, Jr., T. E. (2010). The interpersonal theory of suicide. *Psychological Review, 117*(2), 575–600.

.

23

"NOBODY TALKS ABOUT SUICIDE, EXCEPT IF THEY'RE KIDDING"

Disenfranchised and re-enfranchised grief and coping strategies in peer suicide grievers

Tanetta Andersson

Introduction

Since Durkheim's ([1897]1979) classic study, sociologists have understood that while suicide appears to be a highly personal and private act, it is also a social act. Today, nearly 37,000 Americans die by suicide annually (American Association of Suicidology, 2012). Experts estimate that every suicide intimately affects at least six individuals, both family members and friends, connected to the suicide decedent (Shneidman, 1969). A central question in the field of suicide bereavement is how suicide grief differs from other types of loss (Jordan, 2001). However, this focus has restricted suicide grievers studied to next-of-kin relationships, despite emphasis that suicide grievers constitute several populations (Substance Abuse and Mental Health Services Administration, 2010). By investigating suicide loss in peer relationships through a qualitative study, this study serves to diversify scholarly inquiry of suicide grief. Moreover, employing the disenfranchised grief framework (Doka, 1989; 2002) as a theoretical lens emphasizes the sociality of suicide loss, especially in terms of relational status and stigmatized dimensions of death by suicide (Charmaz & Milligan, 2006).

Drawing on a review of grief literature in general and suicide grief literature in particular, the central study aim of this investigation asks: to what extent do non-family status and/or stigma related to suicide affect the social support outcomes of peer suicide grievers? Indeed, the disenfranchised grief framework posits that grief is disenfranchised when it cannot be openly acknowledged or publicly mourned, thereby inhibiting social support for such grievers (Corr, 1998/1999; Doka, 1989, p. 4; 2002). In *Disenfranchised Grief: Recognizing Hidden Sorrow*, Doka (1989) introduces disenfranchised grief as a concept and proposes that disenfranchised grief may occur along three dimensions: (1) in the context of disenfranchised relationships (friends, colleagues, ex-spouses, or former lovers); (2) disenfranchised losses (i.e., miscarriage and companion animal loss); and (3) disenfranchised grievers (i.e. grandchildren, older adults). A second anthology, *Disenfranchised Grief: New Directions, Challenges, and Strategies for Practice* (Doka, 2002), added two additional dimensions of disenfranchisement to the original typology, including circumstances of the death and ways individuals grieve. Doka asserts that suicide, execution, AIDS-related, or alcohol-related deaths may be understood through this former category of disenfranchised grief (Doka, 2002). Therefore, in each of these realms, grievers might experience their relationship, type of loss, style of mourning, and their age status as socially marginalized, trivialized, or stigmatized by others on an interpersonal and societal level (i.e., workplaces, schools, and the media).

Methods and sample description

Twenty-six peers were identified through nonprobability, chain referral sampling strategies (Berg, 2007) at several recruitment sites including eight suicide bereavement support groups, suicide prevention conferences and fundraising walks, bereavement centers, and suicide prevention advocacy email list servers. Study parameters for inclusion were: (1) two years or greater since bereavement; (2) 16 years of age or older at the time of loss; and (3) participant and decedent were friends for at least two years prior to suicide. In-depth, semi-structured, face-to-face and telephone interviews were conducted with participants from eight states ranging in age from 22 to 66 years of age. Interviews ranged in length from 46 minutes to 2 hours and 11 minutes and were conducted between May, 2008 and November, 2009.

Drawing on the semi-structured interview guide elaborated in Davidman's (2000) work on mother loss, open-ended questions and probes in this study address: general background questions, initial loss and years afterward, friendship prior to loss, relationships with other members of peer network, views of suicide prior to loss, life story after friend's death and, finally, broader representations of friendship and suicide. Data analysis included manual precoding (i.e., circling, highlighting, or underlining significant participant quotes or passages), first cycle coding, and second cycle, categorical coding. First cycle or initial coding generated some 55 general codes which broadly reflected psychological, somatic, and social realms in participants' suicide loss experiences. Analytical memos were developed and maintained by the investigator to stimulate reflexivity about possible conceptual categories signaled by the codes generated during the coding process. Drawing from the investigator's reflections in analytical memos created during the initial coding phase, participants' data cleaved along the concept of grief disenfranchisement and re-enfranchisement (Silverman & Marvasti, 2008).

Seventeen women and eight men participated in the study. Of the male study participants, two self-identified as African American and one female identified as African American, while the rest of sample identified as White. Current age of the participants ranged from 22 years old to late sixties. Occupations of participants included several social workers, two psychologists, two retirees, three Master's students and a college student, a researcher, a high school teacher, a legal aid worker, a suicide awareness organizer, a college football assistant coach, a college residence life administrator, a youth camp advisor. Participants resided in Ohio, Illinois, Wisconsin, New Mexico, New York, Louisiana, and California. In regards to bereavement characteristics, respondents' age at the time of bereavement ranged from as young as 8 years old to mid-sixties. The quality of most friendships was close and went beyond "just friends." Many respondents had met their peers during their school years, church activities, and work settings. Suicides included several by gunshot, and also hanging, drug overdose, immolation, carbon monoxide poisoning, and jumping from a bridge. Finally, four respondents had more than one suicide loss, so they spoke to these multiple losses in their interviews.

Findings

Disenfranchised suicide loss

The following data vignettes highlight several participants' accounts of negotiating relationships in the aftermath of suicide and reveal this as a complex task for peer grievers. Consequently, expectations for social support may be either thwarted or foreclosed by the nature of society's stigma around suicide. Findings identified several new variants of relational and suicide loss disenfranchisement. Because of the limitations on the chapter length, findings are demonstrated through a single vignette to illustrate each finding related to disenfranchised grief. First, this research study identifies stratified relational disenfranchisement, where some but not all of the decedent's family disenfranchise peer suicide grievers. For example, Christy, who is 46 years old, lost her friend, Candace, some 26 years ago during Christy's undergraduate college years. They had been close during childhood and after Christy's family moved away, they kept in touch through letters and would try to see each other a couple times a year. Christy recalls not being able to attend her friend's memorial service because she wasn't made aware of it by Candace's family. Also, Candace was a twin, so Christy is the only co-survivor to which Rachel, her surviving twin, can look to for support:

> I'm not even sure there was one. I'm sure because her mom was . . . A lot of it is their family dynamic, which is very secretive and didn't want to talk about it and to look like she didn't have a daughter. Oh, but sometimes Rachel would say her mom wouldn't talk about it, so it was almost like her mom is not a support for her. It's almost like—I'm Rachel's twin in a way; I'm not Candace's replacement—we are kind of sisters in that and in a way it's kind of hard for me to really describe, I think.
>
> *(Christy)*

Later in her interview, Christy explains that it was probably for the best because Candace's mother would be "very upset and very irritated" with how much Christy "knew." Yet, Christy affirms that being included in a memorial service was still important to her.

Second, reverse relational disenfranchisement captures when peers end their relationships with decedents' families. For example, Andrea is 24 years old and lost one of her best friends, Andrew, seven years ago when she was 17 years old. Andrew was 19 years old when he took his life. Andrea was a seventh grader when her friendship with Clayton (Andrew's best friend) began in an internet chat room. Both Clayton and Andrew lived on the West Coast of the United States. Andrea is quick to say she's aware of how meeting through an internet chat room sounds, but she describes her friendship with the boys as "really good long-distance pen pals." When asked about her friendship with Andrew being validated and supported, she pointed to several instances of relational disenfranchisement with Andrew's family, especially their reluctance to share a suicide letter addressed to her:

> Yeah, he had written to us. Clayton got his letter because he fought for it. Well, his mom fought for it. She went over there and she, like, started yelling at people, his mom, and she was, like, "You know it's meant for them. You need to give it to them." So the boys got their letters, but because I live in Ohio, and his mom didn't think I was worthy of it, so I never got it, and, like, for a long time I was really angry and, like, when I went there I had said something to [my sister] about going over and trying to get it and she's, like, you know, and she's, like, "Just wait. You know what's in that

letter. You know what Andrew had to say and you don't really need to fight with them about it to get it," and I agreed with her on that, like, you know, I didn't push it.

(Andrea)

Third, bilateral relational disenfranchisement refers to peers' experiences of negative support not only from their suicide decedent's family, but also from their own family members. Megan, for example, is 36 years old and lost her best friend, Michelle, nineteen years ago during her early college years. She talks about this kind of disenfranchisement in regards to her own family. She expresses that she sought out college counselors, in part, because her parents did not understand her grief reaction. This was further evidenced by her recollection of her father's angry reaction to her counselor calling their home when Megan was "having a real bad time." Her account follows on the heels of describing a disagreement with Michelle's mother about Michelle's intent to take her life, as Megan believes Michelle's intent was to self-harm and not to take her life:

It was rough and, like I said, my parents just didn't quite understand and, you know,I ended up seeing a counselor at school, which my dad really didn't understand, and that really made him angry. And the counselor called the house one time I was having a real bad time and my dad got on the phone and he was . . . He's a very nice guy, don't get me wrong. He just, I don't think he knew how to handle everything . . . Yeah, and it was, you know, he was "Who are you on the phone with? And you don't need to be doing this," and, you know, it was just basically a "grow up" type of thing and I'm thinking, "This has nothing to do with . . ." It was a lot.

(Megan)

Fourth, secondary relational disenfranchisement reflects disenfranchisement by non-co-survivor friends, as Abby conveys: " I had a lot of them pull away and I think I ended up losing a lot of friends because I needed to talk about it and I was seeking out people to talk to." Abby is 23 years old and a college student; she was 20 years old when her best friend's younger brother, Adam, took his life. Adam was 17 years old at the time of his death.

Fifth, peer co-survivor disenfranchisement reflects relational disenfranchisement by co-survivors who share the same suicide loss. Some participants' experiences reveal that looking to co-survivors for support in suicide loss may prove to be a blocked avenue of support. For example, in an earlier section, Andrea relates instances of relational disenfranchisement upon losing her close friend, Andrew, after becoming close friends over the internet. In the statements below, she describes her concern for Clayton and his well-being. After the loss, he withdrew for weeks and would only communicate about Andrew's loss on days that are symbolically tied to Andrew. Andrea stresses Clayton's deep sense of grief by indicating that Clayton has never visited Andrew's grave. In talking about Clayton, Andrea opens up about the strain in their friendship after Andrew's loss:

I asked if he would be willing to be involved and he said no. When Andrew died, we talked about it the day he died and we talked about it on the day of his funeral, and we talked about it when his ex- . . . Well, when his ex-girl . . . The girl he was dating at the time was pregnant, so when she had his baby, Clayton went to see the baby and that was the last time we talked about it. Otherwise, he's not willing to talk about it. I mean, he feels responsible and he's the one that found him. Yeah. And I mean to this day, like, Clayton won't talk about it. I think he . . . It was really rough for him, and it put a strain on our friendship or what happened with us.

In terms of disenfranchisement related to the mode of death being suicide, participants highlighted numerous occasions in which their loss was trivialized, distorted, or rendered invisible across educational, media, and religious contexts. This new subcategory of disenfranchisement is identified as institutional/bureaucratic disenfranchisement. For instance, Abby describes deep anger at her high school for covering up the role of bullying in Adam's suicide loss. Abby indicates the administrators' attempts to shift blame to a suicide pact instead of understanding the bullying problem in their midst as a source of significant anger:

> I think some of his friends went to talk to them, but I didn't. I was so mad at the school that I sat there gripping my chair to keep myself from yelling because I was so angry that the Principal wouldn't do anything and wasn't comforting his family at all. Like the school just made it into this big mess and tried to cover it.

Further, the media can sensationalize and disenfranchise suicide grievers in a number of ways. In the case of one participant, for instance, who learnt about her friend's suicide while watching the news on her lunch break at place of employment. At the micro-societal level, another pattern of disenfranchising suicide loss was observed by participants in respect to disenfranchising suicide loss through language or gestures. Below, Beth underscores linguistic suicide loss disenfranchisement:

Beth: But I think on a lot of levels or with a lot of different people, suicide is so far out of their realm of even possibilities that it's almost like, "I've got to look that word up in the dictionary," you know.
Interviewer: Right. Right.
Beth: It's not . . . Nobody talks about that except if they're kidding.
Interviewer: Yet 40,000, you know 30 or over 30,000 Americans take their lives every year.
Beth: Yeah.
Interviewer: And yeah, I think, yeah, trying to sort of . . .
Beth: And I always wondered why we had to have that disease, you know, the depression that led into suicide. Why couldn't we have something that lots of Americans have? You know what I'm saying?

In sum, the preceding accounts have illustrated disenfranchised grief, both in terms of peer relational complexity and distorting or stigmatizing forces associated with suicide loss in multiple social contexts. This work provides an explicit analysis of suicide loss in the disenfranchised grief framework which has been pointedly absent from the grief literature. Moreover, Doka (2008) has called for grief scholars to extend the disenfranchised grief framework by studying which experiences might serve to counteract the type of disenfranchisement described above. The following section, then, describes processes and experiences in terms of support and coping in peer suicide grievers at the individual and community levels and, in particular, re-enfranchisement.

Re-enfranchising suicide loss

Surprisingly, few study participants sought counseling for their grief and, of those who did, their experiences were mixed. This pattern is also supported by a handful of studies in the scholarly literature (Provini, Everett, & Pfeffer, 2000). This section addresses key questions such as: Aside from support groups, what does re-enfranchisement look like in peer suicide grief? Where did study participants find such experiences? Is there a relationship between these group-based outreach and advocacy social contexts and the likelihood of identifying as a suicide survivor?

The most recent scholarship on disenfranchised grief emphasizes moving beyond simply cataloguing which losses reflect the disenfranchised grief typology and advancing the framework by delving into the processes and outcomes behind such losses and how grievers can be assisted or 're-enfranchised' (Doka, 2008). Study outcomes demonstrate that participants' supportive behaviors towards others dealing with depression or suicide loss, in either informal and formal social contexts, helps to re-enfranchise grievers and, for some, fosters a suicide survivor identity. Thus, a continuum of intrapersonal, interpersonal, and group-based or extrinsic coping behaviors was developed from study findings to conceptualize and understand participants' varied re-enfranchisement experiences. Briefly, intrapersonal coping strategies include keeping mementoes like photographs (though not always displaying them) and notes from suicide decedents. Further, those participants who advocated for others dealing with depression or suicide loss in their personal networks or work spheres, but who did not engage in group-based coping or re-enfranchising strategies, are understood to be on this continuum with interpersonal coping strategies. These strategies are not viewed as mutually exclusive, so participants could engage in both intrapersonal and group-based coping strategies. Of most significance to Doka's call in the study of disenfranchised grief is the final group of strategies along this continuum. For example, these participants engage in group-based re-enfranchising strategies like suicide prevention fundraising Out of the Darkness Community Walks, and Local Outreach to Survivors of Suicide or LOSS programs (see Chapter 22 in this volume).

For instance, of her participation in an Out of the Darkness Community Walk, Lisa says:

> We did that walk . . . That was the first one. Well, the first that we had heard about it, and it was just kind of, like, a chance thing. It wasn't like an advertisement or anything like that, you know. It's just, like, it was word of mouth. Somebody found out about it in some other town and told my sister, you know, and said, "Hey, they do this . . . So we went and it was good. It was really good, you know . . . Everybody has like shirts and stuff made up and like just looking around at all the people you know that were affected and it's like you've got to think "This is just this one small area in the country in the world, you know, and these are the people that know about the walk and that feel comfortable coming out and doing it." You know it's just a small representation of the people that are out there. It's amazing.

These organized walks began in 2003 with an overnight walk to raise funds for the American Foundation for Suicide Prevention (AFSP). In the following year, 25 community walks took place involving around 4,000 participants. Since then, the number has ballooned with some 230 being held in 49 states across the United States last year. In 2011, the AFSP reports that more than 90,000 participants have walked in their communities, "to raise over $6.5 million to support suicide prevention research, local prevention and educational programs, advocacy, and survivor loss programs" (American Foundation for Suicide Prevention, 2012).

Grief interventions for suicide grievers like psychological counseling, support groups, and even the Out of the Darkness Walks are all still passive in nature because they rely on suicide grievers to initiate the support-seeking process. On the other hand, the LOSS program is an Active Postvention Model (APM) which aims to deliver immediate support to suicide grievers at the time of death through the LOSS volunteer team. Begun in 1999, the LOSS program coordinates with the local Coroner's Office, and when a suicide occurs, the team is alerted and travels to the scene to sit and talk with family and friends after the police and medics have finished their duties. The team consists of a mental health professional and other para-professional volunteers who are veteran suicide survivors:

> The L.O.S.S. team reaches out to survivors to let them know that they are not alone, provides immediate contact and support, informs them of the resources available to them in the community, and provides an installation of hope that they, too, can survive this traumatic loss.
>
> *(Campbell, Cataldie, McIntosh, & Millet, 2004, p. 30)*

Daniel, for example, who is 63 years old and has suffered three suicide loses, including his wife, a girlfriend, and a friend, describes himself as floundering until he found a role in the LOSS program:

> Some of it's hard. Some of it's very hard. I think it gives me a sense of well-being to know that I'm at least offering help to people that I wish I'd had 20 odd years ago. Maybe I wouldn't be sitting here today if I had it 20 years ago. Like I say, some of it's hard. I can very vividly remember some and can't remember others at all . . . But it makes me feel good, like I say, to know that I may be giving some hope to people and letting some people know that there are some options. They don't have to sit on it like I did for 20 years. You can start getting help and not have to live with the shame and the guilt all by yourself.

Other emergent study findings related to the varied salience of a suicide survivor identity among participants. One participant, Carrie, identifies so strongly with this status, she has "survivor" tattooed on her arm. For Carrie, who is 30 years old and lost one of her very best high school friends, Thomas, around nine years ago, her suicide survivor status is extremely salient:

Carrie: I have, yeah, I have a ribbon, "I'm a suicide survivor," so I have "Suicide Survivor" tattooed on my arm, and then on the back of my neck I have a green shamrock with a yellow ribbon tied around it with a little bow, because yellow ribbons was how we started talking about suicide . . .

Interviewer: So they're all tied to Thomas?

Carrie: Those three, yeah.

Moreover, such participants indicated that their identification with this term was fostered by group survivor events or programs. Another participant, Jonathan, describes his identification as a suicide survivor and explicitly links it to both his advocacy in his occupational sphere and group-based coping contexts like the suicide prevention fundraising walks. Jonathan is in his fifties and lost the mother of his son over five years ago (Jonathan was never married to or lived with the mother of his son):

> Well, I do identify. I've had other suicides in my life and I think that they came at really, you know, an earlier life when I was a teenager, and they were very upsetting. I felt very guilty about one of them in particular, that I should've known, should've stopped it, I could've . . . But as I matured and I got older and I could see this as being real and it's my life's work, I more identify as being someone who helps people survive suicide or depression or what have you, but for one day out of the year when I go to that march and I wear a shirt or I have her name on my back, I walk and I identify . . .

On the other hand, the following comments from Bill reflect a number of negative cases of participants for whom a survivor identity held no salience:

> There were, and I don't think of myself as a suicide survivor, which is kind of interesting, 'cause I am a suicide survivor, but there were three key people in my background that did suicide . . . I guess to a certain extent I've kicked these suicides out of my closet, so to speak, and maybe that's why I don't consider myself a suicide survivor even though I clearly am.

Bill is a 60-year-old social worker who has experienced triple suicide loss (homicide-suicide of a close friend, a family friend, and a coworker). Across these cases, participants drew attention to numerous contingencies in respects to this identity. Some participants expressed concerns about identifying as a survivor that were relational in nature (i.e., can a clinician be a survivor?), whereas other concerns addressed temporal dimensions around when one identifies as survivor (i.e., being a survivor indicates having closure), and some were leery about being mistaken for attempting suicide themselves.

Discussion and clinical implications

Overall, this research is consistent with other researchers' observations about ways to build community for survivors. Given the re-enfranchising value these contexts seem to hold for suicide loss survivors, this sociological research deepens our understandings of these suicide prevention advocacy events and programs and illuminates a critical blind spot regarding the suicide prevention movement. At the macro-level, the lens of the health social movement literature within medical sociology sheds light on this impetus towards advocacy for suicide prevention. According to Brown and his co-authors (2004), such organized efforts represent embodied health movements and challenge knowledge and practice concerning etiology, treatment, and prevention of disease (i.e., Gulf War or Chronic Fatigue Syndrome disease groups). Yet, others outside sociology including suicide prevention experts and advocates do not view these fundraising community walks as a significant part of the suicide prevention movement. For example, in a recent publication by Spencer-Thomas and Jahn (2012), which tracks key events in the suicide prevention movement, the Out of the Darkness Community Walks mobilization were excluded from this ranking.

Unlike other sociological social movement thinkers, Klawitter (1999) includes extrinsic expressions such as performances and practices in their definition of social movement culture. For example, in studying the breast cancer movement, Klawitter asks: How is culture, "enacted, enunciated, and emoted" in breast cancer social mobilization? She asserts that such outward expressions of culture build and shape symbolic communities like those reflected in participants' accounts of suicide prevention and advocacy group contexts. Alternatively, at the micro-level, findings from this study suggest that a suicide survivor identity is a collaboratively based identity, whereby group contexts affect how this status is influenced by extrinsic phenomena. To understand the links between identity and group-based suicide loss coping strategies, the concept of subcultural identity work offers many insights (Schwalbe & Mason-Schrock, 1996). This concept unpacks how people work together to create signs, codes, and rites of affirmation that become shared resources of identity and sometimes even function to police shared status. For participants, it is clear that cultural symbols present at fundraising walks including tee shirts, signs, and public discussion of this stigmatized loss contribute to signifying a survivor identity and a community.

What are the clinical implications of these study findings? While the recently proposed changes to the DSM-V rejected medicalizing suicide grief by maintaining the grief exclusion for depression disorder, the push remains (Kleinman, 2012). In the future, growing numbers of individuals with long-term suicide grief may qualify for treatment under their health insurance coverage, subsequently more mental health practitioners may encounter such patients. Increased awareness of the beneficial dimensions found in these suicide loss group-based coping settings is needed among mental health experts. Unlike other types of grief, suicide loss seems to involve an identity process which for some grievers may aid their efforts to overcome suicide loss. Additionally, acknowledging and remedying social factors which aggravate suicide grief may be more effective for long-term prognosis.

References

American Association of Suicidology (2012). Suicide data page, 2009. Available at: http://www.suicidology.org/c/document_library/get_file?folderId=232&name=DLFE-382.pdf (accessed March 18, 2012).

American Foundation for Suicide Prevention (2012, January 31). Community walks nationwide raise needed funds and awareness. Available at: http://www.afsp.org/index.cfm?fuseaction=home.viewPage&page_ID=8A646C2B-E866-F64F-E5E32C885FB71889.

Berg. B. (2007). *Qualitative research methods for the social sciences* (6th ed.) New York: Pearson Education, Inc.

Brown, P., Zaestoski, S., McCormick, S., Mayer, B., Morello-Forsch, R., & Gasior Altman, R. (2004). Embodied health movements: New approaches to social movements in health. *Sociology of Health & Illness, 26*(1), 50–80.

Campbell, F., Cataldie, L., McIntosh, J., & Millet, K. (2004). Clinical insights: An active postvention program. *Crisis, 25*(1), 30–32.

Charmaz, K., & Milligan, M. (2006). Grief. In Jan E. Stets, & Jonathan Turner (Eds.), *Handbook of the sociology of emotions* (pp. 516–543). New York: Springer.

Corr, C. A. (1998/1999). Enhancing the concept of disenfranchised grief. *Omega, 38* (1), 1–20.

Davidman, L. (2000). *Motherloss.* Los Angeles, CA: University of California Press.

Doka, K. (1989). Disenfranchised grief. In K. J. Doka (Ed.), *Disenfranchised grief: Recognizing hidden sorrow* (pp. 3–11). Lexington, MA: Lexington Books.

Doka, K. (2002). *Disenfranchised grief: New directions, challenges, and strategies for practice* (2nd ed.). Champaign, IL: Research Press.

Doka, K. (2008). Disenfranchised grief in historical and cultural perspective. In M. S. Stroebe, R. O. Hansson, H. Schut, & W. Stroebe (Eds.), *Handbook of bereavement research: Advances in theory and intervention* (pp. 223–240). Washington, DC: American Psychological Association.

Durkheim, E. ([1897] 1979). *Le Suicide* (J. Spaulding, & G. Zimmerman, Trans). New York: The Free Press.

Jordan, J. (2001). Is suicide bereavement different? A reassessment of the literature. *Suicide and Life-threatening Behavior, 31*, 91–102.

Klawitter, M. (1999). Racing for the cure, walking women, and toxic touring: Mapping cultures of action within the Bay Area terrain of breast cancer. *Social Problems, 46*, 1, 104–126.

Kleinman, A. (2012). The art of medicine: Culture, bereavement, and psychiatry. *The Lancet, 379*, 608–609.

Provini, C., Everett, J., & Pfeffer, C. (2000). Adults mourning suicide: Self-reported concerns about bereavement, needs for assistance, and help seeking behavior. *Death Studies, 24*(1), 1–19.

Schwalbe, M., & Mason-Schrock, D. (1996). Identity work as group process. *Advances in Group Processes, 13*, 113–147.

Shneidman, E. (1969). Prologue: Fifty-eight years. In E. S. Shneidman (Ed.), *On the nature of suicide* (pp. 1–30). San Francisco: Jossey-Bass.

Silverman, D., & Marvasti, A. (2008). *Doing qualitative research: A comprehensive guide.* Thousand Oaks, CA: Sage Publications:

Spencer-Thomas, S., & Jahn, D. (2012). Tracking a movement: U.S. milestones in suicide prevention. *Suicide and Life-threatening Behavior, 42*, 1, 78–85.

Substance Abuse and Mental Health Services Administration (2010). Suicide prevention dialogue with consumers and survivors, from pain to promise (HHS Pub. No. SMA 10-4589). Available at: http://store.samhsa.gov/shin/content//SMA10-4589/SMA10-4589.pdf.

24

CAN GOOD COME FROM BAD?

Do suicide survivors experience growth from their loss?

Melinda M. Moore

Introduction

In his seminal book, *Man's Search for Meaning*, Viktor Frankl recounts his search for meaning in the suffering he experienced and witnessed while interred at Auschwitz during the Holocaust. He argued that, "Even the helpless victim of a hopeless situation, facing a fate he cannot change, may rise above himself, may grow beyond himself, and by so doing change himself. He may turn a personal tragedy into a triumph" (2006, p. 146). Years before Lawrence Calhoun and Richard Tedeschi pioneered the concept of "Post-traumatic Growth" (1996), Frankl described a process of personal transformation inspired by internal processes initiated under unfair and unjust circumstances. To a person who loses a loved one to suicide, there can be no greater injustice. Unfortunately, it is an experience that occurs more frequently than expected. Every 15.2 minutes an individual in the United States dies by suicide (McIntosh, 2010), leaving behind in the wake of this tragic death loved ones, family, and friends known as "suicide survivors" (Knieper, 1999), also known as the "suicide bereaved." It is estimated that for every death by suicide, there are six individuals profoundly affected (McIntosh, 2010). Others place the number as high as ten (Mitchell, Kim, Prigerson, & Mortimer-Stephens, 2004). Some have suggested that as many as 28 individuals may be touched directly by a suicide death (Knieper, 1999). While it is difficult to calculate the actual number affected directly, when extrapolating from suicide death records from 1983 to 2007 and using the more conservative approach to approximate the number of suicide survivors, it is estimated that 4.6 million Americans have been personally impacted by suicide over this 25-year period. In 2007, the year for which we have the latest data, that number grew by 207,588 individuals (McIntosh, 2010).

Suicide bereavement

While clinicians who work with survivors of suicide agree that the grief process for suicide survivors is different and more difficult than for those mourning a loved one through other causes of death (Jordan, 2001), questions about the nature of suicide bereavement still exist. Historical methodological issues, including small sample sizes, lack of comparison or control groups and sufficient power to be statistically robust have undermined the integrity of the small amount of research on suicide bereavement (Bailley, Kral, & Dunham, 1999; Ellenbogen & Gratton, 2001).

In *Grief After Suicide: Understanding the Consequences and Caring for the Survivors*, a compendium of the existing research, Jordan and McIntosh (2011) argue that more research and clinical attention are needed in order to increase our general understanding of the effects of suicide bereavement, but more importantly, to be able to assist survivors in the aftermath of this devastating loss. Still, what we do know is compelling.

Early suicide bereavement research concluded that suicide survivors tended to experience more guilt, less social support, and were highly motivated to understand why the death occurred (Calhoun, Selby, & Selby, 1982). More recent investigations have cast doubt on empirical differences and suggest more similarities between survivors of suicide and those surviving the loss of loved ones to other causes of death (Clark & Goldney, 2000). In a review of those studies that did contain a control or comparison group, McIntosh (1993) found six general conclusions about the course of suicide bereavement: (1) the bereavement experience is generally nonpathological; (2) there are more similarities than differences compared with those mourning losses due to other modes of death; (3) there may be aspects of grieving that characterize a "survivor syndrome," but they have yet to be defined; (4) the course of suicide survivorship may differ over time, however; (5) after the two-year mark, differences in grief from other forms of bereavement may appear minimal; and (6) relationship to and closeness with the decedent, as well as time passed since the death, may be important factors in the course of bereavement.

Thematic differences may be present as well. Jordan (2001) suggests that survivors experience a greater struggle to find meaning, more intense feelings of guilt, responsibility, and blame, as well as feelings of rejection and abandonment by and anger toward the deceased. A recent qualitative analysis of 41 suicide bereavement studies indicate that survivors may experience higher levels of overall grief distress, shame and stigma, desire to conceal the means, and feelings of blame (Sveen & Walby, 2008). Depending upon the individual personalities and attitudes toward suicide by the survivor and their network, social support may also frequently be different and more difficult (Jordan, 2001). The loss of social support due to the stigmatized nature of suicide may account for both the social isolation and withdrawal from social interaction and comfort. Survivors may also pre-emptively "self-stigmatize" and reject the awkward offerings of help and support from individuals who genuinely wish to help but are uncomfortable and uncertain about how to proceed. Instead, the survivor perceives their discomfort and uncertainty as rejection. Survivors may mirror negative cultural attitudes toward suicide, which then causes them to either fear or assume that others are judging them. Either approach may deprive the survivor of much needed support and understanding from their social network (Jordan, 2001).

Bereavement from suicide has been associated with psychiatric disorders such as Posttraumatic Stress Disorder (PTSD) and Prolonged Grief Disorder (PG) (Latham & Prigerson, 2004; Mitchell et al., 2004). Investigations of emotional memory for trauma reconceptualize the sequelae of traumatic events, like suicide bereavement, as memory for an event that becomes central to the bereaved's identity and personal narrative (Berntsen & Rubin, 2006). It is the appraisal of the memory that causes pathological symptom profiles, such as PTSD (Berntsen & Rubin, 2006), and grief reactions associated with continued preoccupation with the decedent (Safer, Bonanno, & Field, 2001). Newer investigations of "cognitive scarring" that may be associated with identity-level "trait hopelessness" in suicide survivors are also possible outcomes of suicide bereavement (Rudd et al., 2009), but have yet to be investigated.

Posttraumatic growth

While the limited research and literature on suicide bereavement have focused on the psychopathology associated with this experience of loss, a new area of positive psychology offers another vehicle for investigating the possibilities of personal growth within the context of this distressing and traumatic event. Calhoun and Tedeschi (2006) pioneered the concept of post-traumatic growth (PTG), a construct of positive psychological change that occurs as the result of one's struggle with a highly challenging, stressful, and traumatic event. This growth is measured by the Post-traumatic Growth Inventory (PTGI; Tedeschi & Calhoun, 1996), a 21-item instrument for assessing positive outcomes in people who have experienced traumatic events. Five domains or factors are contained within the larger construct of PTG and are measured on subscales within the PTGI. The five factors include Relating to Others (greater intimacy and compassion for others), New Possibilities (new roles and new people), Personal Strength (feeling personally stronger), Spiritual Change (being more connected spiritually), and a deeper Appreciation of Life (Tedeschi & Calhoun, 2004).

Many agree that growth in the midst of crisis is possible, but not necessarily likely (Tedeschi & Calhoun, 2004). What increases the likelihood is one's cognitive engagement with the traumatic event in its aftermath or one's ability to reflectively engage or "ruminate" over elements of the event in order to repair and restructure one's understanding of the world (Calhoun & Tedeschi, 2006). Rumination is defined by Nolen-Hoeksema (2004, p. 107) as "persistent thoughts about one's symptoms of distress and the possible causes and consequences of those symptoms" and is a construct closely associated and predictive of depressive symptoms and dysphoria (Nolen-Hoeksema & Morrow, 1991; Nolen-Hoeksema, 2000; Nolan, Roberts, & Gotlib, 1998). Tedeschi and Calhoun adopt Martin and Tesser's (1996) definition of rumination as thinking that revolves around resolving discrepancies and making sense of one's previous goals and self and one's current reality (Calhoun & Tedeschi, 2006). While the term "rumination" has acquired a negative connotation within the confines of social and behavioral research due to its association with depression (Calhoun & Tedeschi, 2006), posttraumatic growth theory uses this more neutral definition to define the function of rumination. It also distinguishes between an earlier more intrusive, involuntary, "brooding" style of rumination and a later, more deliberate, "reflective" rumination that is associated with posttraumatic growth. While the first kind of rumination may be associated with early sense-making of an untoward event, the second kind of rumination may be conceptualized as a form of cognitive processing in the aftermath of a crisis that leads to recognition that the changes experienced are deeply profound and building of a kind of wisdom.

Posttraumatic growth theory does not suggest that there is an absence of suffering as wisdom builds, but rather that appreciable growth occurs within the context of pain and loss. In fact, some measure of significant distress may be necessary for growth to occur, although too much distress may impair the bereaved and render them unable to engage in the growth process (Butler et al., 2005). Research has demonstrated that higher PTGI scores are correlated with post-traumatic stress disorder (Solomon & Dekel, 2007), suggesting that the disruption caused by the trauma is significant enough to create psychiatric symptoms and "shattering" enough to their "assumptive world view" (Janoff-Bulman, 1992) to generate growth.

Along with growth or wisdom-building, the fruits of PTG may also include a preparedness or "resilience" for future events that may otherwise be traumatic (Calhoun & Tedeschi, 2006; Meichenbaum, 2006). George Bonanno, whose research has been instrumental in challenging our assumption that the bereaved necessarily moves through "stages" of grief, has characterized resilience as an adaptive process that occurs in the wake of a traumatic event, such as the suicide of a loved one, to be able to maintain "healthy levels of psychological and physiological functioning . . . as well as the capacity for generative experiences and positive emotions" (2004, pp. 20–21). Some researchers speculate that PTG is a kind of resilience, while others suggest that resilience plays an important role in the development of PTG (Lepore & Revenson, 2006).

Calhoun and Tedeschi conceptualize a complicated relationship between PTG and resilience. Studies have shown an inverse relationship between PTG and resilience where highly resilient people experience less PTG than less resilient people do (Tedeschi & McNally, 2011). Highly resilient individuals may have stronger coping skills and are less likely to struggle with the psychological consequences of trauma, but are also less likely to experience as many opportunities for change that proceed from the emotional wrestling with trauma.

What makes growth more likely in some individuals and less likely in others? Personality traits and mood states, such as extraversion, optimism, positive affect, openness to experience have been positively associated with PTG, while personality traits, such as neuroticism, have been negatively associated with PTG (Costa & McCrae, 1985; Linley & Joseph, 2004; Stanton, Bower, & Low, 2006). Other demographic variables, including gender and socioeconomic status, are also associated with this process (Calhoun & Tedeschi, 2006). These characteristics may play a central role in how an individual manages the interruption of one's life goals or plans through a personal crisis or a trauma (Tedeschi & Calhoun, 2004).

Posttraumatic growth of parent survivors of suicide

Understanding posttraumatic growth and factors that may contribute to or undermine PTG, such as rumination style, personality traits, mood, prolonged grief, and resilience, have not been studied in the suicide bereaved. In the fall of 2009, a dissertation study at The Catholic University of America to investigate these variables was proposed and data was collected in the spring and summer of 2010. In order to test the PTG theory that growth is likely to occur closer to the traumatic event than farther away (Calhoun & Tedeschi, 2006), parents who had lost a child to suicide within two years were selected to be studied. The participants were recruited through two suicide bereavement organizations, Friends for Survival, Inc., a Sacramento, California, based group that distributes a newsletter to more than 4,000 individuals internationally, and Parents of Suicide, a Chattanooga, Tennessee, based online survivor support community. Participants were directed to the website www.post-traumatic growth.com and data were collected online.

Measures used for this study included the Post-traumatic Growth Inventory (PTGI; Tedeschi & Calhoun, 1996), in order to measure overall PTG as well as measure to what degree an individual experienced growth in the five domains of PTG, Relating to Others, New Possibilities, Personal Strength, Spiritual Change, and Appreciation of Life. Personality traits were measured using three subscales of the NEO Five-Factor Inventory (NEO-FFI; Costa & McCrae, 1989; 1992) for Neuroticism, Extraversion, and Openness to Experience. Optimism was measured using the Life Orientation Test-Revised (LOT-R; Scheier et al., 1994). Mood states were measured using the Positive Affect and Negative Schedule (PANAS; Watson, Clark, & Tellegen, 1988). Rumination and its subtypes, "brooding" and "reflective," were measured using the Ruminative Response Scale (RRS; Treynor, Gonzalez, & Nolen-Hoeksema, 2003). Resilience was measured using the Resilience Scale (RS-14; Wagnild & Young, 2009), a shortened version of the 25-item Resilience Scale (Wagnild & Young, 1993) that assesses adults' trait of resilience. Prolonged Grief was measured using the Prolonged Grief Disorder measure (PG-13; Prigerson, Vanderwerker, & Maciejewski, 2008). Demographic information, including gender, education, and income, was also collected. These variables were analyzed using multiple regression analysis to assess which of these variables predicted PTG.

What were the results and what do they mean?

Of the 154 participants, 15 (9.9%) were male and 137 (90.1%) were female. Two participants did not register a gender. Ninety-nine respondents (65.1%) were married and 37 (24.3%) were divorced. A nearly equal number of the rest were either never married (3.3%), widowed (3.9%), or had an unmarried partner (3.3%). In terms of education, 18 participants (11.8%) had a high school education, high school equivalent, or less; 70 participants (45.7%) had attended college or had an Associate degree; 33 participants (21.6%) had a Bachelor's degree; and 32 (20.9%) had a graduate or professional degree. Income was roughly divided into three groups: 46 (31%) made less than $50,000 per year, 58 (39.2%) reported making $50,000–100,000 per year, and 44 (29.7%) reported making $100,000–200,000 per year. Overall, this group was educated and had incomes exceeding the median income (U.S. Census Bureau, 2009).

Contrary to hypotheses and predictions set forth at the outset of this study, none of the study variables predicted PTG except resilience (Table 24.1). Consistent with previous research (Tedeschi & McNally, 2011), there was as inverse relationship between PTG and resilience (e.g., as PTG scores increased, resilience scores decreased and vice versa), further supporting the idea that highly resilient individuals have stronger coping skills and may not struggle with the psychological consequences of trauma and experience positive life changes as a result. Resilience was also the only predictor of the PTG first factor, Relating to Others (Table 24.2). Resilience demonstrated an inverse relationship with this first domain which suggests an increased sense of closeness to others, especially significant others, and greater compassion and empathy toward others. Factor two, New Possibilities, was predicted by optimism, resilience, and neuroticism (Table 24.3). Optimism had a positive relationship with this domain of new responsibilities and new relationships, while resilience and neuroticism had an inverse relationship with this domain. Optimism scores grew and resilience and neuroticism scores decreased as this second factor's score rose, suggesting that dispositional optimism nurtures this tendency to seek out "new possibilities," even in the midst of trauma and loss.

The suicide bereaved parents' mean total PTGI score (SD) was 46.26 (24.8), indicating a lower degree of posttraumatic growth for the group as a whole. Mean total PTGI scores of individuals who have been exposed to trauma in other studies have fallen within a range. For

Table 24.1 Results of multiple regression predicting posttraumatic growth (PTG)

	Variable	Unstandardized coefficient (standard error)	Standardized coefficient
Gender	−2.38	(6.34)	−0.02
Openness	0.45	(0.38)	0.12
Extraversion	0.10	(0.41)	0.03
Neuroticism	−0.54	(0.43)	−0.20
Optimism	−0.77	(0.49)	−0.19
Positive Affect	0.26	(0.39)	0.09
Negative Affect	−0.08	(0.33)	−0.03
Brooding	−0.36	(1.08)	−0.05
Reflection	−0.20	(0.90)	−0.20
Prolonged Grief	7.62	(6.32)	0.12
Resilience	−0.71	(0.31)★	−0.29

Note: N = 154. R^2 = .08. ★$p < .05$.

example, mean scores were 41.2 for Japanese motor vehicle accident survivors (Nishi, Matsuoka, & Kim, 2010), 51 for cancer patients (Steel, Gamblin, & Carr, 2008), and 62.31 for caregivers bereaved by the death of a loved one to HIV/AIDS (Cadell & Sullivan, 2006). One study characterized total PTGI scores that were equal to or greater than 60 as representing moderate positive life change and those equal to or exceeding a score of 80 indicating a great or very great degree of positive change (Feder et al., 2008). In this study of suicide bereaved parents, 26% of participants registered a score equal to or great than 60, representing moderate growth, and 12% of the scores were equal to or above 80, representing great or very great positive growth. Scores tended to be in the lower range with 31% scoring between 20 and 40 and 27% scoring between 40 and 60.

For the group as a whole, the items endorsed most strongly on the PTGI corresponded to the Relating to Others factor (Figure 24.1). An examination of the factor scores determines that

Table 24.2 Results of multiple regression predicting factor one

	Variable	Unstandardized coefficient (standard error)	Standardized coefficient
Gender	0.10	(2.68)	0.00
Openness	0.08	(0.13)	0.06
Extraversion	0.09	(0.14)	0.07
Neuroticism	−0.15	(0.15)	−0.15
Optimism	−0.11	(0.16)	−0.07
Positive Affect	0.06	(0.13)	0.06
Negative Affect	0.01	(0.12)	0.01
Brooding	−0.28	(0.36)	−0.11
Reflection	−0.02	(0.30)	−0.00
Prolonged Grief	1.86	(2.11)	0.08
Resilience	1.31	(0.11)★	−0.35

Note: N = 154. R^2 = .06. ★p < .05.

Table 24.3 Results of multiple regression predicting factor two

	Variable	Unstandardized coefficient (standard error)	Standardized coefficient
Gender	0.73	(1.90)	0.03
Openness	0.21	(0.09)★	0.21
Extraversion	0.07	(0.09)	0.07
Neuroticism	−0.23	(0.10)★	−0.31
Optimism	−0.23	(0.13)	−0.21
Positive Affect	0.11	(0.10)	0.14
Negative Affect	0.00	(0.08)	0.00
Brooding	0.06	(0.26)	0.03
Reflection	−0.15	(0.23)	−0.07
Prolonged Grief	2.81	(1.56)	0.16
Resilience	−0.20	(0.07)★	−0.30

Note: N = 154. R^2 = .12. ★p < .05.

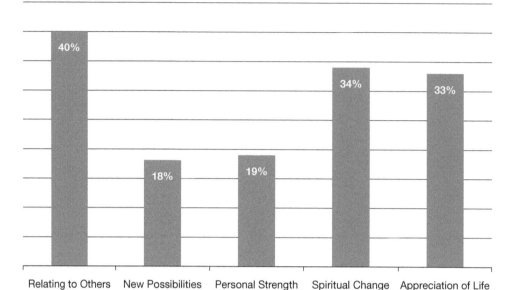

Figure 24.1 Percentage of PTGI factor scores greater than or equal to 3 (moderate growth)

40% of the suicide bereaved parents reflected a mean factor score of 3 or greater, which indicates at least moderate growth. This is flanked by the fourth factor, Personal Strength (34%), and the fifth factor, Appreciation of Life (33%). Much lower percentages of factor scores demonstrating at least moderate growth were signaled on the second factor, New Possibilities (18%), and the third factor, Personal Strength (19%).

Given the lower mean PTGI score of this sample and the low percentages of moderate growth scores on the factors, one must consider the temporality of these responses and the closeness in proximity to the death of the child (within two years of the death of the child) as being a disadvantage rather than an advantage. One of the limitations of this study is its cross-sectional nature. Was time measurement a barrier to measuring true growth from this trauma? The total mean PTGI score in a previous study of parents bereaved by homicide, accident, or illness was 64.66, but was measured a mean number of 7 years from the death of the child (Engelkemeyer & Marwit, 2008). A previous study of Vietnam War POWs (Feder et al., 2008) demonstrates much higher percentages of respondents indicating moderate growth on the five domains of PTG, including 93% on Appreciation of Life and 80% on Personal Strength, but was measured several decades from the event. While Tedeschi and Calhoun (2006) hypothesize that the growth occurs closer to the traumatic event, rather than farther away from it, does this necessarily hold for the suicide bereaved? Marilyn Koenig, founder of Friends for Survival, a California-based suicide bereavement nonprofit that helped recruit participants for this study, has pondered the relationship between length of time from the suicide, the internal processes that this manner of death spurs, and potential growth as a result. "Due to the sheer trauma of this experience, the terrible shock and, sometimes, the PTSD experienced by family and friends, it takes months and years for suicide survivors to gain perspective on this experience. It takes a long time for survivors to appreciate how this death has affected their lives, in both positive and negative ways" (personal communication, June 9, 2011).

Because the current study respondents were asked to participate in future research, perhaps, a longitudinal study of posttraumatic growth of parents bereaved by suicide will render different data including higher growth scores and higher factor scores consistent with previous research. In future research, it is also possible that PTG will vary based upon different relationships that will be taken into consideration, recruited, and carefully studied. Additionally, the quality and closeness of the relationship between the decedent and the bereaved may also be taken into consideration in future research. This will be accompanied by an investigation of the suddenness of the death and whether or not the death was after multiple previous attempts or long struggle with mental and/or physical illness and the suicide was seemingly out of the blue. These questions are for future studies. The current study is the first of its kind among the suicide bereaved and more research, longitudinal in nature, is necessary before any definitive statements can be made about the nature of the relationship between this form of trauma, suicide bereavement, and the potential for growth as a result.

References

Bailley, S. E., Kral, M. J., & Dunham, K. (1999). Survivors of suicide do grieve differently: Empirical support for a common sense proposition. *Suicide and Life-threatening Behavior, 29*, 256–271.

Berntsen, D., & Rubin, D.C. (2006). The centrality of event scale: A measure of integrating a trauma into one's identity and its relation to post-traumatic stress disorder symptoms. *Behaviour Research and Therapy, 44*, 219–231.

Bonanno, G. A. (2004). Loss, trauma, and human resilience: Have we underestimated the human capacity to thrive after extremely aversive events? *American Psychologists, 59*, 20–28.

Butler, L. D., Blasey, C. M., Garlan, R. W., McCaslin, S. E., Azarow, J., Chen, X. H., et al. (2005). Posttraumatic growth following the terrorist attacks of September 11, 2001: Cognitive, coping, and trauma symptom prediction in an Internet convenience sample. *Traumatology, 11*, 247–267.

Cadell, S., & Sullivan, R. (2006). Posttraumatic growth and HIV bereavement: Where does it start and when does it end? *Traumatology, 12*, 45–59.

Calhoun, L., Selby, J., & Selby, L. (1982). The psychological aftermath of suicide: An analysis of current evidence. *Clinical Psychology Review, 2*, 409–420.

Calhoun, L. G., & Tedeschi, R.G. (2006). *Handbook of posttraumatic growth: Research and practice.* New York: Lawrence Erlbaum Associates.

Clark, S. E., & Goldney, R. D. (2000). The impact of suicide on relatives and friends. In K. Hawton, & K. van Heeringen (Eds.), *The international handbook of suicide and attempted suicide* (pp. 467–484). New York: Wiley & Sons.

Costa, P. T., Jr., & McCrae, R. R. (1985). *The NEO personality inventory manual.* Odessa, FL: Psychological Assessment Resources.

Costa, P. T., Jr., & McCrae, R. R. (1992). *Revised NEO personality inventory (NEO-PI-R) and NEO Five Factor Inventory (NEO-FFI) professional manual.* Odessa, FL: Psychological Assessment Resources.

Ellenbogen, S., & Gratton, F. (2001). Do they suffer more? Reflections on research comparing suicide survivors to other survivors. *Suicide and Life-threatening Behavior, 31*, 83–90.

Engelkemeyer, S. M., & Marwit, S. J. (2008). Posttraumatic growth in bereaved parents. *Journal of Traumatic Stress, 21*, 344–346.

Feder, A., Southwick, S. M., Goetz, R. R., Wang, Y., Alonso, A., Smith, B. W., et al. (2008). Posttraumatic growth in former Vietnam prisoners of war. *Psychiatry, 71*, 359–370.

Frankl, V. E. (2006). *Man's search for meaning.* Boston, MA: Beacon Press.

Janoff-Bulman, R. (1992). *Shattering assumptions: Towards a new psychology of trauma.* New York: Free Press.

Jordan, J. R. (2001). Is suicide bereavement different? A reassessment of the literature. *Suicide and Life-threatening Behavior, 31*, 91–102.

Jordan, J. R., & McIntosh, J. L. (2011). Is suicide bereavement different? A framework for rethinking the question. In J. R. Jordan, & J. L. McIntosh (Eds.), *Grief after suicide: Understanding the consequences and caring for the survivors* (pp. 19–42). New York: Taylor & Francis.

Knieper, A. (1999). The suicide survivor's grief and recovery. *Suicide and Life-threatening Behavior, 29*, 353–364.

Latham, A. E., & Prigerson, H. G. (2004). Suicidality and bereavement: Complicated grief as psychiatric disorder presenting greatest risk for suicidality. *Suicide and Life-threatening Behavior, 34*, 350–362.

Lepore, S., & Revenson, S. (2006). Relationships between posttraumatic growth and resilience: Recovery, resistance, and reconfiguration. In L. G. Calhoun, & R. G. Tedeschi (Eds.), *Handbook of posttraumatic growth* (pp. 24–46). New York: Lawrence Erlbaum Associates.

Linley, P. A., & Joseph, S. (2004). Positive change following trauma and adversity: A review. *Journal of Traumatic Stress, 17,* 11–21.

Martin, L. L., & Tesser, A. (1996). Clarifying our thoughts. In R. S. Wyer (Ed.), *Ruminative thought: Advances in social cognition* (pp. 189–209). Mahwah, NJ: Lawrence Erlbaum Associates.

McIntosh, J. L. (1993). Control groups studies of suicide survivors: A review and critique. *Suicide and Life-threatening Behavior, 23,* 146–161.

McIntosh, J. L. (for the American Association of Suicidology) (2010). *U.S.A. suicide 2007: Official final data.* Washington, DC: American Association of Suicidology. Available at: http://www.suicidology.org (accessed May 23, 2010).

Meichenbaum, D. (2006). Resilience and posttraumatic growth: A constructive narrative perspective. In L. G. Calhoun, & R. G. Tedeschi (Eds.), *Handbook of posttraumatic growth* (pp. 355–368). New York: Lawrence Erlbaum Associates.

Mitchell, A. M., Kim.Y., Prigerson, H. G., & Mortimer-Stephens, M. (2004). Complicated grief in survivors of suicide. *Crisis, 25,* 12–18.

Nishi, D., Matsuoka, Y., & Kim, Y. (2010). Posttraumatic growth, posttraumatic stress disorder and resilience of motor vehicle accident survivors. *BioPsychoSocial Medicine, 4.* doi: 10.1186/1751-0759-4-7.

Nolan, S. A., Roberts, J. E., & Gotlib, I. H. (1998). Neuroticism and ruminative response style as predictors of change in depressive symptomatology. *Cognitive Therapy and Research, 22,* 445–455.

Nolen-Hoeksema, S. (2000). The role of rumination in depressive disorders and mixed anxiety/depressive symptoms. *Journal of Abnormal Psychology, 109,* 504–511.

Nolen-Hoeksema, S. (2004). Response styles theory. In C. Papageorgiou, & A. Wells (Eds.), *Depressive rumination: Nature, theory and treatment* (pp. 107–124). New York: Wiley.

Nolen-Hoeksema, S., & Morrow, J. (1991). A prospective study of depression and posttraumatic stress symptoms after a natural disaster: The 1989 Loma Prieta earthquake. *Journal of Personality and Social Psychology, 61,* 115–121.

Prigerson, H. G., Vanderwerker, L. C., & Maciejewski, P. K. (2008). A case for inclusion of prolonged grief disorder in DSM-V. In M. Stroebe, R. Hansson, H. Schut, & W. Stroebe (Eds.), *Handbook of bereavement research and practice: 21st-century perspectives* (pp. 165–186). Washington, DC: American Psychological Association Press.

Rudd, M. D. (2009). Dublin Award Presentation: Individual Vulnerability, Suicide Intent, and Residual Risk. Presented April 17, 2009 at the American Association of Suicidology Annual Conference, San Francisco, California.

Safer, M. A., Bonanno, G. A., & Field, N. P. (2001). "It was never that bad": Biased recall of grief and long-term adjustment to the death of a spouse. *Memory, 9,* 195–204.

Scheier, M. F., Carver, C. S., & Bridges, M. W. (1994). Distinguishing optimism from neuroticism (and trait anxiety, self-mastery, and self-esteem): A re-evaluation of the Life Orientation Test. *Journal of Personality and Social Psychology, 67,* 1063–1078.

Solomon, Z., & Dekel, R. (2007). Posttraumatic stress disorder and posttraumatic growth among Israeli ex-POWs. *Journal of Traumatic Stress, 20,* 303–312.

Stanton, A. L., Bower, J. E., & Low, C. A. (2006). Posttraumatic growth after cancer. In L. G. Calhoun, & R. G. Tedeschi (Eds.) *Handbook of posttraumatic growth* (pp. 138–175). New York: Lawrence Erlbaum Associates.

Steel, J. L., Camblin, T. C., & Carr, B. I. (2008). Measuring posttraumatic growth in people diagnosed with hepatobiliary cancer: Directions for future research. *Oncology Nursing Forum, 35,* 643–650. Doi: 10.1188/08.ONF.643–650.

Sveen, C-A., & Walby, F. A. (2008). Suicide survivors' mental health and grief reactions: A systematic review of controlled studies. *Suicide and Life-threatening Behavior, 38,* 13–29.

Tedeschi, R. G., & Calhoun, L. G. (1996). The Post-Traumatic Growth Inventory: Measuring the positive legacy of trauma. *Journal of Traumatic Stress, 9,* 455–471.

Tedeschi, R. G., & Calhoun, L. G. (2004). The foundations of posttraumatic growth: New considerations. *Psychological Inquiry, 15,* 93–102.

Tedeschi, R. G., & McNally, R. J. (2011). Can we facilitate posttraumatic growth in combat veterans? *American Psychologist, 66,* 19–24.

Treynor, W., Gonzalez, R., & Nolen-Hoeksema, S. (2003). Rumination reconsidered: A psychometric analysis. *Cognitive Therapy and Research, 27,* 247–259.

United States Census Bureau (2009). Median household income. Available at: http://quickfacts.census.gov/qfd/states/00000.html.

Wagnild, G. M., & Young, H. M. (1993). Development and psychometric evaluation of the Resilience Scale. *Journal of Nursing Measurement, 1,* 165– 178.

Wagnild, G. M., & Young, H. M. (2009). The 14-Item Resilience Scale (RS-14). Available at: www.resiliencescale.com (accessed April 20, 2009).

Watson, D., Clark, L. A., & Tellegen, A. (1988). Development and validation of brief measures of positive and negative affect: The PANAS scales. *Journal of Personality and Social Psychology, 54,* 1063–1070.

25

FAMILY NEEDS FOLLOWING THE SUICIDE OF A CHILD

The role of the helping professions

David Miers, Paul R. Springer and Douglas Abbott

Introduction

While suicide and suicide prevention are an important focus of training for mental health providers, little is done to prepare clinicians in working with family members who have survived the suicide of a loved one. In fact, Edwin Shneidman, PhD, the founding President of the American Association of Suicidology stated that survivors of suicide (e.g., family members or friends) represent the largest mental health casualties related to suicide (American Association of Suicidology, 2011). It is estimated that for every suicide there are at least six family members who are left behind to pick up the pieces (American Association of Suicidology, 2011). This equates to over 6 million American survivors in the last 25 years. It is important to understand the impact that suicide has on survivors. Clearly, more needs to be learned about survivors' experiences after a loss of a child, especially given the literature that states that survivors are at an increased risk for suicide (Runeson & Asberg, 2003). However, without effective intervention and support from helping professionals, many families will continue to suffer in silence.

Families who lose a member to suicide face many challenges. For example, Dunne and Morrish-Vidners (1988) studied the psychological and social experiences of suicide survivors and found that survivors face emotional, personal, and adjustment problems. They found that family members (suicide survivors) have a tendency to place blame on others or oneself (guilt) and place their energy into finding answers to "why?" the suicide happened. Unfortunately, suicide survivors report lacking the emotional and moral support from others and even indicate feeling blamed or stigmatized by others. Previous studies by Dunne and colleagues (1987) corroborate these findings, in which they stated, "In addition to the guilt . . . are feelings of being blamed, stigmatized, and unsupported by others" (p. 74).

The stigma and feelings of blame surrounding suicide becomes a barrier for many who should seek professional support. Mitchell, Sakraida, Kim, Bullian, and Chiappetta (2009) found that closely related survivors had significantly higher mean levels of depression and anxiety and had lower levels of quality of life than more distantly related survivors. Brent (1992) and Rudestam (1992) also found that individuals who experience a suicide in the family tend to suffer from a number of prolonged psychological and medical dysfunctions related to their grief process.

Suicide survivors with mental health concerns have a need to turn to someone for support; however, other family members may not function as the best form of support for these individuals. In fact, Lohan and Murphy (2002) found those families who have experienced a suicide struggle to make necessary and healthy changes in their family functioning. Rather, these families tend to experience decreases in family closeness and cohesiveness and are less adaptable in their rules, roles and expectations; which places them at risk for more mental health problems.

Findings from bereavement literature add to the knowledge of how families are affected by suicide. Dyregrov (2002) found that "When young people commit suicide, their parents will suddenly have their lives overturned. Deaths of young people are often unanticipated and out of the developmental order, and the bereaved feel stigmatized" (p. 648). In fact, the death of a loved one from suicide requires a different type of mourning than from other losses. For example, Jordan (2001) reported that suicide bereavement is distinct in three significant ways: (1) the thematic content of grief which means survivors struggle with three questions, "Why did they do it?," "Why didn't I prevent it?," and "How could they do this to me?"; (2) in the social process surrounding the survivor meaning they feel more isolated and stigmatized than other mourners; and (3) in the impact suicide has on the family system in that suicide may be more difficult for the family unit than death from natural causes.

One researcher has argued that families, who lose a loved one as a result of grief, can create a population more at risk for complicated and prolonged grief (Clark, 2001). Because of this, there are certain things that professionals need to be aware of to help families process their grief more fully. These things include: (1) allowing the individual to view the body or be near the body; (2) moving them away from the question of "why;" and (3) normalizing their anger, and helping them find meaning in life.

Findings from research suggest that bereavement from suicide is an ongoing process with many family members experiencing a more prolonged sense of mourning. Consequently, assistance for these family members may need to be repeated many times during the bereavement period to adequately address the needs of this population (Provini, Everett, & Pfeffer, 2000).

Clearly, families are at an increased risk for mental health and relational problems as a result of complicated grief (Jordan, 2001). However, little attention has been given by researchers and clinicians in developing effective prevention and intervention programs when working with family survivors (Jordan & McMenamy, 2004). Despite this fact, Jordan has argued that meeting the immediate needs of families bereaved by suicide "may be one of the most important forms of multigenerational prevention available to mental health professionals" (2001, p. 99). Cerel, Jordan, and Duberstein (2008) further argued that because suicide occurs within families, the focus on the aftermath of suicide with families is an important next step to determine exactly how to help survivors.

Parents' needs following sudden child death

The little research that exists in this area suggests that one of the most important needs of parents is caring, human contact (Miles & Perry, 1985). Often parents are numb with pain after a child's death and are unaware of what to do next. As a result, Miles and Perry suggest that providers help parents in the following way: (1) provide information about the child's situation; (2) support parents in their questions about legal implications; (3) facilitate problem solving with parents; (4) begin discussion with parents about organ donation; (5) provide listening support; and (6) provide support in seeing the child after death and provide information about the grief process.

Other studies indicate that parents who had a child die by homicide, suicide or accidental death experience difficulty with family functioning (Lohan & Murphy, 2002). Consequently, many of these families may not be able to make health-related decisions for themselves and may not be able to provide a supportive environment where family needs are addressed adequately, as a result of the stress.

Suicide survivors' needs

Only a few studies have addressed the question of what types of support services are needed and actually received by suicide survivors. These limited studies suggest that survivors of suicide express a desire for more professional help; and that this help should occur automatically and not occur solely on the request of the family (Provini et al., 2000; Dyregrov, 2002; Davis & Hinger, 2004). Dyregrov (2002) found that survivors believed that professional support should automatically be provided at the scene because families are generally not in a state of mind to ask for help. Provini et al. (2000) and Dyregrov (2002) further reported that exhaustion and loss of energy make many survivors incapable of initiating contact with community services. It is not until at least two weeks have passed since the death of a loved one that survivors begin to feel a need for more formal support such as books, counseling and other support groups (Davis & Hinger, 2004). However, too often survivors indicated that they had to seek out support on their own and it was not easy finding these resources (Davis & Hinger, 2004).

McMenamy, Jordan, and Mitchell (2008) provided further evidence for the need of formal and informal support and suggest who should provide it, especially after the suicide of a loved one. Their study found that formal support of a mental health professional was the most often utilized source of support for these families: around 78%. The study also found that informal supports such as friends and other family members were also used for 85% of these families. These formal and informal supports were all rated as being moderately to highly helpful for families to process and deal with their grief. However, what was surprising was the fact that one-on-one support from a suicide survivor was the one resource for healing identified as being "helpful or highly helpful" in 100% of the cases. This result suggests that suicide survivors may benefit more from talking with other survivors who have experienced what they are going through, and can provide meaningful empathy and advice.

This finding was further supported by Davis and Hinger (2004) in which they found that survivors believed that having a Local Outreach to Suicide Survivors (LOSS) team would have been helpful, especially having someone who had been a survivor themselves involved in the response team with other professionals. They also found that both formal and informal support systems were ill prepared to talk to families who had lost a loved one (Davis & Hinger, 2004). As a result, these support systems often inadvertently made hurtful and insensitive comments to family members. It is clear that more can be done to educate and train families, friends and professionals when working with survivors of suicide.

Additional suicide research

Wong et al. (2007) interviewed 150 Chinese relative survivors of suicide and found that stigma and mental health issues associated with the suicide were significant problem areas in their lives. For example, about half of the informants agreed or strongly agreed that they did not want others to know about the true cause of death which may be related to stigma associated with suicide. Some 31% of the informants indicated that they felt lonely, 43% felt anxious, and 44% felt miserable after the suicide. Despite this, nearly 43% of the participants indicated that they felt comfortable that there was someone who listened to their sharing and 74% reported that they visited with relatives and friends. The authors suggested that some informational support and immediate services be made at an early phase of suicide bereavement as a stress management strategy. The authors support Dyregrov's (2002) suggestion that professional support be made available and went one step further and indicated that supportive care should come from trained counselors, social workers, or psychologists.

Lindqvist, Johansson, and Karlsson (2008) interviewed surviving family members who had lost a teenager by suicide in the northernmost counties of Sweden to increase the understanding of the circumstances these families live under. Parents of the suicide victim described immediate shock, disbelief, confusion, and outrage that lasted for months. Families who reported early support from their extended family, friends, or close members of their church were grateful for this support. Other family members were critical of self-invited professionals who came to lend support. Families indicated that they needed their anxiety to be at a level that would allow them to address the crisis and found themselves alone with the grief too soon after the suicide. Families indicated that their relationship with both friends and community members were, at the time of the interview, dissatisfying. These results indicate that the post-suicidal support was ill-timed and randomly provided.

New research and application to helping professionals

In an attempt to understand the needs of families following the death of a teenager to suicide, Miers, Abbott, and Springer (2012) completed a phenomenological study interviewing parents in the Midwest United States. A total of six parent units were interviewed who had a teenager between the ages of 13–19 who had taken his/her own life. The results of this study led to six themes that have important and compelling application for helping professionals who may work with suicide survivors. The six themes are: (1) support by listening and responding; (2) support from another suicide survivor; (3) support in viewing the deceased teen; (4) support in finding direction; (5) support in remembering the teen; and (6) support in giving back. These themes are presented and explained as well as how the helping professionals can apply these when interacting with suicide survivors.

Support by listening and responding

Helping professionals such as police, fire and rescue, chaplains, mental health professionals, or volunteer support are the first individuals these families encounter. It is important that these professionals understand their role of a listener to these families.

Miers et al.'s (2012) study found that listening is often more important than responding or providing ill-timed suggestions or unsolicited comments. One parent in our original research said, "People say things, meaning well, like they'll say, 'Oh, I know what you're going through', but they've never been through it." Another parent described an example when someone said to them, "They're in a better place." "That's not real helpful. None of it. The worst thing you can hear is 'God only gives you what you can handle.' Well, why us then? Give it to someone else."

The atmosphere of a suicide is often compared to a crime scene. There are many helping professionals walking around each with their own task needing completion. Survivors describe the multitude of people walking around as confusing and chaotic. Often these professionals work independently, rather than collaboratively, which further contributes to the chaos; and rather than providing support, they provide more chaos and work for the family.

Suicide survivors need individuals who will listen to their thoughts and feelings. Parents need individuals available in person versus by the telephone to provide such support. This was consistently articulated by the parents in our study (Miers et al., 2012). One parent said that, "Just having people come . . . just having someone there with me" seemed to make all the difference.

It is recommended that the helping professions assign at the scene of a suicide the task of family support to one of their members. While other members of the team are attending to their

311

assigned tasks, one of the members is attending to the family's needs. One task in attending to the family's needs would be to dispatch a suicide survivor or support team to the scene to provide additional support services. Clearly, family members need a shoulder to cry on, to vent, and to process what has occurred. Without this support, family members will often bury their hurt, and pain in an attempt to "be strong" for others, or to answer the many questions police, clergy and others will have. Without properly processing these emotions, family members place themselves more at risk for more serious mental health conditions later on.

Support from another suicide survivor

Our original study describes the characteristics of an existing model of suicide survivor intervention called the Local Outreach to Suicide Survivors (LOSS Team). The LOSS Team is comprised of two suicide survivors and one mental health professional that go to the scene of a suicide to provide support. In most jurisdictions, these teams are dispatched by local authorities after a death has been identified as a suicide. The team is there to provide support in a listening manner and the mental health professional is on hand to lend professional support in the form of a referral as needed.

Our study provides additional information that we believe strengthens the need for LOSS Teams as well as identifies the needs of families who lose a child to suicide and that could be incorporated into the LOSS Team response. Cerel and Campbell (2008) studied the LOSS Team approach and found that individuals who had contact with an active postvention model such as LOSS sought out services quicker than those who did not have contact with a postvention model. Individuals having contact with a LOSS Team were found to seek out services within weeks versus years. Equipping LOSS Teams with training to help them better understand parents' needs means the better they will be able to support the families in finding helpful sources of support. Individuals in our study were given information about the LOSS Team approach and they unanimously supported families having contact with a LOSS Team following a suicide and indicated a LOSS Team visit to them would have been helpful. One parent said, "The people I was visiting with then, even though they were very helpful and wonderful, they hadn't been through what I was going through." Another parent supported the need for a survivor at the scene when they said, "I don't think anyone gets it the way a survivor gets it."

Communities need to work together to bring first responders and mental health professionals together to develop support services for suicide survivors such as the LOSS Team concept. LOSS Team members would have personal experience in knowing a need they had was to see their loved one for one last time at the scene and could be useful in helping coordinate this at the scene.

Support in viewing the deceased teen

Our research found that survivors have a need to spend time with their teen before the body is taken away. Even following death, parents have a need to ensure that their child is being looked after. It is important that at some point in the process someone from the helping profession explains to the family what is going to take place in terms of the handling of the deceased and parents need to be given time with the deceased before the body is taken away. Protocols should allow parents/survivors time to see the child at the scene.

In some circumstances the suicide happens at a scene away from the parents' home. In these instances parents need to be given time with their child before autopsy. In our original research, one parent described the chance she was given to spend with her child,

So the sheriff called, bless his heart, he called and he got her back to the mortuary . . .
They wouldn't let me touch her . . . Her hair smelled so good, she had just washed her
hair. And she just looked like she was sleeping . . .

Another parent in the Miers et al. (2012) study said:

I got the privilege, and I will always be grateful for this, that they brought her body
back, because I felt like she was still present, her spirit was still present. I had a moment
with her and I got to touch her and hug her and say goodbye. I'll always be grateful
for that.

Parents who were given the chance to see their child were thankful for that opportunity.
Unfortunately, helping professionals often do not recognize this need. Instead they may believe
that by removing the body, or keeping the grieving and often erratic parent away from their
deceased child, that this will somehow calm the parent. Another parent described the initial
resistance she received from personnel at the scene to see her child:

I didn't get to see him until they had cut him down and were getting ready to take him
to the transport vehicle. And I was discouraged from seeing him. And I said, "No, I
need to see him." So the investigators talked some people into preparing me for what
I might see . . . Yeah, I needed to be able to see him.

This helping professional had good intentions, but it was clearly ill founded and could have
resulted in more distress and anxiety for that mother. In a way, it allows the parents to begin the
process of saying goodbye and begin to face the multiple decisions ahead of them in terms of
next steps. Oftentimes it is difficult for families to know what first steps or decisions should be
taken and having someone there or a resource guide to help them is helpful.

Support in finding direction

Families are in a state of confusion and shock at the time of death. The information given to
them at the scene is often forgotten or not even heard because of the intense grief and shock that
family members are feeling. Each day brings new questions for the survivors and oftentimes they
are faced with the unknown because that immediate support provided is gone. Our study found
that survivors wanted something substantive that they could have to review well after the LOSS
team has gone. One parent said:

I just think that parents need a lot of support, because after losing a child, it's devastating.
You don't know which way is up. You don't know what to do. It's just a whole
different feeling. The hours and days immediately after a teen suicide are filled with
confusion. It is during these first few hours and days that many decisions are made. It
is difficult to make decisions when filled with pain and confusion. That first 30 days is
such a blur. There are bits and pieces that I remember, but there's a whole lot I don't.

Several parents recognized that they would have benefited from professional resources, and how
it would have been nice if a social worker or other mental health provider would have come to
their home and helped them realize what they needed to do. Consequently, it is important for
a resource packet to be left with the family during that initial contact the day of the suicide. This

packet should contain the phone contact of the suicide survivor(s) who made the LOSS Team visit, support group information, mental health provider information, suicide prevention materials including the crisis line, grief materials, and a guide giving the families a checklist of items to remember after losing a loved one to suicide. This guide should also include information on the feelings and experiences families who have lost someone to suicide face.

Another mother further described the overwhelming emotions she had when shopping for groceries, and seeing her child's favorite food. "It's the last thing I want to do, going to the grocery store, and it's just terribly painful. You go into the store and see your child's favorite foods. It's one of the worst things to do. It's awful." Having a guide book that could prepare parents for these unexpected events was clearly expressed as useful by our participants.

The guide should also include information for families on ideas for remembering their teen and ideas of how to get involved later in their grieving process. This information can be helpful to mental health professionals who work with suicide survivors in helping them find comfort in remembering their teen and in knowing what supports to search when helping families when they express the desire to give back.

Support in remembering the teen

Family members expressed a desire to have support in remembering their teen at key times. They have a need to be able to talk openly about their teen. In our original research a parent said, "You still have a need to acknowledge their presence, at least like at holidays and stuff; you can't just pretend they didn't exist." Assisting families in remembering their teen through the development of rituals during key times can be helpful to them. Miers et al. (2012) give an example of a parent who indicated they have a candle-lighting ceremony each Thanksgiving in remembrance of their teen. Key times may involve holidays, birthdays, anniversaries, anniversary of the death, and any important time the family identifies.

Mental health providers, support group leaders, and other helping professions can assist families in finding meaningful ways to remember their teen. Families should be assisted with helping remember their teen for who they were as a person before death. Providers need to practice being good listeners and help elicit those memories and capture them so that families have these to call upon. Memories are powerful and cannot be taken away from families and helping them recall and capture these memories is important.

Miers et al. (2012) give an idea on how to capture these memories. They discussed two families who shared photographs that were made as keepsakes. One example was a photo collage that was made showing the teen involved in their favorite activities. Another family created a memory book, and invited the teen's friends to write in this book. One parent said:

> We had books here that the kids wrote stories about my child. Little things like that, which means the world to us. They wrote memories down in those books that gave us a whole new insight, a whole side of our child that we didn't know. It was really heartwarming to see how many people he touched and how he touched them.

Families should be given ideas on resources available to help create these photo memories or memory albums. Helping families find mechanisms to remember their teen will help them in processing their grief.

Support in giving back

A final area of importance for the helping professionals to have available to survivors of suicide are resources on giving back to others in need. In our research, families expressed that at a later point in their grieving process they had a need to give back to others.

Individuals who accessed support groups or had contact with Local Outreach to Suicide Survivor (LOSS) Teams expressed a desire to give back by helping others in the support group or developing or helping with LOSS teams. One parent described this strong need the following way, "My big saving grace now is you can't fix yesterday's problems with today's knowledge. All I can do now is help save someone else's life, so no other mother has to go through this" (Miers et al., 2012).

Regardless of how the parent does this, survivors of suicide need an avenue to support giving back to others in the community, whether it is through volunteer work, facilitating support groups, giving presentations or opening their homes to other teens in need of help.

Many communities have developed Suicide Prevention Coalitions or have local affiliates of some of the national suicide prevention programs. Families who engage in these programs often have access to resources for themselves and often are presented with opportunities to give back in terms of awareness events or fundraisers. Helping professions should have a list of support groups, LOSS and other outreach programs, local coalitions or affiliates, and other opportunities that exist for families to seek support in giving back.

Conclusion

It is important that the findings from our research and the literature be incorporated into existing suicide prevention training for the helping professions. Research without application is often meaningless, especially for survivors who are experiencing the grief, pain and loss of losing a loved one. Therefore, mechanisms that the helping professions can put into place to provide needed support to survivors is critical. Further research in this area will make an impact for families to lead healthier lives and ultimately make a difference by serving as a protective factor against suicide.

References

American Association of Suicidology. *Suicide Survivor Fact Sheet* [Flier]. Available at: www.suicidology.com (accessed March 15, 2011).

Brent, W. (1992). Psychiatric effects of exposure to suicide among the friends and acquaintances of adolescent suicide victims. *Journal of the American Academy of Child and Adolescent Psychiatry, 31*, 629–639.

Cerel, J., & Campbell, F. (2008). Suicide survivors seeking mental health services: A preliminary examination of the role of an active postvention model. *Suicide and Life-threatening Behavior, 38*, 30–34.

Cerel, J., Jordan, J., & Duberstein, P. (2008). The impact of suicide on the family. *Crisis, 29*, 38–44.

Clark, S. (2001). Bereavement after suicide: How far have we come and where do we go from here? *Crisis, 22*, 102–108.

Davis, C., & Hinger, B. (2004). *Assessing the needs of survivors of suicide: A needs assessment in the Calgary Health Region (Region 3), Alberta.* Calgary: Calgary Health Region.

Dunn, R. G., & Morrish-Vidners, D. (1988). The psychological and social experience of suicide. *Omega, 18*, 175–215.

Dunne, E., McIntosh, J., & Dunne-Maxim, K. (Eds.). (1987). *Suicide and its aftermath: Understanding and counseling the survivors.* New York: W. W. Norton,

Dyregrov, K. (2002). Assistance from local authorities versus survivors' needs for support after suicide. *Death Studies, 26*, 647–668.

Jordan, J. R. (2001). Is suicide bereavement different? A reassessment of the literature. *Suicide and Life-threatening Behavior, 31*, 91–102.

Jordan, J., & McMenamy, J. (2004). Interventions for suicide survivors: A review of the literature. *Suicide and Life-threatening Behavior, 34*, 337–349.

Lindqvist, P., Johansson, L., & Karlsson, U. (2008). In the aftermath of teenage suicide: A qualitative study of the psychosocial consequences for the surviving family members. *BMC Psychiatry, 8*, 26.

Lohan, J., & Murphy, S. (2002). Family functioning and family typology after an adolescent or young adult's sudden violent death. *Journal of Family Nursing, 8*, 32–49.

McIntosh, J. L. (for the American Association of Suicidology) (2009). *U.S.A. suicide 2006: Official final data.* Washington, DC: American Association of Suicidology. Available at: http://www.suicidology.org (accessed April 19, 2009).

McMenamy, J., Jordan, J. R., & Mitchell, A. M. (2008). What do suicide survivors tell us they need? Results of a pilot study. *Suicide and Life-threatening Behavior, 38*, 375–389.

Miers, D., Abbott, D., & Springer, P. (2012). Phenomenological study of family needs following the suicide of a teenager. *Death Studies, 36*(2), 118–133.

Miles, M. S., & Perry, K. (1985). Parental responses to sudden accidental death of a child. *Critical Care Quarterly, 8*, 73–84.

Mitchell, A. M., Sakraida, T. J., Kim, Y., Bullian, L., & Chiappettta, L. (2009). Depression, anxiety and quality of life in suicide survivors: A comparison of close and distant relationships. *Archives of Psychiatric Nursing, 23*, 2–10.

Provini, C., Everett, J. R., & Pfeffer, C. R. (2000). Adults mourning suicide: Self-reported concerns about bereavement, needs for assistance, and help-seeking behavior. *Death Studies, 24*, 1–19.

Rudestam, K. E. (1992). Research contributions to understanding the suicide survivor. *Crisis, 13*, 41–46.

Runeson, B., & Asberg, M. (2003). Family history of suicide among suicide victims. *American Journal of Psychiatry, 160*, 1525–1526.

Wong, P. W. C., Chan, W. S. C., & Beh, P. S. L. (2007). What can we do to help and understand survivors of suicide in Hong Kong? *Crisis, 28*, 183–189.

26

SUPPORTING MOTHERS BEREAVED BY SUICIDE IN NORTHERN IRELAND

Integrating research and practice

Chris P. Shields, Kate Russo, Michele Kavanagh and Barry McGale

Introduction

On 8th July 1999, and one month before his twenty-first birthday, the nephew of one of the authors of this chapter took the decision to end his own life by hanging. This seemed to be completely out of the blue. In the weeks, months and years that followed there ensued a complex and difficult process whereby the family searched for understanding and meaning concerning his decision. They struggled to find ways of moving forward. Initially the extended family, friends and wider community rallied around, visited the family home and did what they could. However, this support was soon replaced by a sense of awkwardness and uncertainty concerning the appropriate actions and role of the extended family and wider community.

In Northern Ireland, as around the world, this experience is not unusual. Recent statistics reported by the Northern Ireland Statistics & Research Agency (2012) indicate that in 2011 alone, 289 individuals died by suicide in Northern Ireland. Using Shneidman's (1969) estimation of six people being affected by each suicide, this means that 1,734 people were bereaved by these suicides in 2011 alone. Those bereaved are then faced not only with the emotions associated with loss, but also have to discover a reason for the suicide and try to find ways of understanding which allow them to move forward with their own lives. All of this occurs within a social context which can be problematic for the bereaved (Shields, Kavanagh, Russo, & McGale, in preparation a).

The impact of the problematic social context on those bereaved by suicide may be further complicated, in Northern Ireland, by a lack of service provision. Of the five Health and Social Care Trusts which exist in the region, only one employs a suicide liaison officer whose role is specifically to provide services for those bereaved by suicide. As part of this role the liaison officer can aid the bereaved in the immediate aftermath through individual sessions, but is then able to signpost to a support group for additional support concerning making sense of suicide and moving forward without their loved one. Within this support group, those bereaved by suicide are provided with a space in which they can show their true emotions, start to make sense of the suicide and discuss their difficulties with others who have also been bereaved by suicide. This would appear to be particularly important given that research suggests that those who have been bereaved by suicide only feel understood by others bereaved by suicide.

There appears to be much debate concerning the notion that the bereavement process for those bereaved by suicide is different to those bereaved for other reasons (Jordan, 2001). While mourning following suicide is certainly perceived by those bereaved to be different, research concerning the matter is less clear (Jordan & McIntosh, 2011). For example, Clark (2001) states that there are few quantitative differences between those bereaved by suicide and those bereaved by other forms of death. In a more recent review Sveen and Walby (2008) found no significant differences between those bereaved by suicide and other bereaved groups in relation to general mental health, PTSD, depression, anxiety and suicidal behaviour. However, Sveen and Walby (2008) suggest that when suicide-specific measures were used, those bereaved by suicide experienced higher levels of rejection, blaming, shame and stigma in comparison to other bereaved groups.

Much of the research concerning the bereavement process of those bereaved by suicide has focused on a comparison with other forms of bereavement using quantitative methods. While this research has certainly added to our understanding of the grief process for those bereaved by suicide, qualitative methods may provide different perspectives concerning suicide bereavement. Qualitative methods which allow participants to describe their experiences in their own words may be more suited to investigating and understanding the types of experiences faced by those bereaved by suicide (Neimeyer & Hogan, 2001; Jordan & McIntosh, 2011).

In an attempt to gain greater insight into the bereavement process following death by suicide, this chapter provides an overview of our research program in Northern Ireland which is currently in preparation for publication. Our research team consists of a trainee clinical psychologist, two qualified clinical psychologists with experience of working with those bereaved by suicide and those who engage in suicidal behaviours; and a suicide liaison officer who coordinates the Suicide Support Group as mentioned earlier. The first of our papers is a qualitative systematic review of the bereavement process following suicide (Shields, Kavanagh, Russo, & McGale, in preparation a). This review examined 11 qualitative studies which met defined inclusion/exclusion criteria which shed light on the bereavement process. The second paper is a phenomenological exploration of the experience of mothers bereaved by suicide in Northern Ireland and the role of support groups in the meaning-making process (Shields, Russo, Kavanagh, & McGale, in preparation b).

How is grief experienced following suicide? A review of the literature

Our qualitative systematic review identified a complex interaction between the feelings associated with bereavement by suicide, the process of making meaning of the suicide and the social context within which the suicide occurs.

The feelings of bereavement

We found a number of problematic feelings reported in the qualitative literature related to bereavement by suicide. The most commonly reported were related to guilt and blame. Blame tended to be directed towards others or towards the self. Dunn and Morrish-Vidners (1987) suggest that blaming others represented an attempt to regain control, absolve the self from guilt and redirect anger towards the deceased onto others. Self-blame was also pervasive and was often accompanied by guilt (Dunn & Morrish-Vidners, 1987; Fielden, 2003). Begley and Quayle (2007) suggest that those bereaved by suicide struggle with a sense of personal blame for not having prevented the death, and feelings of guilt. This view is echoed by Sands and Tennant (2010).

These feelings of blame and guilt occur within a plethora of other emotions including fear, responsibility, anger and emptiness. Begley and Quayle (2007) suggest that the early months following suicide are filled with intense pain, distress and fear. Van Dongen (1991) states that those bereaved by suicide are left with an emotional burden and unfinished business concerning the suicide, accompanied by feelings of shock and disbelief. Kalischuk and Hayes (2003) suggest that participants experienced a period of intense grief during which they were forced to deal with the emotional impact of the unwanted change to their life. Kalischuk and Hayes (2003) identified a sense of woundedness, personal violation and trauma following a suicide.

The meaning of bereavement

The ability to navigate a path through these emotions was impacted by the struggle to find meaning related to the suicide. Begley and Quayle (2007) suggest that this meaning-making process is a complex one which involves seeking out the death story, matching prior beliefs about the deceased to a possible cause for the death while protecting their sense of self in the process. Sands and Tennant (2010) suggest that the bereaved are left to "try on the shoes" (p. 106) of the deceased in an attempt to develop an understanding of the state of mind, thoughts, feelings and events that led to the suicide and answer the question of *why* the suicide happened.

If those bereaved by suicide are able to find meaning, they may be able to "move forward" (Sands & Tennant, 2010, p. 111) from feelings of guilt and stigma to a position in which they can experience a continuing bond with the deceased in a more positive way. Smith, Joseph and Das Nair (2011) discuss the role of post-traumatic growth following suicide and suggest that the suicide death of a loved one forces participants to face the question of why someone would choose to die. This aided the development of a greater awareness of aspects of their lives and their place in the world and a greater sense of self. Kalischuk and Hayes (2003) suggest that those bereaved by suicide review their lives and find healing strategies and ways of continuing a bond with the deceased in a more positive way. Dunn and Morrish-Vidners (1987) also suggest that, although those bereaved by suicide experienced terrible feelings of loss, many subsequently developed positive attitudes towards themselves and were able to construct new life meanings.

The context of bereavement

The feelings associated with bereavement by suicide and the process of making-meaning of the death occur within a particular social context. Maple, Edwards, Plummer and Minichiello (2010) discuss the issue of "silenced voices" whereby parents who had lost a child to suicide rarely felt permitted by others to talk about their deceased child. This led to parents feeling isolated at a time when they most needed support. This view was echoed by Dunn and Morrish-Vidners (1987) who suggested that those bereaved by suicide felt a lack of permission to express their grief.

Dunn and Morrish-Vidners locate the reactions of others within the concepts of stigma, normlessness and fear. The authors suggest that there are no social guidelines concerning how to react to death by suicide and that the void gets filled by awkward behaviour on both sides. Dunn and Morrish-Vidners suggest that others often behave as if the suicide had never happened, fail to acknowledge it or act as if the deceased never existed. Van Dongen (1991) suggests that those bereaved by suicide also struggled with how to act in the presence of others. This view is supported by Fielden (2003) who found that telling others of the suicide caused distress, and Begley and Quayle (2007) who suggest that social interactions caused much inner turmoil for the bereaved.

Difficulties with social support led those bereaved by suicide to adopt a public guise which masked their true emotions and gave the impression of functioning (Smith, Joseph, & Das Nair, 2011). According to Smith et al., the bereaved only felt able to drop their masks when with others who had also been bereaved by suicide, and felt that only others who had been bereaved by suicide could understand their experience.

Clinical implications of the review

Our review identified three broad areas of importance for those bereaved by suicide which, while presented separately, interact in a number of important ways. One important interaction is that between the painful feelings associated with suicide and the ability to make sense of the event. Therefore, services should focus on helping those bereaved by suicide make sense of the suicide. One mechanism for aiding the process of meaning-making may be through the use of support groups which allow those bereaved by suicide to interact with, and feel supported by each other.

Generally, given the problematic social context, greater availability of services for those bereaved by suicide in Northern Ireland is needed. These services should involve opportunities for those bereaved by suicide to work on an individual basis with professionals trained in the implications of being bereaved by suicide, as well as a range of group services.

The findings of the systematic review outlined above indicate the importance of the meaning-making process for those bereaved by suicide as a way of helping the bereaved to come to terms with the death and the associated feelings and to move forward with their lives. Despite the importance of this process, Begley and Quayle (2007) suggest that few studies have reported on how those bereaved by suicide describe their experiences in the aftermath of a suicide. Given the importance of the social context of the bereavement and difficulties related to social support, support groups for those bereaved by suicide may play a particularly important role. However, the meaning-making process in the context of support groups is under-investigated.

Given these limitations concerning current research coupled with the suggestion by Hjelmeland and Knizek (2010) that the use of quantitative methods has led research concerning suicide into a dead end, a qualitative investigation was thought to be useful in expanding our understanding of this area. We were particularly interested in identifying the experiences of mothers in the immediate aftermath of suicide, ways in which they make sense of the event, the nature of the social support received and the role of support groups.

The experience of support following suicide: a phenomenological study

The aim of our second study was to investigate the experiences of mothers bereaved by suicide and examine the role of support groups in the meaning-making process. Four mothers who had lost their adult sons by suicide and who attended the specialist suicide support group in Northern Ireland were interviewed for this study. Transcripts were analysed using Interpretative Phenomenological Analysis (IPA). IPA is a qualitative approach which allows the researcher to "go back to the experiences themselves" (Smith, Flowers, & Larkin, 2009, p. 1) and enter the world of each participant to gain a rich and detailed understanding of their experience. Full details of the study can be found in the paper which is currently in the process of publication (Shields et al., in preparation b).

Following in-depth analysis of the rich and moving accounts of mothers bereaved by suicide, we identified four main themes. The first theme relates to the "continuing role of mother". This theme refers to a process whereby mothers who have been bereaved by suicide continued on in the role of mother in the absence of their son. As part of this role, mothers protected their sons from blame, either by internalising the blame onto themselves, or by externalising the blame onto others, services, alcohol or medication. By internalising the blame, mothers were left with a sense of guilt for not being able to identify signs leading to the suicide and questioned their ability as a mother. By externalising the blame, they were left with a sense of anger towards others and services whom they felt should have done more to protect their sons. Interestingly, our mothers did not place any of the blame for the suicide on their sons. This allowed mothers to maintain an idealised image of their son which was free from blame, shame or embarrassment and with which the mothers could continue a bond. This bond was maintained by mothers continuing to talk to their sons, looking at photographs and asking their sons for spiritual help and support in times of need.

The second theme related to a "never-ending quest" and outlined the journey to find meaning and understanding concerning the suicide. This involved searching for an explanation which would enable the mothers to move on with their lives in some way. There was a sense that answers were needed to allow these mothers to move on. The search for answers was not limited to the actual suicide, but also related to the method chosen. Whether those who had completed suicide had drowned or died by hanging, mothers were left asking questions to which the answers were no longer available. This involved a process of reliving the last moments of their son's life in attempt to understand their actions.

There seemed to be a realisation that the answers participants were looking for were not available and the only person who could answer them had died by suicide. This led some participants to seek alternative help, such as contacting mediums in an attempt to answer some of their questions. However, mothers soon came to realise that there were no answers available. Despite acknowledging that they might never get the answers they were seeking, mothers did arrive at an explanation that they could accept and which helped them move forward. Such explanations were often related to their son's mental well-being, the role of alcohol and suggestions that the son was now in a better, more peaceful place. The quest for answers and understanding led the mothers in this study to a support group in which they started to learn how to let go of their pain.

The third theme referred to the process of "finding sanctuary". This theme refers to the fact that mothers felt the need to remain strong for their family despite the emotional upheaval caused by the loss of their child. They reported feeling a sense of responsibility towards their families and suggested that if they showed that they were struggling, the rest of the family would lose strength. The pressure to remain strong had important implications for their ability to seek support. Mothers felt that they could not turn to other family members for support, because they had to show that they were strong. Therefore, they could only turn to friends and members of the wider community for support. However, this support was problematic. Mothers reported that there was support in the immediate aftermath of the suicide, but that this support faded over time. There was a sense that members of the wider community were able to provide practical support such as helping out with shopping, making dinners, etc., but struggled to find ways of providing emotional support.

Given the complications related to seeking support from the family and wider community, mothers in our study turned to the support group. This provided a place where they could take off their masks and show their emotions without feeling the need to remain strong. The group provided a space in which participants felt comfortable and contained and felt that others, who had also been bereaved by suicide, really understood the nature of their difficulties. In this sense, it was important that the support group consisted solely of those who had been bereaved by suicide.

The fourth and final theme refers to "rising from the ashes". This theme outlines the process whereby mothers moved from a feeling of personal disintegration and loss of self to a more positive position of hope and rebuilding themselves. Mothers described a sense of utter devastation when their son died by suicide. This devastation had an almost physical quality with mothers reporting a feeling of losing part of themselves. The pain of this loss was so great that whenever anything else problematic happened, such as the breakdown of a marriage, it appeared to pale into insignificance. However, our mothers, with help from the support group, started to move forward and to rebuild their lives in a meaningful way. Mothers described finding hope in the group by seeing others who were further along in their journey. Mothers also described how the support group helped them to find a way through the pain and guilt they had been experiencing. They reported being more open to others' vulnerability, listening more to others and engaging in charity work in an attempt to help others.

Taken together, our research program helps to shed light on the complex bereavement process following death by suicide. While the area of suicidology appears to be gaining interest, the vast majority of research being carried out in the area is of a quantitative nature (Hjelemand & Knizek, 2010). While this has a valuable role and has added much to the understanding of suicide and the consequences for those left behind, quantitative methods have limitations which may be addressed through the use of qualitative approaches. Hjelemand & Knizek suggest that qualitative research allows the researcher to examine relationships between important factors in a way which is not possible using quantitative methods. The authors argue that quantitative methods focus on explaining rather than understanding and that a focus on understanding is now needed. Hjelemand and Knizek go on to suggest that when focusing on understanding, hermeneutics, the theory of interpretation is essential. As this is a central component of IPA, we believe that this approach may be particularly useful when considering future directions for research.

Our research outlined in this chapter suggests that following bereavement by suicide, those left behind experience a range of problematic feelings, particularly related to issues surrounding blame and guilt. Blame tends to be directed either towards other people, services, medication and alcohol, or is internalised and directed towards the self. However, we found that the only place that blame is not directed towards is the person who has completed suicide.

In order to navigate through these feelings successfully, those bereaved by suicide must be able to find meaning and make sense of the suicide in some way. Park and Folkman (1997) suggest that the main role of finding meaning in death is to reduce the incongruence between the appraised meaning of an event and the individual's global meaning in terms of belief and goals. Therefore, the meaning-making process is considered successful when people achieve reconciliation either by changing the appraised meaning of the event to reconcile it with their global meaning, or by changing their beliefs and goals to accommodate the event. Our review identified that participants sought out the death story and matched prior beliefs concerning the deceased to a possible cause of death. Our phenomenological study identified that mothers tried to find an explanation of their child's suicide that allowed them to move forward. This involved relating their explanations for the suicide to aspects of their child's lives which were outside of their control, and thereby absolving their son of any blame. These reasons included their child's physical health, mental health and the role of others within their child's life.

Overall, it would seem that if the meaning-making process could be successfully negotiated, those bereaved by suicide would be able to move forward and reconstruct their lives in a meaningful way. Smith et al. (2011) refer to post-traumatic growth following suicide and Kalischuk and Hayes (2003) outline the role of healing following suicide. Mothers in our phenomenological study reported finding ways of moving forward and becoming more open to others' vulnerability and engaging in voluntary work to help others.

Both our systematic review and phenomenological study indicate that the social context of the suicide can have an important impact on those bereaved. Given that this social context can be problematic, the role of the support group may be particularly important. We suggest that the support group provides a space in which participants could take off their masks and show their true emotions in a non-judgmental, supportive and containing environment. Our mothers reported finding hope within the support group by being able to interact with others who were at different stages of the grief process and had already started to move forward. Within the support group, participants did not feel the need to remain strong and could seek the support that they needed.

Clinical implications

Our research outlined here indicates that the usual support systems which are available for the bereaved may be problematic for those who have been bereaved by suicide. Within this context a greater range of services may be needed for those bereaved by suicide. In Northern Ireland, availability of services for those bereaved by suicide may be location-specific and may not meet the needs of the bereaved. For example, in Northern Ireland, the Western Health and Social Care Trust (WHSCT) is the only Trust of the five which exist that has an appointed suicide liaison officer offering services for those bereaved by suicide. Many services then need to be provided by voluntary organisations. Given the complex nature of the bereavement process, the implications of the meaning-making process for the ability of those bereaved by suicide to move forward, and the problematic social context, specialist services may be needed.

We found that those bereaved by suicide feel most understood by others who have also been bereaved by suicide. They also appear to gain hope from interacting with others who have come through the process and started to move forward with their lives. Therefore, support groups consisting solely of those who have been bereaved by suicide may be most beneficial and should contain members at different stages of the grief process. These groups should be open and flexible and allow participants opportunities to explore their emotions without feeling the need to remain strong.

Given the "normlessness" (Dunn & Morrish-Vidners, 1987, p. 175) faced by both those bereaved by suicide and those in the wider community, further psycho-education concerning suicide and the bereavement process may be beneficial and should be made widely available within communities and services. It may also be important for practitioners working with those bereaved by suicide to have an awareness of the need for those bereaved by suicide to have the space and time to make sense of the suicide in a way which allows them to move forward. Therefore, brief, focused interventions with limited numbers of sessions may not be most beneficial.

Conclusion

Following my nephew's death by suicide, our family was left in a social vacuum in which others, despite their best intentions, struggled to find ways to provide support. Within this vacuum the family were left to try and to discover why my nephew had taken his life. This led to questions of who, or what, was to blame. Had he been depressed? Had he consumed alcohol? Had he been arguing with anyone? Such questions reflected an intense search for understanding, with no one able to provide answers. We all felt guilt for not identifying the signs, for not acting differently and not providing the support which he obviously needed. However, as the research outlined within this chapter shows, we were not alone in going through this difficult journey.

Despite the fact that many people are bereaved by suicide each year in Northern Ireland, and across the world, Feigelman and Feigelman (2008) suggest that those bereaved by suicide tend to be neglected by research. However, given the complicated bereavement process for those bereaved by suicide and the impact that factors such as the meaning-making process and the social context can have on negative feelings related to suicide, more research is needed. The current publication provides an important contribution to that research but adds an international perspective concerning the difficulties faced by those bereaved by suicide.

Our research in Northern Ireland highlights that the bereavement process following suicide is a complex one which involves a range of difficult emotions, a search for understanding and a complicated social context in which both those who have been bereaved and members of the wider community are unsure of their actions (Dunn & Morrish-Vidners, 1987). Within this context support groups may provide opportunities to discuss their experiences openly without masking their true emotions. Such support groups can help participants make meaning of their experiences and move forward with their lives. The challenge for services involved in the care of those bereaved by suicide is to find ways of providing support and helping the bereaved find meaning in the suicide. Support groups may provide one way in which this could be achieved.

While our phenomenological study focuses on the experiences of mothers bereaved by suicide in Northern Ireland, the findings of that study fit well within the context of research carried out in other countries. This is indicated by the research identified in our systematic review which originated in a range of countries including the USA, the UK, Ireland and Taiwan. It would seem that the intensely difficult emotions faced by those bereaved by suicide, their struggle to make sense of suicide and move forward, and the difficult social context for those bereaved by suicide may be universally experienced regardless of culture.

References

Begley, M., & Quayle, E. (2007). The lived experience of adults bereaved by suicide: A phenomenological study. *Crisis, 28*, 26–34.

Clark, S. (2001). Bereavement after suicide: How far have we come and where do we go from here? *Crisis, 22*, 102–108.

Dunn, R. G., & Morrish-Vidners, D. (1987). The psychological and social experience of suicide survivors. *Omega, 18*, 175–215.

Fielden, J. M. (2003). Grief as a transformative experience: Weaving through different lifeworlds after a loved one has completed suicide. *International Journal of Mental Health Nursing, 12*(1), 74–85.

Hjelemand, H., & Knizek, B. L. (2010). Why we need qualitative research in suicidology. *Suicide and Life-threatening Behavior, 40*(1), 74–80.

Jordan, J. R. (2001). Is suicide bereavement different? A reassessment of the literature. *Suicide and Life-threatening Behavior, 31*(1), 91–102.

Jordan, J. R., & McIntosh, J. L. (2011). Is suicide bereavement different? A framework for rethinking the question. In J. R. Jordan, & J. L. McIntosh (Eds.), *Grief after suicide: Understanding the consequences and caring for the survivors* (pp. 19–43). New York: Routledge.

Kalischuk, R., & Hayes, V. (2003). Grieving, mourning, and healing following youth suicide: A focus on health and well being in families. *Omega: Journal of Death and Dying, 48*(1), 45–67.

Maple, M., Edwards, H., Plummer, D., & Minichiello, V. (2010). Silenced voices: Hearing the stories of parents bereaved through the suicide death of a young adult child. *Health & Social Care in the Community, 18*(3), 241–248.

Neimeyer, R. A., & Hogan, N. S. (2001). Quantitative or qualitative? Measurement issues in the study of grief. In M. S. Stroebe, R. O. Hansson, W. Stroebe, & H. Schut (Eds.), *Handbook of bereavement research* (pp. 89–118). Washington, DC: American Psychological Association.

Northern Ireland Statistics & Research Agency (2012). *The Registrar General's Quarterly Report.* Belfast: NI Govt.

Park, C., & Folkman, S. (1997). The role of meaning in the context of stress and coping. *General Review of Psychology, 2*, 115–144.

Sands, D., & Tennant, M. (2010). Transformative learning in the context of suicide bereavement. *Adult Education Quarterly*, 60, 99–121.

Shields, C. P., Kavanagh, M., Russo, K., & McGale, B. (in preparation a). A qualitative systematic review of the bereavement process following suicide. Manuscript in preparation.

Shields, C. P., Russo, K., Kavanagh, M., & McGale, B. (preparation b). Angels of Courage: The experience of mothers who have been bereaved by suicide. Manuscript in preparation.

Shneidman, E. (1969). Prologue. In E. S. Shneidman (Ed.), *On the nature of suicide* (pp. 1–30). San Francisco: Jossey-Bass.

Smith, A., Joseph, S., & Das Nair, R. (2011). An interpretative phenomenological analysis of post-traumatic growth in adults bereaved by suicide. *Journal of Loss & Trauma*, 16(5), 413–430.

Smith, J. A., Flowers, P., & Larkin, M. (2009). *Interpretative phenomenological analysis: Theory, method and research*. London: Sage.

Sveen, C. A., & Walby, F. A. (2008). Suicide survivors' mental health and grief reactions: A systematic review of controlled studies. *Suicide and Life-threatening Behavior*, 38(1), 13–29.

Van Dongen, C. J. (1991). Experiences of family members after a suicide. *The Journal of Family Practice, 33*, 375–380.

EDITORIAL COMMENTARY

The following is information I received from a colleague Mr. Patrick McGreevy of Northern Ireland, who might be considered a modern-day 'Marco Polo'. He journeys to faraway places and imports practice modalities to create suicide safer communities in his part of the United Kingdom. A trained clinical nurse and two-time recipient of the Florence Nightingale Foundation travel scholarship, Pat has traveled the globe to secure the most relevant models of suicide prevention, intervention and postvention for his country. Following such a voyage he then applies what he learned, using models with cultural sensitivity to the communities with which he works. Being a suicide prevention expert requires that he venture outward securing models and ideas to facilitate downward trends in suicide for his country. His ability to take theoretical and applied research and convert it into a model that is culturally sensitive and relevant in his own sphere of influence is invaluable. The following summary of his trip focuses so clearly what T. S. Eliot meant by "know the place for the first time" and simultaneously captures the key message I wish to convey in this commentary.

Executive summary of Florence Nightingale Foundation Scholar trip, Patrick McGreevy, Northern Ireland, UK

This report is the result of a scholarship that enabled consultation by the scholar visiting the United States of America and Canada to explore current theories of suicide prevention and to consider how they might be applied in England, Scotland, Wales and Northern Ireland.

This scholar visited in 2011: Tallahassee, Florida, USA, to work alongside Dr. Thomas Joiner and his team; Baton Rouge, Louisiana, USA, which is the home base for Dr. Frank Campbell and the LOSS Team; and to the University of Toronto, Canada, to work with and learn from Yvonne Bergmans and Dr. Heather Fiske.

The overview provides a brief description of the lessons learned and consideration of them for implementation in the UK. Rationale for selection of individuals and practices: I believe Dr. Thomas Joiner's interpersonal theory of suicide has the potential to transform how we care for suicidal people. His more recent work on the myths that surround suicide has the potential to demolish the ignorance and misinformation that is held about the topic.

Dr. Heather Fiske has applied solution-focused brief therapy successfully with suicidal people for many years. Yvonne Bergman has used the solution-focused approach and many others in group therapy for those who have made repeated suicide attempts. Dr. Frank Campbell has been a tireless advocate of "active" postvention. In his work he has proved that the active postvention model (APM) enables survivors of suicide to access longer-term help in weeks rather than the years it can take if postvention is provided passively.

Overview of findings

Thomas Joiner has systematically provided the evidence that debunks many of the myths surrounding suicide. A large-scale media campaign would have a major impact on removing the general ignorance of suicide that contributes to the stigma of suicide. The stigma of suicide may mean that suicide prevention is not seen to be as deserving of resources as other life-saving activities such as cancer research or road safety campaigns. A call is made in this report for the issue of suicide to become a major political issue through the influence of high profile political figures being encouraged to "champion" the cause of suicide prevention. The UK countries could and should provide conferences on suicide prevention at least annually in each country and could potentially share international speakers. The USA and Canada both have national organizations that support and challenge the work of their respective governments' efforts to prevent suicide. It is recommended here that similar organizations should be set up in the countries of the UK and this scholar has begun preliminary work to realize this in Northern Ireland.

Mental health promotion is a significant component of suicide prevention. One of the recommendations made here is that campaigns to promote mental health should be oriented away from old evidence and be focused on the latest best evidence. The "Five ways to well-being" from the Foresight's report produced by a government think tank made up of 400 scientists (Government Office for Science, 2006) should be the basis of current mental health promotion campaigns. This scholarship report also recommends that all mental health nurses should be trained in solution-focused brief therapy. This therapy is directly in line with the recovery approach being promoted in mental health care and it has been proven to be effective with the most at risk patients, those who are suicidal. This study tour has reinforced for this scholar the huge contribution volunteers can make to suicide prevention. More use should be made of volunteers in crisis telephone services and in services provided to "survivors" of suicide.

Several recommendations have direct practical potential for those people struggling with suicide. These include use of hope boxes and virtual hope boxes; provision of crisis cards that include individually derived reasons for living; changing the way "low risk" self-harm is considered and managed; transforming the attitudes the Emergency Department staff have towards self-harming persons and those who self-harm and abuse substances; use of Joiner's INQ and ACSS in assessing suicidality and his cognitive ICARE approach in follow up treatment; the provision of "safe places" for those suicidal people who are intoxicated/incapable as the result of alcohol and/or drugs; wider application of the ground-breaking work of the PISA (Psychosocial/Psycho-educational Intervention for Persons with Recurrent suicide Attempts) model for those with recurrent suicidal attempts which has been developed by Yvonne Bergmans and her colleagues in Toronto.

Scholar's recommendations

Based on the learning and analysis this report makes some direct and indirect practice recommendations as well as political and social recommendations that include: whole community prevention programs, intervention programs (i.e., with those at risk of suicide) and postvention programs for those bereaved by suicide. The report also advocates national and international conferences to reduce stigma with the enlistment of influential personalities to champion suicide prevention campaigns in an effort to reduce suicide throughout the UK.

Conclusion

Today we take for granted the imports and products explorers once risked their lives to bring to us. So many lives have been lost to suicide. To ignore research that confirms best practices would compound the tragedy and fail to change the legacy of suicide. What Pat McGreevy has boldly stated in his report supports the reality that suicide is a global problem needing international cooperation to share information about best practices so that the replication of those can be a reality throughout the world.

This section of research into bereavement reveals new knowledge just below the tip of the survivors' iceberg. The frozen truth is much deeper and will take unified international support to explore. Prospective studies are expensive and difficult to launch, requiring long periods of study. Moving beyond the "Acquired Knowledge" (Dr. Edwin Shneidman often called the six survivors for every suicide acquired knowledge) and accepting new research is a powerful goal. An unknown number of people might actually be survivors of suicide. In my own research I have identified over 45 unique relationships to the deceased who sought help at a crisis center following a suicide. However, my research identified a consistent pattern of about 1.5 people per suicide who seek help. In a community where 40 people die by suicide per year, an average of 60 people might seek help. When so few are reached or even aware of services, and services are scarce, the imperative is clear that there is more work to be done if we are ever to truly . . . arrive where we started, and "know the place for the first time."

Acknowledgements

Contact information: Pat McGreevy, email: mcgreevy_pat@yahoo.co.

PART VI

Indigenous peoples

EDITORIAL INTRODUCTION

Suicide among Indigenous people, especially the young, is a hot topic in our society today. Rarely a week goes by where a news story is not written about the epidemic of Indigenous youth suicide or the rash of Indigenous suicides. While all suicides are tragic, we disagree with the characteristics often ascribed to Indigenous suicide and believe that a disservice is being done to indigenous peoples around the world by making grandiose overstatements about suicide in communities when virtually no research exists that would back up claims one way or the other. Part VI, the aboriginal section, seeks to draw attention to developments in this arena and to further the dialogue around suicide in indigenous populations around the world.

Part VI begins with Chapter 27 by Darien Thira examining the transition from suicidal crisis to activism among members of the Kwakwaka'wakw and Coast Salish nations of British Columbia. In the author's research, healing is redefined from the reduction of personal distress to an increased state of harmony within the self/community life-world. Thira posits that individualized interventions are often necessary, but are not sufficient. If, as the results suggests, resistance to the alienation (disconnection), hostile dependency (disempowerment), victim-identity, and anomie promoted by the colonial enterprise is resilience, then community mobilization and the encouragement of activism (i.e., actively increasing available self/community engagements) are a preferred focus of intervention.

In Chapter 28, Rod McCormick, Sharon Thira, Marla Arvay and Sophia Rinaldis report on McCormick's retrospective exploratory study on how to facilitate healing for suicidal Indigenous youth. Given that 13 of the 22 facilitating categories involved cultural/spiritual practices, the results of this study suggest that it is necessary to understand the belief systems and world-views of Indigenous cultures before applying theories and techniques of healing. Belief systems, decision-making strategies, models of problem solving, assumptions about how problems arise, and how change occurs are all connected to how Indigenous peoples see the world. The authors hope that this research will generate an understanding of the value of mobilizing the belief system and natural healing resources of the clients that we serve in order to facilitate healing for them.

Following this, in Chapter 29, Christopher Lalonde provides us with an overview of his research examining identity formation and cultural resilience in Indigenous communities. According to Lalonde, when communities succeed in promoting their cultural heritage and in securing control of their own collective future—in claiming ownership over their past and future—the positive effects reverberate across many measures of youth health and well-being.

Suicide rates fall, fewer children are taken into care, school completion rates rise, and rates of intentional and unintentional injury decrease. Lalonde argues that what is needed instead of the usual top-down forms of "knowledge transfer," is some way to facilitate lateral "knowledge exchange" and the cross-community sharing of those forms of Indigenous knowledge that have already proven their worth in Indigenous communities.

To conclude Part VI, Henry G. Harder, Joshua A. Rash, Travis Holyk, Eduardo Jovel, and Kari Harder provide a systematic review of the scientific literature relevant to Indigenous youth suicide. The evidence suggests that it is not only having a sense of culture that buffers against the negative pathways of suicide but rather the act of engaging in culturally relevant activities with respected others in the community. The authors' review pertaining to Indigenous youth suicide identified a small number of studies that were high in methodological rigor. These studies were mostly epidemiological in nature with very few pertaining to interventions for the prevention of Indigenous youth suicide. Although these studies offer insight into the etiology of Indigenous youth suicide, additional methodologically rigorous intervention studies are needed to promote and develop an effective program for suicide prevention.

27

"AND I LIVE IT"

From suicidal crisis to activism among members of the Kwakwaka'wakw and Coast Salish nations

Darien Thira

Introduction

According to Statistics Canada, individuals self-identified as Aboriginal made up 3% of the overall population in 1996 (Statistics Canada, 2001). However, the Canadian Aboriginal community is over-represented in terms of many indicators of biological, psychological, and social distress (White, Maxim, & Beavon, 2003). The risk of suicide among Aboriginal people in Canada is between 300% (off-reserve) and 600% (on-reserve) that of non-natives (RCAP, 1995; Mussel, Cardiff, & White, 2004). This makes the development of an understanding of Aboriginal suicide-related resilience all the more pressing.

The post-colonial lens

From the post-colonial point of view, a clinical psychological approach renders invisible the impact of history (Kirmayer, Brass, & Tait, 2000; Duran, 2006). Academics and researchers within this paradigm suggest that the dominant psychological discourse serves to maintain the power of the colonizer at the expense of those being colonized (Said, 1993; Battiste, 2000; Harris, 2002). It describes the dominant culture's Aboriginal research as expert researchers studying marginalized human specimens (e.g., Lassiter, 2000). Aboriginal psychopathology and suicide are understood to be a result of the pathologizing of individuals and cultures that suffer from colonial oppression (e.g., White & Lutz, 1992; Lykes, 1996; Satzewich, 1998; Smith, 1998).

In relation to the British Columbian Aboriginal experience, this oppression can be summarized to be the product of four colonial waves: The first, legal wave declared Aboriginal people to be "wards of the state" and the Department of Indian Affairs was created to manage the lives of Aboriginal people, traditional practices were criminalized, ceremonial objects removed, and political, cultural and spiritual leaders were jailed (Furness, 1995). In a parallel administrative wave, the federal government created a reserve system in order to limit Aboriginal movement and their use of the land (Tennant, 1990; Harris, 2002). In a third, ideological wave, the government established a legally enforced Indian Residential School (IRS) system run by several Christian denominations in order to "take the Indian out of the child" and in which conditions were generally very harsh for the children in physical, sexual, psychological and spiritual terms (Milloy, 1999; Sivaraksa, 1999). Finally, the fourth social service wave of colonization as provided by "social services" has provided a method to continue control and exploit the Aboriginal population as effectively as the previous colonial waves (e.g., Chrisjohn et al., 1997; Wade, 2000; Ward, 2001; Smye, 2003). "In the discourse of colonization, Aboriginal persons were violated and displaced because they were seen as deficient. In the discourse of psycholonization, Aboriginal persons are seen as deficient (damaged, disordered, dysfunctional, etc.) because they were violated and displaced" (Stephenson, 1995, p. 201). The impacts of these interventions on Aboriginal communities, families, and individuals have been profound. For example, Aboriginal suicide has been argued to be:

> the expression of a kind of collective anguish—part grief, part anger . . . the cumulative effect of 300 years of colonial history: lands occupied, resources seized, beliefs and cultures ridiculed, children taken away, power concentrated in distant capitals, hopes for honorable co-existence dashed over and over . . .
>
> *(RCAP, 1995, p. 3)*

As a result, the mainstream notion of "healing" is understood as a rhetorical sleight of hand, the experience of "adjustment" within an oppressive context is, ultimately, surrender to assimilation (Prilliltensky, 1994). In this context, any contribution in a community that is struggling with oppression in a manner that challenges the intention of that oppression can be described as activism.

Gaps in the literature

There are three essential gaps in the relevant literature. The first is our lack of a socioculturally-specific Aboriginal model of resilience (van Uchelen, Davidson, Quressette, Brassfield, & Demerais, 1997; Kirmayer & Minas, 2000). Second, the results of research that has been undertaken have not yet been used to formulate a theoretical model of resilience within an Aboriginal community (e.g., McCormick, 1996; Mussel et al., 2004; Indian Residential Schools, 2005). Finally, the Aboriginal resilience literature suggests that the individual and communal challenges of colonial oppression underlie Aboriginal suicide-related resilience (e.g., McCormick, 1996; Chandler & Lalonde, 1998; Kirmayer et al., 2000). As a result, there is a need for research that specifically examines the link between Aboriginal suicide-related resilience and activism. The question that this study sought to answer was: What is the experience of Aboriginal men and women who have been suicidal and have transitioned from their crisis to a pro-social active role in their community?

The rationale for a qualitative research methodology

Just as Traditional stories are woven together into a system that reveals the protocols and core values of an oral culture, the development of a grounded theory is a distillation of narrative themes into a thematic network of core ideas and relationships that reveal the experiences of the participant group in relation to the issue at hand. Josselson (2004) notes:

> [A qualitative] approach is of paramount value when our aim is giving "voice" to marginalized or oppressed groups and thus representing their experiences. Meanings may be assigned between the researcher and researched and understood to be co-constructed through conversation between them.

A qualitative research methodology combines the strengths of the Western academic model of research (i.e., its essentialist focus on the identification and validation of relevant factors) with the Aboriginal methodology of story-telling and contemplation of the narrative's potential significance (Montgomery, Miville, Wointerowd, Jeffries, & Baysden, 2000).

This approach is supported by the Royal Commission on Aboriginal Peoples' (1995) recommendations that research into the experience of being Aboriginal must: (1) reflect Aboriginal perspectives and understanding; (2) allow participants to reassess findings; (3) validate knowledge identified as oral tradition; (4) reflect the multiplicity of viewpoints within the community; and (5) respect the community protocol. Such an approach can be enhanced by considering Aboriginal participants as collaborators in a shared exploration that is of use to the community (Smith, 1998).

Methods and procedure

Four criteria were necessary for each participant to be included in the study: (1) previous suicidality (now resolved); (2) current social activism/community contribution; (3) membership of one of two specific Vancouver Island British Columbia First Nations; and (4) an age of 21 or greater.

The procedure included a six-step research interview process: (1) receive an invitation into the community, based on their interest in the study and facilitate an ethical review by the community; (2) conduct an initial focus group to review the interview data collection instrument; (3) recruit participants (nominators were invited to contact possible participants who were then invited to join the study and given an information sheet by the nominators although knowledge of any suicidality in the potential participant was not a requirement for the nomination), and obtain informed consent from those who approached the researcher as volunteers; (4) undertake the research interview; (5) data analysis and grounded theory development; and (6) follow-up interview in which the participants reviewed the sections of their transcript that were to be included in the dissertation, and to comment upon and/or revise the meanings derived from the quotations selected.

Results: participants

Eight activists engaged in the interview process. They lived through diverse histories (ranging in age from 30–69 years old, with diverse education and employment) and engaged in the six-part interview process in their home communities. However, they were all from either the Coast Salish or Kwakwa-ka'wakw communities on Vancouver Island, and they had all experienced a suicidal crisis (or crises) in their past. The role of an activist is understood as contributing to the well-being of their community in a manner that confronts the impacts of colonization, and all the participants were fulfilling such a role. Table 27.1 summarizes the relevant demographic information.

Analysis

In the same way that Traditional stories intertwine into a system that reveals the protocols and core values of an oral culture, the present development of a grounded theory is a distillation of narrative themes into a thematic network of essential ideas and relationships that reveal the experiences of the participant group regarding the issue in focus. The eight participants' stories were analyzed and the result was the identification of two interconnected central themes:

Table 27.1 Demographic information on the participants

Name	Age	Gender	Nation	Location	Education	Role
Alice	69	Female	Coast Salish	Urban	High School	Elder/Teacher
Barry	55	Male	Coast Salish	Reserve (Urban)	Adult Diploma	Lay Counselor/ Support Worker
Cathy	60	Female	Coast Salish	Reserve (Urban)	Bachelors Degree	Human Service Administrator
Diane	56	Female	Coast Salish	Reserve (Urban)	High School	Human Service Coordinator
Eric	30	Male	Coast Salish	Urban	Professional Diploma	Human Service Coordinator
Felicity	57	Female	Kwakwa-ka'wakw	Reserve (Rural)	Bachelor's Degree	Human Service Coordinator
George	69	Male	Kwakwa-ka'wakw	Reserve (Urban)	High School	Special Advisor
Harold	44	Male	Kwakwa-ka'wakw	Urban	High School	Counselor/Outreach Worker

(1) self/community life-world; and (2) self/community engagements. The former context provides the location for the latter process. Furthermore, the notion of activism and the process of the healing journey emerged as elaborating issues. Overall, the analysis of the interviews suggested three interconnected areas of discussion: (1) within their integrated self/community life-world, (2) mutually reflexive self/community engagements facilitated (3) the healing journey of Aboriginal activists within a colonized context. Each of these three areas of discussion can be understood as the integration of a specific dichotomy within the literature as resolved by the participating activists: namely, (1) self and community; (2) personal resilience and social contribution; and, finally, (3) healing and activism.

Self/community life-world

According to the participants, they live within a self/community life-world—that is, an integration of their biological, psychological, social, cultural, historical, ecological, and spiritual experience of themselves and their context—that simultaneously defines the activists' identity and describes the community in which they live. While an artificial compartmentalization risks the unintended suggestion of a non-integrated model, it was useful to divide the self/community life-world into seven interdependent "spheres"; namely self, family, individuals, community, outside community, nature and spirit.

The sense of an individual self was essential to the participants' descriptions of themselves, while at the same time it was understood to be embedded within their context. The inability to identify with the self was a challenge for all of the participants to overcome during their healing journey. As Alice put it, "My counselor asked me how I was that day. I told her at the time I didn't even know who I was. And I was really down that day."

The integrated nature of the self/community life-world was exemplified by the participants' description of their family sphere. Felicity shared: "Whatever I do is a reflection on my family, my father's family and my mother's family, and all of those before them." The insult of colonization upon the family was identified by every one of the participants.

The individual sphere includes non-familial individuals in their local community whom the participant recognizes or knows by name. The sub-category of Elder was stressed by all of the participants. According to Diane, "Elders are the ones that carry the teachings." They are the living voice of the cultural community.

The local community sphere is the larger-scale social context of the activist's self/community life-world; it is made up of groups and services not identified with a specific individual. Felicity shared, "I remember growing up in, in my community and everyone knew everyone I knew . . . And, you know, everybody helped everyone." However, when the participants spoke of their community they also meant their local "cultural community," that is, its traditions, history, and Traditional land.

The outside community sphere is any collective or individual outside the community that has an impact on a participant. The outside community was split by the participants into two distinct groups: Aboriginal and non-Aboriginal. While a sense of cultural and historical commonality with other Aboriginal communities was common among the participants, the distinction of their own community from others was also consistent. The non-Aboriginal outside community was a locale in which the participants' culture and identity were directly confronted by non-Aboriginal culture.

The natural sphere provided both the environmental container for the community's context and a sacred place separate from the social milieu. According to Cathy, "I really believe that the spiritual way of being for us comes from our belief in nature and the natural." Nature is respected, turned to for assistance and it was thanked.

Finally, the spiritual sphere was understood to embrace and permeate all of the other spheres. According to Eric, "I believe that there's a spiritual aspect to nature and everything on the earth." Traditional Culture was understood by the activists to be linked to Spirit. Ancestors also played a meaningful role in many of the activists' lives: as sources of wisdom and support and as providers of direction, courage, and voice. The participants understood Ancestors to be Elders who have "gone to Spirit." There was a co-existent, although sometimes ambivalent, vision among the participants that allowed for both the notion of a spiritual connection to traditional ceremony, ancestors (Elders who have "gone to Spirit") and nature as well as to a "Creator" or Christian God. "And I finally had a Elder tell me, 'Barry,' he said, 'you know, your higher power can be anything you want it to be, the God of your making. It could be that tree; it could be anything you want. It could be that rock on the ground.'"

These findings support Duran's (2006) liberation psychological recommendation that Aboriginal people be considered within their bio-psycho-socio-historical-cultural-ecological-spiritual "life-world" (e.g., Lykes, 1996; McCormick, 1996; Weaver, 2002; Tsosie, 2003; Mussel et al., 2004). The self/community life-world is both existential (i.e., it exists and defines the activists' self) and experiential (i.e., it is their community as experienced by the activists; Husserl, 1970).

Resolving the individual-collective dichotomy

Engagements were identified by the participants within all seven spheres of the self/community life-world. This is in keeping with many specific factors of resilience previously identified in research within Aboriginal communities (Haig-Brown, 1991; Ladd-Yelk, 2001; Dion Stout &

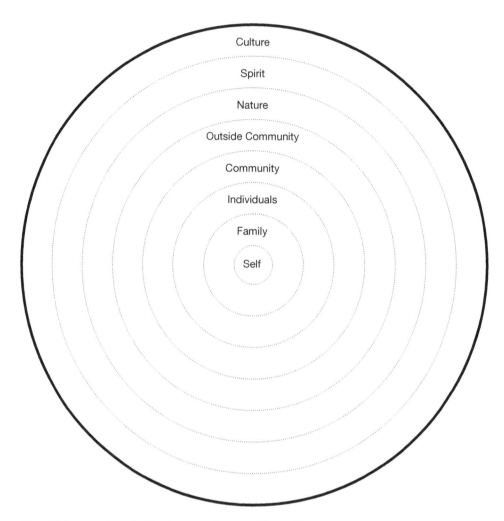

Figure 27.1 Integration of self and community in the life-world

Kipling, 2003). In their complex identity and lived experience, the participants' integration of self and community in their life-world revealed a sense of self that is Culture-driven, holistic, and relational (Figure 27.1). This is a paradigmatic fusion of both an individualist constructivist model of self (Mahoney, 1991) and a collectivist constructionist model (Gergen, 2000) that resolves the tension between individualism and collectivism (Bhargava, 1992).

The cultural life-world

Experiential continuity within the self/community life-world is provided by the participants' Culture. Culture is ubiquitous; it is the lens through which the participants experience their life-world (e.g., Schwartz, 1992). Culture is indivisible from all of the participants' self/community engagements and their activism. It provides many things, including self/community connection and the social encouragement to care for one another, collective empowerment and the demand that respect is maintained, an ego- and time-transcendent identity and set of responsibilities, and a collective vision co-created by the local community into a specific "Culture" (Ross, 1992; Cross, 1998).

Self/community engagements

Self/community engagements are activities and experiences in which the activists "engaged" within their self/community life-world that promoted self/community balance and life-world harmony (van Uchelen, Davidson, et al., 1997; Marsella, Olivira, Plummer, & Crabbe, 1998). There are three types of self/community engagement: grounding engagements (which are activities and experiences that ground the activists in one of the four foundational categories of engagement); activating engagements (which is a motivating form of engagement); and healing engagements (which are activities and experiences that were specifically identified as promoting the participants' healing) (Figure 27.2).

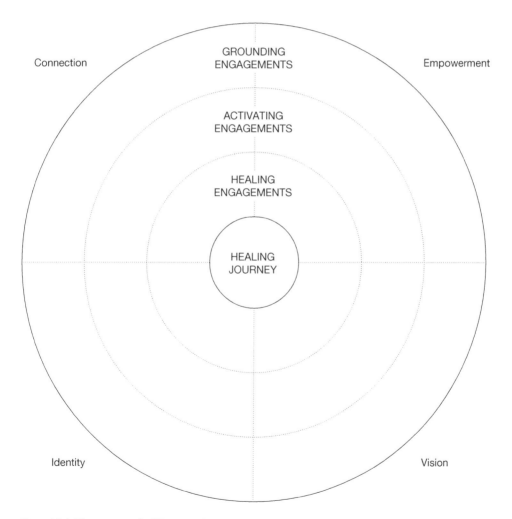

Figure 27.2 Three types of self/community engagement

Grounding engagements

Grounding engagements are opportunities for harmony grounded in the four foundational categories of engagement within the activists' self/community life-world. For this reason, the four grounding engagements are named after the four foundational categories of engagement, themselves:

- *Connection*: The grounding engagement of connection is the experience of connectedness within and across the various spheres of the self/community life-world. As George put it, connection asserts, "You are part of this, you are born to this, you're not alone."
- *Empowerment*: The grounding engagement of empowerment is the experience of agency within the activist's self/community life-world. All of the participants identified the empowerment they felt when they saw the positive changes resulting from their efforts as activists in their self/community life-world. For example, Alice found empowerment through contribution to others as a healer:

    > They would come in with a sore back, headaches and such, and I'd be able to help them! I was doing it myself, healing people through Reiki . . . And I never thought I could do that for somebody. And after that there was no stopping me.

- *Identity*: The grounding engagement of identity is the self-referential description of the self/community life-world. For all of the activists, the recognition of their individual identity was essential to their healing journey. However, their collective identity, in relation to their family and community, was also deemed essential by the participants. George asserted,

    > If you're a Kwakwaka'wakw child, you're a member of a clan; then you know your territory, the roles and responsibilities you have in the family, the roles and responsibilities with the resources around you, and what you need to do to support other people in the clan.

- *Vision*: The grounding engagement of vision is the participants' self/community world-view. Nature was considered the template for the vision of life and how to live for most of the activists. And the terms balance and harmony were identified by the activists as essential to their vision. Vision includes the ethics and principles by which one is to live. Felicity shared:

    > For me, healing is balance in all aspects of the emotional, spiritual, and physical, and mental . . . I know that at times I'm out of balance, and not only healthwise, but out of balance with family or with nature or with community. And so I work towards restoring balance and harmony in whatever it is.

Grounding engagements as resistance

When grounding self/community engagements are expressed in an overtly oppressive context, they can be understood as resistance. This is true whether or not they are confronting internalized colonization (i.e., oppression within themselves or by others in their community) or colonial interventions by the outside non-Aboriginal community.

Activating engagements

Rooted in each of the foundational categories of engagement, the four activating engagements propel the participants into action within their self/community life-world (Figure 27.3). Whether offered to the participants or received from them, these self/community engagements initiate

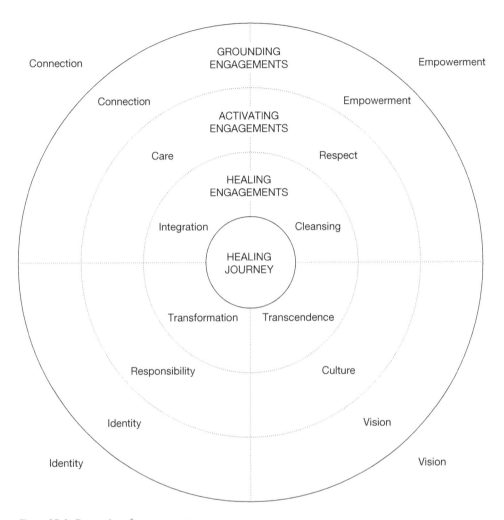

Figure 27.3 Categories of engagement

activity. They are reflexively related to the grounding engagements; they both emerge from them and support and enhance them:

- *Care*: Rooted in the foundational category of connection, care motivates compassionate intervention. Care is the desire to support those with whom one is connected in being happy, healthy, and safe. Socially, care offers those who receive it an experience of connection. Reciprocally, when one feels connected to someone or something in one's self/community life-world, one cares for them. Alice shared:

    So in order to fill that void that I lost, not having a mom, I had to give to others. So I could give to others that didn't have a mom. I'd hug them and love them. I didn't want to see the other children go through what I had to go through.

- *Respect*: Rooted in the foundational category of empowerment, respect is the recognition of capacity and value across the self/community life-world. In relational terms, respect is both the acknowledgment of difference within the self/community life-world and the valuing of the other. It is the recognition of self–other boundaries—the recognition that, at some level, we are as separate from one another as we are connected. Eric described respect when he states his recognition that "I'm not more than you, you're not more than me but, you know, we're both here."

- *Responsibility*: Rooted in the foundational category of identity, responsibility is an activating engagement of relational obligation. Diane shared:

  And my mother-in-law said to me, "Diane, we don't want you to leave us. We want you to: learn the Culture, the language, be our voice, and our legs when we can't do that" . . . So I decided I wasn't going to be a nurse. I followed my mother-in-law and learned the language, learned the history, learned who I am; to be a voice for the Elders.

  Responsibility provides the activists with a role in the community: it is both the product of their identity and a producer of it.
- *Culture*: Culture is an activating engagement that reciprocally emerges from and contributes to the activists' vision. Among the participants, "Culture" was used as a term specific to their own local community vision as well as to differentiate their Aboriginal vision and traditions from the non-native. As George put it, "The real worth of Culture is not in the button blankets or in the mysterious ceremonies—although they are important—it's really in giving expression to one's value and place in the universe."

Balance of activating engagements

Each of the four modes of activating engagements requires the ongoing resolution or balancing of a related tension emerging between self and community spheres of their self/community life-world. The tension emerging from the activating engagement of care requires a balance between self-care and care for community. The tension emerging from empowerment requires a balance of empowered service with respectful non-interference. Emerging from responsibility is a tension that requires a balance between current responsibility and traditional identity. Finally, emerging from Culture is a tension that requires a balancing of Western with Aboriginal cultural traditions.

Healing engagements

Healing engagements are those activities and experiences within the self/community life-world described by the activists that specifically contributed to the paths of transition from pain rooted in past wounds to a healthy present and a hopeful future. (The sub-headings given to the psychosocial and cultural-spiritual paths of each healing engagement ought to be considered a convenience for the sake of organization.)

- *Integration*: Rooted in the foundational category of connection, integration is the re-connection of previously disconnected aspects of the activists' self/community life-world. All of the participants described integration experiences and linked them to their healing journey. In psychosocial terms, growth is the resolution of previously disintegrated states of being, variously modeled by the activists as: a loss of self, alienation from community, detachment from experience, and/or a premature foreclosure of development. For example, Felicity shared, a closing conversation with a therapist:

  "When I came here I was a 5-year-old little girl feeling lost and disconnected from everything and everyone and with no value" I said. And then he said, "So how old are you today?" And I said, "I'm 16, and . . . I have no fear, and believe that I can do and be whoever I'm meant to be."

- *Retraditionalization*: Retraditionalization is the cultural and spiritual integration of the self/community life-world. Felicity's involvement in an annual Tribal Canoe Journey was a result of her role as the coordinator of a program that served the needs of Aboriginal youth. The two-week cultural experience was profound for her healing:

  And when I was on the canoe, every stroke was for the health of my community, and my family, and my self, for me, you know, for all people. And I felt, I felt so full of power. It was very empowering 'cuz it wasn't foreign to me, it was who I am as a First Nations woman, doing something that my grandmother, and her grandmother, and her grandmother before her. It felt that I was working for the health of the past and the future, connecting them.

- *Cleansing*: Rooted in the foundational category of empowerment, cleansing is a process through which distress and imbalance are externalized and removed from the activist's life. The healing engagement of cleansing is a non-integrating form of healing that releases or purges what does not properly "belong" to the person seeking healing. In psychosocial terms, cleansing is the release of the impacts of internalized painful past events. As Alice put it: "When I let go of the past, everything started to work out wonderfully." In cultural-spiritual terms, cleansing is the purging of that which interferes in the participants' desire to live in balance or harmony or which contaminates the spirit within a person. When dealing with the suicide of her son, Cathy experienced ceremonial purging in nature.

  We were taken as a family to a bathing spot and you had to go before daybreak . . . It was winter when we were there, but you didn't feel the cold. Then you came out of the water and . . . brushed yourself with cedar . . . The feeling that you had was one of healing.

- *Transformation*: Rooted in the foundational category of identity, transformation is a healing engagement in which the activists left their "old" identity behind as they took on a "new" one. In psychosocial terms, transformation is a significant change in role—becoming a parent or grandparent was identified as such an event. Transformation resulting from cultural-spiritual ceremony is termed a rebirth. When Diane spoke about her initiation onto the Longhouse, she shared the words of one of her spiritual "mothers," words that marked her rebirth:

  "You've now entered into the Spirit world; you've now entered into a culture that's going to be with you for the rest of your life . . . You have been reborn, given a second chance in life to rebuild yourself, and if you follow that life, you're gonna be strong, you're gonna be positive, and you're going to have your respect back." I'll always remember those words, and that's 18 years ago. And I live it.

- *Transcendence*: Rooted in the foundational category of vision, transcendence described the healing effects of the activists' expansion of their vision from their personal distress to a "larger" experience. In psychosocial terms, transcendence was experienced when the activists were able to contextualize the suffering in their self/community life-world within the impact of colonization—personal and social problems were understood to transcend themselves and their community. Felicity's commentary on "healing" itself offers an example:

  And I think the reason I have difficulty with "healing" is because—I don't know if you want to get political, but that's what it is, politics. You know, with the impacts of contact, colonization and Residential School . . . The government did a really good job of separating the crime of genocide by manipulating our people to believe that they needed to be healed. We are suffering from the legacy of Residential School, but I believe that what happened was a crime.

- Spirituality as a transcendence-oriented healing engagement was a consistent theme among the activists. Harold shared:

> I started Sundancing. And it just got more and more intense. That was where I felt, you know, connected to God. I just finished dragging buffalo skulls and then all of a sudden I felt a feeling that I'd never felt, I just felt, you know, well nobody can describe it, it was just like how you have a mother's love, but it was like a thousand times intensified like the spirits and the grandmothers, the grandfathers and the Creator all love you, right. I just started bawling.

Activism

While self/community engagements often came from the interventions of others across their life-world, receiving from others was insufficient for the activists' healing journey. Central to their suicide-related resilience, every participant perceived the provision of self/community engagements to others to be central to their healing journey. George shared:

> Spiritual awakenings are important, but they are like a turning point. You've gotta nurture that, build on it, continue to look at yourself and improve who you are. I'm grateful for all the things I've been blessed with over the years. I'm so fortunate that I do the work I'm doing. Otherwise I would still be broken, still be harming myself and others . . . The thing that's kept me going though all the years is that I've been able to be of service.

As the activists helped their fellow community members heal their lives, they accomplished their own transition to a greater connection with their fellows, greater empowerment through the change they saw in others at risk, a healthier identity as a helper, and a vision of compassionate hope both for others and, ultimately, for themselves. In the same manner as the other healing engagements, activism can be organized into psychosocial and cultural-spiritual semi-spheres (Figure 27.4).

Psychosocial contribution: community activism

Contribution in a community that is struggling with the oppression of colonization can properly be described as activism. Community activism is a form of resistance in the face of the false generosity (Freire, 2005) of the colonizers' provision of its own sanctioned community services that have followed the impacts of the colonial interventions. The enforced dependency has been internalized in a sense of disempowerment at the community level. Resisting the dependency promoted by colonial interventions, the activists discovered that community mobilization was an important part of their own healing and suicide-resilience—contribution and resilience are indivisible within the activists' self/community life-world.

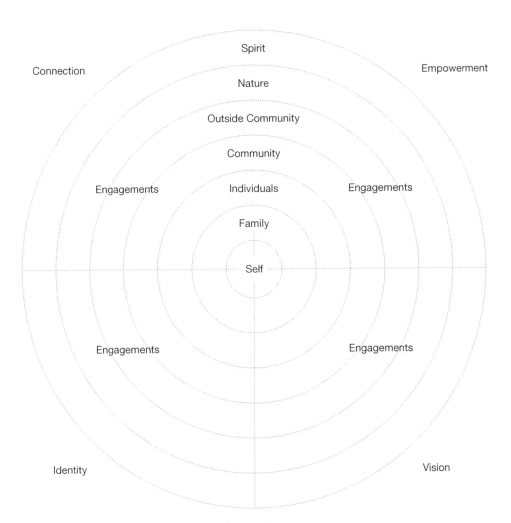

Figure 27.4 Psychosocial and cultural-spiritual semi-spheres

Cultural-spiritual contribution: cultural activism

The activists also contributed to the cultural and spiritual spheres of their self/community life-world in a manner that can be understood to be post-colonial activism, in that their activities challenge the intention of the colonizer to "solve the Indian problem" by assimilation and control. Through their community service (often outside of the market economy and utilizing Traditional methodologies), the activists contribute to the resilience of their Culture. This activism may, at times, directly confront the colonizer: Diane shared about her advocacy on behalf of her Ancestors during a meeting with government representatives about land use after a burial discovery in her community's traditional territory. After first consulting with Elders, she followed their instructions about the protocol required to receive guidance from the Ancestors on how to best be their voice:

> And then I fell asleep and I dreamt and I seen what I had to do. I had to convince the parks people not to make that a park, on the wishes of the spirit people there . . . And I said: "We will never let you make that a park land. I will gather as many people as I

can and sit on that land if I have to, but you will never make it a park land. And I will share my story and my dream and my experience to everyone else who's gonna follow in my footsteps. And that land will always be protected." And that was eight years ago, and it's still the same.

Cultural activism is the antidote to the cultural-spiritual impacts of colonization (i.e., anomie). The role of the activists in ceremony provided them and those who learned from or participated with them a deeper cultural and community connection and vision, a sense of empowerment in their increased cultural knowledge, competence in traditional and ceremonial protocol and role recognition by others, and a new identity.

The healing journey of activism

Described by the model in Figure 27.5, the transition from suicidal crisis to activism by this study's participants can be conceptualized as the result of a process of reciprocal engagements within the activists' self/community life-world, beginning with colonial impacts and ending with positive change through increased self/community life-world harmony. This process enhanced the activists' sense of connectedness and empowerment and developed their identity and vision within it. At the same time as the process supported their resilience, it contributed to the resilience of their community.

The social activism literature has generally defined community activism in specifically focused political terms (Noggle, 1996). There is relatively little written about activism as the general enhancement of individual and community resilience within an oppressive context. Nonetheless, the participants did not identify a "watershed issue" around which they collectively mobilized. Instead, they described an iterative process of change within themselves and their community. Through the activism of its members, the community itself has had the opportunity to transition to a connected and empowered collective with a self-generated identity (rather than one imposed by the colonizer) and a culturally rooted contemporary and hopeful vision of its future. That is, the community's resilience is enhanced.

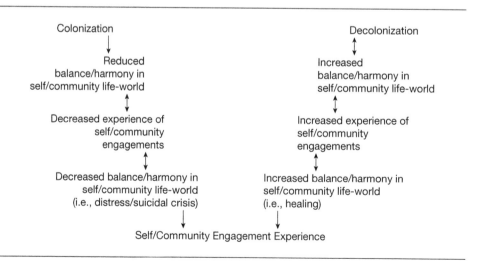

Figure 27.5 The healing journey of activism

Resolving the healing–activism dichotomy

The post-colonial literature's assertion of a necessary dichotomy between personal "healing" and community "activism"—identifying the first with assimilation and the second with resistance (Chrisjohn, Young, & Mauraun,1997)—was not supported by the activists. While many of the participants utilized sanctioned (i.e., mainstream) treatment modalities and services to reduce their immediate distress, there appear to be three reasons for lack of assimilation. First, in several cases resistance was promoted by the sanctioned service providers. Second, all of the activists maintained their self/community integration by taking the techniques they received for their own healing (such as bibliotherapy, Reiki, supportive counseling, etc.) and using them to serve as healers and helpers for others in their self/community. And, third, all of the participants utilized as transcendence engagement—either contextualizing their experience as the product of colonization rather than a sign of pathology (Atleo, 1997; Freire, 2005; Wade, 2000) and/or utilizing local Cultural spirituality to respond to the experience of imbalance within their self/community life-world (which, due to the reflexivity inherent in the self/community life-world) supported their community (Dion Stout & Kipling, 2003; Smith, 1998; Wesley-Esquimaux & Smolewski, 2004). This holistic impact of their engagement resolves the post-colonial dichotomy of personal versus social change.

Limitations

There are four limits to this study that must be identified, and one recommendation that follows from them: (1) this research is intentionally specific to two closely related First Nations; (2) the researcher was a cultural outsider (although his work in the communities extends over two decades); (3) the small sample size (only eight in-depth interviews); (4) this is a pilot study, as there has been little or no research into suicide-related resilience within the population of socially contributing Aboriginals. It is hoped that further research will overcome these challenges.

Implications

There are three main implications that emerge from this study. These implications emerge from (1) the self/community life-world; (2) self/community engagements; and (3) the conflation of healing with activism. First, the self/community life-world model suggests the possible integration of many lines of enquiry into Aboriginal health. For instance, ecological conservation, Cultural tradition, and intergenerational social history are as important as genetics and family dynamics. This implies that any health-promoting assessment or intervention ought to be holistic, and that policies and interventions must consider the entire bio-psycho-socio-historical-cultural-ecological-spiritual community in their approach. For example, the impacts of an intervention at one of the self/community spheres require an outcome assessment across the community's life-world. As a result, evaluations of any intervention in the self/community can be framed in terms of the impact on these engagements across the life-world. Of course, negative "side-effects" and/or positive synergies will require consideration both before interventions are undertaken, as well as in their evaluation.

Second, the identification of self/community engagements provides an opportunity for policy-makers and clinicians to approach the issue of Aboriginal suicide in a manner that is congruent with the experience of the community and its members. Enhancing resilience through focusing attention on each of the grounding, activating, and healing engagements expands the resource base from those often utilized in treatment. The model of self/community engagements offers an opportunity for a strengths-based intervention that simultaneously serves the individual and their community. Likewise, the development of these engagements can be directed at the individual, family, and community level, thereby serving to integrate personal healing with community mobilization.

Third, the conflation of healing with activism suggests a reconsideration of the definition of resilience and healing as it applies to the Aboriginal community. To locate a so-called mental health problem, such as suicide, on the level of self (i.e., as a personal problem) is to ignore its role as an expression of family and community distress and cultural theft. Individualized pathologization not only allows the oppressor to avoid responsibility for the crisis as a natural result of a "national crime," but also blinds us to possible interventions at the family, community and cultural level. Instead, interveners are encouraged to collaborate with the oppressor by defining mental health as congruent to the successful adjustment of an individual (to a life of oppression).

From these findings, healing is redefined from the reduction of personal distress (i.e., individualized pathologization) to an increased state of harmony within the self/community life-world. Individualized interventions are often necessary, but are not sufficient. If, as the results suggest, resistance against the alienation (disconnection), hostile dependency (disempowerment), victim-identity, and anomie promoted by the colonial enterprise is resilience, then community mobilization and the encouragement of activism (i.e., actively increasing available self/community engagements) are a preferred focus of intervention. According to the example provided by the suicide-related resilient activists, the encouragement of activism is a suitable prescription; community and Culture will necessarily impact healing (in both the activist and across the community life-world).

Acknowledgement

This chapter is an adaptation of the author's doctoral dissertation of the same title.

References

Atleo, M. (1997). First Nations healing: Dominance or health. *The Canadian Journal for the Study of Adult Education, 11*(2), 63–67.

Battiste, M. (2000). Unfolding the lessons of colonization. In M. Battiste (Ed.), *Reclaiming Indigenous voice and vision* (pp. xvi–xxx). Vancouver, BC: University of British Columbia Press.

Bhargava, R. (1992). *Individualism in social science: Forms and limits of a methodology.* New York: Oxford University Press.

Chandler, M. J., & Lalonde, C. (1998). Cultural continuity as a hedge against suicide in Canada's First Nations. *Transcultural Psychiatry, 35*, 191–219.

Chandler, M. J., & Lalonde, C. (2004). Transferring whose knowledge? Exchanging whose best practices?: On knowing about Indigenous knowledge and Aboriginal suicide. In J. White, P. Maxim, & D. Beavon (Eds.), *Aboriginal policy research: Setting the agenda for change, Vol. 2.* Toronto, ON: Thompson.

Chrisjohn, R., Young, S., & Mauraun, M. (1997). *The circle game: Shadows and substance in the Indian residential school experience in Canada.* Penticton, BC: Theytus Books.

Cross, T. (1998). Understanding family resiliency from a relational world-view. In H. McCubbin, E. Thompson, A. Thompson, & J. Fromer (Eds.), *Resiliency in Native American and immigrant families* (pp. 143–157). Thousand Oaks, CA: Sage.

Dion Stout, M., & Kipling, G. (2003). *Aboriginal people, resilience, and the residential school legacy.* Ottawa, ON: Aboriginal Healing Foundation.

Duran, E. (2006). *Healing the soul wound: Counseling with American Indians and other native peoples.* New York: Teachers College Press.

Freire, P. ([1970] 2005). *Pedagogy of the oppressed.* New York: Continuum Press.

Furness, E. (1995). *Victims of benevolence: The dark legacy of the William's Lake residential school.* Vancouver, BC: Arsenal Pulp Press.

Gergen, K., & Gergen, M. (2000). Toward a cultural constructionist psychology. Available at: http://www.swarthmore.edu/SocSci/kgergen1/web/page.html (accessed 29 September 2008).

Haig-Brown, C. (1991). *Resistance and renewal: Surviving the Indian residential school.* Vancouver, BC: Arsenal Pulp Press.

Harris, C. (2002). *Making Native space.* Vancouver, BC: University of British Columbia Press.

Husserl, E. (1970). *The crisis of European sciences and the transcendental phenomenology* (Trans. D. Carr). Evanston, IL: Northwestern University Press.

Indian residential schools mental health support program (2005). *Program framework.* Ottawa, ON: Indian Residential Schools Resolution Canada.

Josselson, R. (2004). The hermeneutics of faith and the hermeneutics of suspicion. *Narrative Inquiry, 14*(1), 1–28.

Kirmayer, L., Brass, G., & Tait, C. (2000). The mental health of Aboriginal peoples: Transformations of identity and control. *Canadian Journal of Psychiatry, 45,* 607–616.

Kirmayer, L., & Minas, H. (2000). The future of cultural psychiatry: An international perspective. *Canadian Journal of Psychiatry, 45*(5), 438–436.

Ladd-Yelk, C. (2001). *Resiliency factors of the North American indigenous people.* Stout, WI: University of Wisconsin.

Lassiter, L. (2000). Authoritative texts, collaborative ethnography, and Native American studies. *American Indian Quarterly, 24*(4), 601–614.

Lykes, M. B. (1996). Meaning making in a context of genocide and silencing. In M. B. Lykes, A. Banuazizi, L. Ramsay, & M. Morris (Eds.), *Myths about the powerless: Contesting social inequities* (pp. 159–178). Philadelphia, PA: Temple University Press.

Marsella, A. J., Olivira, J. M., Plummer, C. M., & Crabbe, K. M. (1998). Native Hawaiian culture, mind, and well-being. In H. McCubbin, E. Thompson, A. Thompson, & J. Fromer (Eds.), *Resiliency in Native American and immigrant families* (pp. 93–114). Thousand Oaks, CA: Sage.

McCormick, R. (1996). The facilitation of healing for the First Nations people of British Columbia. *Canadian Journal of Native Education, 21*(2), 249–322.

Milloy, J. (1999). *A national crime: The Canadian government and the residential school system: 1879–1986.* Winnipeg, MB: University of Winnipeg Press.

Montgomery, D., Miville, M., Winterowd, C., Jeffries, B., & Baysden, M. (2000). American Indian college students: An exploration into resiliency factors revealed through personal stories. *Cultural Diversity and Ethnic Minority Psychology, 6*(4), 387–398.

Mussel, B., Cardiff, K., & White, J. (2004). *The mental health and well-being of Aboriginal children and youth: Guidance for new approaches and services.* Chilliwack, BC: British Columbia Ministry for Children and Family Development.

Noggle, D. (1996). Women activists of diverse backgrounds: A qualitative study of self perceived developmental influences and values. Unpublished doctoral dissertation, Fielding Graduate Institute, Santa Barbara, CA.

Prilleltensky, I. (1994). *The morals and politics of psychology: Psychological discourse and the status quo.* New York: State University of New York Press.

Ross, R. (1992). *Dancing with a ghost: Exploring Indian identity.* Markham, ON: Octopus.

Royal Commission on Aboriginal Peoples (RCAP) (1995). *Choosing life: Suicide among Aboriginal people.* Ottawa, ON: Royal Commission on Aboriginal Peoples.

Said, E. (1993). *Cultural imperialism.* London: Chatto and Windus.

Satzewich, V. (1998). Race, racism and radicalization: Contested concepts. In V. Satzwich (Ed.), *Racism and social inequality in Canada: Concepts, controversies and strategies of resistance* (pp. 25–45). Toronto, ON: Thompson Education Publishing.

Schwartz, T. (1992). Anthropology and psychology: An unrequited relationship. In T. Schwartz, G. White, & C. Lutz (Eds.), *New directions in psychological anthropology* (pp. 324–349). Cambridge: Cambridge University Press.

Sivaraksa, S. (1999). *Global healing: Essays and interviews on structural violence, social development, and spiritual transformation.* Bangkok: Thai Inter-Religious Commission for Development.

Smith, L. T. (1998). *Decolonizing methodologies: Research and indigenous peoples.* New York: Zed Books.

Smye, V. (2003). The nature of the tensions and disjunctures between Aboriginal understandings of and responses to mental health and illness and the current mental health system. Unpublished doctoral dissertation, The University of British Columbia, Vancouver.

Statistics Canada (2001). *Aboriginal peoples in Canada*: Canadian Centre for Justice statistics profile series. Ottawa, ON: Ministry of Industry.

Stephenson, P. (1995). *A persistent spirit: Toward understanding Aboriginal health in British Columbia*. Victoria, BC: Western Geographical Press.

Tennant, P. (1990). *Aboriginal people and politics: The Indian land question in British Columbia, 1849–1989*. Vancouver, BC: University of British Columbia Press.

Tsosie, R. (2003). Land, culture, and community: Envisioning Native American sovereignty and national identity in the twenty-first century. In D. Champagne, & I. Abu-Saad (Eds.), *The future of indigenous peoples: Strategies for survival and development* (pp. 3–20). Los Angeles: UCLA American Indian Studies Centre.

van Uchelen, C., Davidson, S., Quressette, S., Brassfield, C., & Demerais, L. (1997). What makes us strong: Urban Aboriginal perspectives on wellness and strength. *Canadian Journal of Community Mental Health, 16*(2), 37–50.

Wade, A. (2000). Resistance knowledges: Therapy with Aboriginal persons who have experienced violence. In P. Stephenson, S. Elliot, L. Foster, & J. Harris (Eds.), *A persistent spirit: Towards understanding Aboriginal health in British Columbia* (Vol. 31). Victoria: University of Victoria, Western Press.

Ward, K. (2001). *Residential Schools in British Columbia: The Journey*. Penticton, BC: Theytus Books.

Weaver, H. N. (2002). Perspectives on wellness: Journeys on the Red Road. *Journal of Sociology and Social Welfare, 24* (1), 5–15.

Werner, E. (1993). Risk, resilience, and recovery: Perspectives from the Kauai longitudinal study. *Development and Psychopathology, 5,* 503–513.

Wesley-Esquimaux, C., & Smolewski, M. (2004). *Historic trauma and Aboriginal healing*. Ottawa, ON: Aboriginal Healing Foundation.

White, G., & Lutz, C. (1992). Introduction. In T. Schwartz, G. White, & C. Lutz (Eds.), *New directions in psychological anthropology* (pp. 1–20). Cambridge: Cambridge University Press.

White, J., Maxim, P., & Beavon, D. (Eds.). (2003). *Aboriginal conditions: Research as a foundation for public policy*. Vancouver, BC: University of British Columbia Press.

28

THE FACILITATION OF HEALING FOR INDIGENOUS YOUTH WHO ARE SUICIDAL

A retrospective exploratory study

Rod McCormick, Sharon Thira, Marla Arvay and Sophia Rinaldis

Introduction

In Canada and the United States, Indigenous people under the age of 25 continue to experience a much higher suicide rate than non-Indigenous people in the same age group (Ferry, 2000; Statistics Canada, 2006). Suicide rates, in Canada, for Indigenous youth steadily increased from the 1960s until the mid-1990s (Kirmayer, Brass, Holton, Paul, Simpson, & Tait, 2007). During this 30-year time frame, analysis revealed that suicide among Indigenous youth in North America living on reserves escalated from 200% to 300% (Berlin, 1987). By the end of the 20th century, rates began to stabilize or slightly decrease for the general Indigenous population. However, for Indigenous youth, the numbers continued to grow (Kirmayer et al., 2007). This was especially the case for male youth. Although very few authors have investigated rates of suicide attempt, it is safe to say that these statistics are also high when compared to youth of the general population. Furthermore, rates of suicide attempt are dangerously high among female youth (Kirmayer et al., 2007). Today, Indigenous people are, generally, between two and five times more likely to commit suicide than non-Indigenous people (Chandler & Lalonde, 2008; Kirmayer et al., 2007); these estimates inevitably vary across communities. The statistics for Indigenous youth between the ages of 15 and 25 are even higher. Indigenous youth in Canada between 10 and 19 years of age are five to six times more likely to commit suicide than non-Indigenous youth of the same age; rates are the highest for youth between the ages of 20 and 29 (Royal Commission Report, 2002).

Empirical research has not yet demonstrated a direct causal link between colonization and suicide rates. However, widespread social conditions resulting from colonization have been identified as important determinants of Indigenous mental health (Kirmayer 2003; King, 2009) and suggest the need for multiple rather than singular responses. Particularly, in the case of suicide, many of the consequences of colonization have been suspected to mediate its relation to suicide rates.

Colonization has imposed assimilationist practices that have impacted Indigenous lifestyles. For example, residential schools have resulted in a breakdown of extended family and community systems, the assault on traditional values as well as serious impact on cultural identity. The imposed settlement of Indigenous people into sedentary communities has disrupted an ongoing connection with the land and environment. In general, the colonization process can be held accountable for damage to culture, tradition, continuity and meaning.

Authors have also put forward hypotheses regarding more specific repercussions. Hodson (1986) and Chandler and Lalonde (2008) connect what they call cultural losses to First Nations youth, frequently leaving them vulnerable to feelings of confusion as well as a sense of alienation from their roots and culture. Other authors have identified the acculturative stress caused by oppressive methods of colonization as a possible mediating factor in this abnormal identity development. Duran and Duran (1995) describe the effects of acculturative stress as a form of intergenerational post-traumatic stress disorder suffered by all Aboriginal peoples consistent with Danieli's (1998) later work on multigenerational stress. Acculturative stress also seems to play a role in the postcolonial increase of mental health problems such as mood and anxiety disorders seen in Indigenous peoples (Kirmayer et al., 2007). Colonization is presumed to be linked to alarming rates of drug and alcohol abuse amongt Aboriginal peoples (Leenaars, Brown, Taparti, Anowak, & Hill-Keddie, 1999). These consequences are all known risk factors for suicide. Therefore, in examining what facilitates healing and recovery for Indigenous youth who are suicidal, de-colonizing methods must be included in the analysis and application of the findings. Such models embed multifactorial causes within singular frameworks or process maps like the medicine wheel in order to conceptualize an Indigenous holistic paradigm (Smylie, 2001; Walker, 2001; MacDonald, 2008).

Despite growing awareness of the issue of suicide, the impacts of colonization and the consequent profusion of mental health problems, Indigenous people tend to under-utilize mental health services provided by the majority culture (Waldram, Herring, & Young, 2006; Gone & Alcantara, 2007). Explanations have often held the patient accountable for his/her resistance or lack of response to treatment although it is becoming increasingly apparent that the larger part of the problem rests in the epistemological and methodological tensions between westernized approaches and traditional Indigenous practices (Duran & Duran, 1995). Research conducted by McCormick (1995) indicated that community-based models of care that utilize the natural healing methods of Indigenous people are more effective in recovery and healing than those utilized in mainstream psychotherapeutic models (Mussel, Cardiff, & White, 2004; Thira, 2009). Duran, Firehammer and Gonzalez (2008) reiterate the need for a liberated approach to counseling through which the proposed methods of healing are congruent with Indigenous world-views and belief systems where health is viewed as holistic and interrelated rather than distinct from other aspects of life (MacDonald, 2008). Given the complex history of Aboriginal peoples, many authors also identify the need for sociological models of analysis and treatment (Durkheim, 1966; Royal Commission on Aboriginal Peoples, 1995; Chrisjohn & Young, 1997). Further research of this nature is needed to explore the natural methods of healing and recovery utilized by Indigenous people who are suicidal.

Very little research has focused on solutions to the problem of suicide among Indigenous people. Katz (2006), while noting that much research exists on the causes of suicide, speaks of the need for evidence-based recovery interventions. Much of the literature on youth suicide recommends teaching self-esteem, communication skills, knowledge on how to handle grief, a sense of community, a sense of one's own value, and how to deal with emotions (Hafen & Frankness, 1986). Of these, limited recommendations for Indigenous suicide reduction exist: teaching positive self-image, exploration of traditional healing practices, and the re-introduction of traditional cultural activities (Cooper, Carlsberg, & Pelletier-Adams, 1991; Kirmayer et al., 2007). Bostick's (2007) study of adolescent youth suicide recovery demonstrates how attachment relationships and experiences of attachment with parents, peers and others developed a sense of connection which served to change self-perceptions. Spirituality also played a role, as noted in a study on Indigenous women in British Columbia for whom reconnection to cultural identity and traditional native spirituality were recovery factors (Paproski, 1997). In grey and academic literature, practitioners are calling for more healing programming that reflects the history of colonization, the need for self-determination and the importance of cultural and traditional activities (Hill, 2009; Crooks, 2009).

The purpose of this research was to examine what facilitates healing and recovery for Indigenous youth who are suicidal, from their point of view. This chapter, then, approached the issue of healing and recovery in a way that included the input of Indigenous youth themselves. Nwachuku and Ivey (1991), in their promotion of culture-specific counseling, argue that counseling research must first start with an exploration of the natural helping styles of a culture before developing theories and approaches for it. Researchers need to explore the insights and experiences of Indigenous youth in order to obtain information to determine the best way to facilitate healing for suicidal Indigenous youth. Furthermore, Duran et al. (2008) recommend that research in this context use research methods that match Indigenous ways of acquiring information.

Method

The study described in this chapter was an exploratory research study that examined what facilitates healing and recovery for suicidal Indigenous youth by eliciting participants' experience through an unstructured critical incident interview. Twenty-five participants in the study provided 280 critical incidents of their own experiences in healing by describing what was done and what action was taken to facilitate healing for them. A scheme of categories was established to organize this data so that it could be of use to both theorists and practitioners. The generic term "healing" was used in this study as no attempt was made to define healing compartmentally, be it physical, mental, emotional or spiritual. Indigenous people tend to see healing from a holistic perspective (Medicine Eagle, 1989), and any effort to differentiate one from another would contradict the belief in the interconnectedness of these inseparable dimensions of the self.

Participants

Potential participants were made aware of the study through the researcher's contacts with the Aboriginal community in Vancouver, British Columbia. The participants in this study ranged in age from 17 to mid-forties, the mean age being late twenties. Geographically, the 25 participants originally came from many different communities in British Columbia and a few from other provinces; however, all had been living in the Vancouver area at the time of the interviews. Eleven of the participants were male and 14 were female. This study focused on the period of life described as "youth". For the purpose of this study, the researcher defined youth as under the age of 30.[1] The researcher chose participants to interview who had experienced being suicidal in the past and had fully recovered from being suicidal. This 'distance' from the event allowed the participants enough time in their lives beyond the event to enable them to reflect upon the recovery experience and make sense of what helped them to recover. This 'retrospective' view proved to be very effective.[2]

Procedure

Critical Incident Technique

The Critical Incident Technique (Flanagan, 1954) is a form of qualitative interview research in which participants provide descriptive accounts of events that facilitate or hinder a particular aim. The aim in this study was to gather descriptions of significant incidents in the lives of First Nations people that helped facilitate their healing and recovery from suicidal ideation during their youth. Study participants were selected from those who had been in a position to experience relevant facilitation or hindrance, and who were capable of articulating their experiences. Upon completion of interviews, critical incidents are extracted from accounts and then grouped by similarity of content to form a set of categories that encompassed the events.

Procedures

In this study the Critical Incident interview involved two parts, namely, an orientation to the purpose of the research (the research aim), and an elicitation of facilitating events or incidents. The orientation clarified the nature of the study and provided time to establish rapport. In particular, the orientation was an attempt to communicate the aim or nature of events to be reported. The second part of this interview was an attempt to elicit events that facilitated healing. Participants were encouraged to describe events clearly and completely. The interviewer was to listen carefully to ensure that the events were complete and accurate. It was necessary to learn what led up to the incident, what actually happened, and what the resulting outcome was. Each participant was asked to "Please describe a particular incident or incidents when you did something or someone did something to help facilitate your healing and recovery from suicide in your youth." The interviewer then asked: "What was the effect of the incident?" The interviewer gained clarity on the responses before continuing to search for other critical incidents. Once the interviews were completed, they were transcribed verbatim.

During data analysis, the events or critical incidents were extracted and put on index cards. Once all interviews were analyzed for critical incidents, two graduate research assistants and the primary researcher independently extracted incidents from the interviews. Initial attempts at extracting incidents were corrected by comparing them with incidents recorded from the researcher's interviews. The process is repeated until all three coders consistently obtained the same incidents. Establishing the categories is an inductive process involving sorting the incidents into clusters that seem to group together. Before categorizing the incidents, we reviewed the information about the context or relationship to which the incident referred by reviewing the interview as a whole. The categories were "worked on" until a sense of "rightness" (Woolsey, 1986) was found. Woolsey (1986) and others (Andersson & Nilsson, 1964; Cohen & Smith, 1976) suggest that an acceptable rate of inter-rater agreement needs to have between 75% to 85% agreement.

The categories were validated in five different ways by answering five different types of questions regarding the soundness and trustworthiness of the category system. The first validation procedure examined the reliability of categorizing the incidents by assessing whether different people could use the categories in a consistent way. Independent judges were asked to place a random sample of the events into the categories (28 events or approximately 10% of the total number of incidents gathered). The independent judges used in this study were graduate students in the Department of Counselling Psychology at the University of British Columbia. The resultant average inter-rater reliability of 91% strongly indicated that the categories were reliable or trustworthy.

The second procedure assessed the soundness of the categories by examining the comprehensiveness of the categories. To assess comprehensiveness or completeness of the categories, another 28 incidents (10%) were previously withheld from the categorization process until after the categories were formed. When category formation was finished, the withheld incidents were easily placed within the categories by the independent judges. If this were not the case, it would have been necessary to form new categories until all of the withheld incidents had been correctly placed.

The third procedure assessed the soundness of the categories by examining the participation rate for categories. It is possible to determine whether a category is sound or well founded by examining the level of agreement among the participants in the study in reporting the same thing. Agreement in this study was gauged by the participation rate for each category (the number of participants reporting a category of events divided by the total number of participants; see Table 28.1). The categories with the highest participation rate are therefore those with the highest level of agreement. Borgen and Amundson (1984) suggest that a significant category is one in which 20–25% of participants identified incidents that fit into a particular category. The participation rates ranged from a low of 4% (Eliminating drugs and alcohol; number of critical incidents = 1) to a high of 88% (Self-esteem/self-acceptance; number of critical incidents = 46) as illustrated in Table 28.1.

The fourth procedure assessed the soundness of the categories by means of expert appraisal. This validation process placed the research findings within the context of counseling psychology by asking expert practitioners in the field to determine whether or not these categories were

Table 28.1 Categories that facilitate healing and recovery for suicidal First Nations youth, in descending order of significance

Factor (in descending order)	Participation rate (%)
Self-esteem/self-acceptance	88
Obtaining help from others	64
Changing thinking	64
Connection with culture/tradition	52
Responsibility to others	48
Expressing emotions/cleansing	44
Future goals/hope	40
Spiritual connection	40
Learning from others/role models	24
Connection to nature	20
Helping others	20
Keeping occupied	20
Exercise/sports	20
Recognize/identify emotions	16
Shutting down emotions	16
Participation in ceremonies	12
Guiding visions/dreams	12
Understanding the problem	12
Humour/perspective	12
Removing self from bad environment	8
Learning problem-solving/communication skills	4
Eliminating drugs and alcohol	4

consistent with what they had found from their own clinical experiences. Interviews with two mental health providers working with First Nations populations did confirm that the categories were valid in the context of their practices.

The fifth procedure assessed the soundness of the categories by examining its agreement with previous research (Royal Commission on Aboriginal Peoples, 1995; Wilson & Wilson, 1995; Strickland, 1997). A comparison of the categories with previous research led to consistent findings of agreement.

Results

Through interviews with 25 participants, 280 critical incidents were elicited reporting what facilitated healing and recovery for First Nations youth who were suicidal. The 280 critical incidents were then placed into 22 categories. Table 28.1 shows the categories with the corresponding participation rate for each category. The participation rate is the number of participants reporting a category of events divided by the total number of participants. A brief description of the categories and examples of incidents in each category will be provided for the top 10 categories that have a participation rate of 20% or greater.

- *Self-esteem/self-acceptance.* In this category, participants describe incidents or events that cause them to feel loved, respected, acknowledged, and valued. Participants also described incidents in which they were: accepting of self, able to recognize their own skills, be genuine, and build their self-confidence. Examples:

  The thing that stopped me from committing suicide was learning that I loved myself and I trusted myself.

  Hurting myself would be disrespect for myself and for the Creator. I learned that respect is the most significant value. Even drugs are disrespectful because it isn't being who you are and who you are supposed to be.

- *Obtaining help from others.* This category describes participants being understood and listened to, being accepted, supported, and encouraged. Helpers ranged from friends to mental health professionals. Example:

  This girl I didn't know that well came up to me and said,"You look so sad, why do you look so sad?" and I told her that I was going to jump in the river and I told her why and she gave me some really simple advice that was the start of the solution. Somebody just had to care enough to come over and ask why I looked so sad.

- *Changing thinking.* In this category, individuals changed their beliefs or outlook concerning their problems in a positive way. This reframing enabled participants to put their problems into perspective and to focus their energies towards constructive action. Examples:

  Changing the way I think of things has helped me to be a stronger person. Back when I was miserable, I was so narrow minded. I saw things with blinders on. I accept things now and everybody the way they are.

  Belief system is so important. I was so angry at white people and the world and that affected my willingness to approach people for help. There was no trust. After being introduced to the belief system that we are all related, and that there is positive in all ways, and that you must use the tools that will help you, I was able to seek the help I needed.

- *Connection with culture/tradition.* This category describes incidents in which participants connected to their culture and tradition. This connection led to empowerment, pride, purpose, and meaning. Examples:

  > My great grandmother taught me about our culture and tradition and that helped me to feel like I belonged.

  > My culture as a practicing winter spirit dancer has been very good. I can feel the power, the universal knowledge, the strength. I feel the goodness of the Creator by practicing my culture, it saved me.

  > Receiving an Indian name created a sense of belonging which was lacking.

- *Responsibility to others.* This category refers to participants deciding not to commit suicide due to their commitment or sense of responsibility to family, community, ancestors and others. Examples:

  > My brother had committed suicide and I couldn't see putting my parents through that again. I couldn't imagine how devastating that would be. Identifying with what it would be like to lose a child helped stop me.

  > Seeing the pain and suffering that other people in the village experienced and how it hurt me made me think about how my death would hurt the people that I respected. Respect for others really stopped me. I thought about the consequences.

  > Having a baby sister helped me to decide to live because I wanted to be a part of her growing up, a sense of responsibility as a brother. Wanting to see the joy in her growing up gave me some optimism for the future.

- *Expressing emotions/cleansing.* In this category, individuals describe incidents in which they were able to let go of their pain, get rid of bad feelings, and cleanse themselves. Examples ranged from crying to writing. Examples:

  > The process of writing my feelings out was very helpful. It was cleansing.

  > I pick sharing circles and ceremonies where people feel it's okay to crumble because there were a lot of times when I crumbled and was able to just let go of the pain.

  > Being able to cry really helped because I was able to get the pain out.

- *Future goals/hope.* In this category, participants were able to set short- or long-term goals that helped them to recover from feeling suicidal. Examples ranged from finishing their education to learning about their culture. Example:

  > Having goals helped me a lot with the depression. To get up every morning and know that I'm going to do something that's constructive to my future was so important.

- *Spiritual connection.* This category refers to participants gaining strength and guidance through spiritual connection. Examples range from praying to communication with spirit guides. Examples:

  > I went to the Indian cemetery and talked to the people there because I was so lonely and they were Indian people. It was a spiritual connection and this helped me to go on.

  > The realization that the spirits of my grandmother and grandfather and my ancestors are with me has helped me because I know that they are always there and I just have to ask them to come. Knowing that I'm not alone helped me to want to live.

- *Learning from others/role models.* This category describes the healing benefits of learning from others such as role models and family. Examples:

> I got to know more people, people who were going through the same thing that I wanted to go through. That made it a lot easier too, the fact that some were succeeding at the same struggle.

> What kept me going was the knowledge that what I was going through had been felt by other native people before and they survived. I just waited because everyone told me it would pass, and it did.

- *Connection to nature.* In this category participants described the healing benefits they obtained by connecting to nature. Examples:

> The thing that helped a lot was water. I would go to the river or to the lake or something. I would just sit by the river and watch the water flow. The water was continuously flowing whatever happened even if there was a snag or something it would just flow around it. If a rock was sticking out of the surface the water would flow around it. It made me feel that's how I should be and that I should carry on.

> Mountains have helped me. One time I was really anxious in remembering the sexual abuse I had experienced as a kid. I was at my Dad's house and feeling sad and I looked out the window at this snowcapped mountain. It was beautiful and it was solid and it had been there a long, long time. At different times of the year it looks different, sometimes it is mostly snow and other times it is mostly green. That helped me that day to think about that mountain that was put there by the Creator. Sometimes we are given a huge problem to deal with for a reason. Without seeing that mountain, I don't think I would have survived that day. I wanted to be like that mountain. The mountain will always be there, it doesn't go anywhere but it changes how it looks. It has strength and beauty. The problem I have with those memories will always be there but some days it will look a lot better than other days. I am learning to be like that mountain.

Discussion and implications

The results of this study confirm and extend the research pertaining to the facilitation of healing and recovery for suicidal Indigenous youth as expressed in the review of the literature. The most important implication is that it provides an empirical basis for what has previously amounted to opinions from researchers. Previous scholars have stressed a number of factors that they believed facilitated healing and recovery for suicidal Indigenous youth. Those factors are: teaching self-esteem and communication skills, providing knowledge on how to handle grief, a sense of community, a sense of one's own value, and how to deal with emotions. These factors were empirically supported in this research by the following categories: self-esteem and self-acceptance, learning problem-solving and communication skills, connection with culture, recognizing/identifying emotions, and expressing emotions/cleansing.

Furthermore, this research building on suicide recovery work around attachment relationships, changing self-perceptions and cultural identity and native spirituality expands the existing categories by adding the categories of: obtaining help from others, responsibility to others, learning from others/role models, helping others, changing thinking, establishing future goals/hope, understanding the problems, spiritual connection, participation in ceremony, connection to nature, guiding visions/dreams, keeping occupied, exercise/sports, shutting down emotions, humor/perspective, removing self from the bad environment, and eliminating drugs and alcohol. All 22 categories therefore represent ways to facilitate healing and recovery for Indigenous youth who are suicidal.

Given that colonization has been implicated in suicide and suicidal ideation in Indigenous peoples, the 22 categories begin to address the conditions created by colonization in a holistic manner. Participants mention emotional factors such as releasing and understanding emotions; spiritual factors such as connection to ancestors, physical factors such as sport or being in nature; and mental factors such as changing thoughts or guiding dreams/visions.

Implications for theory and research

The 22 categories also indicate areas of potential research both in the identified categories and in ones that are absent. Future research needs to be conducted to determine the generalizability of the results of this research, perhaps utilizing a survey instrument that could be developed for that purpose. It would be productive to replicate this study with other Indigenous youth in countries such as New Zealand and Australia. Additional research might also replicate this study to determine if new information and healing categories could be obtained. Replication might help to refine, extend, or revise these categories to further our understanding of healing and recovery for suicidal American Indian youth.

Given that 13 of the 22 categories involved cultural/spiritual practices, the results of this study suggest that it is necessary to understand the belief systems and world-views of Indigenous cultures before applying theories and techniques of healing. Belief systems, decision-making strategies, models of problem-solving, assumptions about how problems arise, and how change occurs are all connected to how we see the world (Ibrahim, 1984; Torrey, 1972). It is hoped that this research will generate an understanding of the value of mobilizing the belief system and natural healing resources of the clients that we serve in order to facilitate healing for them. To ignore these belief systems or to impose a contrary one is to potentially overlook important healing resources and undermine the working relationship between our clients and ourselves as therapists.

Implications for practice

In addition to the categories themselves, this study has specific implications for practice. Conceptualization of the data in the form of a process map (Figure 28.1) not only essentializes the findings into a more recognizable Indigenous healing format (the medicine wheel) but also a tool with implications for treatment planning, counseling, counselor training, program development, and community-based initiatives. The medicine wheel, adapted as it has been by many Indigenous people and programs, as a theoretical paradigm with four constituent parts (mental, physical, spiritual, emotional) is a widely accepted and recognizable health model (Dapice, 2006). While the process map is not strictly a medicine wheel, its similar format suggests a similar usage. Individuals or groups could tailor the map, adding or removing categories or groupings based on relevance. The map could be used as a theoretical framework in a culturally relevant program design. Programs could be developed to include some or all of the 22 categories that facilitate healing. A treatment program, for example, might provide options for participants based on individual needs and preferences: participation in healing ceremonies or connection with nature or emotional expression, for example. The use of the map may be considered in terms of work with individuals, small groups or large groups.

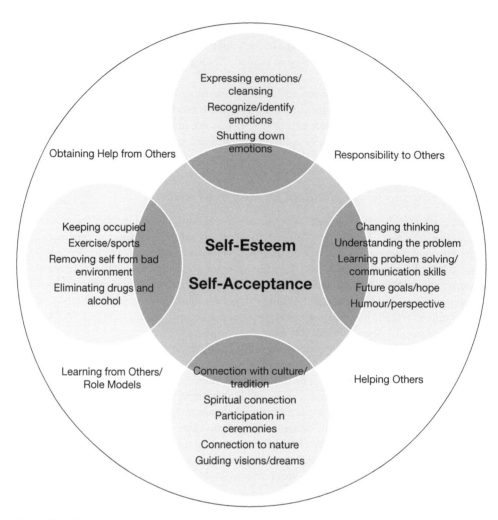

Figure 28.1 The process map

Through the factors presented in this research, the map further indicates that an abundance of potential healing resources exist for Indigenous youth who are suicidal. This finding has the potential to significantly re-orient the way Indigenous communities and practitioners view the nature and source of mental health services provided to them. In recognizing that the natural healing resources of youth themselves can be effective sources of healing, Indigenous community leaders may feel empowered to start examining ways to utilize these methods of healing in addressing youth suicide in their communities.

Limitations

There are a number of factors that limit this investigation. A primary limitation of the study is that the results cannot easily be generalized at this time. It should be noted that the majority of the participants were Indigenous youth from British Columbia and did not represent a wide range of Indigenous communities from Canada. This could also be described as delimitation because it was known at the onset that this study would only provide an initial set of categories that describe healing and recovery and not a definitive description of effective and ineffective healing/recovery techniques for all Indigenous youth. Future studies will be needed to explore the generalizability of the categories with other Indigenous communities. Another limitation of the study is that the categories were derived from self-reporting rather than by observation. Critical incidents obtained through self-reporting are limited to the events that people are able to remember during the interview. It is likely that some events were not mentioned because they had been forgotten by the participant. Another limitation of the use of self-reporting is that participants could only report what they could articulate. This may have excluded some events from being revealed. The focus on healing events as opposed to healing relationships is also a limitation of the study because relationships are more enduring than events. This study did not focus on the question of who was helpful in facilitating healing but on the action taken to facilitate healing for the participant.

Recommendations

The following recommendations are intended for Indigenous leaders and health service providers. Many recommendations could be made for non-Indian service providers as well but as Indigenous mental health service providers, we strongly believe that the solution to youth suicide can best be found within our own communities and youth themselves. It is understandable how Indigenous communities have become disempowered to believe that we are unable to deal with the problem of suicide, but as we gain awareness of the problem and some of the solutions, our communities need to start dealing with the suicide problem. An important place to start is to increase awareness of the problem and mobilize as many community members as possible to brainstorm available strategies that will address youth suicide. Communities must find out what works to prevent suicide by asking those who have recovered from being suicidal because it is important to acknowledge the coping/healing resources that exist within the individual, the community, and the culture. This would serve to develop the connections that youth in this study have indicated are necessary in recovery. Public education strategies in which youth are trained to teach community members about crisis intervention techniques, the warning signs and predictors of suicide, and knowledge of the grief process following a suicide are also recommended. This is indicated in the categories of "responsibility to others" and "helping others". Communities can enlist the assistance of schools and outside mental health resources to jointly develop programs for youth that deal with: positive self-esteem, self-awareness, cultural identity, communication skills, life skills such as problem-solving, decision-making, values clarification, relationship skills and stress management. What is most important is that youths be involved with the development and operation of these programs to ensure a sense of ownership. Many Indigenous communities have historically held community events and ceremonies that assist youth in reinforcing their personal and cultural identity and their connection to the community and culture. Other communities that do not use these ways are encouraged to consider such approaches along with the healing effects on youth of talking circles, traditional ceremonies, and the involvement of healthy elders.

Notes

1   According to Canada, Parliament (2003):

    Statistics Canada defines youth as those between the ages of 15 to 24 years. Aboriginal organizations have their own categories for defining youth: The National Association of Friendship Centres, the

Congress of Aboriginal Peoples and the Metis National Council all define youth as being between the ages of 15 to 24. The Inuit Tapiriit Kanatami employs a broader range. They define youth as those between 13 to 29 years. Finally, the Assembly of First Nations, the Native Women Association of Canada and the Aboriginal Healing Foundation all define youth as age 18 to 24.

2   To limit or minimize the risks inherent in suicide research and specifically with youth (Fisher, 2003; Mishara, 2005; King, 2008), this study utilized participants who had experienced suicidal crises as youth but at the time of the research had fully recovered from their youth crisis. This was confirmed by risk assessments conducted by the researcher prior to each participant's interview.

References

Andersson, B., & Nilsson, S. (1964). Studies in the reliability and validity of the critical incident technique. *Journal of Applied Psychology, 48*, 398–403.

Berlin, I. N. (1987). Suicide among Aboriginal American Indian adolescents: An overview. *Suicide and life-threatening Behavior, 17*(3), 218–232.

Borgen, W. A., & Amundson, N. E. (1984). *The experience of unemployment*. Toronto, ON: Nelson Canada.

Bostick, K. E., & Everall, R. D. (2007). Healing from suicide: Adolescent perceptions of attachment relationships. *British Journal of Guidance and Counselling, 35*(1), 79–96.

Canada, Parliament, Senate. Standing Senate Committee on Aboriginal Peoples (2003). *Urban Aboriginal Youth: An action plan for change*. 37th Parl., 2nd sess. Final Report. Available at: http://www.parl.gc.ca/Content/SEN/Committee/372/abor/rep/repfinoct03-e.pdf.

Chandler, M. J., & Lalonde, C. E. (2008). Cultural continuity as a protective factor against suicide in First Nations Youth. *Horizons* (Special issue on Aboriginal Youth, hope or heartbreak: Aboriginal Youth and Canada's future), 10(1), 68–72.

Chrisjohn, R., & Young, S. (1997). *The circle game: Shadows and substance in the Indian residential experience in Canada*. Penticton, BC: Theytus Books.

Cohen, A., & Smith, R. (1976). *The critical incident in growth groups*. La Jolla, CA: University Associates.

Cooper, M., Karlberg, A., & Pelletier-Adams, L. (1991). *Aboriginal suicide in British Columbia*. Burnaby, BC: Institute on Family Violence Society

Crooks, C. V., Chiodo, D., & Thomas, D. (2009). *Engaging and empowering Aboriginal youth: A toolkit for service providers*. Victoria, BC: Trafford.

Danieli, Y. (1998). *International handbook of multigenerational legacies of trauma*. New York: Springer.

Dapice, A. N. (2006). The medicine wheel. *Journal of Transcultural Nursing, 17*(3), 251–260.

Duran, E., & Duran, B. (1995). *Native American post-colonial psychology*. Albany, NY: SUNY Press.

Duran, E., Firehammer, J., & Gonzalez, J. (2008). Liberation psychology as the path toward healing cultural soul wounds. *Journal of Counseling and Development, 86*, 288–295.

Durkheim, E. ([1897] 1966). *Suicide: A study in sociology*. Toronto: Maxwell McMillan.

Ferry, J. (2000). No easy answer to high Native suicide rates. *Lancet, 355*(9207), 906–909.

Fisher, C. B. (2003). Adolescent and parent perspectives on ethical issues in youth drug use and suicide survey research. *Ethics & Behavior, 13*(4), 303–332.

Flanagan, J. (1954). The critical incident technique. *Psychological Bulletin*, 51(4), 327–358.

Gone, J. P., & Alcantara, C. (2007). Identifying effective mental health interventions for American Indians and Alaska natives: A review of the literature. *Cultural diversity and ethnic minority psychology, 13*(4), 356–363.

Hafen, B. Q., & Frandsen, K. J. (1986). *Youth suicide: Depression and loneliness*. Colorado: Cordillera Press Inc.

Hill, D. (2009). Traditional medicine and restoration of wellness strategies. *Journal of Aboriginal Health, 5*(1), 26–42.

Hodson, D. (1986). The Native belief system: Explaining suicide. In *Proceedings of the conference Suicide: Helping Those at Risk*, pp. 185–192.

Ibrahim, F. A., (1984). Cross-cultural counseling and psychotherapy: An existential-psychological approach. *International Journal for the Advancement of Counselling, 7*(3), 159–169.

Katz, L. Y., Elias, B., O'Neil, J., Enns, M., Cox, B. J., Belik, S. L., & Sareen, J. (2006). Aboriginal suicidal behaviour research: From risk factors to culturally sensitive interventions. *Journal of the Canadian Academy of Child and Adolescent Psychiatry*, 15(4): 159–167.

King, C. A., & Kramer, A. C. (2008). Intervention research with youths at elevated risk for suicide: Meeting the ethical and regulatory challenges of informed consent and assent. *Suicide and Life-threatening Behavior, 38*(5), 486–497.

King, M., Smith, A., & Gracey, M. (2009). Indigenous health, Part 2: The underlying causes of the health gap. *The Lancet, 374*(9683), 76–85.

Kirmayer, L., Simpson, C.,& Cargo, M. (2003). Healing traditions: Culture, community and mental health promotion with Canadian Aboriginal peoples. *Australasian Psychiatry,* 11(s1), S15–S23.

Kirmayer, L. J., Brass, G. M., Holton, T., Paul, K., Simpson, C., & Tait, C. (2007). *Suicide among Aboriginal people in Canada.* Ottawa: The Aboriginal Healing Foundation research series.

Kirmayer, L., Simpson, C., & Cargo, M. (2003). Healing traditions: Culture, community and mental health promotion with Canadian Aboriginal peoples. *Australasian Psychiatry, 11*(s1), S15–S23.

Leenaars, A. A., Brown, C., Taparti, L., Anowak, J., & Hill-Keddie, T. (1999). Genocide and suicide among Indigenous People: The North meets the South. *The Canadian Journal of Native Studies, 14*(2), 337–363.

MacDonald, C. (2008). Using components of the medicine wheel to develop a conceptual framework for understanding Aboriginal women in the context of pap smear screening. *Pimatisiwin: A Journal of Aboriginal and Indigenous Community Health, 6*(3), 95–108.

McCormick, R. M. (1995). The facilitation of healing for the Indigenous people of British Columbia. *Canadian Journal of Native Education, 21*(2), 249–322.

Medicine Eagle, B. (1989). The circle of healing. In R. Carlson & J. Brugh (Eds.) *Healers on Healing* (pp. 58–62). San Francisco: Harper & Row.

Mishara, B. L., & Weisstubb, D. N. (2005). Ethical and legal issues in suicide research. *International Journal of Law and Psychiatry, 28*(1), 23–41.

Mussel, B., Cardiff, K., & White, J. (2004). *The mental health and well-being of Aboriginal children and youth: Guidance for new approaches and services.* Chilliwack, BC: British Columbia Ministry for Children and Family Development.

Nwachuku, U. T., & Ivey, A. E. (1991). Culture-specific counseling: An alternative training model. *Journal of Counseling and Development, 70,* 106–111.

Paproski, D. L. (1997). Healing experiences of British Columbia First Nations women: Moving beyond suicidal ideation and intention. *Canadian Journal of Community Mental Health, 16*(2), 69–89.

Royal Commission on Aboriginal Peoples (1995). *Choosing life: Suicide among Aboriginal people.* Ottawa, ON: Royal Commission on Aboriginal Peoples.

Smylie, J., Lessard, P., Bailey, K., Couchie, C., Driedger, M., Eason, E. L., Goldsmith, W. J., Grey, R., O'Hearn, T., & Seethram, K. (2001). A guide for health professionals working with Aboriginal peoples: Health issues affecting Aboriginal peoples. *Journal of Society of Obstetricians and Gynecologists of Canada, 23*(1), 54–68.

Strickland, C. J. (1997). Suicide among American Indian, Alaskan Native and Canadian Aboriginal youth: Advancing the research agenda. *International Journal of Mental Health, 25*(4), 11–32.

Thira, D. T. (2009). And I live it: From suicidal crisis to activism among members of the Kwakwaka'Wakw and Coast Salish Nations. Unpublished doctoral dissertation, University of British Columbia, Vancouver.

Torrey, E. F. (1972). *Witchdoctors and psychiatrists: The common roots of psychotherapy and its future.* Toronto: Fitzhenry & Whiteside.

Waldram, J. B., Herring, A., & Young, T. K. (2006). *Aboriginal health in Canada: Historical, cultural and epidemiological perspectives* (pp. 201–235). Toronto: University of Toronto Press.

Walker, P. (2001). Teaching and learning journeys around the medicine wheel: A story of indigenous research in a western university. *The Australian Journal of Indigenous Education, 29* (2), 18–21.

Wilson, S., & Wilson, P. (1995). Communities and culture at risk: Searching for the invisible. In *Executive summaries: Focus group on suicide prevention* (pp. 36–40). Regional Medical Services Branch. Ottawa, ON: Health Canada.

Woolsey, L. K. (1986). The critical incident technique: An innovative qualitative method of research. *Canadian Journal of Counselling, 20*(4), 242–254.

29

IDENTITY FORMATION AND CULTURAL RESILIENCE IN ABORIGINAL COMMUNITIES

Christopher E. Lalonde

The program of research that I and my colleagues[1] have been engaged in, and that I will go on to describe in the pages that follow was never meant to be about resilience. Nor was it meant to be about children in care. It began with studies of identity formation, moved on to encompass studies of youth suicide, and has increasingly come to focus on youth suicide in Aboriginal[2] cultures. Having admitted to all of that at the outset, the reader might feel in need of something by way of assurance that this chapter actually belongs in the current volume. First, I really do have data to report on children in care. Second, the research that we have been engaged in—while not expressly about resilience in the usual sense—actually addresses issues of resilience at a cultural rather than an individual level.

Getting from here to there, that is, from our work on identity formation and Aboriginal suicide to our data on children in care, will demand stretching the concept of resilience to try to explain not individual coping in the face of adversity, but the ability of whole cultural groups to foster healthy youth development. There are some who harbour strong doubts about the value of the concept of resilience, however, and it is best to put these doubts on the table before we begin tugging at the concept and testing its elasticity for the job at hand.

The concept of resilience has, of late, found itself living in an increasingly rough neighbourhood. The early excitement—prompted by the work of Garmezy (1970) and Werner (1971)—about the prospect of identifying and studying those "resilient individuals who have defied others' expectations and survived or surmounted daunting and seemingly overwhelming dangers, obstacles and problems" (Leshner, 1999, p. 2), seems to have lapsed somewhat. As Luthar, Cicchetti, and Becker (2000) put it, there are "growing concerns about the rigor of theory and research in the area, misgivings which have sometimes culminated in assertions that overall, this is a construct of dubious scientific value" (p. 543). Liddle (1994), for example, asks: "Does resilience qualify as an organizing concept with sufficient logical and emotional resonance to yield systematic theoretical and research inquiry that will make a lasting contribution?" (p. 167). For Tarter and Vanyukov (1999), the answer is clear: "based on both theoretical and practical considerations . . . it is becoming increasingly evident that this construct not only lacks denotative meaning but has obscured thinking about the etiology and prevention of psychopathology, behavior disorder, and substance abuse" (p. 100). If Tarter and Vanyukov pull no punches, for Bartelt, the gloves are off:

Frankly, I feel that we are imbuing resilience with the same overarching powers that early chemists attributed to phlogiston, the mystical substance that was ostensibly released during combustion and, being contained within the object being consumed enabled it to successfully burn, Resilience, as a psychological trait, that is seen as a component of the self that enables success in the face of adversity, and may either be consumed or, paradoxically, reinforced by adversity.

In short, I make the case that resilience, as a concept is difficult, if not impossible to empirically specify, and is too easily conflated with measures of situational success or failure. It suffers from its roots in subjective interpretations of biographical events, and it is too closely dependent on observer-imputed stresses and resources for dealing with stressors.

(1994, pp. 98–99)

If resilience really does live in what is quickly becoming the dodgy part of town, we might all wonder, along with Tolan who asks in the title of his 1996 article "How resilient is the concept of resilience?" Taking the two-part definition provided by Luthar, Cicchetti, and Becker (2000), it meets the test of being exposed to "significant threat or adversity" (p. 543). The open question is whether it can go on to achieve "positive adaptation despite major assaults on the developmental process" (Luthar, Cicchetti, & Becker, 2000, p. 543). Perhaps I am predisposed to root for the underdog, but I believe the concept of resilience will, to use Garmezy's words, "manifest competence despite exposure to significant stressors" (Rolf, 1999, p. 7). There is much to do, of course, to improve the neighbourhood (if I have not pushed this metaphor too far already), and the work needs to begin with an examination of what might be called 'the trait trap'.

A common criticism of research on resilience is that it aims to identify those "at-risk" children who, when their peers are falling by the wayside, are seen to have "the right stuff" to shoulder the weight of adversity, if not with a smile, then at least without buckling to the pavement. The search for such "resilient children" who remain standing in the most crippling of environments fosters the mistaken and dangerous notion that resilience is a characteristic located somewhere within the child. This view of resilience as a trait was understandable given that early research reports referred to "invulnerability" (Anthony, 1974), or "stress resistance" (Garmezy, 1985), or "hardiness"—all of which have been taken to mean that some children "possess the phenotype of high resilience" (Tarter & Vanyukov, 1999, p. 87). This 'trait trap' view is mistaken because even those researchers who were 'first on the block' understood resilience to be a process rather than a trait (e.g., Werner & Smith, 1982; Werner 1984), and whole armies of researchers have worked to establish the fact that resilience is not a feature of children, but a process that involves interactions between attributes of children, their families, neighbourhoods, and wider social and cultural environments. And it is dangerous because traits are rarely taken to be malleable and if resilience can only be identified but not fostered (you either have what it takes to overcome adversity or you don't), and if risk factors are ubiquitous and inevitable (poverty will be with us until the meek inherit the earth), then we are left with little in the way of real motivation or useful tools to design prevention and intervention strategies for children facing adversity. For those interested in the welfare of whole populations of children who are, almost by definition, taken to be "at-risk of adversity"—children growing up in care, Aboriginal children—the shackling effect of this narrow view of resilience is simply intolerable.

And here is where I want to begin. At the interface of child and culture and with our own attempts to better understand the interplay of risk and protective factors in development. My purpose will be to frame our research in a way that speaks to the issue of resilience in indigenous communities in Canada. I scrupulously avoided the phrase "resilient indigenous communities" both to steer myself clear of the trait trap that I have just warned against, and also to emphasize the point that, just as it is dangerous to imagine that resilience is a feature of children, so too, it would be ill-advised to use a phrase that implies that only some indigenous communities are resilient. Still, I will be presenting results from an ongoing program of research that shows that within the "context of significant adversity" that faces all Aboriginal communities in Canada, differences between communities regularly appear in what resilience researchers would call "positive adaptation". Some communities seem to be "adapting to" or overcoming adversity better than others. As our data show, some First Nations communities have exceedingly high rates of youth suicide, for example, while in others suicide is entirely absent. Some communities have no children and youth living in care, whereas in others, almost 1 in 10 children are placed in care each year. It would be tempting to label some of these communities 'resilient' or to talk of differences in 'levels of resilience'. That is, we have what appear to be similar levels of risk or adversity but large differences in outcome—the same phenomenon that continues to fuel research on resilience in child development—but expressed here at a cultural or community level.

If this is the same phenomenon, and if the detractors are correct, then we have every right to wonder whether the embattled concept of resilience is up to the task of explaining variability in rates of youth suicide or in rates of children in care across diverse groups of Aboriginal communities. In other words, can a concept developed for explaining individual differences be made to work at the level of whole cultural communities? And if resilience can be bumped upstairs to this higher level of analysis, can it be done in ways that avoid the trait trap—that resist the application of global judgments about whether or not a particular community is or is not resilient? Of course, I believe that it can, and if the task of stretching the concept is done carefully enough, I believe there is some potential theoretical clarity to be gained that can better capture the influence of culture on youth development. The sort of care that will be required comes in two forms. First, I will need to be careful to avoid what is sometimes called "the psychologist's fallacy"—a kind of category error in which one applies psychological causes and explanations to every event in sight. My attempt to use the psychological concept of "resilience" at a sociological or cultural level, if not executed properly, threatens to become just this sort of embarrassing error.

The second kind of caution concerns, not the folly of *attempting* to use resilience in this way, but the dangers of actually *succeeding*. If the similarities between individual resilience and cultural resilience are more than just analogous, then (theoretically at least) all of the promise and all of the problems that have attended the history of resilience research will be seen to apply more or less directly to the study of entire cultures. The most pointed dangers—but also the most promising benefits—will come from applying the lessons of research on resilience in children to intervention efforts meant to minimize the effect of risk factors and maximize the effect of protective factors for whole cultural groups. In the current case, our work has identified a set of cultural or community practices and forms of indigenous knowledge that are associated with "better" youth outcomes. These findings threaten to set in motion a well-intentioned, but potentially disastrous, application of the standard knowledge transfer model. What I have in mind here is a variation on the trait trap that would see these findings taken as licence to begin a strip-mining operation bent on extracting some set of cultural "best practices" from beneath the feet of "resilient" communities for processing at some central plant and eventual export to those poor "non-resilient" communities. Though that may seem a harsh characterization, in the context of research and policy as it has been applied "to" indigenous communities in Canada and elsewhere, it is a well-founded fear.

These long-winded introductory remarks—largely a list of doubts and dangers—though a necessary part of mapping out the terrain, have done little to point the route ahead. Belatedly, then, here is how I plan to proceed. Part I begins with a set of definitions common to research on resilience in childhood, and an attempt to show that the situation of contemporary Aboriginal cultures in Canada meets what will amount to the twin conditions of risk and competence that constitute the concept of resilience. This will be accomplished in two steps. The first examines the level of risk faced by Aboriginal and non-Aboriginal persons in Canada—and works to establish the fact that a higher burden of risk is borne by the Aboriginal population. The second step will focus on outcome rather than risk and, as noted above, will include the presentation of data on rates of youth suicide that illustrate wide variability in community-level adaptation or success within a shared climate of heightened risk.

Having established at least a *prima facie* case for using of notion of resilience at this higher level of abstraction, I will go on in Part II to describe how our studies of individual identity formation have led us to use measures of cultural identity as the key to understanding variability in suicide rates and the issues surrounding children in care within First Nations communities. This will, again, be accomplished in two steps. Step one will open with a brief discussion of the concept of 'self-continuity' and will be devoted to making the point that acquiring a working sense of one's own personal persistence in time, an understanding that, despite all the changes that life and time has in store, you can claim confident ownership of your own past and feel a strong commitment to your own future is a crucial part of the identity formation process. In fact, as I will go on to show, failures in the process of constructing or maintaining this sense of self-continuity are strongly associated with the risk of suicide.

Step two—and this is the tricky part where the threat of committing the psychologist's fallacy looms large—will concern the 'levels of analysis' problem that arises whenever one attempts to use a concept developed at one level of analysis (in this case, at the level of individual persons) to explain phenomena at some higher level (communities, or cultures). The case that I will present involves drawing parallels between the continuity of persons and the continuity of cultures. The essential argument is this: In our day-to-day experience, both selves and cultures are commonly understood to both change and yet remain the same. We experience ourselves and others as temporally stable or continuous, yet we also expect people to change—and often strive to bring about change in ourselves and others. In much the same fashion, we understand that cultures must change and yet, if they are to survive pressures of assimilation, or colonization, or conquest, must somehow remain 'the same'. Both persons and cultures, then, are obliged to find some procedural means of preserving identity (personal identity and cultural identity) across time and through change. Just as threats to personal continuity are associated with individual acts of suicide, our research has shown that threats to cultural continuity are associated with rates of suicide within cultural communities. More importantly, efforts to promote culture are associated with increased resilience as evidenced by data that will be presented on the relation between rates of children in care and rates of youth suicide.

The point to be made in all of this is that, if one is as careful as I will try to be, one can sometimes commit the psychologist's fallacy and get away with it. The concept of resilience *can* be applied at a group level. But more than that, the conclusion that I will work toward, is that the process of creating and maintaining a strong sense of collective cultural identity not only promotes the continuity or resilience of the culture itself, but also acts to support and protect young persons in their efforts to build a commitment to their own future that is able to withstand and overcome periods of adversity.

Part I: Applying definitions of resilience to Aboriginal communities

In everyday usage, the term "resilient" can apply to almost anything. Militias and markets can be said to "recover quickly after a setback", and everything from contortionists to camisoles can "spring back quickly into shape after being bent, stretched or deformed". In the social sciences, however, a more precise meaning is intended. Here the term is reserved for those cases (i.e., children) in which exposure to risk or adversity fails to produce the usual or expected degree of negative effect, or the magnitude of recovery is greater than anticipated. In studies of child development, one can refer to a general hardiness in response to adversity—"manifest competence despite exposure to significant stressors" (Rolf, 1999, p. 7)—or to a more distributed and "dynamic process encompassing positive adaptation within the context of significant adversity" (Luthar, Cicchetti, & Becker, 2000, p. 543). Common language and scientific definitions of resilience both refer to a relation between risk and outcome but differ in the way this relation is characterized. In social science, risk is typically defined as that which commonly produces (or is statistically associated with) a negative outcome. Poverty, abuse, illness, etc. are all said to be risk factors in childhood because the population of children exposed to these factors is known to have a lower average score on some outcome measure than the average score for the population of children who were spared such adversities. The term "resilient" is used to describe any at-risk child who exhibits an outcome score that is higher than expected. Just how high one needs to score is a matter of serious scholarly debate. The score can be measured statistically relative to one's at-risk peers (e.g., scoring somewhere above the at-risk mean = resilient), or to scores in the non-risk group (scoring within the non-risk range = resilient), or to the total population (scoring in the top 10% = resilient). Masten, Best, and Garmezy (1990), for example refer to three forms of resilience: (1) positive outcome despite adversity; (2) sustained competence under stress; and (3) successful recovery from trauma. Resilience can also be measured by the presence or absence of certain conditions—at-risk children can be judged resilient if they graduate from high school (presence of positive outcome) or if they fail to develop a mental illness (absence of negative outcome).

My purpose in rehearsing all of this is to highlight the key elements of the concept of resilience as it is commonly employed and to point out the fact that risk and outcome are often conflated. To determine whether or not the concept can be applied to the Aboriginal population, we will need to show that there is a special burden of risk or adversity within this population. This much is relatively straightforward. In a history that is shared with aboriginal people across the Americas, following contact with Europeans, the Aboriginal peoples of Canada have endured a series of sustained assaults upon their cultures. Communities have been forcibly relocated, access to resources and lands has been blocked, and traditional ways of living have been rendered all but impossible to sustain. In Canada, this history has included the official prohibition of religious practices and traditional forms of government, as well as the systematic removal of children from their parents care to be "educated" in residential schools. Such policies (as the Canadian government now admits) were "intended to remove Aboriginal people from their homelands, suppress Aboriginal nations and their governments, undermine Aboriginal cultures, [and] stifle Aboriginal identity" (Report of the Royal Commission on Aboriginal Peoples, 1996). And these policies were undeniably effective: Aboriginal groups continue to struggle to maintain the "matrix of stories, beliefs and values that holds a society together, allows individuals to make sense of their lives and sustains them through the trouble and strife of mortal existence" (Eckersley & Dear, 2002, p. 1592). While no one, perhaps, needs to be especially reminded of this shameful history of "colonial entrapment" (Carsten, 2000), the point of my recounting it is that the difficulties faced by contemporary Aboriginal communities need to be understood within this historical context. The legacy of these policies can be found on any number of indicators of risk status—from infant mortality, injury and disease rates, to life expectancy, school performance and drop-out rates, and almost any measure of health, economic or social disadvantage one cares to choose.

For our present purpose, however, establishing a higher burden of risk satisfies only the first part of the preconditions for cultural resilience. If it were the case that rates of ill health, or social disadvantage were uniformly high in each and every Aboriginal community or group, then there would be no hope for demonstrating resilience. That is, where risk and outcome are conflated, one needs to demonstrate that risk and outcome varies not by individual, but across communities. Because resilience requires a positive outcome amid a climate of increased risk, we need to locate a community, or a set of communities, that have somehow managed to beat the odds. The odds to beat that form the focus for this example will be rates of youth suicide.

Since 1987, we have been monitoring the suicide rates in all of the 196 First Nations communities located in British Columbia. These monitoring efforts reveal two clear trends. First, the rate of suicide for First Nations youth is much higher than for non-Native youth. By our calculations, the risk of suicide (i.e., the burden of risk) is 5 to 20 times higher for First Nations youth as a group. Within this climate of increased risk, however, there is huge variability in the rates of suicide at the level of communities. This might be expected given that suicide is a rare event, and that many of these communities have small populations. For that reason, it is important to measure suicide rates over larger populations and for long periods of time. To date, we have data covering the years 1987 to 2000. With the names of particular First Nations communities (or bands) removed, the rates of youth suicide for this time period are displayed in Figure 29.1.

While it might be natural for the eye to linger on those especially sharp spikes in Figure 29.1, on those communities that exhibit tragically high rates of youth suicide, it should be noted that the line also touches the axis at the zero point. That is, there are communities with youth suicides of zero. To highlight the importance of this phenomenon, the same data are sorted in Figure 29.2 from lowest to highest. As can be clearly seen in this figure, more than half of all communities suffered no youth suicides during the 14-year study window. By this reckoning, the heaviest burden of risk is borne by a tiny fraction of the communities.

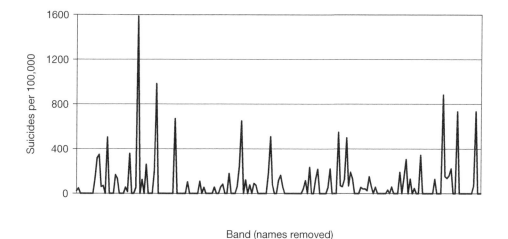

Figure 29.1 Youth suicide rate by band, 1987–2000

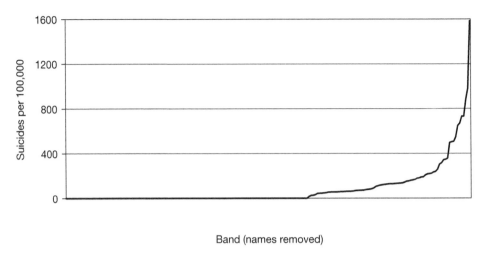

Figure 29.2 Youth suicide rate by band, 1987–2000, sorted from lowest to highest

It might be the case that these differences in community level rates of suicide, while dramatic and apparently stable across time, are nonetheless essentially random. That is, even though the differences between communities persist, there is nothing that would help us distinguish high suicide communities from their low suicide neighbours. But our work has shown that there are ways of making sense of this variability and indeed of predicting which communities will have the lowest (or highest) rates, not just of suicide, but of other good and bad youth outcomes. The business of explaining why some communities manage to thrive in an environment of general adversity—why some communities are resilient—is taken up in the section to follow.

Part II: Personal persistence and cultural resilience

For more than a decade, my research colleagues and I have been struggling to understand how it is that young persons—first of different ages (Chandler, Boyes, Ball, & Hala, 1987), and then of mental health statuses (Chandler & Ball, 1990; Lalonde & Ferris, 2005), and, most recently, of different cultures (Chandler, Lalonde, Sokol, & Hallett, 2003; Lalonde & Chandler, 2004)— differently comprehend their own personal persistence in the face of inevitable developmental and social change. The problem—the paradox—of personal persistence arises from the fact that our ordinary understanding of the concept of "person" or "self" contains two fundamentally contradictory features: selves "embody both change and permanence simultaneously" (Fraisse, 1963, p. 10). On the one hand, we understand that persons change—often dramatically so—yet, on the other, persons must somehow persist as continuous or numerically identical individuals, and be understood, as Locke ([1694] 1956) famously put it, "as the same thinking thing in different times and place". If persons were not understood to persist in this way, then the concept of self would be stripped of its usual meaning. Routine matters of everyday life—such as identifying individual persons at different moments in time—would become impossible, and any hope of maintaining a legal and moral order would collapse if persons could not be held responsible for their own past actions or compelled to follow through on future promises. A conception of the self that did not encompass personal persistence, or that otherwise failed to meet Flanagan's "one self to a customer rule" (1996, p. 65), would be unrecognizable as an instance of what we ordinarily take selves to be (Cassirer, 1923).

Though persistence or continuity is foundational to any workable definition of self, we are not born with arguments at the ready concerning how we ourselves (or anyone else) ought to be understood to change and yet remain "the same" person. It seemed clear enough to us at least, that there is a developmental story to be told here—a story about how young persons come to defend notions of their own continuity in the face of inevitable change. Before going on to briefly outline some of the findings or our own research on this topic, however, a few words need to be said about how it is that adolescents can be prompted to seriously consider matters of self-continuity and to offer up their own best solutions to the paradox of sameness in change.

What does *not* work (or more rightly did not work for us) is to outright ask young people how it is that they should be understood to persist through time. The more roundabout and more productive method of engaging adolescents with the problem is to begin by asking them to discuss instances of particularly dramatic personal change in the lives of fictional story characters. We managed this by presenting them with various "Classic Comic Books" (e.g., Victor Hugo's *Les Misérables* and Charles Dickens's *A Christmas Carol*), that depict examples of persistent identity in the face of personal change, and then pressed them for their own reasons for believing that, despite dramatic transformations, Jean Valjean or Ebenezer Scrooge still deserve to be counted as the self-same continuous and numerically identical person. We followed this by asking them to describe themselves at some time in the past (typically 5–10 years in the past, depending on the age of the participant), and then to describe themselves in the present. Drawing out their thoughts on continuity in their own life involved pointing out the contrasts between these two self-descriptions and repeatedly asking them how such different descriptions could apply to the same person. In following these procedures with upwards of 600 young persons we have found that even the youngest of typically developing adolescents can be counted on to engage the problem of personal persistence with serious attention and to work hard to construct what they take to be convincing arguments in favour of self-continuity.

Before recounting some of the details of our findings, it is important to consider the fact that, although we must each find *some* means of understanding our own persistence in time, there is no reason to suppose that everyone would arrive at precisely the *same* solution strategy. Developmental psychologists, for example, have every right to suspect that persons of different ages would process this problem differently. We might even predict that something like a developmental sequence of solution strategies would emerge. In some similar (though perhaps less clear-cut) fashion, cultural psychologists or anthropologists might predict that even if the problem of self-continuity turned out be one of those rare universals of human development, the procedural means for accomplishing personal persistence might still be free to vary considerably from one culture to the next. As it happens, both groups turn out to be right.

In brief, what we have found is that, as young persons themselves become more complex, so too do the arguments they offer up. In late childhood, for example, most employ simple physicalistic arguments concerning aspects of themselves that have managed to withstand the ravages of time: "My name/appearance/fingerprints are still the same." By the end of their teen years, the form of their reasoning has typically become almost excruciatingly abstract: "I am the ship that sails through the troubled waters of my life." Changes in the sophistication of their reasoning are associated (as every developmentalist has a right to expect) with increasing age and level of cognitive development. Between the ages of 12 and 18, our research suggests, the average young person can be expected to step through a series of up to five different and increasingly complicated ways of warranting their own persistence in time.

In addition, cutting across the different levels of reasoning, we have identified two general strategies for approaching this problem that appear to be associated with the participants' cultural background. One of these aims to preserve continuity through time by denying that real change has taken place and by seeking sameness in those features or aspects of the self that have managed to endure despite surface change in other quarters. These "Essentialist" strategies range from simple claims about physical features remaining the same (my eye colour, my birthmark) to increasingly abstract notions of personality traits and enduring souls. Though such claims can be made at different levels of abstraction, they all share in the idea that beneath a changing surface, more enduring aspects of self can remain untouched by time and change. The second strategy is more "Narrative" and fully abandons the idea that change can be denied. Instead, these "Narrative" accounts find continuity by creating a followable story that stitches together the various and changing parts of their life. Of course, some of these stories are more sophisticated than others. Young adolescents, for example, typically offer a simple chronology of events that rarely amounts to anything like a real plot. Older adolescents can express the more poetic conviction that the only real 'plot' to one's life is that of an endless series of attempts to interpretively re-read the past in light of the present.

Understanding why some adolescents choose the Essentialist approach and others are more Narrative turns out to depend on matters of culture. Some 80% of the culturally mainstream Canadian youth we have tested employ an Essentialist view of personal persistence. Among Aboriginal youth, more than 70% are Narrative in their view. This dissimilarity results from certain deep-seated differences between Euro-American and Aboriginal cultural and intellectual traditions. Where contemporary Western culture routinely sees truth as hidden beneath an obscuring surface and where hidden essences need to be separated from mere appearances, Aboriginal cultures see a need for interpretation and the creation of meaning. Polkinghorne (1988) contrasts these views as a "metaphysics of substance" and a "metaphysics of potentiality and actuality". What adolescents drawn from these groups have to say about personal persistence largely reflects these contrasting cultural traditions.

In arguing that continuity or persistence is constitutive of what it means to be a person, I noted that without it, no one could be held accountable for their own past actions nor obliged to carry through on future commitments. Without this, no society could hope to maintain law and order and good government. But on an individual level, what would it mean to somehow fail or falter in the process of developing a persistent identity? What would it mean to lose a sense of personal persistence? If you had no way to weave together your own remembered past with any anticipated future, what would give you any sense of enduring identity worth caring about? If we are invested in our own well-being precisely because we understand that we persist, or, if Flanagan is right that, "As beings in time, we are navigators. We care how our lives go" (1996, p. 67), then without a sense of self-continuity, what would stop anyone from acting on those transient thoughts of self-destruction that occasionally haunt us all?

All of this would suggest that the costs of failures in personal persistence can be measured in individual acts of suicide. And this is precisely what we have found in our studies. Of the nearly 600 individual young people we have tested to date, the only ones who come up empty-handed when asked to defend notions of persistence in themselves and others are patients in psychiatric settings whom we know to have been actively suicidal at the time of the interview. Unlike all of our other participants—and unlike their non-suicidal ward-mates—those who are without a working sense of self-continuity are marked by being suicidal. Read in the opposite direction, roughly 85% of suicidal participants utterly fail to produce reasons for personal persistence.

As compelling as such data may be, we are not, of course, free to conclude that losing a sense of self-continuity *causes* one to become suicidal. Other explanations are possible. But the kernel idea that we have been exploring is that the same natural developmental process that drives young persons forward through a series of different solutions to the paradox of their own persistence also works to create the possibility of awkward transitions between earlier and later ways of framing this problem and so threatens to leave them, if only temporarily, in the dangerous position of having no working conception of their own enduring identity and no ready care and concern for their own future. One of the special merits of this approach, at least in our own view, is that it provides the basis for a developmental account of why it is that adolescence should prove to be the fraction of the lifespan with the highest attendant risk of suicide.

If the usual course of development can be seen to put adolescents at higher risk of suicide, then what would explain the fact that Canadian Aboriginal youth suffer rates of suicide that are 5–10 times higher than the already elevated rates of their non-Aboriginal peers (Chandler & Lalonde, 1998)? Two possibilities immediately present themselves. First, it might be that the usual constellation of socio-economic and psychological risk factors (inadequate income, education, housing, health care, etc.) simply cluster more tightly around Aboriginal communities. That much is true enough of many Canadian Aboriginal groups—but is not especially true of those communities in Figure 29.2 that are marked by high suicide rates. Alternately, and in keeping with my earlier claim that Aboriginal youth tend to take a different approach to the problem of personal persistence, it might be that their preferred Narrative strategies are somehow inherently defective and fail to adequately sustain self-continuity, or otherwise operate to more often put them in harm's way. There is nothing in our data to suggest that a Narrative approach is any less effective than its Essentialist counterpart at actually solving the problem of personal persistence. Both yield solutions that preserve a sense of connection to one's past and present, and a reasoned commitment to one's future. In fact, it is only among those who have entirely lost the thread of their own continuity that we find increased suicide risk. If one can mount an argument of any kind—whether Essentialist or Narrative, simple or complex, one is insulated from risk.

To understand why suicide risk seems to be so unevenly distributed across communities, we need to look more carefully at the relation between personal and cultural continuity. Our claim is that just as the loss of personal continuity puts individual young persons at risk, the loss of cultural continuity puts whole cultural groups at risk. Given the history of Aboriginal peoples in Canada, no one could seriously doubt that the continuity of Aboriginal culture has been compromised. Indeed, this is part of the climate of adversity argument outlined in Part I. Still, although all Aboriginal cultures have suffered and had much of their culture stolen from them, they have not all responded to these assaults in identical ways. Some communities have been able to rebuild or rehabilitate a connection to their own cultural past with more success than others. Perhaps differences in suicide rates between communities are associated with differing levels of success in their struggles to resist the sustained history of acculturative practices that threaten their very cultural existence.

To test this idea, we needed some way to measure the extent to which these communities have taken active steps to preserve and promote their own cultural heritage and to regain control over various aspects of their communal life. Our measures of cultural continuity include efforts to regain legal title to traditional lands and to re-establish forms of self-government, to reassert control over education and the provision of health care, fire, and policing services, as well as steps to erect facilities within the community devoted to traditional cultural events and practices. More recently, we have added measures of the participation of women in government, and control over the provision of child and family services. Though this handful of items might not be among the first to leap to mind when searching for indexes of cultural continuity, they do reliably capture concrete steps that communities can take to wrest control of their lives from the hands of government overseers, and to reintroduce their own culture into their children's schools and their own communal spaces. The balance of my remarks will (as promised) focus on the relation that these measures of cultural continuity have with rates of youth suicide and the number of children in care.

What we have consistently observed, using suicide data that now covers a 14-year period, is that success on each and every one of these measures is associated with a decrease in the rate of youth suicide. For example, within Aboriginal communities that succeed in their efforts to restore systems of self-government, the relative risk of suicide among youth is 85% lower than in communities that have not. The risk is 52% lower within communities that control education— and the list goes on like this for each one of our measures. More important than the effect of these single variables, however, is the cumulative effect of such successes. When one counts the number of factors present in each community and then calculates the suicide rates separately for those communities with 0, 1, 2 . . . etc. factors present, a clear step-wise pattern emerges. When none of these marker variables are present, the youth suicide rate is 10 times the provincial average; when all six are present, the rate falls to zero (see Figure 29.3). As Figure 29.3 clearly shows, investing in activities that further cultural goals pays dividends in dramatically lowering rates of youth suicide in these communities.

This same relation between cultural continuity and youth suicide holds when one examines the level of control that communities exert over the provision of child and family services. As with suicide, a disproportionate number of children in care are Aboriginal. Just as with suicide rates, there is wide variability from one community to the next in the number of children in care. And, just as we have seen with suicide, this variability is not random but instead attaches itself to community efforts to promote culture and regain control of services. As part of a continued 'devolution' of power, provincial agencies are in the process of returning control of these services to First Nations communities. Some First Nations are farther along in this process than others. Within those communities that have assumed control and implemented plans for their children in care, the youth suicide rate is 25% lower than in communities that still lack control over children and family services. Although when one casts an eye across the whole of the province, there is no direct relation between youth suicide and the number of children in care (see Figure 29.4, r = .115), a closer inspection of the data reveals that, within the group of communities that experience no youth suicide, the number of children in care is 25% lower.

Resilience implies transcendence. While there is perhaps no happy ending to be found in the story told by these data, there is hope. Within a population that suffers the highest rate of suicide in any culturally identifiable group in the world (Kirmayer, 1994), and that even after the "60's

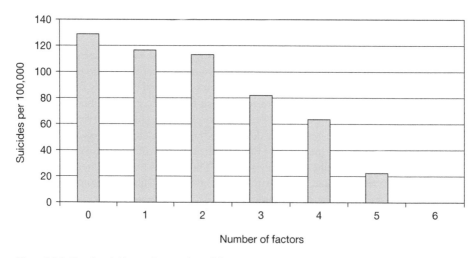

Figure 29.3 Youth suicide rate by number of factors present

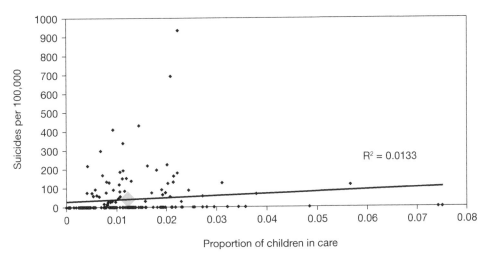

Figure 29.4 Youth suicide and numbers of children in care

scoop" continues to see a disproportionate number of children taken into care, there is evidence of resilience. The surprising outcomes—the transcendence—is not found in the single 'hardy' or 'invulnerable' child who manages to rise above adversity, but in the existence of whole communities that demonstrate the power of culture as a protective factor. When communities succeed in promoting their cultural heritage and in securing control of their own collective future—in claiming ownership over their past and future—the positive effects reverberate across many measures of youth health and well-being. Suicide rates fall, fewer children are taken into care, school completion rates rise, and rates of intentional and unintentional injury decrease.

In contrast to the critics, this cultural resilience is not simply a "situational success or failure" (Bartelt, 1994). The association between community efforts and outcome shows that instances of success are not random. And rather than working to "obscure thinking about the etiology and prevention" (Tarter & Vanyukov, 1999), the success that these communities have achieved has clear implications for policy-makers and service providers. The most important implication follows from the source of the success: the First Nations themselves. If there is any take-home message to be found in our research efforts, it is that some communities have evidently already found solutions to the problems faced by Aboriginal youth. As we have argued elsewhere (Chandler & Lalonde, 2004), the parachuting of solution strategies into Aboriginal communities from far-off university campuses or government offices, is not just disrespectful but also bound to fail. What is needed instead of the usual top-down forms of 'knowledge transfer', is some way to facilitate lateral 'knowledge exchange' and the cross-community sharing of those forms of indigenous knowledge that have already proven their worth in First Nations communities. If the concept of resilience can be stretched to apply to First Nations, as I believe that it can, then the best chances for success lie in the efforts of First Nations to reassert cultural sovereignty and to expand the indigenous knowledge base that has allowed them to adapt to, and in some cases, overcome the climate of adversity.

Acknowledgement

This chapter was first prepared for: Flynn, R.J., Dudding, P., & Barber, J. (Eds.) *Promoting Resilient Development in Young People Receiving Care: International Perspectives on Theory, Research, Practice & Policy*.

Notes

1 The program of research described in this chapter has a long history and has included a shifting set of contributors all of whom are (or were) graduate students working with Michael Chandler at the University of British Columbia. These include: Lorraine Ball, Michael Boyes, Suzanne Hala, Darcy Hallett, Bryan Sokol, and myself.

2 The term "aboriginal" refers to indigenous people in general, while "Aboriginal" is meant to reference specific groups within Canada. The Aboriginal peoples of Canada consist of three distinct groups: First Nations, Inuit, and Métis. The First Nations were once termed "Indian". The Inuit were formerly referred to as "Eskimo". The Métis trace their origins to marriages between the First Nations and European settlers.

References

Anthony, E. J. (1974). Introduction: The syndrome of the psychologically vulnerable child. In E. J. Anthony, & C. Koupernik (Eds.), *The child in his family: Children at psychiatric risk* (vol. 3, pp. 3–10). New York: Wiley.

Bartelt, D. W. (1994). On resilience: Questions of validity. In M. C. Wang, & E. W. Gordon (Eds.), *Educational resilience in inner-city America* (pp. 97–108). Hillsdale, NJ: Erlbaum.

Carsten, J. (2000). *Cultures of relatedness: New approaches to the study of kinship*. Cambridge: Cambridge University Press.

Cassirer, E. (1923). *Substance and function*. Chicago: The Open Court Publishing Company.

Chandler, M. J., & Ball, L. (1990). Continuity and commitment: A developmental analysis of the identity formation process in suicidal and non-suicidal youth. In H. Bosma, & S. Jackson (Eds.), *Coping and self-concept in adolescence* (pp. 149–166). New York: Springer-Verlag.

Chandler, M. J., Boyes, M., Ball, S., & Hala, S. (1987). The conservation of selfhood: Children's changing conceptions of self-continuity. In T. Honess, & K. Yardley (Eds.), *Self and identity: Perspectives across the life-span* (pp. 108–120). London: Routledge & Kegan Paul.

Chandler, M. J., & Lalonde, C. E. (1998). Cultural continuity as a hedge against suicide in Canada's First Nations. *Transcultural Psychiatry, 35*(2), 193–211.

Chandler, M. J., & Lalonde, C. E. (2004). Transferring whose knowledge? Exchanging whose best practices?: On knowing about Indigenous knowledge and Aboriginal suicide. In J. White, P. Maxim, & D. Beavon (Eds.), *Aboriginal policy research: Setting the agenda for change, Vol. 2*. Toronto, ON: Thompson.

Chandler, M. J., Lalonde, C. E., Sokol, B., & Hallett, D. (2003). Personal persistence, identity development, and suicide: A study of Native and non-Native North American adolescents. *Monographs of the Society for Research in Child Development*, Serial No. 273, Vol. 68, No. 2.

Eckersley, R., & Dear, K. (2002). Cultural correlates of youth suicide. *Social Science & Medicine, 55*(11), 1891–1904.

Flanagan, O. (1996). *Self expressions: Mind, morals and the meaning of life*. New York: Oxford University Press.

Fraisse, P. (1963). *The psychology of time*. New York: Harper & Row.

Garmezy, N. (1970). Process and reactive schizophrenia: Some conceptions and issues. *Schizophrenia Bulletin, 2*, 30–74.

Garmezy, N. (1985). The NIMH-Israeli high-risk study: Commendation, comments, and cautions. *Schizophrenia Bulletin, 11*, 349–353.

Kirmayer, L. (1994). Suicide among Canadian aboriginal people. *Transcultural Psychiatric Research Review, 31*, 3–57.

Lalonde, C. E., & Chandler, M. J., (2004). Culture, selves, and time: Theories of personal persistence in Native and non-Native Youth. In C. Lightfoot, C. Lalonde, & M. Chandler (Eds.), *Changing conceptions of psychological life* (pp. 207–229). Mahwah, NJ: Laurence Erlbaum & Associates.

Lalonde, C. E., & Ferris, J. M. (2005). Reasoning about self-continuity and self-unity among psychiatrically ill adolescents. Unpublished manuscript, University of Victoria, Victoria.

Leshner, A. (1999). Introduction. *Resilience and development: Positive life adaptations* (pp. 1–5). New York: Kluwer Academic/Plenum Publishers.

Liddle, H. A. (1994). Contextualizing resilience. In M. Wang, & E. Gordon (Eds.), *Educational resilience in inner-city America* (pp. 167–177). Hillsdale, NJ: Erlbaum.

Locke, J. (1956). *Essay concerning human understanding*. Oxford: Clarendon Press.

Luthar, S. S., Cicchetti, D., & Becker, B. (2000). The construct of resilience: A critical evaluation and guidelines for future work. *Child Development, 71*(3), 543–562.

Masten, A., Best, K., & Garmezy, N. (1990). Resilience and development: Contributions from the study of children who overcame adversity. *Development and Psychopathology. 2,* 425–444.

Polkinghorne, C. (1988). *Narrative knowing and the human sciences.* Albany, NY: SUNY Press.

Rolf, J. (1999). Resilience: An interview with Norman Garmezy. In M. Glantz, & J. Johnson (Eds.), *Resilience and development: Positive life adaptations* (pp. 5–17). New York: Kluwer Academic/Plenum Publishers.

Royal Commission on Aboriginal Peoples (1996). *Report.* Hull, Quebec: Canada Communications Group Publishing.

Tarter, R. E., & Vanyukov, M. (1999). Re-visiting the validity of the construct of resilience. In M. Glantz, & J. Johnson (Eds.), *Resilience and development: Positive life adaptations* (pp. 85–100). New York: Kluwer Academic/Plenum Publishers.

Tolan, P. T. (1996). How resilient is the concept of resilience? *The Community Psychologist, 29,* 12–15.

Werner, E. E. (1984). Resilient children. *Young Children, 1,* 68–72.

Werner, E. E., & Smith, R. (1982). *Vulnerable but invincible: A study of resilient children.* New York: McGraw-Hill.

Werner, E. E., Bierman, J. M., & French, F. E. (1971). *The children of Kauai Honolulu.* Honolulu, HA: University of Hawaii Press.

30

INDIGENOUS YOUTH SUICIDE

A systematic review of the literature

Henry G. Harder, Joshua A. Rash, Travis Holyk,
Eduardo Jovel and Kari Harder

Introduction

This chapter presents a systematic review of the literature surrounding suicide in Indigenous youth populations. The aim of this research is to make sense of the literature surrounding Indigenous Youth Suicide (IYS) in order to advance knowledge that will stimulate and inform future research in this area.

Suicide is an important and tragic public health concern and IYS has been called a crisis and an epidemic. According to the World Health Organization (WHO, 1999), every year, about one million people die from suicide and 10 to 20 million attempt suicide around the world. The global mortality rate from suicide is 16 per 100,000, which equates to about one death every 40 seconds (WHO, 2010).

Historically, suicide rates have not been as prominent as today. In the 1950s, the mortality rate attributable to suicide was around 10 per 100,000. This rate has increased by more than 60% in the past 45 years (WHO, 2010), and likely has not yet reached its plateau.

Once predominant among the elderly, suicide is fast becoming a youth phenomenon localized among those between the ages of 15 to 24. Young people all over the world are committing suicide at unprecedented rates, replacing unintentional injuries as the number one cause of death among this age group (WHO, 2010). This so-called epidemic of youth suicide is most prominent among Indigenous peoples, who are over-represented in every suicide statistic (WHO, 2009).

Between 1987 and 1991, the rate of suicide among the Inuit of Canada was 3.9 times greater than that of the general population (Royal Commission, 1995). This rate was drastically higher among the Inuit youth of Quebec who were some 20 times more likely to commit suicide than their majority counterparts (Kirmayer, 1994). During this same period, Aboriginal youth of British Columbia complete suicide nearly 4.5 times more often than the majority of the youth population (104.8 per 100,000 vs. 24.0 per 100,000; Chandler & Lalonde, 1998).

Indigenous populations in the United States, New Zealand, and Australia also exhibit uncharacteristically high levels of suicidal behaviour. According to statistics from the Centers for Disease Control (CDC) between 2002 and 2006, American Indian/Alaskan Native (AI/AN) have the highest suicide rates among all ethnic groups in the United States at 16.25 suicides per 100,000, which is 1.8 times the national average (CDC, 2009). The Maori of New Zealand have had higher rates of suicide than their non-Maori peers each year from 1996 to 2005 (Beautrais & Fergusson, 2006). Similarly, Indigenous Torres Strait Islanders of Australia complete suicide at a higher rate than the remaining age group from the state as a whole (Hunter & Harvey, 2002).

The etiology of these trends is still poorly understood and few theories have attempted to elucidate it. One of the most promising is the Cultural Continuity theory, which postulates that lack of cultural connectedness may explain why Indigenous youth commit suicide at such alarming rates (Chandler & Lalonde, 1998). This theory proposes that a tight-knit and productive cultural community may buffer against IYS. However, little research has examined cultural continuity theory in the social context in which Indigenous populations are embedded.

The aim of this chapter was to systematically assess IYS using peer-reviewed articles that met set criteria for scientific rigor and quality. Two main objectives were addressed through this review process: (1) the methodological rigor present in the current IYS literature was assessed in hopes of guiding the design of future studies in this area; and (2) the relative importance of risk and protective factors across studies of IYS was examined with a particular emphasis placed on culture.

Methods

Literature search

Research databases available at the University of Northern British Columbia and the University of British Columbia were reviewed: PsychInfo (EBSCO), Web of Sciences (ISI), Academic Search Premier (EBSCO), Science Direct (Elsevier), Highwire Press, and Medline (OVID). Examples of search terms used include: Aboriginal youth suicid★★, Inuit adolescent suicid★★, Maori youth suicid★★.

Review process

Two review authors assessed the studies for eligibility and methodological rigor without consideration of the results. Trials were not blind assessed as author name, institution, and source of publication were known. Throughout this process, any disagreements were resolved until consensus was reached. A third review author decided eligibility in the event that consensus could not be reached.

Inclusion and exclusion criteria for the selection of articles

For this systematic review, the inclusion and exclusion criteria were met if the article had the following characteristics: (1) the sample consisted exclusively of Indigenous youth (aged 13 to 25), or the article contained a specifically defined sub-sample of Indigenous youth; (2) the study was empirical, offering quantitative data; (3) the outcome measure was suicidal behavior of all types including suicide, suicide attempt, or suicidal ideation; (4) the study was published in English; and (5) the article was published after 1996 or was deemed to make a meaningful contribution to the review.

Quality assessment

Evaluation guidelines for rating the quality of a study

Quantitative studies meeting inclusion criteria were assessed for methodological quality using six methodological criteria developed by the authors' consensus. These six methodological criteria

Table 30.1 Checklist for inclusion/exclusion and data integrity rating criteria

Checklist for study inclusion:

1. Deals with indigenous youths (aged 13–25)   ❑

2. Contains quantitative data   ❑

3. Measures suicide or attempted suicide as an outcome   ❑

Data Integrity Rating Criteria

4. Contains multiple measures of suicide = 2; contains one measure of suicide = 1; does not contain or quantify suicide = 0

5. Reports from primary data = 1; Reports from secondary data sources = 0

6. Precautions are taken to ensure the accuracy of the data = 1; Data accuracy is not confirmed or validated = 0

7. Employs a randomized longitudinal design = 2; Employs a longitudinal design = 1; Employs a randomized design = 1; Employs a nonrandomized, nonlongitudinal design = 0

8. Sample size with adequate power ($n > 300$) = 1; Sample size < 300 = 0

9. Controls or otherwise restricts potential confounds (e.g., history of trauma, exposure to suicide, gender, etc.) = 1; No control or measurement of potential confounds = 0

were similar to the criteria used by Wulsin et al. (1999) but tailored towards the assessment of suicide research. These criteria were developed into a rating of rigor assessing suicide research on a scale from 0 to 8. The rating of rigor can be found in Table 30.1. The methodological quality of studies scored was on the basis of rigor as follows: high = a score of 5 or greater, medium = a score of 3 to 4, or low = a score of 1 to 2. A study was selected for data extraction if its rating of rigor was 4 or greater.

Data extraction

While some studies sampled both Indigenous and majority youth, only data pertaining exclusively to Indigenous youth were extracted. Standardized forms were developed by the authors to independently assign each article to one, or a combination, of the following three categories: (1) data integrity; (2) risk and protective factors; and (3) emphasis on culture. Data extracted under each category included: (1) study design, variables of interest, population characteristics, methodological strengths, methodological weaknesses; (2) risk and protective factors for each of the following: suicide, attempted suicide, and suicidal ideation; and (3) definition of culture, country of origin, and effect of culture on suicide. Definitions of constructs can be found in Table 30.2.

Quantification of risk and protective factors

All influences that increased or decreased the risk of suicidality (e.g., depression, social support, culture, substance abuse) were converted into standardized effect sizes as Cohen's d. Cohen's d is a measure of the difference between the means of two groups and by convention ds of .80, .50, or .20 are considered large, medium, and small effects, respectively (Cohen, 1988). Influences

Table 30.2 Definition of terms and constructs used

Definition of terms and constructs used	
Culture	Highly variable systems of meaning which are learned are shared by an identifiable group of people (Betancourt & Lopez, 1993; Rohner, 1984). It represents designs and ways of life that are transmitted across generations.
Enculturation	The process by which individuals learn about and identify with their ethnic minority cultures (Zimmerman et al., 1996). It can also be thought of as a lifelong learning experience in which cultural awareness and understanding develops (Wilbert, 1976).
Indigenous	Any ethnic people who inhabit a geographic region in which they have a historical continuity to the land and to pre-colonial and pre-invasion societies (Cobo, 1987). They form non-dominant sectors of society and are determined to preserve, develop and transmit to future generations their ancestral territories, and their ethnic identity, as the basis of their continued existence as peoples, in accordance with their own cultural patterns, social institutions and legal system (Cobo, 1987).
Internal Locus of Control	Having a tendency to believe that one is personally responsible for, or has control over, the outcomes of their actions (Lefcourt, 1982).
PanIndian	A strategy comparing across all Indigenous groups. The prefix pan is Greek for all.
Self-esteem	An important aspect of self-concept, the broadest evaluation of the self. Perceptions of the self as good or bad or mediocre (Baumeister, 2005).
Suicidal ideation	Having conscious suicidal intent such as self-destructive thoughts or wishes or uttering suicidal threats (Beck, Kovacs, & Weissman, 1979).

that increased the risk of suicidality were given effect sizes that were positive in value whereas influences reducing the risk of suicidality were given effect sizes that were negative in value. Converting risk and protective factors into Cohen *d* effect sizes places all effects onto the same metric allowing for the analysis and comparison of effects. Both significant and non-significant risk and protective factors were maintained in the analysis, owing to the consideration that null findings may still prove important when comparing across studies.

Thematic categorization

Once all the risk and protective factors were standardized, variables were thematically reviewed and categorized using a process of consensus. Variables such as age and gender were considered stand-alone variables that needed no categorization. However, most variables were single item questions such as "family cares about feelings" that could be subsumed by a larger variable of family support. Thematic categories can be found in Table 30.3.

Evidence synthesis

The nature of research in this area is marked by highly heterogeneous study designs, units of analysis, statistical methods, and populations sampled. Consequently, a large net was cast to include the full range of study designs used to evaluate IYS.

Table 30.3 Thematic categorization of risk and protective factors

Thematic category	Variables subsumed
Age	Stand alone
Gender	Stand alone
Depression	Stand alone
Other psychiatric condition	PTSD, anxiety, having a family history of other psychiatric diagnosis, eating disorder
Alcohol abuse	Stand alone
Substance abuse	Substance abuse, marijuana use, inhalant use, other substance abuse
Conduct disorder	Violent behaviour, aggression, violent ideation, anger, delinquency, antisocial behaviour
Family history	Family member or relative who attempted or committed suicide
Friend attempt	Having a friend who has attempted or committed suicide
Social support	Having caring friends, high perceived social support
Family support	Having a caring family, both parents present and supportive, perceived parental support, family connectedness
Physical abuse	Self-reported childhood physical abuse, physical or vicarious
Sexual abuse	Self-reported childhood sexual abuse
Self-esteem	Stand alone
Internal locus of control	Stand alone
Uncomfortable in one's culture	Alienation, discomfort in cultural surroundings
Cultural factors	Involvement in traditional activities, high traditional and spiritual orientation, traditional importance, church attendance

Results

Our systematic review evaluated 771 articles for inclusion (see Figure 30.1 for an illustration of the review process). Only 23 articles met our quality appraisal criteria and were used for data extraction. Information on methodological integrity, risk and protective factors, and cultural influences was extracted from 23, 14, and 6 articles, respectively. Only one article implemented an intervention program. Characteristics of the studies proceeding to data extraction are summarized in Table 30.4.

Description of studies selected for data integrity

Sample

Two articles assessed the Sami people of Scandinavia; two examined the Maori of New Zealand, one looked at Native Hawaiians, and 18 sampled Aboriginal populations of North America and New Mexico. All of the articles used large samples recruited through analysis of communities or populations. Specifically, three studies sampled tribes, four used retrospective data obtained from coroner reports and 18 utilized large-scale epidemiological-type designs.

Outcomes considered

Of the 23 articles deemed methodologically rigorous, eight (34.8%) measured suicidal ideation, 18 (78.3%) assessed attempted suicide and six (26.1%) examined suicide, see Table 30.4. Suicidal ideation and attempted suicide were measured by way of self-report. Suicide was mainly assessed

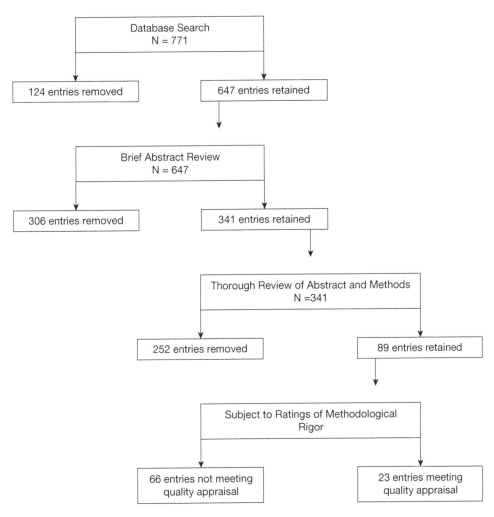

Figure 30.1 Literature review process and decisions

through Coroner Service data. This data was often mapped onto population estimates using an epidemiological approach, and was occasionally substantiated with police reports and medical history (see Boothroyd et al., 2001).

Data integrity analysis

Only 23 (2.9%) out of the 771 articles reviewed were deemed eligible for inclusion in the review. Clearly, there is a paucity of methodologically sound research examining IYS and further research is required to address the issue in any scientifically rigorous way.

Eight studies assessed more than one facet of suicidal behaviour (e.g., suicidal ideation, suicide attempts and completed suicides), with only one of these studies assessing all three facets, see Table 30.4. Although suicidal ideation is private by nature, no study assessed validity of ratings by obtaining third party reports from a family member or close friend. Due to the private nature of suicidal behavior, future studies should implement multiple measures, or use multiple items capturing suicidal behaviour and wherever possible utilize multiple sources of inquiry.

Table 30.4 Characteristics of studies included in the systematic review

Author	Variables of interest	Variables assessed	Sample size	Age range	Data source	Methodological strengths	Population	Use in review
Beautrais & Fergusson (2006)	Suicide attempt	Gender	Population	<15 15–24	New Zealand Health Services	Large sample Self classified Ethnicity Compare Maori and non-Maori attempters.	Maori	Data Integrity
Boothroyd et al. (2001)	Suicide	Attempts Psychiatric diagnosis depression Conduct disorder Personality disorder Psychiatric history Hospital admission	50/71 4/71 17/71	15–24 12–14 25+	Coroner of Quebec from Nunavik Public Health Department	Case control design Matched participants on sex, community, and age. Validated coroner data using medical and police records	Inuit of Nunavik	Data Integrity RF/PF
Borowsky et al. (1999)	Suicide attempt	Age Friend attempt Family attempt Somatic symptoms Sexual abuse Physical abuse Health concerns Drug use Gang involvement Family connectedness	11,666	Grade 712	1990 National American Indian Adolescent Health Survey (NAIAHS)	Compare attempters to non-attempters Statistically adjusts confounds Large sample Involved pretesting, trained researchers, and monitored administration	AI/AN	Data Integrity RF/PF
Chandler & Lalonde (1998)	Suicide	Language Self governance Land claims Education Health Cultural facilities Fire/Police	Population of British Columbia	15–24	BC Coroner 1986–1991 BC Census	Substantiated coroner reports Large sample Unique operational definition of culture	B.C. Native Americans	Data Integrity Culture

Study	Outcome	Predictors	N	Age	Survey	Methods	Population	Theme
Clark (2007)	Suicide attempt	Depression, Age, Gender, Anxiety, Vicarious childhood abuse, Friend or family suicide, Alienation, Social support	2340	12–18	New Zealand Youth 2000 Health Survey	Consultation with community members, Pilot testing, Cognitive testing as pre-screening, Statistically adjusts confounds, Large sample	Maori	Data Integrity RF/PF
Dinges & Duong-Tran (1994)	Suicide attempt, Suicidal ideation	Gender, Depression, Drinking, Drug Use	291	14–18	Boarding school	Instruments tested for cultural language, content, and administration, Instruments validated through interviews, Intensive interviewer training	AI	Data Integrity RF/PF
Freedenthal et al. (2004)	Suicide attempt	Alcohol abuse, Family attempt, Social support, Age, Gender, Income	314	13–20	American Indian Multi-sector Help Inquiry	Intensive field supervisor and interviewer training, Statistically adjusts confounds	AI	Data Integrity RF/PF
Garroutte et al. (2003)	Suicide attempt	Importance of cultural and spiritual beliefs	Population	15–54	American Indian Service Utilization, Psychiatric Epidemiology, Risk and Protective Factors (AISUPERPFP)	Large sample, Statistically adjusts confounds, Interviewers were community members, Administrations was standardized and reliable, Stratified random sampling	AI	Data Integrity Culture

Table 30.4 Continued

Author	Variables of interest	Variables assessed	Sample size	Age range	Data source	Methodological strengths	Population	Use in review
Grossman et al. (1991)	Suicide attempt	Physical abuse Sexual abuse Gender Family history Friend attempt Physical health Mental health Alienation Alcohol abuse	7241	Grade 6–12	Navajo Adolescent Health Survey	Large sample Compare attempters and non-attempters Pilot testing Subjects were pre-screened	Navajo	Data Integrity RF/PF
Hallet et al. (2007)	Suicide	Aboriginal language knowledge	Population of British Columbia	15–24	BC Coroner 1986–1991 BC Census	Substantiated coroner reports Large sample	B.C. Native	Data Integrity Culture
LeMaster et al. (2004)	Suicide attempt Suicide ideation	Gender Age Depression PTSD Substance abuse Violence	403	15–24	AISUPERPFP	Interviewers were trained community members Tribal approval Quality control procedures used to ensure standard and reliable implementation	AI	Data Integrity RF/PF
Malus (1994)	Suicide attempt Suicide ideation	Gender Friend attempt Alienation Age Family psychiatric history Physical abuse Drug use Church attendance	99	14–25	Community sample	Case control design True random sampling Instruments were linguistically checked Assessed seriousness of suicide attempts Used quantitative and qualitative methodologies.	Inuit of Quebec	Data Integrity Culture

Study	Outcome	Predictors	Sample	Age/Grade	Setting	Methodology	Population	Themes
May et al. (2005)	Suicide attempt Suicide ideation	Family attempt Friend attempt Intervention led changes in suicidality	in 1990 = 769 in 2000 = 829	10–19	Tribal community	Interviewed participants in their language Longitudinal Large sample Carefully documented training methods, measurement tools, and intervention policies Designed and implemented in collaboration with tribal officials Regular interactive community workshops	O'Odham Tribe	Data integrity Intervention
Novins et al. (1999)	Suicide ideation	Age Gender Friend attempts Nuclear family Locus of control Self esteem Social support Depression Antisocial behaviour	1378	Grade 9–12	Tribal Communities VOICES project	Longitudinal Large sample Several tribes Designed through focus groups, pretesting, and scientific review of results	AI	Data Integrity RF/PF Culture
Pharris et al. (1997)	Suicide ideation	Cultural factors Family support Involvement in traditional activities	13,929	Grade 7–12	NAIAHS	Large sample Used pretesting, carefully trained researchers, and carefully monitored administration	AI/AN	Data Integrity RF/PF

Table 30.4 Continued

Author	Variables of interest	Variables assessed	Sample size	Age range	Data source	Methodological strengths	Population	Use in review
Rutman et al. (2008)	Suicide attempt Suicide ideation	Ethnic differences	513	Grade 9–12	Youth Risk Behavior Survey	Large sample Longitudinal 3-stage cluster design ensuring nationally representative sample	AI/AN	Data Integrity
Silviken (2009)	Suicide Suicide attempt	Ethnic differences	2691	15–21	Northern Norwegian Youth Study (NNYS)	Large national sample Longitudinal design	Sami	Data Integrity
Silviken & Kvernmo (2007)	Suicide attempt	Suicide ideation Depression Anxiety Single parent family Alcohol abuse Gender Eating disorder	591	15–21	NNYS	Compared suicide attempters to non-attempters Large nationally representative sample Statistically adjusts confounds	Sami	Data Integrity RF/PF
Walls (2007)	Suicide ideation	Gender Age Remote living Discrimination Negative life events Traditional importance Enculturation Self esteem Alcohol use Anger	746	10–12	Community sample	Longitudinal Focus group interviewing Community involvement Employed community members. Statistically adjusts confounds	AI/ Canadian	Data Integrity RF/PF Culture

Study	Outcome	Factors	N	Age	Sample	Notes	Population	Category
		Delinquency Depression						
Walls et al. (2007)	Suicide attempt Suicide ideation	Depression Discrimination Drug use Negative emotionality Coercive parenting	721	10–12	Community sample	See above	AI/ Canadian	Data Integrity
Yuen et al. (1996)	Suicide attempt	Gender Depression Substance abuse Family support	1779	Grade 9–12	Community sample	Large sample Longitudinal and cross sectional Developed in collaboration with the National Center for AI/AN Mental Health Research	Native Hawaiian	Data Integrity RF/PF
Zitzow & Desjarlait (1994)	Suicide Suicide attempt Suicide ideation	Mental confusion Relationship problems Loss due to death Disability	130	12–24	Suicide registry for rural plains	Substantiated suicide registry with medical and police records Full spectrum of suicide behaviour Examined protocol for face, content and construct validity	AI/ Ojibwa	Data Integrity
Centers for Disease Control and Prevention	Suicide attempt	Age	3225	15–19	CDC	Large national sample	AI Western Athabaskan Tribes	Data Integrity

Note. AI = American Indian, AN = Alaskan Native, RF/PF = Analysis of Risk and Protective Factors.

Finally, although many studies used population data with large samples, only three implemented longitudinal or case-control designs (Boothroyd et al. 2001; Malus et al., 1994; May et al., 2005). Such designs are good for determining causation because they allow for repeated observations of the same individual over longer periods of time, and are excellent at making allowances for confounding factors while maintaining adequate statistical power.

Methodological strengths

Each study offered information on the ways in which future research exploring IYS can be strengthened, refer to Table 30.4. Four methodological strengths to emerge were: (1) community involvement; (2) pilot testing; (3) ensuring accuracy of data; and (4) controlling for, or limiting, the presence of extraneous influences.

Community involvement

Community involvement at every level of study design and implementation proved one of the most useful methodological strengths. Many of the population or community-level studies made it a priority to gain involvement and support of the participating community during study implementation. Community involvement ranged in degree. Some studies obtained minimal community involvement by attaining tribal approval prior to implementation (Chandler & Lalonde, 1998) while others obtained significantly more community involvement through the construction of cultural advisory groups that were consulted during every step of study design and implementation (May et al., 2005; Clark, 2007). Some researchers went one step further in hiring and training community members as research assistants (Freedenthal & Stiffman, 2004; LeMaster et al., 2004; Walls, 2007).

Attaining community involvement and support is important to show respect for both the individual and the culture, and to ensure validity of the findings (Tchacos & Vallence, 2004). The Canadian Institute of Health Research (CIHR) promotes participatory-research approaches at all stages in the research process (CIHR, 2007).

One particular intervention study summarized by May and colleagues (2005) illustrates just how active involvement from key community constituencies – tribal leadership, health care providers, parents, elders, youth, and clients – can be effective. This intervention took place between the years 1988 and 2003 and served a tribal population of approximately 3,000 residents. More than 50 active community workgroup sessions were held addressing questions about problem issues in the community (May et al., 2005). This process resulted in a document forming the foundation for the program components.

The results of this intervention study were promising. Suicidal gestures and suicide attempts decreased throughout the course of the program. Annual averages dropped from 15 gestures and 19.5 attempts before 1988 down to 4 gestures and 4 attempts in 2002 (May et al., 2005). The annual average for self-destructive acts was also reduced from 36 to 14. The only form of suicide that remained impervious to the intervention was completed suicides, which remained at 1 to 2 incidents per annum.

Pilot testing

Many of the studies performed pilot testing prior to commencement of the larger research project. For example, researchers involved in the 2000 New Zealand Health Survey conducted pilot projects and cognitive testing prior to implementation in order to ensure that the questions were appropriate and easy to understand across a wide range of literacy levels (Clark, 2007). Other authors pre-tested their tools to ensure that the language, content, and administration were appropriate for the culture being studied (Dinges & Duong-Tran, 1994; Malus et al., 1993; Novins et al., 1999).

Accuracy and validity

Accuracy and validity of the statistical analyses form another important issue addressed by most studies. Limiting confounding factors often enhanced validity of statistical analysis. For example, epidemiological studies employed case-control designs by comparing individuals who experienced problems with suicide to those who did not have such problems (Boothroyd et al., 2001; Borowsky et al., 1999; Malus et al., 1993; Silviken & Kvernmo, 2007). In another example, researchers using Coroner Service data removed extraneous variability by validating such reports with medical records and police reports (Boothroyd et al., 2001; Zitzow & Desjarlait, 1994).

Controlling for extraneous influences

Finally, only seven studies included in this review attempted to control for potential confounding influences by measuring and statistically controlling relevant variables using fully adjusted models (Borowsky et al., 1999; Clark, 2007; Freedenthal & Stiffman, 2004; Garroutte et al., 2003; Silviken & Kvernmo, 2007; Walls, 2007; Walls et al., 2007). Variables that were controlled for include demographic information such as age, gender, marital status, socioeconomic status, employment and education.

Analysis of risk and protective factors

Fourteen of the 23 articles (61%) measured and supplied enough information regarding risk and protective factors to merit inclusion in this analysis. Standardized measures of effects coded for each study were imported into SPSS version 18.0 for analysis. However, the data points in the thematic categories were too few to permit statistical analysis. Owing to this consideration, the average effect and standard error were computed for each of suicidal ideation, suicide attempts, and completed suicides. Results of this process can be found in Figures 30.2–30.4.

Figures 30.2–30.4 show the risk and protective factors related to suicidal ideation, attempts, and completions. Any effect size whose standard error does not bisect zero was viewed as exerting a significant influence on IYS. Effects that are greater than zero were interpreted as variables increasing the likelihood of suicidal behaviour (risk factors), whereas effects less than zero were interpreted as variables reducing it (protective factors).

This form of analysis only allows for the interpretation of risk and protective factors in isolation. It is not possible to identify the combined or interactive effects between risk and protective factors due to small sample size of effects. However, wherever possible, effects were used from fully adjusted models in which combined effects were statistically controlled and parsed out.

Interpretation of risk and protective factors analysis

A comparison of risk factors predisposing suicidal ideation, attempts, and completions identifies remarkable consistency in the variables of importance. First, the two strongest risk factors consistently emerging are depression and having a friend attempt or commit suicide. The next strongest predisposing factors were conduct disorder and substance or alcohol abuse. Finally, having a psychiatric disorder, other than depression, and suffering from previous childhood abuse also increase the likelihood of attempting suicide.

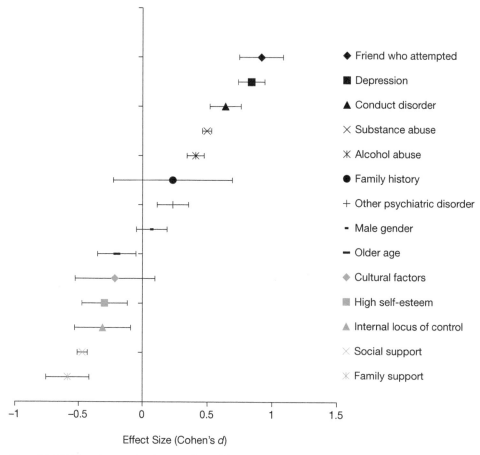

Figure 30.2 Risk and protective factors of suicidal ideation

Although no study explicitly examined the protective factors of completed suicides, a breakdown of the protective factors of suicide ideation and attempts show similar patterns. The variable most strongly buffering against suicide was high support, whether social or familial. The importance of culture was more profound for suicide attempts than for suicidal ideation. Personality variables of high self-esteem and having an internal locus of control further reduced the risk of suicide. Finally, the natural process of aging reduced the associated risk of suicide only minimally. The importance of these variables across the spectrum of suicide is suggestive of some underlying common process.

Emphasis on culture as a protective factor

The current review focuses on trends present across a broad range of Indigenous populations due to a lack of studies in the extant literature. Only six of the articles reviewed presented enough data to examine the effects of culture on IYS (Chandler & Lalonde, 1998; Garroutte et al., 2003; Hallet, Chandler, & Lalonde, 2007; Malus, Kirmayer, & Boothroyd, 2004; Novins et al., 1999; Walls, 2007). Operational definitions of culture can be found in Table 30.5. All of the studies examined various Indigenous populations in North America. Some interesting details emerged

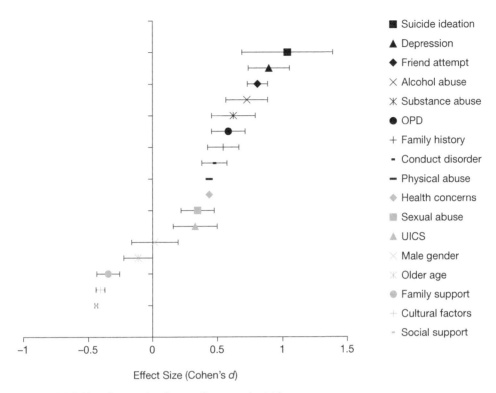

Effect Size (Cohen's *d*)

Figure 30.3 Risk and protective factors of attempted suicide

that merit attention. The three main trends to emerge were: (1) a lack of empirical research; (2) the need for a unified definition of culture; and (3) the effects of culture depended upon which level the construct was analyzed.

Lack of empirical research

Very few studies have examined culture as a protective factor of IYS in a methodologically sound manner. A lack of evidence makes it difficult to ascertain the true importance of culture in IYS.

Need for a unified definition of culture

The influence of culture was also difficult to determine, in part because the operational definitions of culture used in the selected studies were ambiguous and lacked consensus. No study gave a formal definition of what they believed culture to be at the outset, and only a few studies gave an adequate operational definition of culture during implementation. Furthermore, not a single study assessed the construct of validity by mapping participants' perceptions of culture onto the researcher's notion of the construct. Assessing face and construct validity is of particular importance when working with Indigenous population who could have different meanings of inter-tribal culture.

Culture was assessed through an amalgam of cultural activities, spiritual beliefs, self-governance, and knowledge of cultural language that proved highly variable across studies. This degree of variability made culture a ubiquitous construct.

Broadly speaking, culture was analyzed at two levels. One group of researchers evaluated culture as a group process. For example, Chandler and Lalonde (1998) measured cultural

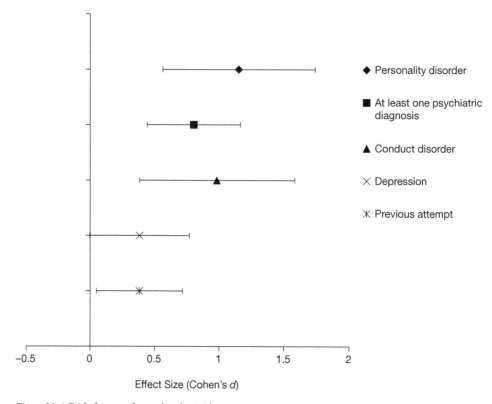

Figure 30.4 Risk factors of completed suicide

continuity operationalized as degree of self-governance using today's Chief and Council structure rather than Indigenous governance systems. This was designed to reflect the degree that groups have maintained societal integration by using their traditional culture to build a collective future. Hallett et al. (2007) included Aboriginal language knowledge as a proxy measure of culture and re-analyzed this data. The idea being that language maps reality in culture-specific ways and that traditional knowledge is an essential way to transfer and learn about culture. These were the most objective uses of culture.

The remaining authors assessed individual perceptions of culture with an implicit assumption that participants have a cogent internal definition of this construct. Garroutte and colleagues (2003) defined culture as the orientation, value, and commitment that people experience towards their cultural heritage. This definition of culture was similar to that of Novins et al. (1999) who measured level of cultural orientation to both Indian and Caucasian cultures. Malus and colleagues (2004) did not directly measure culture but did ascertain indexes of spirituality, which they likened to cultural history. Finally, Walls (2007) assessed level of participation in traditional cultural activities (e.g., participation in traditional pow-pow among 19 other traditional activities, and knowledge and use of traditional language), comfort in cultural surroundings, and cultural identification. These conceptualizations differ markedly from those put forward by Chandler and colleagues in that they focus measurement on the individual.

Table 30.5 Definition and measures of culture

Author/country	Cultural construct assessed	Cultural measures	Findings and implications
Chandler & Lalonde (1998) Canada	Cultural continuity Cultural fragmentation and dislocation	Self-governance Land claims Cultural amenities available	Suicide was 102.8, 60.5, 45.4, 36.1, 29.3, and 24.7 per 100,000 fewer for bands containing self-governance, land claims, education services, health services, cultural facilities, and police and fire services, respectively The effects of cultural continuity factors are additive
Garroutte et al. (2003) United States	Commitment to spiritual beliefs Cultural importance and connectedness	Importance of cultural beliefs Cultural orientation Cultural commitment	Suicide attempts were highest (12.1%) among those reporting cultural beliefs as unimportant Those reporting a high commitment to cultural and spiritual beliefs had the fewest suicide attempts (4.3%)
Hallett, Chandler & Lalonde (2007) Canada	Cultural continuity/ fragmentation	Knowledge and use of aboriginal traditional language	Suicide rates were six times lower among bands in which more than half of the members have a conversational knowledge of an aboriginal language
Malus, Kirmayer & Boothroyd (2004) Canada	Importance of spirituality	Participation in spiritual activities Feelings of alienation	Suicide ideation and attempts were lower among those who attended church every Sunday Youth with suicide ideation and who attempted suicide suffered greater alienation
Novins et al. (1999) United States	Bicultural ethnic identity compared across three tribal groups	Connection with Native and Caucasian cultures	Ethnic identity was not associated with suicide among any of the three tribal groups
Walls (2007) Canada and United States	Cultural continuity, involvement and identification	Discrimination Enculturation Cultural identification Participation in traditional and spiritual activities	Traditional spirituality and enculturation in the preteen and early adolescent years show indirect, life course relevant, relations to suicidality Greater endorsement of the importance of traditional spirituality was negatively related to suicidality through lessened levels of depressive symptoms, anger, and alcohol use, and greater reports of self-esteem

Effects of culture

The effects of culture depended upon how the construct was measured. The influence of culture on IYS was most pronounced when culture was examined as a group process, and it was more diffuse when measured as individual perception or participation.

Two studies measured cultural continuity as the degree to which bands along the west coast of British Columbia have been able to fight for and maintain a strong sense of culture by challenging the government to allow them to live in, govern, and perform cultural rituals on their native lands (Chandler & Lalonde, 1998; Hallett et al., 2007). The idea is that bands undertaking an active role in maintaining and preserving their culture will reduce youth suicide by providing a thread between self and culture, thus promoting the development of a strong sense of self. While difficult to quantify and evaluate empirically, their general findings suggest that this is the case.

Valuing, maintaining, and participating in traditional cultural and spiritual practices had mixed effects on buffering against suicide. Three studies assessed the effectiveness of identifying with one's culture at buffering against suicide (Garroutte et al., 2003; Novins et al., 1999; Walls, 2007). One study (Novins et al., 1999) found no relationship between ethnic identity and youth suicide, while two studies found that identifying and committing to one's culture buffers against suicide (Garroutte et al., 2003; Walls, 2007). Garroutte et al. (2003) found that youth scoring higher in cultural spiritual orientation made fewer attempts at suicide. Interestingly, this relationship was only found for youth scoring in the highest one-third on a measure of cultural spiritual orientation. Walls (2007) found that being embedded within one's culture and valuing traditional spirituality led to less suicidality over time, however, this relationship was complex and most pronounced when cultural identification was endorsed at an earlier age. Similarly, actively participating in spiritual practices on a regular basis was found to buffer against suicide (Malus et al., 1993).

Only one study assessed the developmental pathway of enculturation on IYS. Importantly, Walls (2007) was able to assess the influence of enculturation while taking into account causal pathways. Walls found that enculturation and endorsement of traditional spirituality led to lower levels of suicidality, however, this relationship was complex. The endorsement of enculturation and traditional spirituality at age 10, but not at subsequent assessments, was found to decrease the risk of current and future suicidality suggesting that the beneficial effects of culture on suicidality may be limited to certain developmental stages. Importantly, this effect was partially explained by reductions in depression, negative life events, anger and alcohol use, and through an enhanced sense of self-worth. It is worth noting that the majority of youth assessed by Walls (2007) came from isolated and socially disadvantaged reserves across North America. This study indicates the need to assess pathways to suicidality among Indigenous youth. A life-course perspective needs to be adopted in order to better understand how culture attenuates the risk of suicidality conferred by factors such as poverty, genetics, psychopathology, social disadvantage, discrimination, and stressful events. Only once the pathways to IYS are understood can interventions be implemented that properly address risk and protective factors identified by epidemiological research.

Discussion

Assessment of methodologies

Designing methodologically sound research with a lens focused on IYS is by no means an easy task. This review highlighted many of the difficulties in the current literature. For example, few studies utilized multiple measures of suicidal ideation or verified the accuracy of these measures. It also became apparent that research in this area is reliant on large-scale populations data often obtained from Coroner reports and other secondary sources in which the researcher had no decision-making control.

Since acts of suicide are relatively low with estimates ranging between 48 per 100,000 to 108 per 100,000 (Beautrais & Fergusson, 2006; Chandler & Lalonde, 1998), large-scale community and population-based samples of Indigenous youth are required to ensure that findings are meaningfully interpretable rather than statistical artifacts. Large aggregate samples offer the benefit of easily identifying and tracking universal trends in IYS. However, such samples do not permit a detailed analysis of the factors impacting Indigenous youth at the local or geographic level. Thus, while the use of population sampling seems like a necessity in this research area, it comes at the cost of detecting more subtle influences.

A heavy focus was placed on data obtained from the Coroner's Office. As noted by Chandler and Lalonde (1998), relying on data from the Coroner Service allows for two significantly potential sources of error. First, a death may be labeled accidental unless there is compelling reason for classification as a suicide; this can lead to a misunderstanding about the true incidence and factors preceding a suicide. Second, Indigenous populations may seek to under-report deaths as suicides in an attempt to reject a perception of themselves as being particularly prone to suicide. Unfortunately, the best source of data for assessing suicides is Coroner Service data, imposing a limitation on suicide research.

This review also uncovered some successes in the IYS literature. Cultural relevance was often obtained by pilot testing instruments before study implementation. A high degree of community involvement further ensured that data was reported accurately. In addition, potential confounds were often measured and statistically controlled using fully adjusted models. However, only one intervention was found that utilized these strengths indicating a relative lack of support for youth to maintain their overall resilience. Future research examining the efficacy of intervention elements is sorely needed.

Application to theories on Indigenous youth suicide

Some preemptive findings into the etiology of IYS emerged from our systematic review that could be of benefit to future studies. As suggested by Chandler et al. (2003), the common element underlying the pathways to IYS could be an inability to form a sense of identity and purpose in life. This theoretical framework could explain the influences of IYS identified in the present review.

Individuals are likely to search for identity during developmental crises where psychological growth can be triggered through the experience of stressful life events (e.g., having a friend attempt suicide or contemplating the inevitability of death; Anthis, 2002). If such meaning cannot be located and the struggle for identity cannot be resolved, then a serious period of hopelessness or depression would occur (Duran & Duran, 1995). Being unable to find continuity and a sense of belonging in the self, individuals devoid of an identity often adopt and cling to an addictive lifestyle; such a lifestyle can include problematic use of drugs and alcohol, gambling, and sex (Alexander, 2006). This myriad of negative effects resulting from discontinuity in the self is believed to precede suicide (Ball & Chandler, 1989; Chandler et al., 2003). Such negative effects are believed to be more abundant among Indigenous populations.

Indigenous populations have become fragmented and suffer acculturation and oppression as a result of colonization. The effects and presence of acculturation are still evident in today's reality, which includes poverty, discrimination, racism, and the history of assimilation (e.g., being forced to attend residential schools; Berry, 1997). Such fragmentation and dislocation of culture negatively affect the formation of identity, self-esteem, and purpose among Indigenous populations.

The maintenance of culture and formation of social and familial supports are ingredients that may offset IYS. Social and family support positively influences the development of relational, occupational, and self-identity (Meeus & Dekoviic, 1995), and it was found to be the strongest protective factor reducing the risk of suicide among the studies examined. The assessment of culture as a protective factor for IYS presented in other studies (e.g., Chandler & Lalonde, 1998; Walls, 2007) is but one of many necessary interventions. We agree that connection with one's culture of origin is an important preventive factor for reducing the incidence of suicide among Indigenous peoples. However, this needs to be put into the ongoing context of the realities that Indigenous peoples face today including crippling poverty, unequal access to health and wellness services as well as ongoing issues with access to social services, and education.

Culture-connectedness may well be a useful measure of resilience among Indigenous populations, but this review has shown that such effects are far more complex than originally believed. For instance, the intervention study summarized by May et al. (2005) shows that while culture is important, it is the integration of social, family, education and training, job creation and other elements that bring cohesion to a community. Indigenous youth suicide must be addressed as a community by forming community cohesion (see also Middlebrook et al., 2001).

Conclusion

This systematic review of the scientific literature relevant to Indigenous youth suicide indicates that suicidal behavior among Indigenous youth is a complex issue. The evidence suggests that it is not only having a sense of culture that buffers against the negative pathways of suicide, but rather the act of engaging in culturally relevant activities with respected others in the community. This larger process can be theoretically likened to how Indigenous youth search for and develop a sense of meaning and purpose in their lives. However, there is little to no data that speak to this theoretical assertion – at present it will have to remain a theoretical speculation.

This stringent search of the literature pertaining to IYS identified a small number of studies that were high in methodological rigor. These studies were mostly epidemiological in nature with very few pertaining to interventions for the prevention of IYS. Although these studies offer insight into the etiology of IYS, additional methodologically rigorous intervention studies are needed to promote and develop an effective program for suicide prevention.

Recommendations and future directions

Indigenous youth suicide is a poorly-researched area in which further investigation is urgently needed. The present review has identified several risk and protective factors of IYS but cannot indicate how these influences interact to culminate in suicidality among Indigenous youth. Future research examining the interactive nature of the risk and protective factors identified in this review in a longitudinal manner is required. Particularly, research examining pathways to IYS that evaluate the interactions between demographics (e.g., poverty, social disadvantage), psychopathology (e.g., depression, substance abuse), social support, life stress, cultural connection, and future occurrences of suicide among this population is of vital importance. Such studies are critical to determine the impact of culture on youth suicide and determine the underlying mechanisms involved. This is a necessary step if epidemiological research is to be translated into effective interventions.

Unexpectedly, not one study gave an explicit definition of culture at the outset. This came as quite a surprise considering six studies attempted to measure the influence of culture on suicide among Indigenous populations. Beyond that, studies assessing culture poorly defined and operationalized the construct. A unified definition of culture is required in order to evaluate operational definitions to ensure that accurate interpretations can be made across studies.

Finally, further research is needed into the effects of community involvement. Studies that utilized higher degrees of community involvement appeared to fare well but this conclusion is difficult to substantiate without empirical assessment into its unique contributions.

Limitations and potential biases

All systematic reviews require that the process focuses on the commonalities across studies at the expense of features that are unique to each study. We have attempted to reduce this limitation by referencing details of each study whenever possible.

This review used a scale of quality assessment that may be overly rigorous given the difficulties of performing research on suicide with Indigenous populations. In an attempt to overcome this problem, we performed a systematic evaluation of all articles deemed moderately rigorous (i.e., all articles scoring a 3 or a 4) and included only those that were found to make an adequate contribution to this review.

Selection bias may also have occurred when choosing articles to be cited; this is a problem in systematic review methodologies. To minimize the potential selection bias we added a third review author, who acted as an independent evaluator to resolve disagreement between other reviewers.

Curiously, the literature search did not return a single article that utilized Indigenous methodologies. One possibility is that such manuscripts exist, but may not be published in English. Thus, they were missed by our database searches as only studies written in English were included. Similarly, the databases searched may not carry more obscure Indigenous journals, which are likely candidates to publish articles that utilize Indigenous methodologies.

Finally, the studies reviewed often used a pan-Indian approach in amalgamating evidence across a large and heterogeneous group of Indigenous peoples. Localized Indigenous populations may be distinct and it is unclear how well such findings could be generalized at a local level.

Acknowledgement

This systematic review is used by permission and was first published in *Pimatisiwin: A Journal of Aboriginal and Indigenous Community Health*, *10*(1), 2012.

References

Alexander, B. K. (2006). Beyond Vancouver's "four pillars". *International Journal of Drug Policy, 17*(2), 118–123.

Anthis, K. S. (2002). On the calamity theory of growth: The relationship between stressful life events and changes in identity over time. *Identity, 2*(3), 229–240.

Ball, L., & Chandler, M. J. (1989). Identity formation in suicidal and nonsuicidal youth: The role of self-continuity. *Development and Psychopathology, 1*, 257–275.

Baumeister, R. F. (2005). Self-concept, self-esteem, and identity. In V. J. Derlega, B. A. Winstead, & W. H. Jones (Eds.), *Personality: Contemporary theory and research* (3rd ed., pp. 246–280). Toronto: ON: Thoomson Wadsworth.

Beautrais, A. L., & Fergusson, D. M. (2006). Indigenous suicide in New Zealand. *Archives of Suicide Research, 10*(2), 159–168.

Beck, A. T., Kovacs, M., & Weissman, A. (1979). Assessment of suicidal intention: the Scale for Suicide Ideation. *Journal of Consulting Clinical Psychology, 47*(2), 343–352.

Berry, J. W. (1997). Immigration, acculturation, and adaptation. *Applied Psychology, 46,* 5–68.

Betancourt, H., & Lopez, S. R. (1993). The study of culture, ethnicity, and race in American psychology. *American Psychologist, 48*(6), 629–637.

Boothroyd, L. J., Kirmayer, L. J., Spreng, S., et al. (2001). Completed suicides among the Inuit of northern Quebec, 1982–1996: A case-control study. *Cmaj, 165*(6), 749–755.

Borowsky, I. W., Resnick, M. D., Ireland, M., et al. (1999). Suicide attempts among American Indian and Alaska native youth: Risk and protective factors. *Archives of Pediatrics & Adolescent Medicine, 153*(6), 573–580.

Centers for Disease Control and Prevention (CDC) (1998). Suicide prevention evaluation in a Western Athabaskan American Indian Tribe–New Mexico, 1988–1997. *MMWR, Morb Mortal Weekly Report, 47*(13), 257–261.

Centers for Disease Control and Prevention (CDC) (2009). *Suicide: Facts at a glance.* Available at: http://www.cdc.gov/ViolencePrevention/pdf/Suicide-DataSheet-a.pdf (accessed March 25, 2011).

Chandler, M. J., & Lalonde, C. (1998). Cultural continuity as a hedge against suicide in Canada's First Nations. *Transcultural Psychiatry, 35*(2), 191–219.

Chandler, M. J., Lalonde, C. E., Sokol, B. W., et al. (2003). Personal persistence, identity development, and suicide: A study of Native and Non-native North American adolescents. *Monographs of the Society for Research in Child Development, 68*(2), vii–viii, 1–130; discussion 131–138.

CIHR (Canadian Institute for Health Research) (2007). *CIHR guidelines for health research involving Aboriginal peoples.* Available at: http://www.cihr-irsc.gc.ca/e/documents/ethics_aboriginal_guidelines_e.pdf. (accessed January 12, 2010).

Clark, T. C. (2007). *Factors associated with reduced depression and suicide risk among Maori high school students New Zealand.* ProQuest Information & Learning, US.

Cobo, J. M. (1987). *Study of the problem of discrimination against indigenous populations.* New York: United Nations.

Cohen, J. (1988). *Statistical power analysis for the behavioral sciences* (2nd ed.). Hillsdale, NJ: Lawrence Earlbaum Associates.

Dinges, N. G., & Duong-Tran, Q. (1994). Suicide ideation and suicide attempt among American Indian and Alaska Native boarding school adolescents. *American Indian and Alaska Native Mental Health Research, 4,* 167–188.

Duran, E., & Duran, B. (1995). *Native American postcolonial psychology.* Albany, NY: SUNY Press.

Freedenthal, S., & Stiffman, A. R. (2004). Suicidal behavior in urban American Indian adolescents: A comparison with reservation youth in a southwestern state. *Suicide and Life-Threatening Behavior, 34*(2), 160–171.

Garroutte, E. M., Goldberg, J., Beals, J., et al. (2003). Spirituality and attempted suicide among American Indians. *Social Science & Medicine, 56*(7), 1571–1579.

Grossman, D. C., Milligan, B. C., & Deyo, R. A. (1991). Risk factors for suicide attempts among Navajo adolescents. *American Journal of Public Health, 81*(7), 870–874.

Hallett, D., Chandler, M. J., & Lalonde, C. E. (2007). Aboriginal language knowledge and youth suicide. *Cognitive Development, 22*(3), 392–399.

Hunter, E., & Harvey, D. (2002). Indigenous suicide in Australia, New Zealand, Canada, and the United States. *Emerg Med (Fremantle), 14*(1), 14–23.

Kirmayer, L. J. (1994). Suicide among Canadian Aboriginal peoples. *Transcultural Psychiatry, 31*(1), 3–58.

Lefcourt, H. M. (1982). *Locus of control: Current trends in theory and research.* London: Routledge.

LeMaster, P. L., Beals, J., Novins, et al. (2004). The prevalence of suicidal behaviors among Northern Plains American Indians. *Suicide and Life-threatening Behavior, 34*(3), 242–254.

Malus, M., Kirmayer, I. J., & Boothroyd, L. J. (1994). *Risk factors for attempted suicide among Inuit youth: A community survey* (No. 3). Montreal: Culture & Mental Health Research Unit: Institute of Community & Family Psychiatry.

May, P. A., Serna, P., Hurt, L., et al. (2005). Outcome evaluation of a public health approach to suicide prevention in an American Indian Tribal Nation. *American Journal of Public Health, 95*(7), 1238–1244.

Meeus, W., & Dekoviic, M. (1995). Identity development, parental and peer support in adolescence: Results of a national Dutch survey. *Adolescence, 30*(120), 931–944.

Middlebrook, D. L., LeMaster, P. L., Beals, J., Novins, D. K. & Manson, S. M. (2001). Suicide prevention in American Indian and Alaskan Native communities: A critical review of programs. *Suicide and Life-threatening Behavior, 31,* 132–149. doi: 10.1521/suli.31.1.5.132.24225.

Novins, D. K., Beals, J., Roberts, R. E., et al. (1999). Factors associated with suicide ideation among American Indian adolescents: Does culture matter? *Suicide and Life-threatening Behavior, 29*(4), 332–346.

Pharris, M. D., Resnick, M. D., & Blum, R. W. (1997). Protecting against hopelessness and suicidality in sexually abused American Indian adolescents. *Journal of Adolescent Health, 21*(6), 400–406.

Rohner, R. P. (1984). Towards a conception of culture for cross-cultural psychology. *Journal of Cross-Cultural Psychology, 15*(2), 111–138.

Royal Commission on Aboriginal Peoples (1995). Choosing life: A special report on suicide among Aboriginal people. *The Commission, Cat no. Z1-1991/1-41-4E.*

Rutman, S., Park, A., Castor, M., et al. (2008). Urban American Indian and Alaska Native youth: Youth Risk Behavior Survey 1997–2003. *Maternal & Child Health Journal, 12*, 76–81.

Silviken, A. (2009). Prevalence of suicidal behaviour among Indigenous Sami of Northern Norway. *International Journal of Circumpolar Health, 68*(3), 204–211.

Silviken, A., & Kvernmo, S. (2007). Suicide attempts among indigenous Sami adolescents and majority peers in Arctic Norway: Prevalence and associated risk factors. *Journal of Adolescence, 30*(4), 613–626.

Tchacos, E., & Vallence, R. J. (2004). Research in aboriginal communities: Cultural sensitivity as a prerequisite. Paper presented at the AARE.

Walls, M. L. (2007). *A mixed methods examination of indigenous youth suicide.* ProQuest Information & Learning, US.

Walls, M. L., Chapple, C. L., & Johnson, K. D. (2007). Strain, emotion, and suicide among American Indian youth. *Deviant Behavior, 28*(3), 219–246.

WHO (1999). Figures and facts about suicide. Geneva. Available at: http://whqlibdoc.who.int/hq/1999/WHO_MNH_MBD_99.1.pdf (accessed 10 January 2010).

WHO (2009). World Suicide Prevention Day 2009: Suicide prevention in different cultures. Available at: http://www.who.int/mental_health/prevention/suicide/wspd_2009_statement.pdf (accessed 10 February 2010).

WHO (2010). Suicide prevention (SUPRE). Available at: http://www.who.int/mental_health/management/en/SUPRE_flyer1.pdf (accessed 10 February 2010).

Wilbert, J., & UCLA Latin American Center (1976). *Enculturation in Latin America: An anthology.* Los Angeles: UCLA Latin American Center Publications, University of California.

Wulsin, L. R., Vaillant, G. E., & Wells, V. E. (1999). A systematic review of the mortality of depression. *Psychosomatic Medicine, 17*, 6–17.

Yuen, N., Andrade, N., Nahulu, L., et al. (1996). The rate and characteristics of suicide attempters in the native Hawaiian adolescent population. *Suicide and Life-threatening Behavior, 26*(1), 27–36.

Zimmerman, M. A., Ramirez-Valles, J., Washienko, K. M., et al. (1996). The development of a measure of enculturation for Native American youth. *American Journal of Community Psychology, 24*(2), 295–310.

Zitzow, D., & Desjarlait, F. (1994). A study of suicide attempts comparing adolescents to adults on a Northern Plains American Indian reservation. *American Indian and Alaska Native Mental Health Research, 4*, 35–69.

EDITORIAL COMMENTARY

A systematic review first published in *Pimatisiwin: A Journal of Aboriginal and Indigenous Community Health*, by Harder et al., examined methodological rigor in the current literature of indigenous youth suicide and further examined the importance of risk and protective factors. From 771 papers, only 23 were of sufficient quality to be included in the review. Identified risk factors included depression and having a friend attempt and/or successfully kill themselves. An example of a protective factor was high levels of support. Further risk and protective factors are presented but a major finding of this review (Chapter 30) was the lack of academic rigor in much of the available research, indicating a need for increased efforts for researchers to conduct and present more rigorous research. One example of the problems within the research was the lack of any consistent definition of the concept of culture and how the term is used in research.

In Chapter 27, Darien Thira takes us into the world of lived experience and the resilience of those who lived under the influences of colonization that resulted in feelings of depression and suicidal behaviours, and who are now in leadership positions. Using qualitative research methods, he gives voice to those who have experienced oppression by others and who now have to ensure that they do not in turn oppress those whom they are responsible for. Further, his findings give voice to the importance of healing both the individual and the community as a precursor to creating healthy communities.

In Chapter 28, McCormick et al. examine which factors facilitate healing in indigenous youth who have suicidal ideation or who have attempted suicide. They focus on the impact of colonization as well as showing an absence of research in this area. The first five factors that facilitated healing included self-esteem, self-acceptance, obtaining help from others, changing thinking and connection with culture and traditions. McCormick et al. also developed a process map that shows how the factors interact with parts of the medicine wheel which has been adopted in many indigenous communities. The focus is holistic healing, taking into account the indigenous views/beliefs of each individual and community.

Christopher Lalonde, in a book chapter first published in *Promoting Resilient Development in Young People Receiving Care: International Perspectives on Theory, Research, Practice & Policy*, identifies the importance of identity formation and cultural resilience in indigenous communities. He defines cultural resilience and shows how critical it is to the health of communities and youth in particular. He stresses the critical nature of empowering the community to reassert cultural sovereignty and to expand the indigenous knowledge base if they are to overcome the overall climate of adversity.

Indigenous suicide is a phenomenon different from suicide in the dominant culture. Indigenous suicide often takes place in remote, isolated areas where the person's whole identity may be associated only with that community. This increases the need for the entire community to be healthy, not just individuals within a community. This kind of singular identity of and within a community rarely happens in southern, larger or less isolated communities. The phenomenon puts pressure on an entire community and the leadership of that community for the prevention of suicide among many other things.

Research in the area of Indigenous suicide is woefully lacking. There is an overall lack of research and an even greater lack of methodologically rigorous research. This is ably demonstrated in the systematic review as well as literature reviews that are part of the other chapters. Why should this be so? There is a shortage of journals that will publish indigenous research as well as qualitative research. Indigenous world-views often are a better fit with qualitative research methods and the scope of journals available that will publish qualitative work reduces the opportunity to publish. One of the editors of this section has personal experience of trying to get an article published that was rejected by various American journals as being too qualitative, being too Indian, and the research taking place in Canada, for example. Although funding for research with indigenous communities has been more available in recent years, the knowledge translation or knowledge transfer from this research has proven to be difficult. It is evident that publishers of journals focused on health need to become more open to publishing such research, and researchers as well as other interested parties need to create new journals focusing on indigenous health.

Indigenous suicide is an important component of suicide in general and deserves high quality researchers and high quality research. It is our hope that future research will arise out of a caring for community and individuals as well as scientific curiosity.

INDEX

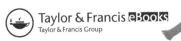